NEUROONCOLOGY - NEWER DEVELOPMENTS

Edited by **Amit Agrawal**

Neurooncology - Newer Developments
http://dx.doi.org/10.5772/61724
Edited by Amit Agrawal

Contributors

Judith Marcela Duenas-Jimenez, Anne Santerre, Irene Aguilar-García, Sergio Horacio Dueñas-Jiménez, Luz María Galván Ramírez, Erika Priscilla Domínguez Rangel, Jorge David Rivas-Carrillo, Jesus Pastor, Lorena Vega-Zelaya, Rafael G Sola, Jer-Yen Yang, Sherri Huang, Eric Trieu, W. Phillip Law, Giulia Cossu, Mahmoud Messerer, Fabrice Parker, Marc Levivier, Roy Daniel, Takashi Sasayama, Kazuhiro Tanaka, Eiji Kohmura, Karen Wonders, Scott Turner, Jens Schittenhelm, Marco Skardelly, Massimo Miscusi, Stefano Forcato, Antonino Raco, Mohamed Saad Zaghloul, Heloisa Moser, Eshini Panditharatna, Roger Packer, Javad Nazarian, Zhong-Ping Chen, Ke Sai, Shu-Xin Sun, Davide Schiffer, George Alexiou, Anastasia Zikou, Maria Argyropoulou, Maleeha Ahmad, Ali Kafadar, Ilhan Yaylim, Sumeyya Azam, Ammad Ahmad Farooqi, Muhammad Ismail, Ozlem Kucukhuseyin, Romana Richterová, Mohammad Abu-Hegazy, Hend El-Hadaad, Alireza M. Mohammadi

Published by InTech

Janeza Trdine 9, 51000 Rijeka, Croatia

Publishing Process Manager Dajana Pemac

Technical Editor SPi Global

Cover InTech Design team

First published July, 2016

Printed in Croatia

Additional hard copies can be obtained from orders@intechopen.com

Neurooncology - Newer Developments, Edited by Amit Agrawal

p. cm.

Print ISBN 978-953-51-2425-2
Online ISBN 978-953-51-2426-9

For EU product safety concerns:
IN TECH d.o.o., Prolaz Marije Krucifikse Kozulić 3, 51000 Rijeka, Croatia,
info@intechopen.com or visit our website at intechopen.com.

Meet the editor

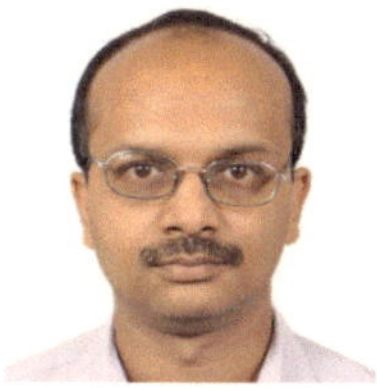

Dr Agrawal completed his neurosurgery training from the National Institute of Mental Health and Neurosciences, Bangalore, India, in the year 2003. Dr Agrawal is self-motivated, enthusiastic, and result-oriented professional with over 12 years of rich experience in research and development, as well as teaching and mentoring in the field of neurosurgery. He is proficient in managing and leading teams for running successful process operations and has experience of developing procedures and service standards of excellence. He has attended and participated in many international and national level symposiums and conferences and delivered lectures on vivid topics. He has published more than 500 articles in the medical field covering various topics in various national and international journals. His expertise is in identifying training needs, designing training modules and executing the same while working with limited resources. He has excellent communication, presentation and interpersonal skills with proven abilities in teaching and training for various academic and professional courses. Presently he is working at the Narayana Medical College and Hospital, Nellore, AP, India.

Contents

Preface

The present book "Neurooncology: Newer Developments" contains the information of various aspects of newer developments and recent advances in the field of central nervous system (CNS) tumor molecular biology, tumor progression, clinical presentation, imaging and management. The authors from different reputed institutions shared their knowledge on this open access platform to disseminate their knowledge at global level. As it is obvious in the current text, the field of neurooncology is heterogeneous and under continuous development with addition of new knowledge and information on regular basis. The collective contributions from experts attempt to provide updates regarding ongoing research and developments pertaining to CNS tumor genetics and molecular aspects and their applied aspect in reference to patient management. I believe that the presented information shall be successfully conveyed to the readers and researchers and they shall find the text to be a valuable guide to further develop their understanding about complicated field of neurooncology.

I am thankful to all the authors who have vast experience in their respective fields and wish that these experts from world-class institutions shall be successful in their attempt in providing the best of neurooncologic fundamentals to improve patient care including outcome and ongoing research. I would also like to thank all of our InTech colleagues for their excellent job to complete this project and provide the best information to the world.

Dr Amit Agarwal
Narayana Medical College and Hospital,
Nellore, AP, India

Section 1

Neuropathology

Chapter 1

Molecular Advances in Glioblastoma Neuropathology

Jens Schittenhelm and Marco Skardelly

Additional information is available at the end of the chapter

http://dx.doi.org/10.5772/62670

Abstract

Glioblastoma is the most frequent and malignant brain tumor with a wide variety of morphological appearances. For a long time, the tumors were classified either as primary ("de novo") glioblastomas that develop rapidly in elderly patients or as secondary glioblastomas with clinical or histological progression from low-grade diffuse astrocytoma or anaplastic astrocytoma. Recent data from the comprehensive genetic characterization of these tumors identified a number of common and diverging alterations and pathways that allow future stratification of glioblastomas into several age-dependent biological subgroups. While the histological classification of diffuse gliomas based on the WHO grading scheme is still necessary, the use of additional meaningful immunohistochemical (and mutation-specific) markers, such as IDH R132H, ATRX, and H3F3A K27M, has improved routine diagnosis. In recent years, the spectrum of clinically relevant molecular markers has expanded. The utility of MGMT, ATRX, TERT, H3F3A and LOH 1p/19q in predicting prognosis and response to therapy in routine diagnostic settings is discussed.

Keywords: neuropathology, histopathology, immunohistochemistry, molecular classification, glioma

1. Introduction

Gliomas are diffusely growing neoplasms of the central nervous system that present high rates of morbidity and mortality. They are the most frequent CNS neoplasms, accounting for approximately 29% of all CNS neuroepithelial tumors [1]. In contrast to almost all other brain tumors, such diffuse gliomas are characterized by extensive, diffuse infiltration of tumor cells into the brain parenchyma—the neuropil. This infiltration is so extensive that even past attempts with radical resection of a hemisphere were not successful, as the tumors reemerged on the contralateral hemisphere [2]. Because of their similarity with non-neoplastic glial cells, these tumors are considered to be of astrocytic and/or oligodendroglial lineage and do not include the biologically different group of ependymomas [3]. The most common primary and malignant brain tumor among this group is glioblastoma, widely known by its acronym "GBM." The tumor was originally designated as "glioblastoma multiforme" because of the extensive variability of tumor histologies. However, some specific (and rare) entities have been isolated from this umbrella term, and individual glioblastomas can also appear quite monomorphic in histology. For this reason, the term "multiforme" is no longer in use following the WHO 2007 classification [4].

Glioblastomas are preferentially located in the subcortical or deep white matter of the cerebral hemispheres, but they may be observed in any other region of the brain, including the cerebellum and spinal cord [3]. Upon initial presentation, less than 2% of the tumors show multiple, clearly distant lesions [5]. In our institution, we prefer to use the term "multifocal" for such lesions without apparent MRI and histological continuum and the term "multicentric" for tumors with radiologically or macroscopically visible distinct tumor centers that have developed from a single lesion. Conventional radiological modalities tend to underestimate the extent of diffuse infiltrative glioma growth. Tumor cells are usually present even outside the peritumoral areas of low density in CT and hyperintensive regions on T2-weighted images in MRI [6]. Not surprisingly, the radiological distinction between multifocal and multicentric gliomas is slightly uncertain. The most extreme example of diffuse infiltrative glioma growth is represented by gliomatosis cerebri. This diagnosis requires the involvement of at least three cerebral lobes, usually bilaterally [3]. Because gliomatosis lacks molecular differences between more circumscribed tumors, this entity will most likely be removed in the next WHO revision. Unlike secondary/metastatic brain tumors, gliomas usually respect the blood-brain barrier, and extraneural metastasis, which is extremely rare, occurs due to ventriculo-peritoneal shunts [6]. In contrast, cerebrospinal fluid spread of glioblastoma cells is occasionally observed, but it is still far less common than in ependymomas or childhood primitive neuroectodermal tumors. Common routes of spread of glioblastoma include the fornix, corpus callosum, anterior commissure, and radiatio optica because of the high affinity of tumor cells to myelinated structures [7]. Symmetric tumors spread across the corpus callosum are called "butterfly gliomas." Tumors that reach the dura often show marked desmoplasia, leading to a firm texture that resembles gliosarcoma or meningioma [8].

2. Clinicopathological parameters of glioblastoma

Glioblastomas represent approximately 65% of all astrocytic or oligodendroglial neoplasms [1]. Incidence rates, estimated to be up to 4.6 per 100,000 people, tend to vary by region, with generally higher numbers in developed countries, increasing with patients' age and showing a slight predominance for males [9]. The vast majority of tumors are observed in adults, with a mean age at diagnosis of 61 years. However, GBM can be found in children, and due to their lower incidence, these tumors are often grouped together with anaplastic astrocytomas and intrinsic pontine gliomas as high-grade (i.e., WHO grade III and IV) tumors. As a matter of fact, comparing clinical and molecular data from such cohorts with adult tumors is difficult. Generally, a younger age of onset in non-pediatric GBM is one of the strongest predictive factors of prolonged survival [10]. Despite this fact, surprisingly, many publications do not include patients' age in multivariate analysis when analyzing biomarkers of patient survival. While almost all GBM occur sporadically, in individuals with Lynch syndrome, a constitutional mismatch repair defect results in an increase of brain tumors, including GBM, among families [11]. Glioblastomas have been reported in other inherited tumor syndromes, including neurofibromatosis type 1, Li-Fraumeni and Turcot-Syndrome and multiple enchondromatosis [3].

Because diffuse astrocytomas show a tendency to progress to a more malignant phenotype during disease progression, these tumors end up as the so-called secondary glioblastomas, (10–15% of all glioblastomas). However, the vast majority of glioblastomas (85–90%) develop without a precursor lesion—the so-called "de novo" or primary glioblastoma [12]. Based purely on histology, primary and secondary glioblastomas cannot be distinguished and it is expected will be rather separated in future WHO classification that glioblastomas will be separated by their molecular profile, than their clinical history (this will be discussed in more detail below). While there is no doubt that oligodendrogliomas undergo a similar malignant tumor progression as astrocytic neoplasms, there is still debate about how many of these truly develop into glioblastomas. As there is some overlap in preoperative imaging of GBM with solitary metastases or lymphomas, intraoperative cytology and frozen sectioning may help in the rapid diagnosis and decision making in neurosurgical procedures. In many cases, nuclear atypia, uneven cell distribution, and the presence of fibrillary processes should guide diagnosis. However, cellularity in frozen sections is often underestimated as a result of artifactual spaces (**Figure 1**).

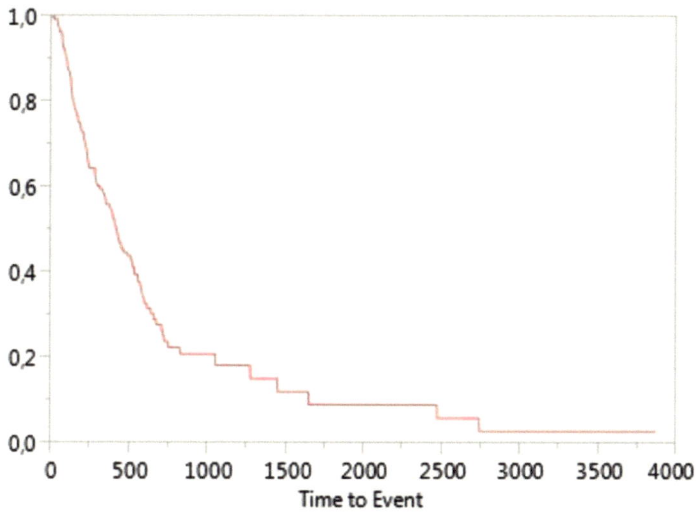

Figure 1. Glioblastomas have a poor prognosis. Kaplan–Meier overall survival Tübingen glioblastoma cohort (n = 205, median survival: 417 days, all cases IDH-wild-type, age <45 years, primary cases).

In newly diagnosed glioblastoma, current therapeutic strategies include surgery (from biopsy to gross total resection, depending on location, which itself is a prognostic marker [13]) followed by concomitant radiotherapy with temozolomide (TMZ) and up to 6 cycles of TMZ maintenance therapy in patients ≤65 years with a median overall survival (OS) of 14.6 months [14].

In addition to the well-established prognostic factors of survival in GBM patients, such as age, extent of resection (EOR), Karnofsky performance scale (KPS), and the treatment modality, molecular alterations (i.e., IDH mutation and MGMT gene promoter methylation, which we will discuss in more detail below) represent not only new significant prognostic factors of survival but also predictors of therapeutic responses in subgroups of GBM. MGMT gene promoter methylation status is a strong prognostic marker of survival in GBM with a median OS of 12.6 months in unmethylated and 23.4 months in methylated GBM treated by concomitant radio-chemotherapy with TMZ. Moreover, MGMT gene promoter methylation status also serves as a predictor of the response to TMZ therapy. In patients >65 years of age exclusive radiotherapy or chemotherapy is indicated according to the MGMT gene promoter methylation status. Patients with methylated GBM most benefit from monotherapy with TMZ, and patients with unmethylated GBM demonstrated the highest survival profit by exclusive radiotherapy [15, 16]. Recurring tumors with a methylated MGMT promoter (i.e., the silencing of the antagonistic effect of this repairing enzyme on alkylating chemotherapy) may thus benefit from a second round of treatment with TMZ [17]. Approximately 30–35% of glioblastoma samples contain a methylated MGMT promoter [18]. However, tumor treatment in diffuse gliomas lacks a persistent therapy response [19], which is why there is an increase of studies with direct ("personalized") targeting of driver mutations in glioblastomas. Alternative treatment approaches include the application of oncolytic parvoviruses to induce tumor cell cycle arrest and cell death [20], the application of low-energy alternating electric fields that affect dividing cells' viability [21], and the application of local hyperthermia induced by superparamagnetic iron oxide nanoparticles coated with hydrophilic polymers subjected to an alternating magnetic field [22].

One of the primary mechanisms related to treatment failure and tumor recurrence in GBM, even in targeted therapies, might be attributed to intratumoral molecular heterogeneity [23] and the presence of a subpopulation of cancer stem cells that contribute to tumor propagation and tumor maintenance through their ability to self-renew and differentiate [24].

2.1. Histologic tumor classification

Although serious advances in the neuroimaging of glioblastomas have been made in the past, histopathologic evaluation of neurosurgically removed tumor specimens is still required for definite classification and subsequent molecular stratification. In 1979, the World Health Organization (WHO) issued a publication for the classification of tumors of the central nervous system. This included a grading scheme based on the malignancy of tumor behavior. The grading of CNS tumors is performed with a four-tiered score, which ranges from grade II to grade IV in astrocytic/oligodendroglial tumors, to separate the histologic continuum of diffuse gliomas according to their expected clinical behavior. Grade IV has the worst prognosis and is reserved for glioblastoma [3].

On macroscopic view, the necrotic center of the tumor is often surrounded by a macroscopically visible gray rim and surrounded by yellowish-grayish texture blending into the surrounding white matter. Black hemorrhagic streaks and thrombosed veins are typically observed in glioblastomas [4]. Glioblastomas' tumor borders are usually diffuse, but rare cases (especially giant cell glioblastomas and gliosarcomas) can be very circumscribed, mimicking a carcinoma metastasis.

The astrocytic heritage of the glioblastoma is best appreciated in cases with prominent eosinophilic cytoplasm of pleomorphic tumor cells resting on a fibrillary background, but this is not the rule for all tumors [25]. As expected in a malignant tumor, marked nuclear atypia and elevated mitotic activity is common. The presence of microvascular proliferations, necrosis or both are required to determine the diagnosis of GBM [3, 4]. Intraoperative consultation with cryosection and smears can provide an initial histological diagnosis and the grade of malignancy. Therefore, intraoperative consultation is useful for neurosurgeons to a) confirm the region of interest in stereotaxic surgery, to b) decide the EOR in relation to the risk of developing new neurological deficits in patients with tumors in eloquent regions, and to c) distinguish between tumor infiltration and reactive astrocytosis.

In absence of these hallmarks, tumors must be classified as anaplastic astrocytomas, even when subsequent molecular data indicates that such tumors are underclassified glioblastomas [26]. On average, three pseudopalisading necroses are present in a glioblastoma specimen. Pseudopalisading cells are usually less proliferative and exhibit higher rates of apoptosis due to hypoxic conditions. More than half of the palisades show a central vascular lumen, and in approximately 20%, intravascular thrombosis is also observed [27]. The presence and extent of necrosis is an adverse prognostic factor [3]. Vascular proliferation in the form of glomeruloid bodies in glioblastomas is observed more frequently than in tumors from any other organ system [28]. Vascular proliferations tend to accumulate in the peripheral region of high cellularity corresponding to the contrast-enhancing ring observed in radiological images [3]. In addition to intrinsic tumor growth, the so-called secondary properties ("Scherer signs") indicate the presence of glioblastoma: perineuronal satellitosis, subpial growth along cortical surfaces and perivascular and intrafascicular growth along myelinated fibers in white matter tracts, mostly characterized by small undifferentiated cells [29]. In the spinal cord, tumor cells might extend into the subarachnoid space [4].

Tumor appearance can be so heterogeneous that diagnosis is often based on tissue patterns rather than individual tumor cell morphology. The 2007 WHO classification recognizes two distinct morphological variants, the giant cell glioblastoma and the gliosarcoma. The giant cell glioblastoma is often subcortically located, and the aptly named cells are regarded as a type of regressive change and harbor a high frequency of Tp53 mutations [3]. Diagnosis requires the presence of giant, often multinucleated cells in more than 50% of tumor cells that can be associated with reticulin deposits [30]. These tumors need to be distinguished from the more benign subependymal giant cell astrocytoma or pleomorphic xanthoastrocytoma. Gliosarcoma consists of often densely interwoven malignant glial and mesenchymal components and account for up to 2% of all glioblastoma samples. The alternating reticulin-free glial and reticulin-containing mesenchymal deposits can be additionally visualized through GFAP immunohistochemistry [3]. While the OS in giant cell glioblastoma is somewhat better, data from a large retrospective study (and others) did not show significant differences for gliosarcomas [31]. Currently considered as a pattern, not a morphological variant, gliomas can show focal areas of epithelial differentiation that range from the positive immunoreactivity of epithelial antigens to adenoid or squamous formations, leading to the misdiagnosis of carcinoma [32]. Among this group, the epithelioid GBM stands out with a younger age of onset and a high percentage of therapeutically relevant BRAF V600E hotspot mutations, and it is very likely that this tumor will become a third glioblastoma variant in the upcoming 2016 WHO classification [32]. These closely packed tumors have variably lipidized, small- to medium-sized cells with rounded cytoplasmic profiles, eosinophilic cytoplasm without stellate processes, and the absence of interspersed neuropils [33].

Small cells with little cytoplasm can appear so monomorphous that small cell glioblastomas mimic anaplastic oligodendrogliomas. Such tumor cells intermingled with gemistocytes are more likely observed in glioblastomas developing from a previous lower-grade gemistocytic astrocytoma. However, the tumors show the same aggressive course as primary GBM [34]. In some tumors, the nucleus-to-cytoplasm ratio is so high that sharply demarcated hypercellular tumor nodules with evidence of neuronal differentiation are present. These clonally expanded, often myc-amplified, so-called PNET components have a high risk of cerebrospinal fluid dissemination [35]. Some tumors may show prominent perivascular rosettes resembling anaplastic ependymomas but usually lack the more uniform roundness of ependymal tumor cells. Tumor cells can be elongated and arranged in fascicles so that upon first viewing them, a sarcoma comes to mind. In up to 15% of the tumors, perinuclear halos around nuclei in glioblastomas may resemble oligodendrogliomas on first viewing; however, the tumor nuclei usually lack the monotonous roundness of true oligodendrogliomas. Such tumors are often called glioblastoma with oligodendroglial component because initial studies suggested that these tumors might have a better prognosis than standard glioblastoma. Comprehensive reviews, including molecular analysis, indicated a pathogenetically heterogeneous group (including misdiagnosed oligodendrogliomas) without a prognostic role [36]. Another occasionally encountered pattern is the presence of adipocyte-like tumor cells that are clearly of astrocytic origin. These tumors are not genetically distinct from conventional glioblastoma [37]. In some cases, the xanthomatous/lipomatous changes are so prominent that the glial nature of these tumors is obscured [38]. Other morphologic variants include granular cell astrocytoma, which is characterized by large, PAS-positive cells with a degenerative granular lysosomal content. These look similar to the benign granular cell tumor of the pituitary stalk [39]. Metaplastic transformation can be so strong that chondroid and osseous formations in gliomas are possible [40]. Rare cases may show melanotic differentiation [41] or a rhabdoid phenotype with focal loss of INI-1 as observed in atypical teratoid/rhabdoid tumors (**Figure 2**) [42].

http://dx.doi.org/10.5772/62670

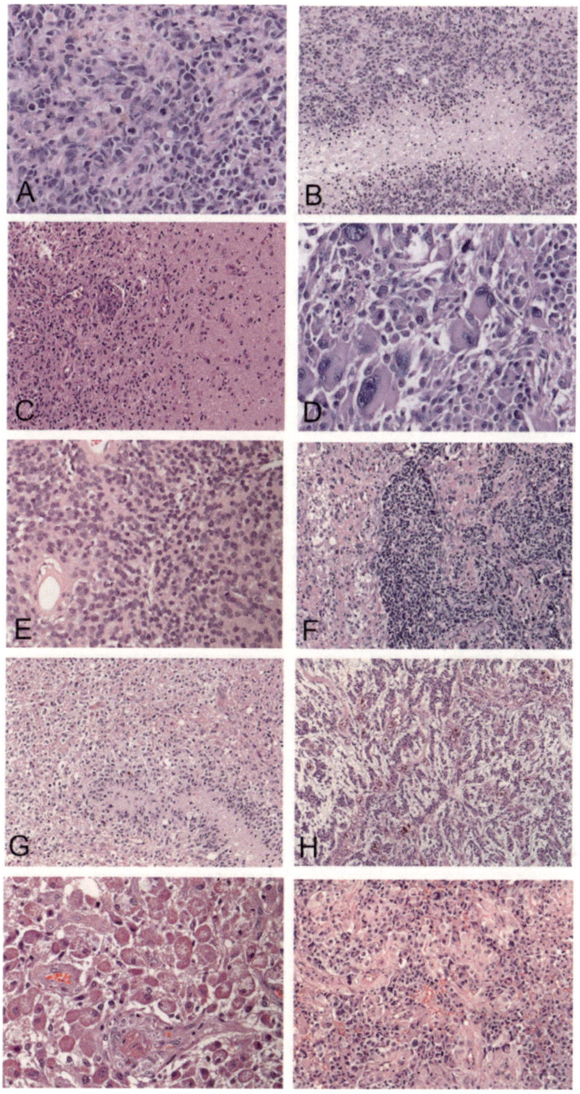

Figure 2. Glioblastoma histology consists of an anaplastic glial tumor with increased cellularity and mitotic activity (A), areas of pseudopalisading necrosis (B). The tumor diffusely invades the brain and has proliferating vessels (C). Morphological variants include giant cell glioblastoma (D), small cell glioblastoma (E), glioblastoma with PNET component (F), with oligodendroglial component (G), with adenoid features on a myxoid background (H), granular cell glioblastoma (I), and epithelioid glioblastoma (K).

2.2. Immunohistochemistry

In many instances, the diagnosis of GBM is straightforward in histology. However, confirmation of the diagnosis with a routine immunohistochemistry panel is mandatory for laboratory quality and improves diagnostic accuracy. Furthermore, some stains have not only diagnostic but also a prognostic role, and their results should be communicated back to clinicians.

The immunoprofile of the glial markers GFAP and EAAT1 in GBM is similar to astrocytomas [43]. In the vast majority of glioblastomas, these antigens are strongly expressed in the cytoplasm of the tumor cells, but they may be occasionally lacking (especially in small cell glioblastomas). The alternatives S-100, WT1, and MAP2 are less specific. Strong MAP2 and WT1 immunoreactivity in cytoplasmatic cell processes is observed in 90% of glioblastomas and is helpful in discriminating GBM from oligodendrogliomas [44, 45]. Vimentin is very unspecific and has no diagnostic value in brain tumors. Cytokeratin expression in glioblastomas (especially in giant cell glioblastomas and glioblastomas with epithelial differentiation) is an important diagnostic pitfall and should not lead to the erroneous diagnosis of carcinoma metastasis [32]. Dot-like EMA immunoreactivity is less frequently observed in GBM than in ependymomas, where usually more than 5 EMA-positive dots per high-power field are observed [46].

Identifying axons with neurofilament stains within the tumor can support the diffuse growth of GBM. In gliosarcomas, GFAP is lacking in reticulin-rich, sarcomatous areas. Usually 15–25% of the nuclei are MIB-1 positive, but the tumor proliferation rate varies greatly between individual GBM. We have observed gemistocytic tumors with less than 5% positive cells and small cell glioblastomas with 90% proliferating cells [25]. Recurrent tumors with history of previous radiation may show little proliferating activity. Because of inconsistent laboratory techniques and varying evaluation methods, MIB-1 immunoreactivity has little prognostic relevance. Nuclear Tp53 immunoreactivity in primary GBM is less present than in astrocytomas and their GBM recurrences, but it may be considerably high in giant cell glioblastomas. Tp53 expression alone is not an independent prognostic marker, but in combination with a methylated MGMT promoter, p53 nuclear staining in more than 50% of tumor cells indicates a less favorable course, similar to GBM with an unmethylated MGMT promoter [47]. It is noteworthy, that not all p53 immunoreactive tumors contain mutations in the Tp53 gene [48] and molecular determination of p53 mutation status in GBM does not correlate with patients' outcome [49]. Several studies have attempted to obtain the MGMT status by immunohistochemistry for MGMT protein expression, but results are hampered by diverging cut-off values and poor correlations with clinical outcome. MGMT immunohistochemistry therefore should be avoided unless there is a consensus with clinical data [50]. Microglial markers, such as CD68- and CD163-positive cells, are regularly found in GBM and can be very widespread, especially in tumors with granular cell components, and must be distinguished from demyelinating lesions.

The NADP-dependent enzymes IDH1 and IDH2 catalyze the conversion from isocitrate to alpha-ketoglutarate. Mutations of the catalytic center in brain tumors result in the accumulation of the oncogenic metabolite D-2-hydroxyglutarate [51]. Because IDH1 mutations are associated with a significantly more favorable outcome in GBM, confirmed in several independent studies, IDH analysis has become the major biomarker in neuropathology practice [52, 53]. The prognostic role of IDH1/2 mutations becomes obvious in WHO grade IV IDH-positive glioblastomas because they show a better prognosis than WHO grade III IDH-negative anaplastic astrocytomas [54]. The upcoming 2016 WHO tumor classification therefore separates glioblastomas according their IDH status. The vast majority of IDH1 hotspot mutations lead to a distinct amino acid substitution on codon 132 (Arg132His), for which a mutation-specific antibody is available [55]. This antibody, however, does not recognize other non-canonical IDH1 and IDH2 mutations, and negative staining results do not imply an IDH wild-type status. IDH1 R132H antibody expression is found in 4% of primary and in 71% of glioblastomas with a lower-grade precursor [55]. In elderly GBM patients above 65 years, the incidence of IDH mutations is rare—one study reported only 2 positive cases out of 167 samples, accounting for the unfavorable prognosis of this age class [56]. Another important clinical aspect is the association of epileptic seizures in IDH1 mutant tumors (**Figure 3**) [57].

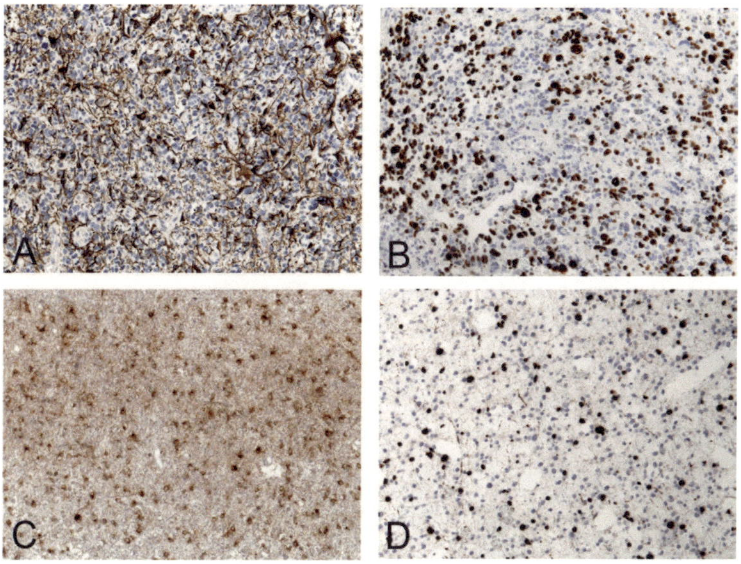

Figure 3. Immunohistochemistry: (A) Limited GFAP expression in a glioblastoma with an oligodendroglial component. The absence of an IDH mutation and partial 19q deletion excluded pure oligodendroglioma in this case. (B) Elevated proliferative activity (MIB-1 index) in the same case. (C) Prognostically relevant IDH1 R132H expression in a glioblastoma arising from a grade II astrocytoma seven years ago. The same case shows nuclear ATRX loss in tumor cells (D).

Some studies aimed to identify antigens to detect the tumor subpopulation with stem cell-like properties, i.e., the cells that have a marked capacity for proliferation, self-renewal, and differentiation. In glioblastoma, the most widely propagated marker for cancer stem cell ability is CD133 along with SOX2 and nestin [58]. However, recent studies indicate that CD133-negative tumor cells may also have stem cell abilities and that different subtypes associated with divergent molecular glioblastoma profiles, discussed below, may exist [59].

2.3. The genetic landscape

Like other tumors, GBM shows an accumulation of several epigenetic and genetic alterations in neoplastic cells within the brain. Recent data from the comprehensive multiplatform genomic characterization of GBM samples identified a number of common and diverging alterations and indicate that glioblastoma consists of biologically heterogeneous subgroups with similar histological appearances. The pilot project of The Cancer Genome Atlas Consortium in 2008 analyzed more than 20000 genes in 90 primary glioblastomas and identified the most common somatic genetic alterations/mutations: Tp53 (42% of the tumors mutated), PTEN (33%), NF1 (21%), EGFR (18%), RB1 (11%), and PI3K-pathway genes (7–10%) [60]. Interestingly, Tp53 mutations are found in almost all GBM with a giant cell component [61]. In addition, pediatric glioblastomas also show a high frequency of Tp53 mutations, as in up to 60% of tumors examined [62].

The most surprising finding was the discovery of isocitrate dehydrogenase (IDH) mutations that occurred in younger patients; these mutations are always heterozygous and are associated with an increase in OS [63, 64]. So far, several hotspot mutations were identified in the catalytic active centers in IDH1 R132, IDH2 R140, and R172 codons, and the most common, R132H, comprises over 80% of all mutations observed to date. The IDH1/2 mutations are present in 50–88% of the so-called secondary glioblastomas (the same point mutation is always present in lower grade precursor tumors, and in cases of a IDH1 R132C mutation, strongly associated with an astrocytoma phenotype). In contrast, IDH1 mutations are observed in only 3–7% of primary glioblastomas and gliosarcomas [54, 65]. In these tumors, IDH2 mutations are virtually absent, except for a single reported case. There is ongoing discussion of whether anaplastic astrocytomas that are IDH1/2 wild-type should be considered glioblastomas without vascular proliferation and/or necrosis because they show the same clinical course and also contain similar genomic alterations as primary GBM. Because IDH1 R132H also represents a tumor-specific antigen, immunotherapy trials currently aim at vaccination to induce antitumor immunoreactions [66].

The activation of receptor tyrosine kinases (RTKs) and the associated RAS/PI3K signaling pathway are common events in GBM. Approximately 45–50% of all primary GBM show high-level genomic amplification of epidermal growth factor receptor (EGFR). Among 30–50% of these amplified cases, intragenic rearrangements with the deletion of exons 2–7, the EGFRvIII variant is detected as a late event. The resulting overexpression leads to the constitutive activity of the receptor in the absence of its ligand and trigger the downstream pathways, resulting in increased cellular proliferation and radiation resistance of the tumor [67]. GBM with small cell morphology are often EGFRvIII-positive tumors [34]. Another important fact is that EGFR mutations in GBM significantly differ from those mutations found in other cancer types, such as non-small-cell lung cancer, where mutations are often located in the intracellular domain [26].

Like EGFR, other RTKs, such as PDGFR and MET, are often amplified in GBM. Platelet-derived growth factor receptor α amplification is significantly enriched for pontine tumors and the pediatric GBM cohort. These tumors are often grouped by the German Cancer Research Center (DKFZ) tumor methylation profiles as RTK class I tumors, while EGFR amplified tumors are classified as RTK-II tumors [68]. Approximately 40% of all PDGFR amplified tumors contain an intragenic deletion of exons 8 and 9 in PDGFRA, which induces an aggressive growth phenotype. Detailed cellular analysis in GBM samples showed that independent focal amplification of PDGFR α and EGFR could coexist in the same tumor [69].

Other common oncogenic alterations in GBM involve the extended PI3K-AKT-mTor and RAS-MAPK pathways. Mutations of the important primary negative regulator PTEN are found in up to 30% of GBM, and the RAS antagonist neurofibromin 1 (NF1) is mutated in 15% of all primary tumors. NF1 germline mutations result in neurofibromatosis type 1, and although rare in comparison to the prevalence of pilocytic astrocytoma, the occurrence of GBM in NF1 syndrome has been reported in a handful of cases [70]. The loss of NF1 is usually associated with concomitant Tp53 mutations, and the additional deletion of PTEN results in the progression of astrocytoma to GBM [48]. Interestingly, PTEN loss and subsequent PI3K-AKT pathway activation results in increased expression of the programmed death ligand-1 (PD-L1), which in turn contributes to GBM immunoresistance and immune escape [71]. Consequently, studies with immune-checkpoint inhibitor treatment in GBM are currently ongoing, although there are conflicting data on the prognostic role and predictive role of PD-L1 gene and protein expression in glioblastoma [72].

Up to 78% of GBMs show alterations of the retinoblastoma (Rb)/CDKN2A-p16^{ink4a} pathway [73]. This pathway plays a central role in proliferation and cell cycle regulation, and alterations include deletions and point mutations in several involved genes. Interestingly, the Rb promoter is far less methylated in primary GBM than in secondary GBM, consistent with the observation that the CDKN2A-p16^{ink4a} gene is affected by the commonly observed chromosomal 9q loss in primary GBM [74]. Although CDKN2A deletion is associated with tumor progression of astrocytomas to GBM and is one of the key molecular marker used to determine a "classical GBM," its prognostic role remains to be elucidated.

Mutations in the promoter region of the telomerase reverse transcriptase (TERT), the catalytic subunit of the telomerase complex, are found in 70–80% of GBM. Similar high frequencies in brain tumors are only observed in oligodendrogliomas [75]. The presence of a TERT mutation in IDH1/2 wild-type tumors is associated with poor outcome and indicates underdiagnosed glioblastoma in a small specimen with otherwise low-grade glioma [76]. TERT itself may also contribute to glioma genesis, as there is evidence that the TERT SNP genetic rs2736100 may influence glioma risk, although it is not a prognostic marker itself [77]. Glioblastomas that do not carry a TERT mutation were recently designated as "triple negative" tumors, i.e., lacking, IDH mutation, 1p/19q codeletion and TERT mutation, again highlighting the importance of these three markers for tumor stratification. TERT mutations are rare in pediatric glioblastomas, where whole exome sequencing recently identified H3F3A mutations, often combined with Tp53 and ATRX/DAXX alterations [78]. The H3F3A mutations are concentrated on two hotspots, K27M and G34V/R, which are mutually exclusive. Both show distinct clinicopathological tumor profiles. H3F3A K27M mutations alter the di- and tri-methylation state of endogenous histone H3 at the Lys27 position and are mainly found in pontine and thalamic tumors [79]. In contrast, the mainly supratentorially located H3F4A G34 mutant tumors presented as a histopathologically heterogeneous group of neoplasms, overlapping classical GBM with central nervous system primitive neuroectodermal tumors (CNS-PNET) [80]. There is growing evidence that G34 mutations may have an alternative mechanism to drive MCYN overexpression for tumor growth [68]. While K27M mutant tumors show a very unfavorable course, the three-year survival rate without this mutation in the pediatric cohort is approximately 70% [81]. Alpha-thalassemia C-linked mental retardation (ATRX) mutations are found in approximately 30% of pediatric GBM and in 6% of adult glioblastoma. Interestingly, in pediatric GBM, ATRX mutations occur around a hotspot near the carboxy-terminal helicase, while they are widely distributed across the gene in adult GBM [82].

ATRX and its binding partner DAXX (death-associated protein) belong to a complex with a role in regulating chromatin remodeling, nucleosome assembly and telomere maintenance. ATRX mutant tumors are associated with alternative lengthening of telomeres, the so-called ALT phenotype [78]. Because nuclear ATRX is diminished in tumors with the ALT phenotype, ATRX immunohistochemistry has become useful in identifying potential IDH mutants, H3F3A alterations or secondary GBM (usually showing ATRX loss and being mutually exclusive of LOH 1p/19q) [83]. Furthermore, retrospective analysis of ATRX in samples from the NOA-04 clinical trial showed a survival benefit of ATRX mutant tumors [84].

2.4. Epigenetics and molecular profiling

The DNA repair enzyme O-methylguanine-DNA methyltransferase (MGMT) removes alkyl groups from the O^6 position. Methylation of the MGMT promoter region results in decreased MGMT activity, which in turn results in decreased tumor resistance to alkylating agent therapy with TMZ, and is therefore a predictive molecular marker [36]. Usually, MGMT is determined in formalin-fixated paraffin-embedded specimens, and approximately 40% of all primary GBM carry a methylated promoter [18]. Less than 15% of gliosarcomas have a methylated phenotype [65]. In pediatric glioblastomas, approximately half of the tumors are methylated, mainly due to the association between H3F3A mutations and the methylated MGMT profile, but the prognostic and predictive role of MGMT methylation in children remains a matter of controversy [62, 68]. MGMT analysis is essential for almost all clinical studies and one of the most requested molecular analyses in routine neuropathology practice.

Unsupervised hierarchical clustering of GBM identified four tumor subclasses called proneural (characterized by mostly IDH/Tp53 mutations, PDGFRα amplifications, PI3K pathway dysregulation), classic (large-scale EGFR amplification, PTEN, and CDKN2A loss), mesenchymal (NF1, Tp53, and CDKN2A alterations), and neuronal (currently no specific genetic alterations). As expected from the IDH mutation data, the patients with a proneural tumor profile were younger and showed the best outcome [60]. The proneural group exhibited a robust hypermethylated glioma-CpG island methylator phenotype (G-CIMP) that is also present in most secondary GBM indicating a common gliomagenesis for IDH-mutated GBMs [85]. Glioma stratification according the IDH status therefore has widely replaced the previous clinic-based separation of primary and secondary GBM. Computational modeling to predict the temporal sequence of driver events during tumorigenesis indicates that most non-GCIMP mesenchymal GBMs arise from a PDGFA-driven proneural-like precursor though additional NF1 loss [86]. However, assignment with established glioblastoma subtype classifiers becomes difficult in cases with substantial tumor heterogeneity and may change further during patient treatment [73].

Glioblastoma intratumoral heterogeneity contributes to therapy resistance. This is exemplified in a whole genome sequencing report that showed not only extensive mutational and copy-number heterogeneity within the primary tumor but also uncovered the recurrence of a double-minute chromosome converging on the KIT/PDGFRA/PI3K/mTOR axis, superseding the IDH1 mutation in dominance in a mutually exclusive manner [87]. Despite targeted therapy with imatinib, the patient succumbed to progressive disease. Another good example is the recent discovery that EGFRvIII mutant cells are expressed only in a fraction of GBM cells of EGFR amplified tumors and enhance the proliferative activity of their neighboring EGFR wild-type tumor cells though cytokine secretion [88]. Because the majority of GBMs exhibit the activation of three or more RTKs, this highlights the need for the combined approach of several specific inhibitors for successful treatment.

Although there is increasing knowledge of divergent molecular alterations in histologically similarly appearing glioblastoma specimens, clinical decision-making on molecular alterations of glioblastoma subtypes is still limited. Notable exceptions include the determination of chromosomal allelic losses in 1p/19q in younger GBM patients, as such tumors respond far better to a combined Procarbazine-CCNU-Vincristine (PCV) therapy regimen [89]. The 1p/19q co-deletion is strongly associated with oligodendroglial tumor morphology and will become a diagnostic marker to be reassigned in future glioblastoma with this signature into the anaplastic oligodendroglioma group [26]. Up to 75% of co-deleted tumors also show either additional IDH1 or IDH2 mutations [90]. This combined molecular signature is so robust and remains visible in tumor recurrences, even in cases with increased intratumoral heterogeneity, and overlaps with "proneural" expression profile of the TCGA genomic landscape [91].

2.5. Conclusion

Glioblastomas have an extensive variety of histological appearances and divergent immunohistochemical and molecular profiles, making diagnosis somewhat difficult for those who are not familiar in working with brain tumors. The histological classification of diffuse gliomas based on the latest WHO grading scheme is a prerequisite to optimal decision-making regarding patient treatment. In addition to core features (microvascular proliferations, necrosis, and secondary structures of Scherer), the clinically relevant pattern and variants (gliosarcoma, giant cell glioblastoma, epithelioid, small cell GBM, and GBM with PNET component) should be clearly depicted in neuropathology reports. Immunohistochemistry and molecular biology have contributed to an improved classification and were shown in some cases to be of prognostic value. A panel of different antibodies is very helpful in securing the diagnosis and avoids potential differential diagnostic pitfalls. The advantages and limitations of the most commonly used antibodies, such as GFAP, WT1, MAP2, MIB-1, P53, IDH1R132H, and ATRX, in GBM have been outlined. The GBM subtype, patient's age, tumor location, and staining results subsequently guide a staged approach to therapeutically relevant molecular analysis, such as the 1p19q codeletion, MGMT promoter methylation, H3F3A screening, TERT promoter and IDH hotspot mutations. The classic concept of primary and secondary glioblastomas has been challenged by the discovery of clinically divergent molecular GBM cohorts, providing a good example of "convergent evolution showing a similar phenotype of genotypically different tumor cells" [92]. The implementation of these additional molecular markers into routine diagnoses has already started, including the routine determination of

MGMT gene promoter methylation status to guide therapy and the re-classification of tumors for appropriate treatment according to LOH1p/19q analysis, and it is expected to further evolve. The heterogenous landscape within and across GBMs underscores the difficulty in developing multimodal targeted therapies and is also a challenge to stratify patients for clinical trials. However, the recent identification of recurring driver mutations as illustrated here provides a rationale to identify tumor-specific peptides and antibody targets that may improve glioblastoma treatment.

Acknowledgements

The authors thank their colleagues at the Department of Neuropathology and Neurooncology for valuable feedback in discussion rounds.

Author details

Jens Schittenhelm[1,2*] and Marco Skardelly[1,2]

*Address all correspondence to: jens.schittenhelm@med.uni-tuebingen.de

1 Department of Neuropathology, Institute of Pathology and Neuropathology, Germany

2 Department of Neurosurgery, University Medical Clinic, University of Tübingen, Germany

References

[1] Ostrom QT, Gittleman H, Fulop J, Liu M, Blanda R, Kromer C, Wolinsky Y, Kruchko C, Barnholtz-Sloan JS. CBTRUS Statistical report: primary brain and central nervous system tumors diagnosed in the United States in 2008–2012. Neuro Oncol. 2015;17(Suppl. 4):iv1–iv62. DOI: 10.1093/neuonc/nov189

[2] Dandy W. Removal of right cerebral hemisphere for certain tumors with hemiplegia. JAMA 1928;90:823–825.

[3] Louis DN, Ohgaki H, Wiestler OD, Cavenee WK, editors. WHO Classification of Tumours of the Central Nervous system, 4th ed. Lyon: IARC Press; 2007.

[4] Burger PC, Scheithauer BW, editors. Tumors of the Central Nervous System. AFIP Atlas of Tumor Pathology Series 4. Washington, DC: ARP Press; 1994.

[5] Barnard RO, Geddes JF. The incidence of multifocal cerebral gliomas. A histologic study of large hemisphere sections. Cancer 1987;60:1519–1531. DOI: 10.1002/1097-0142(19871001)60:7<1519::AID-CNCR2820600719>3.0.CO;2-1

[6] Elena A, Melina C, Raffaele N, Carlo B, Vittoria N, Francesco A, Gaetano F, Marica E. Extraneural metastases in glioblastoma patients: two cases with YKL-40-positive glioblastomas and a meta-analysis of the literature. Neurosurg Rev. 2016;39:37–46. DOI: 10.1007/s10143-015-0656-9

[7] Ganslandt O, Stadlbauer A, Fahlbusch R, Kamada K, Buslei R, Blumcke I, Moser E, Nimsky C. Proton magnetic resonance spectroscopic imaging integrated into image-guided surgery: correlation to standard magnetic resonance imaging and tumor cell density. Neurosurgery 2005;56:291–298. DOI: 10.1227/01.NEU.0000156782.14538.78

[8] Burger PC, Dubois PJ, Schold SC, Smith KR, Odom GL, Crafts DC, Giangaspero F. Computerized tomographic and pathologic studies of the untreated, quiescent, and recurrent glioblastoma multiforme. J Neurosurg. 1983;58:159–169.

[9] Ohgaki H, Kleihues P. Population-based studies on incidence, survival rates, and genetic alterations in astrocytic and oligodendroglial gliomas. J Neuropathol Exp Neurol. 2005;64:479–489. DOI: 10.1093/jnen/64.6.479

[10] Kita D, Ciernik IF, Vaccarella S, Franceschi S, Kleihues P, Lütolf UM, Ohgaki H. Age as a predictive factor in glioblastomas: population-based study. Neuroepidemiology 2009;33:17–22. DOI: 10.1159/000210017

[11] Therkildsen C, Ladelund S, Rambech E, Persson A, Petersen A, Nilbert M. Glioblastomas, astrocytomas and oligodendrogliomas linked to Lynch syndrome. Eur J Neurol. 1995;22:717–724. DOI: 10.1111/ene.12647

[12] Ohgaki H, Kleihues P. Genetic pathways to primary and secondary glioblastoma. Am J Pathol. 2007;170:1445–1453. DOI: 10.2353/ajpath.2007.070011

[13] Marko NF, Weil RJ, Schroeder JL, Lang FF, Suki D, Sawaya RE. Extent of resection of glioblastoma revisited: personalized survival modeling facilitates more accurate survival prediction and supports a maximum-safe-resection approach to surgery. J Clin Oncol. 2014;32:774–782. DOI: 10.1200/JCO.2013.51.8886

[14] Hegi ME, Diserens AC, Gorlia T, Hamou MF, de Tribolet N, Weller M, Kros JM, Hainfellner JA, Mason W, Mariani L, Bromberg JE, Hau P, Mirimanoff RO, Cairncross JG, Janzer RC, Stupp R. MGMT gene silencing and benefit from temozolomide in glioblastoma. N Engl J Med. 2005;352:997-1003. DOI: 10.1056/NEJMoa043331

[15] Malmström A, Grønberg BH, Marosi C, Stupp R, Frappaz D, Schultz H, Abacioglu U, Tavelin B, Lhermitte B, Hegi ME, Rosell J, Henriksson R, Nordic Clinical Brain Tumour Study Group (NCBTSG). Temozolomide versus standard 6-week radiotherapy versus hypofractionated radiotherapy in patients older than 60 years with glioblastoma: the

Nordic randomised, phase 3 trial. Lancet Oncol. 2012;13:916–926. DOI: 10.1016/S1470-2045(12)70265-6

[16] Wick W, Platten M, Meisner C, Felsberg J, Tabatabai G, Simon M, Nikkhah G, Papsdorf K, Steinbach JP, Sabel M, Combs SE, Vesper J, Braun C, Meixensberger J, Ketter R, Mayer-Steinacker R, Reifenberger G, Weller M, NOA-08 Study Group of Neuro-oncology Working Group (NOA) of German Cancer Society. Temozolomide chemotherapy alone versus radiotherapy alone for malignant astrocytoma in the elderly: the NOA-08 randomised, phase 3 trial. Lancet Oncol. 2012;13:707–715. DOI: 10.1016/S1470-2045(12)70164-X

[17] Weller M, Tabatabai G, Kästner B, Felsberg J, Steinbach JP, Wick A, Schnell O, Hau P, Herrlinger U, Sabel MC, Wirsching HG, Ketter R, Bähr O, Platten M, Tonn JC, Schlegel U, Marosi C, Goldbrunner R, Stupp R, Homicsko K, Pichler J, Nikkhah G, Meixensberger J, Vajkoczy P, Kollias S, Hüsing J, Reifenberger G, Wick W, DIRECTOR Study Group. MGMT promoter methylation is a strong prognostic biomarker for benefit from dose-intensified temozolomide rechallenge in progressive glioblastoma: the DIRECTOR trial. Clin Cancer Res. 2015;21:2057–2064. DOI: 10.1158/1078-0432.CCR-14-2737

[18] Tabatabai G, Stupp R, van den Bent MJ, Hegi ME, Tonn JC, Wick W, Weller M. Molecular diagnostics of gliomas: the clinical perspective. Acta Neuropathol. 2010;120:585–592. DOI: 10.1007/s00401-010-0750-6

[19] Stupp R, Hegi ME, Mason WP, van den Bent MJ, Taphoorn MJ, Janzer RC, Ludwin SK, Allgeier A, Fisher B, Belanger K, Hau P, Brandes AA, Gijtenbeek J, Marosi C, Vecht CJ, Mokhtari K, Wesseling P, Villa S, Eisenhauer E, Gorlia T, Weller M, Lacombe D, Cairncross JG, Mirimanoff RO, European Organisation for Research and Treatment of Cancer Brain Tumour and Radiation Oncology Groups; National Cancer Institute of Canada Clinical Trials Group. Effects of radiotherapy with concomitant and adjuvant temozolomide versus radiotherapy alone on survival in glioblastoma in a randomised phase III study: 5-year analysis of the EORTC-NCIC trial. Lancet Oncol. 2009;10:459–466. DOI: 10.1016/S1470–2045(09)70025-7

[20] Marchini A, Bonifati S, Scott EM, Angelova AL, Rommelaere J. Oncolytic parvoviruses: from basic virology to clinical applications. Virol J. 2015;12:6. DOI: 10.1186/s12985-014-0223-y

[21] Swanson KD, Lok E, Wong ET. An overview of alternating electric fields therapy (NovoTTF Therapy) for the treatment of malignant glioma. Curr Neurol Neurosci Rep. 2016;16:8. DOI: 10.1007/s11910-015-0606-5

[22] Legendre C, Garcion E. Iron metabolism: a double-edged sword in the resistance of glioblastoma to therapies. Trends Endocrinol Metab. 2015;26:322–331. DOI: 10.1016/j.tem.2015.03.008

[23] Ellis HP, Greenslade M, Powell B, Spiteri I, Sottoriva A, Kurian KM. Current challenges in glioblastoma: intratumour heterogeneity, residual disease, and models to predict disease recurrence. Front Oncol. 2015;5:251. DOI: 10.3389/fonc.2015.00251

[24] Sundar SJ, Hsieh JK, Manjila S, Lathia JD, Sloan A. The role of cancer stem cells in glioblastoma. Neurosurg Focus 2014;37:E6. DOI: 10.3171/2014.9.FOCUS14494

[25] Schittenhelm J. Diagnostic Evaluation of Diffuse Gliomas, Advances in the Biology, Imaging and Therapies for Glioblastoma, Prof. Clark Chen (Ed.). Rijeka: InTech; 2011. DOI: 10.5772/24225

[26] Aldape K, Zadeh G, Mansouri S, Reifenberger G, von Deimling A. Glioblastoma: pathology, molecular mechanisms and markers. Acta Neuropathol. 2015;129:829–848. DOI: 10.1007/s00401-015-1432-1

[27] Brat DJ, Castellano-Sanchez AA, Hunter SB, Pecot M, Cohen C, Hammond EH, Devi SN, Kaur B, Van Meir EG. Pseudopalisades in glioblastoma are hypoxic, express extracellular matrix proteases, and are formed by an actively migrating cell population. Cancer Res. 2004;64:920–927.

[28] Plate KH. Mechanisms of angiogenesis in the brain. J Neuropathol Exp Neurol. 1999;58:313–320. DOI: 10.1097/00005072-199904000-00001

[29] Scherer HJ. Structural development in gliomas. Am J Cancer 1938;34:333–351.

[30] Palma L, Celli P, Maleci A, Di Lorenzo N, Cantore G. Malignant monstrocellular brain tumours. A study of 42 surgically treated cases. Acta Neurochir (Wien) 1989;97:17–25.

[31] Ortega A, Nuño M, Walia S, Mukherjee D, Black KL, Patil CG. Treatment and survival of patients harboring histological variants of glioblastoma. J Clin Neurosci. 2014;21:1709–1713. DOI: 10.1016/j.jocn.2014.05.003

[32] Rodriguez FJ, Scheithauer BW, Giannini C, Bryant SC, Jenkins RB. Epithelial and pseudoepithelial differentiation in glioblastoma and gliosarcoma: a comparative morphologic and molecular genetic study. Cancer 2008;113:2779–2789. DOI: 10.1002/cncr.23899

[33] Fuller GN, Goodman JC, Vogel H, Ghorbani R. Epithelioid glioblastoma: a distinct clinicopathologic entity. J Neuropathol Exp Neurol. 1998;57:501. DOI: 10.1097/00005072-199805000-00145

[34] Perry A, Aldape KD, George DH, Burger PC. Small cell astrocytoma: an aggressive variant that is clinicopathologically and genetically distinct from anaplastic oligodendroglioma. Cancer 2004;101:2318–2326. DOI: 10.1002/cncr.20625

[35] Perry A, Miller CR, Gujrati M, Scheithauer BW, Zambrano SC, Jost SC, Raghavan R, Qian J, Cochran EJ, Huse JT, Holland EC, Burger PC, Rosenblum MK. Malignant gliomas with primitive neuroectodermal tumor-like components: a clinicopathologic

and genetic study of 53 cases. Brain Pathol. 2009;19:81–90. DOI: 10.1111/j.1750-3639.2008.00167.x

[36] Hegi ME, Janzer RC, Lambiv WL, Gorlia T, Kouwenhoven MC, Hartmann C, von Deimling A, Martinet D, Besuchet Schmutz N, Diserens AC, Hamou MF, Bady P, Weller M, van den Bent MJ, Mason WP, Mirimanoff RO, Stupp R, Mokhtari K, Wesseling P, European Organisation for Research and Treatment of Cancer Brain Tumour and Radiation Oncology Groups; National Cancer Institute of Canada Clinical Trials Group. Presence of an oligodendroglioma-like component in newly diagnosed glioblastoma identifies a pathogenetically heterogeneous subgroup and lacks prognostic value: central pathology review of the EORTC_26981/NCIC_CE.3 trial. Acta Neuropathol. 2012;123:841–852. DOI: 10.1007/s00401-011-0938-4

[37] Rickert CH, Riemenschneider MJ, Schachenmayr W, Richter HP, Bockhorn J, Reifenberger G, Paulus W. Glioblastoma with adipocyte-like tumor cell differentiation--histological and molecular features of a rare differentiation pattern. Brain Pathol. 2009;19:431–438. DOI: 10.1111/j.1750-3639.2008.00199.x

[38] Kepes JJ, Rubinstein LJ. Malignant gliomas with heavily lipidized (foamy) tumor cells: a report of three cases with immunoperoxidase study. Cancer 1981;47:2451–2459.

[39] Schittenhelm J, Psaras T. Glioblastoma with granular cell astrocytoma features: a case report and literature review. Clin Neuropathol. 2010;29:323–329.

[40] Schittenhelm J, Erdmann T, Maennlin S, Will BE, Beschorner R, Bornemann A, Meyermann R, Mittelbronn M. Gliosarcoma with chondroid and osseous differentiation. Neuropathology 2007;27:90–94. DOI: 10.1111/j.1440-1789.2006.00747.x

[41] Jaiswal S, Agrawal V, Vij M, Sahu RN, Jaiswal AK, Behari S. Glioblastoma with melanotic differentiation. Clin Neuropathol. 2010;29:330–333. DOI: 10.1002/1097-0142(19810515)47:10<2451::AID-CNCR2820471024>3.0.CO;2–5

[42] Kleinschmidt-De Masters BK, Alassiri AH, Birks DK, Newell KL, Moore W, Lillehei KO. Epithelioid versus rhabdoid glioblastomas are distinguished by monosomy 22 and immunohistochemical expression of INI-1 but not claudin 6. Am J Surg Pathol. 2010;34:341–354. DOI: 10.1097/PAS.0b013e3181ce107b

[43] Waidelich J, Schittenhelm J, Allmendinger O, Meyermann R, Beschorner R. Glutamate transporters in diagnostic neurooncology. Brain Pathology 2010;20(Suppl. 1):1–99.

[44] Blümcke I, Müller S, Buslei R, Riederer BM, Wiestler OD. Microtubule-associated protein-2 immunoreactivity: a useful tool in the differential diagnosis of low-grade neuroepithelial tumors. Acta Neuropathol. 2004;108:89–96. DOI: 10.1007/s00401-004-0873-8

[45] Schittenhelm J, Beschorner R, Simon P, Tabatabai G, Herrmann C, Schlaszus H, Capper D, Weller M, Meyermann R, Mittelbronn M. Diagnostic value of WT1 in neuroepithelial

tumours. Neuropathol Appl Neurobiol. 2009;35:69–81. DOI: 10.1111/j.1365-2990.2008.00957.x

[46] Hasselblatt M, Paulus W. Sensitivity and specificity of epithelial membrane antigen staining patterns in ependymomas. Acta Neuropathol. 2003;106:385–388. DOI: 10.1007/s00401-003-0752-8

[47] Ogura R, Tsukamoto Y, Natsumeda M, Isogawa M, Aoki H, Kobayashi T, Yoshida S, Okamoto K, Takahashi H, Fujii Y, Kakita A. Immunohistochemical profiles of IDH1, MGMT and P53: practical significance for prognostication of patients with diffuse gliomas. Neuropathology 2015;35:324–335. DOI: 10.1111/neup.12196

[48] Kwon CH, Zhao D, Chen J, Alcantara S, Li Y, Burns DK, Mason RP, Lee EY, Wu H, Parada LF. Pten haploinsufficiency accelerates formation of high-grade astrocytomas. Cancer Res. 2008;68:3286–3294. DOI: 10.1158/0008-5472.CAN-07-6867

[49] Weller M, Felsberg J, Hartmann C, Berger H, Steinbach JP, Schramm J, Westphal M, Schackert G, Simon M, Tonn JC, Heese O, Krex D, Nikkhah G, Pietsch T, Wiestler O, Reifenberger G, von Deimling A, Loeffler M. Molecular predictors of progression-free and overall survival in patients with newly diagnosed glioblastoma: a prospective translational study of the German Glioma Network. J Clin Oncol. 2009;27:5743–5750. DOI: 10.1200/JCO.2009.23.0805

[50] Preusser M, Charles Janzer R, Felsberg J, Reifenberger G, Hamou MF, Diserens AC, Stupp R, Gorlia T, Marosi C, Heinzl H, Hainfellner JA, Hegi M. Anti-O6-methylguanine-methyltransferase (MGMT) immunohistochemistry in glioblastoma multiforme: observer variability and lack of association with patient survival impede its use as clinical biomarker. Brain Pathol. 2008;18:520–532. DOI: 10.1111/j.1750-3639.2008.00153.x

[51] Dang L, White DW, Gross S, Bennett BD, Bittinger MA, Driggers EM, Fantin VR, Jang HG, Jin S, Keenan MC, Marks KM, Prins RM, Ward PS, Yen KE, Liau LM, Rabinowitz JD, Cantley LC, Thompson CB, Van der Heiden MG, Su SM. Cancer-associated IDH1 mutations produce 2-hydroxyglutarate. Nature 2010;462(7273):739–744.

[52] Nobusawa S, Watanabe T, Kleihues P, Ohgaki H. IDH1 mutations as molecular signature and predictive factor of secondary glioblastomas. Clin Cancer Res. 2009;15:6002–6007. DOI: 10.1158/1078–0432.CCR-09-0715

[53] Sanson M, Marie Y, Paris S, Idbaih A, Laffaire J, Ducray F, El Hallani S, Boisselier B, Mokhtari K, Hoang-Xuan K, Delattre JY. Isocitrate dehydrogenase 1 codon 132 mutation is an important prognostic biomarker in gliomas. J Clin Oncol. 2009;27:4150–4154. DOI: 10.1200/JCO.2009.21.9832

[54] Hartmann C, Hentschel B, Wick W, Capper D, Felsberg J, Simon M, Westphal M, Schackert G, Meyermann R, Pietsch T, Reifenberger G, Weller M, Loeffler M, von Deimling A. Patients with IDH1 wild type anaplastic astrocytomas exhibit worse prognosis than IDH1-mutated glioblastomas, and IDH1 mutation status accounts for

the unfavorable prognostic effect of higher age: implications for classification of gliomas. Acta Neuropathol. 2010;120:707–718. DOI: 10.1007/s00401-010-0781-z

[55] Capper D, Weissert S, Balss J, Habel A, Meyer J, Jäger D, Ackermann U, Tessmer C, Korshunov A, Zentgraf H, Hartmann C, von Deimling A. Characterization of R132H mutation-specific IDH1 antibody binding in brain tumors. Brain Pathol. 2010;20:245–254. DOI: 10.1111/j.1750-3639.2009.00352.x

[56] Wiestler B, Claus R, Hartlieb SA, Schliesser MG, Weiss EK, Hielscher T, Platten M, Dittmann LM, Meisner C, Felsberg J, Happold C, Simon M, Nikkhah G, Papsdorf K, Steinbach JP, Sabel M, Grimm C, Weichenhan D, Tews B, Reifenberger G, Capper D, Müller W, Plass C, Weller M, Wick W, Neuro-oncology Working Group (NOA) of the German Cancer Society. Malignant astrocytomas of elderly patients lack favorable molecular markers: an analysis of the NOA-08 study collective. Neuro Oncol. 2013;15:1017–1026. DOI: 10.1093/neuonc/not043

[57] Skardelly M, Brendle E, Noell S, Behling F, Wuttke TV, Schittenhelm J, Bisdas S, Meisner C, Rona S, Tatagiba MS, Tabatabai G. Predictors of preoperative and early postoperative seizures in patients with intra-axial primary and metastatic brain tumors: a retrospective observational single center study. Ann Neurol. 2015;78:917–928. DOI: 10.1002/ana.24522

[58] Singh SK, Clarke ID, Terasaki M, Bonn VE, Hawkins C, Squire J, Dirks PB. Identification of a cancer stem cell in human brain tumors. Cancer Res. 2003;63:5821–5828.

[59] Stopschinski BE, Beier CP, Beier D. Glioblastoma cancer stem cells—from concept to clinical application. Cancer Lett. 2013;338:32–40. DOI: 10.1016/j.canlet.2012.05.033

[60] Verhaak RG, Hoadley KA, Purdom E, Wang V, Qi Y, Wilkerson MD, Miller CR, Ding L, Golub T, Mesirov JP, Alexe G, Lawrence M, O'Kelly M, Tamayo P, Weir BA, Gabriel S, Winckler W, Gupta S, Jakkula L, Feiler HS, Hodgson JG, James CD, Sarkaria JN, Brennan C, Kahn A, Spellman PT, Wilson RK, Speed TP, Gray JW, Meyerson M, Getz G, Perou CM, Hayes DN, Cancer Genome Atlas Research Network. Integrated genomic analysis identifies clinically relevant subtypes of glioblastoma characterized by abnormalities in PDGFRA, IDH1, EGFR, and NF1. Cancer Cell 2010;17:98–111. DOI: 10.1016/j.ccr.2009

[61] Srivastava A, Jain A, Jha P, Suri V, Sharma MC, Mallick S, Puri T, Gupta DK, Gupta A, Sarkar C. MGMT gene promoter methylation in pediatric glioblastomas. Childs Nerv Syst. 2010;26:1613–1618. DOI: 10.1007/s00381-010-1214-y

[62] Meyer-Puttlitz B, Hayashi Y, Waha A, Rollbrocker B, Boström J, Wiestler OD, Louis DN, Reifenberger G, von Deimling A. Molecular genetic analysis of giant cell glioblastomas. Am J Pathol. 1997;151:853–857.

[63] Parsons DW, Jones S, Zhang X, Lin JC, Leary RJ, Angenendt P, Mankoo P, Carter H, Siu IM, Gallia GL, Olivi A, Mc Lendon R, Rasheed BA, Keir S, Nikolskaya T, Nikolsky Y, Busam DA, Tekleab H, Diaz LAJr, Hartigan J, Smith DR, Strausberg RL, Marie SK,

Shinjo SM, Yan H, Riggins GJ, Bigner DD, Karchin R, Papadopoulos N, Parmigiani G, Vogelstein B, Velculescu VE, Kinzler KW. An integrated genomic analysis of human glioblastoma multiforme. Science 2008;321:1807–1812. DOI: 10.1126/science.1164382

[64] Yan H, Parsons DW, Jin G, Mc Lendon R, Rasheed BA, Yuan W, Kos I, Batinic-Haberle I, Jones S, Riggins GJ, Friedman H, Friedman A, Reardon D, Herndon J, Kinzler KW, Velculescu VE, Vogelstein B, Bigner DD. IDH1 and IDH2 mutations in gliomas. N Engl J Med. 2009;360:765–773. DOI: 10.1056/NEJMoa0808710

[65] Lee D, Kang SY, Suh YL, Jeong JY, Lee JI, Nam DH. Clinicopathologic and genomic features of gliosarcomas. J Neurooncol. 2012;107:643–650.

[66] Schumacher T, Bunse L, Pusch S, Sahm F, Wiestler B, Quandt J, Menn O, Osswald M, Oezen I, Ott M, Keil M, BalßJ, Rauschenbach K, Grabowska AK, Vogler I, Diekmann J, Trautwein N, Eichmüller SB, Okun J, StevanovićS, Riemer AB, Sahin U, Friese MA, Beckhove P, von Deimling A, Wick W, Platten M. A vaccine targeting mutant IDH1 induces antitumour immunity. Nature 2014;512:324–327. DOI: 10.1038/nature13387

[67] Hatanpaa KJ, Burma S, Zhao D, Habib AA. Epidermal growth factor receptor in glioma: signal transduction, neuropathology, imaging, and radioresistance. Neoplasia 2010;12:675–684.

[68] Sturm D, Bender S, Jones DT, Lichter P, Grill J, Becher O, Hawkins C, Majewski J, Jones C, Costello JF, Iavarone A, Aldape K, Brennan CW, Jabado N, Pfister SM. Paediatric and adult glioblastoma: multiform (epi)genomic culprits emerge. Nat Rev Cancer 2014;14:92–107. DOI: 10.1038/nrc3655

[69] Szerlip NJ, Pedraza A, Chakravarty D, Azim M, Mc Guire J, Fang Y, Ozawa T, Holland EC, Huse JT, Jhanwar S, Leversha MA, Mikkelsen T, Brennan CW. Intratumoral heterogeneity of receptor tyrosine kinases EGFR and PDGFRA amplification in glioblastoma defines subpopulations with distinct growth factor response. Proc Natl Acad Sci U S A 2012;109:3041–3046. DOI: 10.1073/pnas.1114033109

[70] Jeong TS, Yee GT. Glioblastoma in a patient with neurofibromatosis type 1: a case report and review of the literature. Brain Tumor Res Treat. 2014;2:36–38. DOI: 10.14791/btrt.2014.2.1.36

[71] Parsa AT, Waldron JS, Panner A, Crane CA, Parney IF, Barry JJ, Cachola KE, Murray JC, Tihan T, Jensen MC, Mischel PS, Stokoe D, Pieper RO. Loss of tumor suppressor PTEN function increases B7-H1 expression and immunoresistance in glioma. Nat Med. 2007;13:84–88. DOI: 10.1038/nm1517

[72] Preusser M, Berghoff AS, Wick W, Weller M. Clinical Neuropathology mini-review 6-2015: PD-L1: emerging biomarker in glioblastoma? Clin Neuropathol. 2015;34:313–321.

[73] Patel AP, Tirosh I, Trombetta JJ, Shalek AK, Gillespie SM, Wakimoto H, Cahill DP, Nahed BV, Curry WT, Martuza RL, Louis DN, Rozenblatt-Rosen O, SuvàML, Regev A,

Bernstein BE. Single-cell RNA-seq highlights intratumoral heterogeneity in primary glioblastoma. Science 2014;344:1396–1401. DOI: 10.1126/science.1254257

[74] Appin CL, Brat DJ. Molecular genetics of gliomas. Cancer J. 2014;20:66–72. DOI: 10.1097/PPO.0000000000000020

[75] Koelsche C, Sahm F, Capper D, Reuss D, Sturm D, Jones DT, Kool M, Northcott PA, Wiestler B, Böhmer K, Meyer J, Mawrin C, Hartmann C, Mittelbronn M, Platten M, Brokinkel B, Seiz M, Herold-Mende C, Unterberg A, Schittenhelm J, Weller M, Pfister S, Wick W, Korshunov A, von Deimling A. Distribution of TERT promoter mutations in pediatric and adult tumors of the nervous system. Acta Neuropathol. 2013;126:907–915. DOI: 10.1007/s00401-013-1195-5

[76] Labussière M, Boisselier B, Mokhtari K, Di Stefano AL, Rahimian A, Rossetto M, Ciccarino P, Saulnier O, Paterra R, Marie Y, Finocchiaro G, Sanson M. Combined analysis of TERT, EGFR, and IDH status defines distinct prognostic glioblastoma classes. Neurology 2014;83:1200–1206. DOI: 10.1212/WNL

[77] Mosrati MA, Malmström A, Lysiak M, Krysztofiak A, Hallbeck M, Milos P, Hallbeck AL, Bratthäll C, Strandéus M, Stenmark-Askmalm M, Söderkvist P. TERT promoter mutations and polymorphisms as prognostic factors in primary glioblastoma. Oncotarget 2015;6:16663–166673. DOI: 10.18632/oncotarget.4389

[78] Schwartzentruber J, Korshunov A, Liu XY, Jones DT, Pfaff E, Jacob K, Sturm D, Fontebasso AM, Quang DA, Tönjes M, Hovestadt V, Albrecht S, Kool M, Nantel A, Konermann C, Lindroth A, Jäger N, Rausch T, Ryzhova M, Korbel JO, Hielscher T, Hauser P, Garami M, Klekner A, Bognar L, Ebinger M, Schuhmann MU, Scheurlen W, Pekrun A, Frühwald MC, Roggendorf W, Kramm C, Dürken M, Atkinson J, Lepage P, Montpetit A, Zakrzewska M, Zakrzewski K, Liberski PP, Dong Z, Siegel P, Kulozik AE, Zapatka M, Guha A, Malkin D, Felsberg J, Reifenberger G, von Deimling A, Ichimura K, Collins VP, Witt H, Milde T, Witt O, Zhang C, Castelo-Branco P, Lichter P, Faury D, Tabori U, Plass C, Majewski J, Pfister SM, Jabado N. Driver mutations in histone H3.3 and chromatin remodelling genes in paediatric glioblastoma. Nature 2012;482:226–231. DOI: 10.1038/nature10833

[79] Chan KM, Han J, Fang D, Gan H, Zhang Z. A lesson learned from the H3.3K27M mutation found in pediatric glioma: a new approach to the study of the function of histone modifications in vivo? Cell Cycle 2013;12:2546–2552. DOI: 10.4161/cc.25625

[80] Korshunov A, Capper D, Reuss D, Schrimpf D, Ryzhova M, Hovestadt V, Sturm D, Meyer J, Jones C, Zheludkova O, Kumirova E, Golanov A, Kool M, Schüller U, Mittelbronn M, Hasselblatt M, Schittenhelm J, Reifenberger G, Herold-Mende C, Lichter P, von Deimling A, Pfister SM, Jones DT. Histologically distinct neuroepithelial tumors with histone 3 G34 mutation are molecularly similar and comprise a single nosologic entity. Acta Neuropathol. 2016; 131: 137-146. DOI: 10.1007/s00401-015-1493-1

[81] Korshunov A, Ryzhova M, Hovestadt V, Bender S, Sturm D, Capper D, Meyer J, Schrimpf D, Kool M, Northcott PA, Zheludkova O, Milde T, Witt O, Kulozik AE,

Reifenberger G, Jabado N, Perry A, Lichter P, von Deimling A, Pfister SM, Jones DT. Integrated analysis of pediatric glioblastoma reveals a subset of biologically favorable tumors with associated molecular prognostic markers. Acta Neuropathol. 2015;129:669–678. DOI: 10.1007/s00401-015-1405-4

[82] Jiao Y, Killela PJ, Reitman ZJ, Rasheed AB, Heaphy CM, de Wilde RF, Rodriguez FJ, Rosemberg S, Oba-Shinjo SM, Nagahashi Marie SK, Bettegowda C, Agrawal N, Lipp E, Pirozzi C, Lopez G, He Y, Friedman H, Friedman AH, Riggins GJ, Holdhoff M, Burger P, Mc Lendon R, Bigner DD, Vogelstein B, Meeker AK, Kinzler KW, Papadopoulos N, Diaz LA, Yan H. Frequent ATRX, CIC, FUBP1 and IDH1 mutations refine the classification of malignant gliomas. Oncotarget 2012;3:709–722. DOI: 10.18632/oncotarget.588

[83] Reuss DE, Sahm F, Schrimpf D, Wiestler B, Capper D, Koelsche C, Schweizer L, Korshunov A, Jones DT, Hovestadt V, Mittelbronn M, Schittenhelm J, Herold-Mende C, Unterberg A, Platten M, Weller M, Wick W, Pfister SM, von Deimling A. ATRX and IDH1-R132H immunohistochemistry with subsequent copy number analysis and IDH sequencing as a basis for an "integrated" diagnostic approach for adult astrocytoma, oligodendroglioma and glioblastoma. Acta Neuropathol. 2015;129:133–146. DOI: 10.1007/s00401-014-1370-3

[84] Wiestler B, Capper D, Holland-Letz T, Korshunov A, von Deimling A, Pfister SM, Platten M, Weller M, Wick W. ATRX loss refines the classification of anaplastic gliomas and identifies a subgroup of IDH mutant astrocytic tumors with better prognosis. Acta Neuropathol. 2013;126:443–451. DOI: 10.1007/s00401-013-1156-z

[85] Noushmehr H, Weisenberger DJ, Diefes K, Phillips HS, Pujara K, Berman BP, Pan F, Pelloski CE, Sulman EP, Bhat KP, Verhaak RG, Hoadley KA, Hayes DN, Perou CM, Schmidt HK, Ding L, Wilson RK, Van Den Berg D, Shen H, Bengtsson H, Neuvial P, Cope LM, Buckley J, Herman JG, Baylin SB, Laird PW, Aldape K, Network Cancer Genome Atlas Research. Identification of a CpG island methylator phenotype that defines a distinct subgroup of glioma. Cancer Cell 2010;17:510–522. DOI: 10.1016/j.ccr.2010.03.017

[86] Ozawa T, Riester M, Cheng YK, Huse JT, Squatrito M, Helmy K, Charles N, Michor F, Holland EC. Most human non-GCIMP glioblastoma subtypes evolve from a common proneural-like precursor glioma. Cancer Cell 2014;26:288–300. DOI: 10.1016/j.ccr.2014.06.005

[87] Favero F, Mc Granahan N, Salm M, Birkbak NJ, Sanborn JZ, Benz SC, Becq J, Peden JF, Kingsbury Z, Grocok RJ, Humphray S, Bentley D, Spencer-Dene B, Gutteridge A, Brada M, Roger S, Dietrich PY, Forshew T, Gerlinger M, Rowan A, Stamp G, Eklund AC, Szallasi Z, Swanton C. Glioblastoma adaptation traced through decline of an IDH1 clonal driver and macro-evolution of a double-minute chromosome. Ann Oncol. 2015;26:880–887. DOI: 10.1093/annonc/mdv127

[88] Inda MM, Bonavia R, Mukasa A, Narita Y, Sah DW, Van den berg S, Brennan C, Johns TG, Bachoo R, Hadwiger P, Tan P, Depinho RA, Cavenee W, Furnari F. Tumor

heterogeneity is an active process maintained by a mutant EGFR-induced cytokine circuit in glioblastoma. Genes Dev. 2010;24:1731–1745. DOI: 10.1101/gad.1890510

[89] Cairncross G, Wang M, Shaw E, Jenkins R, Brachman D, Buckner J, Fink K, Souhami L, Laperriere N, Curran W, Mehta M. Phase III trial of chemoradiotherapy for anaplastic oligodendroglioma: long-term results of RTOG 9402. J Clin Oncol. 2013;31:337–343. DOI: 10.1200/JCO.2012.43.2674

[90] Kim YH, Nobusawa S, Mittelbronn M, Paulus W, Brokinkel B, Keyvani K, Sure U, Wrede K, Nakazato Y, Tanaka Y, Vital A, Mariani L, Stawski R, Watanabe T, De Girolami U, Kleihues P, Ohgaki H. Molecular classification of low-grade diffuse gliomas. Am J Pathol. 2010;177:2708–2714. DOI: 10.2353/ajpath.2010.100680

[91] Riemenschneider MJ, Jeuken JW, Wesseling P, Reifenberger G. Molecular diagnostics of gliomas: state of the art. Acta Neuropathol. 2010;120:567–584. DOI: 10.1007/s00401-010-0736-4

[92] Basanta D, Scott JG, Rockne R, Swanson KR, Anderson AR. The role of IDH1 mutated tumour cells in secondary glioblastomas: an evolutionary game theoretical view. Phys Biol. 2011;8:015016. DOI 10.1088/1478-3975/8/1/015016

Chapter 2

The Roles of MicroRNAs in Glioblastoma Biology and Biomarker

Takashi Sasayama, Kazuhiro Tanaka and
Eiji Kohmura

Additional information is available at the end of the chapter

http://dx.doi.org/10.5772/63243

Abstract

MicroRNAs (miRNAs) are small, noncoding RNAs transcribed from DNA that are 18–24 nucleotides in length. A single miRNA has the capacity to regulate a large number of target messenger RNAs (mRNAs), and the main function of miRNAs is to downregulate gene expression. A large set of miRNAs is overexpressed or downregulated in various human cancers compared with normal tissues, and gene silencing by miRNAs enhances tumor malignancies.

In glioblastomas (GBMs), a number of miRNAs are reported to display aberrant expression patterns, and miRNAs have been shown to strongly influence cell viability, cell proliferation, invasiveness, angiogenesis, metabolism, and microenvironment. Since early findings, the number of studies published on this subject has steadily increased, elucidating numerous interesting miRNA-mediated mechanisms in the tumorigenesis of GBM.

A number of studies have recently suggested that circulating miRNAs could be potential biomarkers for cancer diagnosis. Not only the role of miRNAs in glioma development but also their specificity makes them important candidate biomarkers that could provide important characteristic information about a tumor and improve treatment and prognosis. This review summarizes current progress and future directions in this exciting and steadily expanding field.

Keywords: glioblastoma, microRNA, hallmarks, biomarker, circulating

1. Introduction

Glioblastomas (GBMs) are the most common and intractable primary neoplasms of the central nervous system (CNS). Gross total surgical excision followed by radiotherapy up to a total dose of 60 Gy was the only accepted GBM management for decades because no chemotherapeutic agents significantly improved the survival of patients with GBM until the introduction of temozolomide, an oral alkylating agent (1). Despite aggressive treatments, recurrence is inevitable and fatal in GBMs. In a recent clinical study, the median survival was up to approximately 20 months and the two-year survival rate was approximately 30~40% (2, 3). Therefore, more efforts need to be made to change the poor prognosis of patients with GBM.

MicroRNAs (miRNAs) are small (18–24 nt), noncoding RNAs that are transcribed from the intergenic or intronic regions of DNA. miRNAs regulate the expression levels or translational levels of messenger RNAs (mRNAs) post-transcriptionally and affect to various biological processes, such as cell proliferation, cell survival, differentiation, and metabolism (4). Primary miRNAs (pri-miRNAs), transcribed from DNA and have short stem-loop structures (SLSs), are processed into premature miRNAs (pre-miRNAs) and then finally processed into mature miRNAs (5). A single miRNA has many targets of mRNAs, binding its target sites mostly in the 3′ untranslated region (3′-UTR) of the mRNA. The main function of miRNAs is to down-regulate gene expression, and miRNAs can function either as tumor suppressors or as oncogenes (6).

A number of miRNAs are reported to display aberrant expression patterns in GBMs (7). In 2005, the first miRNA dysregulation was identified in GBMs (8). miR-21 detected by northern blot was overexpressed in GBM tissues when compared with non-neoplastic control tissues. On the other hand, a systemic screen for miRNA aberrations by miRNA microarray in GBM was performed by other researchers (7). Using miRNA microarray analysis, we previously reported that miR-10b, miR-21, miR-183, miR-92b, and miR-106b are highly expressed in GBMs compared with normal brain tissue (9). Several other reports have also identified these miRNAs as being upregulated in GBMs (8). Recently, we reported that the expression of miR-183 involved in HIF-1α expression and its downstream molecules (10). Since then, it has been documented that miRNA dysregulation could play an important role in development and progression.

2. MicroRNA expression in glioblastoma

Similar to other malignant tumors, GBM has the hallmarks of cancer: biological capabilities of sustaining proliferative signaling, inducing angiogenesis, evading growth suppressors, resistance to apoptosis, activating invasion and metastasis, genomic instability, reprogramming energy metabolism, limitless replicative potential, and evading immune destruction. It is generally accepted that hallmark features of GBM are not only a reflection of genetic abnormalities and aberrant signal transition but also the dysregulation of miRNA-mediated translational control. The miRNA-mRNA interactions transform the short "nonsense" sequences into endogenous oncogenes or tumor suppressors. miRNA expression patterns could define a tumor type, implying that certain changes in miRNAs might drive the malignant transformation to a particular tumor. Therefore, whether a miRNA acts as an oncomiR or tumor suppressor-miRNA depends on the regulated genes and cellular context.

The first report on altered miRNA expression in GBMs was published in 2005 (8). In this report, miR-21 was shown to be highly upregulated and to have antiapoptotic capabilities in GBM cells. These findings suggest that overexpressed miR-21 may function as an oncogene in GBMs by blocking expression of key apoptosis-enabling genes (8). In the same year, Ciafre et al. analyzed the global expression levels of 245 microRNAs in both GBM cell lines and patient biopsies (7). A systemic screen for miRNA aberrations by microarray identified a set of dysregulated miRNAs in GBM tissues, including the upregulation of miR-10b, miR-21, and miR-25 and downregulation of miR-128 and miR-181a/181b-/181c (7). Since then, miRNA expression in GBMs has been evaluated in several profiling studies. We previously reported that miR-10b, miR-21, miR-183, miR-92b, and miR-106b are highly expressed in GBMs compared with normal brain tissue, and miR-134, miR-302c, miR-324, miR-379, and miR-368-3p are downregulated in GBMs (9). In 2008, Silber et al. reported 13 miRNAs to be downregulated and three miRNAs to be upregulated in anaplastic astrocytomas and GBMs (11). Furthermore, they revealed that expression levels of miRNA-124 and miRNA-137 were significantly decreased compared with non-neoplastic brain tissue, and both of them induce differentiation of adult neural stem cells. Another study carried out by Godlewski et al. found 8 microRNAs to be upregulated and 11 downregulated when analyzing 245 microRNAs in the setting of GBM (12). A microarray-based study by Rao et al. analyzing 756 microRNAs identified another 55 upregulated and 29 downregulated microRNAs in primary and secondary GBMs and anaplastic astrocytoma compared with controls (13). This study not only validated the role of several deregulated microRNAs but also provided data for the development of a 23 microRNA signature pattern for distinguishing between anaplastic astrocytoma and GBM (13).

3. Hallmarks of glioblastoma and microRNAs

3.1. Growth signal activation and microRNAs

Cell proliferation in GBM could be triggered by somatic alterations within the receptor tyrosine kinase (RTK)-signaling pathways. The most important pathways in GBM are the phosphatidylinositide 3-kinase (PI3K)/AKT and RAS/mitogen-activated protein kinase (MAPK) pathways (14). Abnormally augmented signals downstream from RTKs enable tumor cells to sustain proliferation that is under tight control in normal cells. At least 90% of GBM cases harbor genetic alterations in RTK pathways. Epidermal growth factor receptor (EGFR), platelet-derived growth factor receptor alpha polypeptide (PDGFRA), MET proto-oncogene (MET), and fibroblast growth factor receptor (FGFR) are among the most commonly dysregulated RTKs in GBM (15). EGFR and PDGFRA are well-established oncogenes in GBM (16), and thus, identification of their miRNA regulators following the discovery of functional implications of miRNAs in GBMs is warranted.

miR-7 is a common regulator of the PI3K/ATK and MAPK pathways, both of which are launched by EGFR through its two direct targets, the transcription factors PI3K and Raf-1, respectively (17). Human EGFR mRNA 3′-untranslated region contains three miR-7 target sites (18). Transient expression of miR-7 in GBM cells strongly inhibited *in vivo* GBM xenograft growth (17). Decreased expression of miR-128 correlates with aggressive human glioma subtypes, and miR-128 represses growth and mediates differentiation by targeting oncogenic EGFR and PDGFRA (19). The authors demonstrated that miR-128 suppresses glioma formation in a glioma mouse model, suggesting miR-128 as a glioma tumor suppressor that targets RTK signaling to repress gliomagenesis. miR-218 targets multiple components of RTK-signaling pathways, including the EGFR pathway, and miR-218 repression increases the abundance and activity of multiple RTK effectors (20). The expression of miR-218 is significantly decreased in the mesenchymal subtype of GBM, and the miR-218-RTK-HIF2α-signaling axis promotes GBM cell survival and tumor angiogenesis (20). A large-scale, genomewide miRNA expression analysis revealed miR-219 was downregulated in GBM, and exogenous overexpression of miR-219 in glioma cells inhibited proliferation and soft agar colony formation (21). In addition, overexpression of miR-219-5p reduced the activity of PI3 kinase and MAP kinase in glioma cell lines by targeting to EGFR (21). Moreover, overexpression of miR-133 decreased GBM cell growth and increased cell apoptosis, whereas depletion of miR-133 increased cell growth (22). The protein translation inhibition of EGFR by miR-133 was confirmed by a dual luciferase reporter assay (22). miR-340 overexpression suppressed several oncogenes, including EGFR (23). miR-340 induces glioma cells toward terminal differentiation and regulates glioma cell development by downregulating ROCK1 expression (23). miR-491 directly targets EGFR, CDK6, and Bcl-xL (24). Importantly, miR-491 is commonly codeleted with its adjacent CDKN2A on chromosome 9p21.3 in GBM. As a negative regulator of EGFR expression, miR-491 is a tumor suppressor gene. On the other hand, miR-148a expression was elevated in GBM specimens compared with normal human brain and astrocytes (25). miR-148a is a prognostic onco-miRNA that targets MIG6 and BIM to regulate EGFR and apoptosis in GBM (25). By inhibiting MIG6 expression, miR-148a reduced EGFR trafficking to Rab7-expressing compartments, including late endosomes and lysosomes. This process coincided with reduced degradation and elevated expression and activation of EGFR (25). Furthermore, the protein expression of EGFR decreased in cells with forced overexpression of miR-34a (26). Yin et al. reported that both deletion of miR-34a and amplification of EGFR were associated with significantly decreased overall survival of patients with GBM (26).

PDGFRA is a direct target of miR-34a, a downregulated miRNA in the proneural subtype compared with the mesenchymal subtype of GBM (27, 28). miR-34a specifically affects the growth of proneural glioma cells *in vitro* and *in vivo* (28). miR-34a repression in proneural gliomas is only modestly dependent on p53. Derepression of PDGFRA by the downregulation of miR-34a in the proneural subtype that results in a more proliferative phenotype may be responsible for the difference in response to clinical treatment for GBM. Gene mutation or amplification in MET is a relatively rare event in GBM (29). However, miR-34a expression inhibited c-Met reporter activities in glioma cells. In addition, miR-34a levels in human gliomas were inversely correlated with c-Met levels. Transient transfection of miR-34a into gliomas strongly inhibited cell proliferation, cell cycle progression, cell survival, and cell invasion (30).

MET is highly expressed in the mesenchymal subtype of GBM (31). miR-182 sensitized glioma cells to TMZ-induced apoptosis, promoted glioma initiating cell (GIC) differentiation, and reduced tumor cell proliferation via knockdown of c-Met, Bcl2L12, and HIF2A (32). miR-144-3p specifically bound to the MET 3′-untranslated region (3′ UTR) and inhibited its expression. miR-144 strongly repressed GBM cell proliferation and invasion by suppressing MET *in vitro* and *in vivo* (33).

RAS signaling, upstream of MAP kinase, is reported to be regulated by miRNAs. Although only 1% of GBMs have a RAS mutation or amplification, 10% of GBMs contain neurofibromin 1 (NF1) inactivating genetic alterations that lead to hyperactive RAS activity by enhancing the intrinsic GTPase activity (29). Two recent reports focused on miRNAs targeting RAS in GBMs and showed that miR-143 directly targets N-RAS (34) and that let-7a directly targets K-RAS (35). Low expression of let-7a was correlated with a poor prognosis of primary GBM patients (35). In addition, miR-124 governs glioma growth and angiogenesis and enhances chemosensitivity by targeting R-RAS and N-RAS (36). In addition, miR-124 inhibits the MAP kinase pathway by repressing SOS1 mRNA (37). Moreover, these miRNAs are all downregulated in GBM specimens, underlying the malignant transformation.

Phosphatase and tensin homolog (PTEN) and NF1 are the most important negative regulators of cell proliferative pathways. The inactivated genetic mutations of NF1 and PTEN are found in 10 and 41% of GBM cases, respectively (29). NF1 is targeted by miR-9, which is an miRNA upregulated in GBM and promotes the proliferation and migration of glioma cells (38, 39). In addition, NF1 is a direct target of miR-514a, and over-expression of miR-514a inhibited NF1 expression, which correlated with increased survival cells (40). The protein phosphatase activity of PTEN is involved in cell proliferation, preventing cells from growing. miR-26a, frequently amplified at the DNA level in human gliomas, is identified as a direct regulator of PTEN expression (41). miR-26a-mediated PTEN repression in a murine glioma model enhances *de novo* glioma formation (41). Overexpression of miR-26a in PTEN-competent and PTEN-deficient GBM cells promoted tumor growth *in vivo* and further increased growth in cells overexpressing CDK4 or CENTG1 (42). Guo et al. reported that c-Myc modulates genes associated with oncogenesis in GBM through deregulation of miRNAs via the c-Myc-miR-26a-PTEN-signaling pathway (43). CREB, a proto-oncogenic transcription factor that is overexpressed in gliomas, can promote gliomagenesis by modulating the expression of oncogenic miR-23a, which represses PTEN directly (44). miR-23a-mediated suppression of PTEN led to the activation of AKT/ERK pathways and epithelial-mesenchymal transition (EMT) (45). miR-17-5p (46), and miRNA-1908 (47) directly target PTEN in GBMs. Overexpression of miR-17 prolongs GBM cell survival and increases cell motility, and induces HIF-1α activation in response to stress by targeting PTEN. (46). miR-1908 promotes proliferation, invasion, and sphere formation in GBM cells by targeting PTEN, and PTEN levels are inversely correlated with miR-1908 levels in GBM tissues (47). The expression of PTEN-targeting miR-17-5p, miR-19a, miR-19b, miR-21, miR-130b, miR-221, and miR-222 was significantly higher in irradiated glioma cells than in nonirradiated cells, and the PTEN expression levels were lower in the irradiated glioma cells than in the nonirradiated cells (48).

In recent years, molecular target therapy-targeting RTK pathways has been one of the most exciting developments in cancer therapy, and certain molecular targeted drugs have been clinically validated. However, for GBMs, no effective molecular targeted drug has yet been developed. By understanding the roles of miRNAs in growth signal activation, miRNA-based treatments should also be taken into consideration either alone or in combination.

3.2. Sustained angiogenesis and microRNAs

New growth in the vascular network is important because the proliferation, as well as metastatic spread, of tumor cells depends on an adequate supply of oxygen and nutrients and the removal of waste products. GBMs have a strong angiogenetic property because GBMs possess glomeruloid microvascular proliferation, a hallmark of GBMs (49). GBMs stimulate new blood vessel formation through processes driven primarily by vascular endothelial growth factor A (VEGF-A), the most established proangiogenic protein in the VEGF family. The overexpression of VEGF-A, and subsequent activation of its receptors, is an important event during glioma progression (50).

miRNA-205, an miRNA significantly downregulated in GBMs, can specifically suppress expression of VEGF-A directly (51). Moreover, miRNA-205 induces apoptosis and depresses the invasion of glioma cells *in vitro* (51). VEGF-A upregulation can be induced by hypoxia inducible factor 1 alpha subunit (HIF-1α), which is negatively regulated by the von Hippel-Lindau (VHL) tumor suppressor (52). HIF-1α levels were upregulated in glioma cells following transfection with miR-183 mimic RNA, and VEGF-A and glucose transporter 1 (GLUT1), which are downstream molecules of HIF-1α, were upregulated in cells transfected with miR-183 (10). miR-21, miR-23b, and miR-566 are reported to target VHL and decrease the production of the VHL protein, upregulating VEGF-A expression. miR-21 directly targets VHL and peroxisome-proliferator-activated receptor a (PPARa), and miR-21 regulates EGFR/AKT signaling through VHL/β-catenin and the PPARa/AP-1 axis (53). miR-21 significantly colocalized with the hypoxia- and angiogenesis-associated markers HIF-1α and VEGF (54). Downregulation of miR-23b triggered growth inhibition, induced apoptosis, and suppressed invasion of glioma *in vitro* (55). miR-23b deletion decreased HIF-1α/VEGF expression and suppressed β-catenin/Tcf-4 transcription activity by targeting VHL (55). Inhibition of miR-566 expression increases the expression levels of VHL, decreases the expression levels of VEGF, and inhibits the invasive and migratory abilities of GBM cells (56). Moreover, miR-7 downregulates the expression of O-linked *N*-acetylglucosamine transferase (OGT) involved in the VEGF-signaling pathway, leading to a profound reduction in vascularization, similar to the antiangiogenic drug sunitinib (57).

miR-101 is downregulated in GBMs and targets EZH2, a histone methyltransferase affecting gene expression profiles in an epigenetic manner. Inhibition of EZH2 by miR-101 attenuated GBM cell growth, migration, and GBM-induced endothelial tubule formation (58). Ectopic expression of miR-137 inhibited angiogenesis in a SCID mouse xenograft model. EZH2 was identified as a direct target of miR-137, and EZH2 overexpression can rescue the inhibitory effect of miR-137 on cell proliferation and angiogenesis (59). A key step in angiogenesis is the upregulation of growth factor receptors on endothelial cells. miR-296 level is increased in primary tumor endothelial cells isolated from GBM tissues (60). Overexpressed miR-296 enhances angiogenesis by directly targeting the hepatocyte growth factor-regulated tyrosine kinase substrate (HGS), results in upregulation of the VEGF receptoe-2 and PDGF receptor-β (60). miR-93 promotes angiogenesis by suppressing integrin-β8 (61). *In vivo* studies revealed that miR-93-expressing cells induced blood vessel formation, allowing blood vessels to extend to tumor tissues in high densities (61). Angiogenesis promoted by miR-93 in return facilitated cell survival, resulting in enhanced tumor growth. miR-17~92 promotes angiogenesis and tumor growth by downregulation of clusterin (62). Specifically, miR-17-5p and miR-20 reduce the expression of the type-II TGFβ receptor and miR-18 limits the expression of Smad4, namely miR-17~92 attenuates the TGFβ-signaling pathway to shut down clusterin expression, thereby stimulating angiogenesis and tumor cell growth.

Because angiogenesis is a hallmark of GBM, targeting therapies against angiogenesis using the VEGF antibody was previously considered to be promising in GBM. However, recently, two phase-III studies revealed that the addition of the VEGF antibody bevacizumab to radiotherapy-temozolomide did not improve survival in patients with GBM, although improved progression-free survival and maintenance of baseline quality of life and performance status were observed with bevacizumab (2, 3). Therefore, new therapeutic targets or strategies need to be developed. To make progress, a better understanding of the miRNAs contributing to angiogenesis will lead to more effective antiangiogenic therapy for patients with GBM.

3.3. Insensitivity to antigrowth signals and microRNAs

To proliferate without limit, GBM cells must circumvent biologically programmed pathways that negatively regulate cell proliferation. There are two major tumor suppressor genes, retinoblastoma 1 (RB1) and tumor protein p53. Similarly, a better understanding of the dysfunction of the RB1 and p53 pathways should also implicate the roles of dysregulated miRNAs. The mutation of p53 results in the inability to stop further cell-cycle progression triggered by oncogenic signals (63). miR-10b, one of the most studied miRNAs in GBMs, is highly upregulated in human GBM and pleiotropically regulates invasion, angiogenicity, and apoptosis of GBM cells. The pleiotropic effect of miR-10b is caused by its suppression of multiple tumor-suppressive genes, including p53 (7, 64, 65). miR-10b directly targets p53 in GBM, giving the tumors a way to evade growth control and enable persistent cell proliferation by perturbing the miRNAs expression.

Moreover, p53 signaling is under the precise control of the negative regulator mouse double minute 2 (MDM2). MDM2 regulates the ubiquitin-dependent degradation and transcriptional activity of p53 (66). MDM2 mRNA is upregulated in both GBM cell lines and samples (67), and the upregulation could be a consequence of the downregulation of miR-17, miR-181b, miR-25, or miR-32, which directly target MDM2 gene expression (46, 67, 68). It is worth noting that miR-25 and miR-32 are two miRNAs repressed by p53, suggesting a feedback circuit between p53 and MDM2 mediated by miRNAs (67). The feedback circuit can explain the overexpression of miR-25 in GBM reported by several separate studies, in which the miRNA is meant to be downregulated to increase MDM2 expression and thus inactivate p53 (7, 39, 69). In addition, miR-181b is downregulated in GBM samples, further indicating that miRNA contributes to the complexity of the pathological progression of gliomas (68).

Another key tumor suppressive is p16INK4a, an important inhibitor of RB pathway (70), namely p16INK4a can bind specifically to CDK4/6 and inhibit the catalytic activity of CDK4/6-cyclin D complexes (71). Approximately, 80% of GBMs have one or more alterations affecting the RB1 function. In addition to targeting p53 in GBMs, miR-10b also targets p16INK4a, and the inhibition of miR-10b leads to cell cycle arrest (65). miR-26a also targets RB1 in GBMs. Additionally, CDK-cyclin complex-mediated phosphorylation is one of the main mechanisms by which RB1 protein is inactivated (72). The frequent gain-of-function mutations on CDK4/6-cyclin D complexes underscore their importance and potential in the development and progression of GBM. miR-124 is reported to radiosensitize human glioma cells by downregulating CDK4 (73), whereas CDK6 is a direct target of miR-138 (74) and miR-491-3p/5p (24). miR-195 inhibited glioma cell proliferation by downregulating expression of cyclin D1 and cyclin E1, via directly targeting cyclin D1 and cyclin E1 mRNA (75). Notably, those miRNAs that target cyclin-CDK complexes are all downregulated in GBM samples (69).

3.4. Invasion in the brain and microRNAs

The invasive propensity of glioma cells remains the major obstacle to improving the poor outcomes of patients with GBM. GBM cells prefer to migrate through the tortuous extracellular spaces of the brain. Therefore, it is supposed that the interaction of invading glioma cells with the extracellular matrix (ECM) is crucial in the initiation of invasion and migration. Generally, cell attachment is mediated by interactions between cell-cell and cell-ECM receptors, including integrins and cadherins, and degradation of ECM components by metalloproteinases is essential for cell detachment (76). The matrix metalloproteinases (MMPs) and a disintegrin and metalloproteinases (ADAMs) are two distinct types of metalloproteinases secreted by glioma cells to overcome the dense matrix, and the proteolytic activity can be blocked by endogenous metalloproteinase inhibitors, such as tissue inhibitors of metalloproteinase (TIMPs) and reversion-inducing-cysteine-rich protein with kazal motifs (RECK) (76).

miR-218 expression has been found to be significantly downregulated in GBM tissue samples (77). Several studies have shown that miR-218 is a negative regulator of invasion in GBM through various pathways (77, 78). miR-218 has been reported to target the mRNA of Lef1, the transcription factor that is upregulated by β-catenin (77). Suppression of Lef1 leads to the reduction of MMP-2, MMP-7, and MMP-9 activity and inhibition of invasion *in vitro* (79). Another mechanism through which miR-218 negatively regulates GBM invasion is targeting IKKβ mRNA along with reducing the transcription of NF-kB. NF-kB is a transcription factor that is important in many cellular processes and has been strongly linked to the migration and invasion of various cancer cells (78). NF-kB's target genes include MMP-9; therefore, its inhibition by miR-218 causes a decrease in invasion.

MMP-9 is a direct target of miR-491-5p, which is upregulated in GBM (24). miR-491-5p expression has been reported to reduce cell proliferation and invasion by targeting MMP9 (80). miR-491-3p also reduces the invasiveness of GBM cells by targeting the mRNA of insulin-like growth factor-binding protein 2 (IGFBP2). MMP-9 is also a direct target of miR-211 (81). MMP-3 is targeted by miR-152 (82). Additionally, ADAM17, a non-MMP, is under the direct regulation of miR-145 (83). It is clear that if glioma cells lose the control of MMPs and ADAMs by miRNAs, ECM homeostasis is compromised and the combined activity of these proteases remodels the ECM to favor tumor invasion. miR-101 is a tumor suppressor that is downregulated in GBM, as well as other cancers. (58). It has been shown to downregulate the invasion of glioma cells, as well as proliferation and migration, by targeting the transcription factor Kruppel-like factor 6 (KLF6). This suppression of KLF6 reduced the expression of chitinase-3-like protein 1 (CHI3L1) and inactivated MEK1/2 and PI3K signaling (72). miR-101 downregulation has been shown to result in EZH2-induced proliferation, migration, and angiogenesis in GBM (74).

Similarly, miR-152 is a tumor suppressor that is often downregulated in cancers, including in GBM. It was shown to suppress the invasion of glioma stem cells, as well as cell proliferation, migration, invasion, and apoptosis. It has been reported that miR-152 exerts its tumor-suppressing effects by targeting the transcription factor Kruppel-like factor 4 (KLF4). This suppression of KLF4 causes the transcriptional downregulation of galectin-3 (LGALS3) and the inactivation of MEK1/2 and PI3K signaling (75).

Because the MMPs and ADAMs each comprises more than 20 members, targeting a single target appears to be nonessential in cancerous diseases, which provides miR-21 with an opportunity to broadly inhibit metalloproteinase function. miR-21 regulates multiple genes associated with glioma cell migration and invasion, including the RECK and TIMP3 genes, which are inhibitors of matrix metalloproteinases (84).

In addition, interactions with the ECM are mostly mediated by integrins, which enable cells to sense the extracellular environment and adjust their behavior to environmental cues. miR-124, frequently downregulated in GBM, targets β1 integrin and is shown to affect glioma cell migration and invasion *in vitro* (85). PPP1R13L (protein phosphatase 1, regulatory subunit 13 like), an inhibitory member of the apoptosis-stimulating protein of p53 family (IASPP), was found to be a direct target of miR-124 in GBM cells. miR-124-mediated PPP1R13L regulates invasion of GBM cells (86). Cai et al. found that miR-542-3p expression was decreased in GBM cells, and miR-542-3p suppressed GBM cell invasion by not only targeting AKT1 but also directly downregulating its two important upstream regulators, ILK (integrin-linked kinase) and PIK3R1 (87). miR-181 family is downregulated in GBM and is inversely correlated with activities of NF-kB-targeting genes. Furthermore, miR-181b was shown to suppress epithelial-mesenchymal transition (EMT) by targeting KPNA4 (88). miR-181c overexpression inhibits TGF-β signaling by downregulating TGFBR1 (transforming growth factor, beta receptor 1), TGFBR2 and TGFBRAP1 (transforming growth factor, beta receptor-associated protein 1) expression. miR-181c expression levels are correlated with poor prognosis of patients with GBM.

miR-125a are downregulated in GBMs and directly target the 3′-UTR of podoplanin (PDPN) and inhibit invasion, apoptosis, and proliferation of GBMs. In addition, miR-125a inhibits Nrg1, one of the most active members of the EGF-like family, and suppresses the proliferation and migration of GBM cells *in vitro* and *in vivo* (89). miR-203 expression is decreased in anaplastic astrocytoma and GBM tissues. Forced expression of miR-203 was shown to suppress glioma cell proliferation, migration, and invasion, by disrupting the Robo1/ERK/MMP-9-

signaling axis (90). In addition, miR-203 inhibits the proliferation and invasion by directly targeting phospholipase D2 (PLD2) (91). miR-29b expression, downregulated in GBMs, was inversely proportional to that of BCL2-like 2 (BCL2L2) mRNA or protein (92). Interestingly, BCL2L2 mRNA is highly expressed in the mesenchymal type of GBM. BCL2L2 repression is of central importance to miR-29b antitumor activity in migration, invasion, and angiogenesis. Moreover, miR-29b regulates PDPN, which promotes glioma invasion.

miR-10b is overexpressed in GBM and induces glioma cell invasion by modulating expression of RhoC, MMP-14, and uPAR (urokinase-type plasminogen activator receptor) via HOXD10 (93). Multifocal lesions of malignant gliomas were associated with higher expression levels of miR-10b (9). Dong et al. reported that not only miR-10b inhibition but also miR-21 inhibition could exert synergistic inhibition of the invasion of glioma cells. miR-10b pleiotropically regulates invasion, angiogenicity, and apoptosis of glioma cells by the suppression of multiple tumor suppressors, including p53, FOXO3, HOXD10, and NOTCH1 (64). miR-155 has been identified to be an oncomiR and is highly expressed in several solid cancers, including GBM. Knockdown of miR-155 sensitizes glioma cells to the chemotherapy of temozolomide by targeting p38 isoforms of mitogen-activated protein kinase 13 (MAPK13) and MAPK14 (94).

In sum, the roles of miRNAs in glioma cell invasion or migration further our understanding of the genesis of the aggressive glioma phenotype. Some of these miRNAs have been discovered, whereas more still remain to be found. The blockade of excessive pro-invasive miRNAs or the restoration of weakened anti-invasive miRNAs will provide extra treatment options for advanced-stage gliomas that are marked by poor prognoses for decades (**Table 1**).

Hallmarks of glioblastoma	miRNAs	Targets	Expression	Function	Ref
Growth signal activation	miR-7	EGFR, PI3K, Raf-1	down	downregulate PI3K/ATK and MAPK pathways	Liu (17), Webster (18)
	miR-128	EGFR, PDGFRA	down	downregulate PI3K/ATK and MAPK pathways	Papagiannakopoulos (19)
	miR-218	EGFR	down	downregulate PI3K/ATK and MAPK pathways	Mathew (20)
	miR-219	EGFR	down	downregulate PI3K/ATK and MAPK pathways	Rao (21)
	miR-133	EGFR	down	downregulate PI3K/ATK and MAPK pathways	Xu (22)
	miR-340	EGFR	down	induce terminal differentiation	Huang (23)

Hallmarks of glioblastoma	miRNAs	Targets	Expression	Function	Ref
	miR-491	EGFR, CDK6, Bcl-xL	down	inhibit cell proliferation, negative regulator of EGFR	Li (24)
	miR-148a	MIG6, BIM	up	reduce EGFR trafficking	Kim (25)
	miR-34a	PDGFRA	down	inhibit cell proliferation and cell cycle progression inhibit cell survival invasion	Genovese (27), Silber (28)
	miR-182	MET, Bcl2L12, HIF2A		promote glioma initiating cell differentiation	Kouri (32)
	miR-144-3p	MET	down	repress GBM cell proliferation and invasion	Lan (33)
	let-7a	K-RAS	down	downregulate PI3K/ATK and MAPK pathways	Wang (35)
	miR-143	N-RAS	down	inhibit cell proliferation	Wang (34)
	miR-124	SOS1, R-RAS	down	inhibit cell proliferation	Shi (36), Lv (37)
	miR-9	NF1	up	inhibit cell proliferation	Tan (38)
	miR-26a	PTEN	up	promote tumor growth	Huse (41)
	miR-23a	PTEN	up	activate of AKT/ERK pathways and EMT	Tan (44), Tian (45)
	miR-17-5p	PTEN	up	formation of colonies and neurospheres	Li (46)
	miRNA-1908	PTEN	up	promote the tumor forming potential and anchorage-independent growth	Xia (47)
	miR-19a	PTEN	up	promote tumor growth	Tokudome (48)
	miR-19b	PTEN	up	promote tumor growth	Tokudome (48)
	miR-21	PTEN	up	promote tumor growth	Tokudome (48)
	miR-130b	PTEN	up	enhance stem cell-like phenotype	Tokudome (48)
	miR-221	PTEN	up	promote tumor growth	Tokudome (48)
	miR-222	PTEN	up	promote tumor growth	Tokudome (48)
Sustained angiogenesis	miR-205	VEGF-A	down	inhibit expression of VEGF-A induce apoptosis and depress the invasion	Yue (51)
	miR-183	IDH2	up	increase HIF1 expression	Tanaka (10)
	miR-21	VHL, PPARa	up	regulate EGFR/AKT signaling	Harmansen (54)

Hallmarks of glioblastoma	miRNAs	Targets	Expression	Function	Ref
	miR-23b	VHL	up	inhibit tumor growth and invasion, induce apoptosis	Chen (55)
	miR-566	VHL	up	inhibit invasion and migration	Xiao (56)
	miR-7	OGT	down	reduce vascularization	Babae (57)
	miR-101	EZH2	down	attenuate GBM growth and migration/invasion	Smits (58)
	miR-137	EZH2	down	inhibit cell proliferation and angiogenesis	Sun (59)
	miR-93	Integrin-β8	up	promote tumor growth and angiogenesis	Fang (61)
Insensitivity to antigrowth signals	miR-10b	p53, p16INK4a	up	promote cell cycle	Gabriely (65)
	miR-17-3p	MDM2		inhibit tumor progression	Li (46)
	miR-181b	MDM2	down	inhibit tumor progression	Suh (67)
	miR-25-3p	MDM2, p53	up	inhibit cellular proliferation	Suh (67)
	miR-32-5p	MDM2, p53	up	inhibit cellular proliferation	Suh (67)
	miR-26a	RB1	up	promote cell proliferation	Lundberg (72)
	miR-124	CDK4	down	cell cycle arrest	Deng (73)
	miR-138	CDK6	down	cell cycle arrest	Qiu (74)
	miR-491-3p/5p	CDK6	down	cell cycle arrest	Li (24)
	miR-195	cyclin D1, cyclin E1	down	cell cycle arrest	Hui (75)
Invasion and metastasis	miR-218	IKKβ, Lef1	down	inhibit cell invasion	Liu (77), Song (78)
	miR-491	IGFBP2, MMP9	down	reduce cell proliferation and invasion	Yan (80)
	miR-211	MMP9	down	reduce cell invasion	Asuthkar (81)
	miR-101	KLF6, EZH2	down	reduce invasion of glioma stem cells	Smits (58), Qiu (74)
	miR-152	MMP3, KLF4	down	reduce cell invasion and angiogenesis suppress invasion of glioma stem cells	Zheng (82), Hui (75)

Hallmarks of glioblastoma	miRNAs	Targets	Expression	Function	Ref
	miR-145	ADAM17	down	reduce glioma cell invasion and angiogenesis	Lu (83)
	miR-21	TIMP3, RECK	up	promote cell invasion	Gabriely (84), Zhao (86)
	miR-124	β1 integrin, IASPP	down	suppress cell migration and invasion	Fowler (85)
	miR-542-3p	AKT1	down	suppress cell invasion	Cai (87)
	miR-181b	KPNA4	down	inhibit cell invasion and proliferation	Wang (88)
	miR-181c	TGFBR1, TGFBR2, TGFBRAP1	down	inhibit cell invasion and proliferation	Wang (88)
	miR-125a	PDPN, Nrg1	down	inhibit invasion and proliferation	Yin (89)
	miR-203	PLD2	down	suppress cell proliferation and invasion,disrupt the Robo1/ERK/MMP-9 signaling axis	Dontula (90), Chen (91)
	miR-29b	BCL2L2, PDPN	down	inhibit glioma invasion	Chung (92)
	miR-10b	HOXD10, FOXO3, NOTCH1	up	induce glioma cell invasion	Sun (93)
	miR-155	MAPK13, MAPK14	up	regulates glioma cells invasion and chemosensitivity	Liu (94)
Antiapoptosis	miR-21	PDCD4, HNRPK, TP53BP2, p63	up	antiapoptosis	Corsten (95), Gaur (96)
	miR-92a	BCL2L11	up	antiapoptosis	Papagiannakopoulos (97)
	miR-92b	NLK	up	antiapoptosis	Niu (98)
	miR-93	ITGB8	up	antiapoptosis	Fang (61)
	miR-221	p27, p57	up	antiapoptosis	Medina (100)
	miR-222	p27, p57	up	antiapoptosis	Medina (100)
Genome instability and mutation	miR-106a		up	DNA replication and mitosis	Liu (101)
	miR-106b	RBL1, RBL2	up	DNA replication and mitosis	Liu (101)

Hallmarks of glioblastoma	miRNAs	Targets	Expression	Function	Ref
	miR-17-92		up	DNA replication and mitosis	Liu (101)
	miR-20			DNA replication and mitosis	Liu (101)
	miR-221	p27	up	Cell cycle chechpoint regulation	Gillies (103)
	miR-222	p27	up	Cell cycle chechpoint regulation	Gillies (103)
	miR-155	MLH1, MSH2, MSH6	up	DNA mismatch repair	Liu (94)
	miR-125b	p53, MXD1	down	cell cycle arrest to repair damaged DNA spindle assembly checkpoint	Wan (104), Le (105)
	miR-29	PIK3R1, CDC42	down	upregulate p53	Park (106)
	miR-34	CCND1, CCNE2, CDK4, MET, MYC, SNAI1, and SIRT1	down	DNA damage response upregulate p53 downstream molecules	He (107)
	miR-101	ATM, PRKDC	down	DNA repair regulate non-homologous end joining of DNA double strand breaks	Yan (109)
					Li (111)
Tumor-promoting inflammation	miR-21	LRRFIP1	up	regulate NF-kB signaling pathway	
	miR-146a	TRAF6, IRAK1		regulate NF kB activation	Taganov (112), Park (113)
	miR-124		down	inhibit STAT3 pathway	Wei (117)
Reprogramming energy metabolism	miR-451	CAB39	up	regulate LKB1/AMPK signaling activity	Godlewski (124)
	mir-145	c-Myc, Sox9, ADD3	down	reduce Lin28/Lin28b transcription	Rani (130), Gan (132)
	miR-34c	c-Myc		regulate c-Myc mRNA stability and translation	Masui (134)

Hallmarks of glioblastoma	miRNAs	Targets	Expression	Function	Ref
	let-7	RAS, Myc, CCND1, LIN28, HMGA2	down	regulate glucose metabolism	Boyerinas (135)
	let-7a	K-ras	down	regulate glucose metabolism	Boyerinas (135)
	miR-326	PKM2, NOB1	down	regulate glucose metabolism RNA metabolism	Kefas (136), Zhou (137)
Evading immune destruction	miRs-29b		down	differentiation of tumor-associated macrophage	Graff (140)
	miR-125a		down	differentiation of tumor-associated macrophage	Graff (140)
	miR-146a		down	differentiation of tumor-associated macrophage	Graff (140)
	miR-155	C/EBPβ	up	lead to and inversion of M2 into M1 macrophages	Graff (140)
	miR-221	STAT1,2	up	phosphorylation of STAT1 and STAT2	Zhang (143)
	miR-222	STAT1,2	up	phosphorylation of STAT1 and STAT2	Zhang (143)
	miR-20a	NKG2DL	up	immune evasion of glioma cells at the level of the NKG2D recognition pathway	Codo (146)
	miR-93	NKG2DL	up	immune evasion of glioma cells at the level of the NKG2D recognition pathway	Codo (146)
	miR-106b	NKG2DL	up	immune evasion of glioma cells at the level of the NKG2D recognition pathway	Codo (146)
	miR-138	CTLA-4, PD1	down	tumor regression	Wei (147)

Table 1. Hallmarks of glioblastoma and microRNAs.

3.5. Antiapoptosis and microRNAs

Among the tumor-associated miRNAs, miR-21 is frequently overexpressed in various types of tumors, including GBMs (7, 9), and plays a critical role in cell death and apoptosis. Knockdown of miR-21 in cultured GBM cells triggered activation of caspases and led to increased apoptotic cell death (8). miR-21 knockdown disrupts glioma growth *in vivo* and displays synergistic cytotoxicity when combined with the agent tumor necrosis factor-related apoptosis (s-TRAIL), leading to an increase in caspase activity (95). In particular, it was reported that the downregulation of miR-21 in GBM-derived cell lines resulted in an increased expression of a specific target, PDCD4 (programmed cell death 4), a known tumor suppressor gene, with a consequent decrease in proliferation and increase in apoptosis (96). Furthermore, miR-21 regulated a network of p53, TGF-b, and mitochondrial apoptosis tumor suppressor genes in GBM cells, targeting HNRPK (heterogeneous nuclear ribonucleoprotein K), TP53BP2 (tumor protein p53-binding protein 2), and p63, a member of the p53 family of genes (97).

miR-92a and miR-92b, upregulated in glioma, target BCL2L11 (98) and NLK (99), respectively. Their inhibition promotes tumor-suppressive phenotypes through the induction of apoptosis. In addition, miR-93 was found to be upregulated in glioma specimens and resulted in an enhancement in cell survival, promoting sphere formation, and augmenting tumor growth by suppressing the expression of ITGB8 target (61).

miR-221 and 222 were extensively investigated in glioma. These miRNAs were found to be upregulated in this cancer, and both were reported to target the cell growth-suppressive cyclin-dependent kinase inhibitors p27 and p57 (100).

3.6. Genome instability and microRNAs

Genomic instability is defined as a high frequency of mutations within the genome, including changes in nucleic acid sequences, chromosomal rearrangements, or aneuploidy. The stability of the human genome is maintained by multiple mechanisms such as the cell cycle checkpoint, DNA damage response, and mitotic separation machinery. Defects in the DNA damage response could cause genomic DNA mutations, deletions, insertions, or gross chromosomal gains and losses upon cell division and subsequently lead to cancer. Genomic instability is present in GBM and affects the prognosis of patients.

Several members of the miR-106b-25 cluster and its paralog miR-17-92 cluster were associated with DNA replication and mitosis. Overexpression of miR-106b-5p in glioma tumor cells significantly promoted cell proliferation, suggesting a role of this miRNA in cell cycle regulation (101). A mechanistic study revealed that two target genes, retinoblastoma-like 1 (RBL1) and RBL2, were involved in miR-106b-5p's regulation of cell proliferation (101). RBL proteins were involved in genomic instability, coinciding with decreased DNA methylation and increased acetylation of histone H3.

p27, one of the cyclin-dependent kinase inhibitor, inhibits cell cycle progression at the G1 phase by blocking the activation of cyclin-CDK complexes (102). The downregulation of p27 expression by miRNAs could abrogate the cell cycle checkpoints and could increase DNA damages in GBM cells. The regulatory effect of miR-221/222 on p27 and the subsequent effect on cell proliferation were also demonstrated in GBM cells (103). Moreover, p27 inhibition abrogated the growth advantage of cells with miR221/miR-222 downregulation (103).

DNA mismatch repair (MMR) is a system for recognizing and correcting insertions, deletions, and misincorporated bases at DNA replication and recombination. Deficiency of MMR system can be a cause for the development and progression of GBMs. There are two essential members of the DNA MMR genes, MutS homologs and MutL homologs. Computational algorithms predicted, and subsequently *in vitro* studies confirmed, several essential MMR genes, including MLH1, MSH2, and MSH6, as potential binding sites for miR-155. miR-155 is known to elevate its expression levels in primary and secondary GBMs (94).

As an important sensor in the DNA damage response, p53 functions to block the cell cycle to repair damaged DNA. Several miRNAs affect p53 or p53-regulated genes via different mechanisms. For instance, miR-125b, which has been shown to play a potential role in the development of glioma stem cells (104), directly targets p53 by binding to 3′-UTR of p53 and negatively regulates p53 expression (105). In addition, miR-125b negatively regulates MXD1 expression, an adaptor protein for MAD2L2 in the spindle assembly checkpoint. Moreover, miR-29, commonly downregulated in GBMs, indirectly upregulates p53 by targeting PIK3R1 and CDC42 (106). Previous studies have shown that miR-34 is directly regulated by p53 and represses various oncogenes, such as CCND1, CCNE2, CDK4, MET, MYC, SNAI1, and SIRT1. However, these miR-34-targeting oncogenes are upregulated in GBM, because miR-34 is usually downregulated (107). Several studies have shown that miR-34 is indispensable for the DNA damage response, and miR-34a-regulated genes are strongly related with DNA repair and apoptosis (108).

Ataxia telangiectasia mutated (ATM) is an important mediator in connecting DNA damage signals to downstream events, including damage repair. miR-101, a miRNA downregulated in GBM, could directly target ATM via the canonical action mechanism (109). In addition, miR-101 also targets PRKDC (protein kinase, DNA activated, catalytic polypeptide) to regulate nonhomologous end joining of DNA double-strand breaks (109).

3.7. Tumor-promoting inflammation and microRNAs

NF-kB is a transcription factor with pleiotropic activity owing to its central roles in inflammatory processes. A critical regulator of NF-kB activation is the IkB kinase (IKK-β) complex (110). Ectopic expression of miR-218, which is downregulated in GBM, reduced NF-kB activity, whereas inhibition of miR-218 enhanced the transcriptional activity of NF-kB (78). miR-218 could inactivate NF-kB signaling by directly targeting the 3′-UTR of the IKK-β (78). miR-21 was revealed as another regulator involved in the NF-kB-signaling pathway in GBM. Li et al. confirmed LRRFIP1 (leucine-rich repeat interacting protein 1) as a direct target of miR-21 (111). LRRFIP1 is a transcriptional repressor that preferentially binds to the GC-rich consensus sequence and regulates expression of TNF, EGFR, and PDGFA signaling. miR-21 contributes to drug resistance through the depression of LRRFIP1 expression, leading to the reduction of cytotoxicity of chemotherapeutic drugs through the activation of the NF-kB pathway (111).

miR-146a is known as miRNA associated with the innate immune response to microbial infection (112). Promotor analysis revealed that miR-146a is a NF-kB-dependent miRNAs (112). miR-146a has complementary sequences in the mRNA of the TNF receptor-associated factor 6 (TRAF6) and IL-1 receptor-associated kinase 1 (IRAK1), key adaptor molecules downstream of toll-like and cytokine receptors (113). miR-146a overexpression enhanced apoptosis and suppressed NF-kB activation in TMZ-treated GBM cells (114). Increased expression of miR-146a was observed in glioneuronal lesions (115), and miR-146a expression in human glial cells was strongly induced by IL-1β (115). miR-146a expression by transfection in astrocytes regulated many mRNA expression levels, including those of IRAK-1, IRAK-2, and TRAF-6. In addition, the expression of IL-6 and COX-2 was suppressed by miR-146a (115).

Recent evidence suggests that the signal transducer and activator of transcription (STAT) family proteins play a crucial role in selectively inducing and maintaining a procarcinogenic inflammatory microenvironment, both upon the initiation of malignant transformation and during cancer progression (116). Upon upregulating miR-124, a miRNA downregulated in GBM, specifically in glioma cancer stem cells (gCSC), the STAT3 pathway was inhibited, and miR-124 reversed gCSC-mediated immunosuppression of T cell proliferation and induction of regulatory T cells (Treg) (117). Systemic administration of miR-124-transfected T cell transfers exerted potent antiglioma therapeutic effects in murine models of GBM (117).

Human glioma immune activation is potently elicited by a cytokine combination. Cytokines such as IL-1β and TNFα induce the expression of miR-155 and miR-155*, the miRNAs crucial in immunity and inflammation-induced oncogenesis, and this expression is dose dependently suppressed by IRF3. Importantly, IRF3 also inhibits glioma proliferation, migration, and invasion (118).

3.8. Reprogramming energy metabolism and microRNAs

Cellular metabolism of malignant tumor is considerably different from that of normal cell, because of limitless proliferation and motility. (119). GBM cells uptake a large amount of glucose, and aerobic glycolysis generates various substrates, such as fatty acids and nucleotides that are required for rapidly proliferating cells, and is associated with a survival advantage in the tumor cells (Warburg effect). MR spectroscopy analyses have shown that as much as 90% of the glucose converts into lactate by aerobic glycolysis in GBM cells. Clinically, it is known that the levels of lactate are elevated in GBM tissue compared with those in contralateral normal brain tissue. In addition, lactate was shown to be high-grade gliomas than for low-grade gliomas, and glutamate levels were significantly elevated for GBMs. Pretreatment F^{18}-2-fluoro-2-deoxy-D-glucose (FDG)-PET provides significant additional prognostic information in high-grade gliomas (120).

In normal cells, the 5′-adenosine monophosphate-activated protein kinase (AMPK) pathway is the major cellular sensor of energy availability (121), but its function in cancer is not clear. AMPK is activated by metabolic stress to promote energy conservation and glucose uptake, allowing cells to survive periods of low-energy availability. Allosteric interaction with elevated intracellular AMP, which acts to inhibit dephosphorylation of AMPK (122), and phosphorylation at Thr172 by the protein kinase LKB1 are necessary for AMPK activation under conditions of bioenergetic stress (123).

Godlewski et al. identified miR-451 as a glioma-expressed miRNA that regulates the balance of proliferation and migration in glioma cells in response to changes in glucose levels (124). miR-451 regulates LKB1 activity through direct targeting of CAB39, a component of the active LKB1 complex. Glucose deprivation was shown to reduce miR-451 levels (124). Thus, miR-451 plays an essential role in LKB1/AMPK signaling in glioma cells. When glucose is sufficient, elevated miR-451 levels lead to reduced LKB1/AMPK pathway activation, which facilitates cell proliferation by allowing unrestrained mTOR activity and reducing apoptosis. In contrast, when glucose is limiting, miR-451 levels decline, allowing for increased CAB39 expression and activation of AMPK by LKB1-mediated phosphorylation. This effect promotes cell survival in response to metabolic stress and activates pathways involved in glioma motility.

Previous reports indicate that Myc is frequently upregulated or amplified in gliomas. As a transcriptional factor, Myc interacts with many tumor-related oncogenes in glioma cells, such as SPARC (125), GAS1 (126), and VEGF (127). c-Myc has been shown to stimulate glutamine metabolism by increasing the expression of amino acid transporters and glutaminase (128). Mechanistically, c-Myc expression has been shown to be suppressed by miR-145, which results in reduced Lin28/Lin28b transcription (129). miR-145 is one of the miRNAs significantly downregulated during malignant transformation in GBMs (130). miR-145 overexpression suppresses the activity of oncogenic proteins Sox9, leading to reduction of cell proliferation and invasion of GBM cells (130). Reduced levels of miR-145 may lead to metabolic remodeling in glioma cells via Sox9, because Sox9 is known as a regulator of c-myc.

mTORC2 regulates c-Myc and glycolysis through FoxO acetylation, and mTORC2 controls FoxO acetylation through class IIa HDACs, independently of Akt. FoxOs antagonize c-Myc (131) by increasing the expression of miR-145 (132) and miR-34c (133), limiting c-Myc mRNA stability and translation. In GBM cells, miR-34c levels were suppressed by FoxO1/FoxO3 knockdown, and miR-34c regulated c-Myc levels in GBM cells (134). The let-7 family has nine members, and previous studies have identified the let-7 miRNA as a tumor suppressor that regulates many important target genes during tumor development (135), such as RAS, Myc, CCND1, LIN28, and HMGA2, which are involved in cell cycle progression and cell stemness. The majority of let-7a miRNA functions in glioma malignancy are believed to involve K-Ras, suggesting that let-7a-mediated manipulation of K-Ras may also be involved in regulating glucose metabolism and GBM cell growth. The M2 isoform of pyruvate kinase (PK) is upregulated in most cancers, including GBM. The regulation of PKM2 was shown to occur via miR-326 (136). There are four isoforms of PK in mammals, and PKM2 is highly expressed in undifferentiated tissues and tumors. Because PKM2 is regulated by tyrosine phosphorylation and is overexpressed in malignant tumors, PKM2 is considered as key molecule of aerobic glycolysis. In addition, Zhou et al. reported that the human Nin one binding protein (NOB1), which is required for the biogenesis and function of the 26S proteasome and plays a role in RNA metabolism, is a direct target of miR-326 (137).

3.9. Evading immune destruction and microRNAs

In the past, the infiltration of innate and adaptive immune cells into the tumor microenvironment was considered an immune attack against tumors. However, now, it is widely accepted that immune cells also promote tumor initiation, progression, and metastasis (138). Tumor-associated macrophages (TAMs) control the majority of immunological processes within tumors exerting both regressive (M1) and progressive (M2) effects on tumor development (139). However, the majority of TAMs exhibit an M2-like phenotype. Remarkably, miRs-29b, miR-125a, miR-146a, and miR-155 are involved in the differentiation of TAMs (140). Overexpression of miRNA-155 was shown to attenuate the production of cytokines (IL-6 and TNF-α) by suppressing C/EBPβ expression, which led to an inversion of M2 into M1 macrophages (141). M2 TAMs are capable of releasing anti-inflammatory cytokines such as the immunosuppressive cytokine IL-10, which promotes tumor growth (142).

Natural killer T (NKT) cells are a subfraction of T cells. A large number of published studies have demonstrated that NKT cells have miscellaneous functions in immune regulation, one of which is that NKT cells are tumor cell killers, based on the production of antitumor cytokines. In addition to contributing to immune protection, NKT cells are involved in immune tolerance in the body. Tang et al. showed that glioma cells can induce immune-tolerant IL-6+ and IL-10+ NKT cells via miR-92a.

Another study revealed miR-221 and miR-222 as possible regulators of IFN pathways. Type-I IFN receptor activation triggers the JAK-mediated tyrosine phosphorylation of STAT family proteins. Zhang et al. found that STAT1 and STAT2 expression and phosphorylation were upregulated after repression of miR-221/222 in U251 cells (143). Upregulation of STAT pathway is controlled by the IFN-α activation after knockdown of miR-221/222 cluster in U251 glioma cells (143).

NKG2D is one of the major activating receptors of natural killer (NK) cells and binds to several ligands (NKG2DL). NKG2D recognizes different MHC class I-homologous ligands (NKG2DL), including the MHC class I-chain-related molecules A (MICA) and B (MICB) and the UL16- binding proteins (ULBP)1-6 (144), which are also present on the surface of glioma cells (145). Codo et al. reported that miR-20a, miR-93 or miR-106b regulates NKG2DL expression in glioma cells (146), suggesting that the expression of miRNA-targeting NKG2DL may contribute to the immune evasion of glioma cells at the level of the NKG2D recognition pathway.

In addition, miRNA regulates immunocheckpoint molecules. miR-138 could bind the 3′-UTR of CTLA-4 and PD-1, and transfection of human CD4+ T cells with miR-138 suppressed expression of CTLA-4 and PD-1 (147). *In vivo* treatment in immunocompetent mice using miR-138 revealed marked tumor regression and prolonged survival time. Moreover, inoculated tumors showed decrease in intratumoral regulatory T cell, CTLA-4, and PD-1 expression (147). miR-138 exerts antiglioma efficacy by targeting immune checkpoints that may have rapid translational potential as novel immunotherapeutic agents.

On the other hand, miRNA expression is transcriptionally regulated by various cytokines. Ohno et al. analyzed the effect of IFN-β treatment on miR-21 expression in glioma cells and intracranial glioma xenografts (148). Systematic delivery of IFN-β markedly reduced the level of miR-21 in glioma cells 6 hours after the addition of IFN-β.

4. Circulating microRNA in glioma patients

In 2008, Chim et al. firstly demonstrated the existence of placental miRNAs in maternal plasma (149). In the same year, several miRNAs were detected in the serum of the tumor patients. Quantitative real-time polymerase chain reaction (RT-PCR) analyses revealed sera levels of miR-155, miR-210, and miR-21 are higher in diffuse large B-cell lymphoma patient sera than healthy controls (150). To prevent degradation in the circulation, miRNAs are released by cells in both exosomes and miRNA/protein complexes. Exosomes are lipid vesicles ranging between 50 and 100 nm in size and contain a range of molecules, including mRNA, miRNA, DNA, and proteins. The detection of biomarkers within serum is attractive because of the relatively non-invasive process of collection (**Figure 1**).

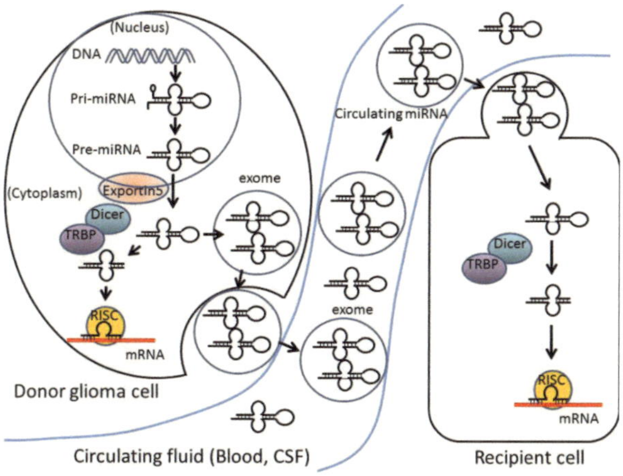

Figure 1. Cell-cell communication through circulating microRNAs. MicroRNAs contained in exosomes are released from glioma cells where they can enter the blood-stream or CSF-stream and circulate through the body to distant sites. These exosomal miRNAs are taken up by recipient cells, where the miRNAs can then suppress target genes in the recipient cells. Circulating miRNAs released by glioma cells may involve in growth signal, angiogenesis, anti-apoptosis, tumor metabolism, and immunoregulation.

Over the past few years, researchers have investigated the capability of using miRNAs as blood biomarkers for the diagnosis of tumors. Circulating miRNAs can be isolated from serum or plasma, but recent studies have indicated plasma to be a more adequate source for miRNA extraction (150). However, depending on plasma preparation, the level of circulating miRNA can be altered. Cheng et al. showed that processing differences resulted in a variation in residual platelet contamination in plasma and significant differences in miRNA abundance (151). Consequently, supplementary centrifugation, the refusal of samples with platelet counts above a certain limit and the quantification of hemolysis are mandatory in accurately determining miRNA levels in plasma.

Cerebrospinal fluid (CSF) is another useful biofluid and is in direct contact with the extracellular fluid of the brain. CSF has various functions, such as protecting the brain, transporting biological substances, and excreting toxic and waste substances. Although the composition of CSF reflects that of the blood plasma, active transport and secretions from the brain tissues contribute to the composition of CSF. Therefore, the analyses of CSF can suggest biological brain processes and is indispensable for understanding disorders of brain (152).

Clinically, histopathological examinations have been widely used to diagnose glioma, but they are invasive because microsurgical resection or stereotactic biopsy is needed to acquire specimens. In this context, it is of great interest to develop novel biomarkers for glioma. Currently, several miRNAs have been identified as noninvasive biomarkers for the diagnosis of cancers, including breast, lung, and gastric cancer. Previous studies have reported that miRNAs can be detected in circulating exosomes in the serum or CSF of glioma, suggesting that miRNAs might be useful biomarkers for glioma diagnosis. However, to effectively apply these findings to clinical detection, further studies must be conducted (**Table 2**).

No.	Authors	Year	Source	Number of glioma	Number of control	microRNA
Blood						
1	Skog	2008	serum	2 (GBM)	none	let-7a, miR-15b, miR-16, miR-19b, miR-21, miR-26a, miR-27a, miR-92, miR-93, miR-320, miR-20
2	Roth	2011	blood	20 (GBM)	20 (Healthy controls)	miR-128(↑), miR-342-3p(↓)
3	Wang	2012	plasma	50 (GBM)	10 (Healthy controls)	miR-21(↑), miR-128(↓), miR-342-3p(↓)
4	Yang	2013	serum	122 (Astro cytoma)	123 (Healthy controls)	miR-15b*(↓), miR-23a(↓), miR-133a(↓), miR-150*(↓),miR-197(↓), miR-497(↓), miR-548b-5p(↓)
5	Dong	2014	serum	3 (GBM)	3 (Healthy controls)	miR-576-5p(↑), miR-340(↑), miR-626(↑), miR-320(↓), let-7g-5p(↓), miR-7-5p(↓)
6	Manterola	2014	serum	25 (GBM)	25 (Healthy controls)	miR-320(↑), miR-574-3p(↑)
7	Shao	2015	plasma	70 (Glioma)	70 (Healthy	miR-454-3p(↑)

No.	Authors	Year	Source	Number of glioma	Number of control	microRNA
					controls)	
8	Wu	2015	serum	83 (Glioma)	69 (Healthy controls)	miR-29b(↓)
9	Liu	2015	serum	120 (Glioma)	120 (Healthy controls)	miR-29b(↓)
10	Lai	2015	blood	136 (GBM)	50 (Healthy controls)	miR-210(↑)
11	Sun	2015	serum	151 (Glioma)	53 (Healthy controls),52 (Meningioma)	miR-128(↓)
12	Yue	2016	serum	20 (Glioma)	5 (Healthy controls)	miR-205(↓)
13	Wei	2016	serum	33 (Glioma)	33 (Healthy controls)	miR-125b(↓)
Cerebrospinal fluid (CSF)						
1	Baraniskin	2012	CSF	10 (Glioma)	10 (Neurologic disorders), 23 (CNS lymphoma), 7 (Metastatic tumor)"	miR-15b(↑), miR-21(↑)
2	Teplyuk	2012	CSF	19 (GBM)	15 (Non-neoplastic control),44 (Metastatic tumor), "	miR-10b(↑), miR-21(↑), miR-200 family(↑)
3	Akers	2013	CSF	13 (GBM)	13 (Non-neoplastic control)	miR-21(↑)
4	Shi	2015	CSF	8 (Astro cytoma), 25 (Epen dymoma), 45 (GBM)	none	miR-21(↑)

Table 2. Circulating microrna in glioma patients.

4.1. Serum and plasma

The first analysis of exosomes in serum identified the presence of 11 miRNAs in the samples from two different patients with primary GBM in 2008 (153). However, the levels were generally lower in exosomes but correlated well with the tumor profile (153). In 2011, Roth et al. analyzed miRNA profiles from the blood of 20 patients with GBM and 20 matched healthy controls (154). Among 1158 tested miRNAs, 52 were significantly deregulated, and of these, two candidates, miR-128 (upregulated) and miR-342-3p (downregulated), remained the most significant miRNAs. The altered expression of these two miRNAs was confirmed in a validation cohort by RT-PCR. In this model, the discrimination between blood samples of patients with GBM and healthy controls reached an accuracy of 81%, specificity of 79%, and sensitivity of 83%. In 2012, Wang et al. determined the plasma miRNA levels of 50 patients with glioma and 10 healthy donors using RT-PCR (155). The plasma level of miR-21 was increased and the levels of miR-128 and miR-342-3p were significantly decreased in the patients with glioma compared with those in normal controls. These miRNAs were able to discriminate patients with glioma from healthy controls with high specificity and sensitivity. However, there were not significant differences between patients with glioma and other brain tumors such as meningioma or pituitary adenoma. Yang et al. performed genomewide serum miRNA analysis using serum samples of 122 untreated astrocytoma patients and 123 normal controls (156). The seven-miRNA panel (miR-15b*, miR-23a, miR-133a, miR-150*, miR-197, miR-497, and miR-548b-5p) demonstrated a high sensitivity (88.00%) and specificity (97.87%) for malignant astrocytoma prediction (156). These identified miRNAs also exhibited a global decrease in tumor tissues relative to normal tissues. Interestingly, these miRNAs in serum were markedly elevated after tumor removal.

In miRNA microarray analysis of the serum of patients with GBM and normal controls, 115 miRNAs were upregulated in the GBM group and 24 miRNAs were downregulated (157). In these microRNAs, a six-membered serum miRNA expression profile (upregulated miRs; miR-576-5p, miR-340, and miR-626, downregulated miRs; miR-320, let-7g-5p, and miR-7-5p) could serve as a noninvasive biomarker for GBM diagnosis (157). Manterola et al. found that the serum expression levels of miR-320 and miR-574-3p were significantly altered in the patients with GBM (158). In addition, small noncoding RNA (RNU6-1) was an independent predictor of a diagnosis of GBMs. Shao et al. compared the expression levels of miR-454-3p between preoperative plasmas from 70 patients with glioma and 70 healthy controls and between these preoperative and postoperative plasmas (159). The expression levels of miR-454-3p in plasma in patients with glioma were significantly higher, and the area under receiver operating characteristic (ROC) curve (AUC) of the expression of miR-454-3p for glioma diagnosis was 0.9063. In addition, the expression levels of miR-454-3p in the postoperative plasmas were significantly downregulated relative to the preoperative plasmas. Wu et al. analyzed serum from 83 patients with glioma and 69 healthy controls and evaluated the availability of the serum miR-29 family in the screening of glioma (160). The predictive value of the serum miR-29 family for glioma was moderate (AUC = 0.74), but that in high-grade glioma detection was sufficient (AUC = 0.81). Another study also showed that the expressions of miR-29b in blood were significantly different compared with those of a healthy control (161).

miR-125b is widely considered a tumor suppressor-miRNA and an ideal biomarker for clinical diagnosis in various human cancers. The study of serum miR-125b from 33 gliomas and 33 healthy controls revealed that the serum miR-125b level was significantly lower in patients with glioma (162). The ROC curve analysis yielded an AUC value of 0.839 (162). Furthermore, a meta-analysis was conducted to assess the diagnostic accuracy of miR-125b in cancer diagnosis, and the results revealed that employing miR-125b as a biomarker for cancer detection achieved a sensitivity of 82% and a specificity of 77% (162).

miR-210 is reported to be another potentially useful biomarker in the serum of patients with glioma. Lai et al. analyzed blood samples collected from patients with glioma (n=136) and healthy controls (n=50) and revealed that an approximately sevenfold increase in miR-210 expression was detected in serum samples from patients with GBM relative to healthy controls (163). miR-210 has been found to be upregulated in a variety of other solid tumor types and potentially influences cellular function through diverse pathways; the miRNA has also been correlated with hypoxia (164). A number of targets of miR-210 have been reported, including VEGF (165), BCL2 (166), and E2F transcription factor 3 (167). Sun et al. analyzed the expression levels of miR-128 in serum samples from 151 gliomas, 52 meningiomas, and 53 normal donors and showed that miR-128 expression was significantly decreased in glioma preoperative serum compared with others. ROC analyses showed that serum miR-128 levels were reliable in distinguishing patients with glioma from normal controls and patients with meningioma, with AUC values of 0.9095 and 0.8283, respectively (168). Although the mechanism has not yet been clarified, the study demonstrated that serum miR-128 expression was significantly elevated after surgery. miR-128 functions as a vital suppressor of tumorigenesis in glioma cells and is reported to downregulate p70S6K1 and its downstream signaling molecules, including VEGF and HIF-1. Another study showed that serum miR-205 expression was significantly lower in patients with glioma than in healthy controls ($p < 0.001$) (169). Interestingly, serum miR-205 expression levels were inversely correlated with pathological grades (169).

4.2. Cerebrospinal fluid

Baraniskin et al. (170) reported the first investigation of microRNA expression in CSF from patients with glioma in 2012. The results demonstrated that miR-15b and miR-21 were differentially expressed in CSF samples from patients with glioma compared with control subjects with various neurologic disorders, including CNS lymphoma and carcinomatous brain metastases. The combination of miR-15b and miR-21 resulted in increased diagnostic accuracy, with 90% sensitivity and 100% specificity in distinguishing patients with glioma from control subjects. Interestingly, miR-15 levels were significantly higher in glioma than in CNS lymphoma or metastatic tumor; however, miR-21 levels were significantly lower in glioma than in CNS lymphoma or metastatic tumor.

Teplyuk et al. (171) determined the CSF levels of several cancer-associated miRNAs for 118 patients diagnosed with different types of brain cancers. The levels of miR-10b and miR-21 were significantly increased in the CSF of patients with GBM and brain metastasis of breast and lung cancer compared with non-neoplastic conditions. Members of the miR-200 family were useful markers for discriminating between GBM and metastatic brain tumors. In addition, quantification of as few as seven microRNAs in CSF (miR-10b, miR-21, miR-125b, miR-141, miR-200a, miR-200b, and miR-200c) enabled differential recognition of GBM and metastatic brain tumor with high accuracy (91%–99%) (171).

Akers et al. analyzed extracellular vesicles (EVs) containing miRNAs in the CSF from patients with GBMs. The EV fraction was isolated by differential centrifugation. Although the analytic algorithm for quantitatively assessing EV miRNA remains underdeveloped, the authors showed that the CSF miR-21 levels of patients with GBM were 10-fold higher than those in the CSF of nononcologic patients (172).

Recently, another study reported results to those of Akers and coworkers. Exosomal miR-21 levels in the CSF of patients with glioma were found to be significantly higher than in controls, although no difference was detected in serum-derived exosomal miR-21 expression. Interestingly, the CSF-derived exosomal miR-21 levels correlated with a level of dissemination and a location of recurrence. Therefore, exosomal miR-21 in CSF may be a predictive marker for the early stages of tumor recurrence or metastasis (173).

5. Future prospects

Over the past decade, our understanding of genetic alterations and the tumor-specific signal pathways in glioma has been made, although this knowledge to date has not been translated into the prognosis of the patients with glioma. However, a better understanding of key pathways associated with gliomagenesis and malignant transformation could promise further improvements in glioma therapy. Maximum safe resection followed by radiotherapy up to a total dose of 60 Gy and TMZ-based chemotherapy have been established as a standard therapy, but new molecular targeting drugs, including small-molecule cell cycle inhibitors and biological and immune-based therapies have begun to yield promising results in clinical studies.

Over the past two decades, miRNAs have emerged as molecules central to glioma biology. miRNAs represent an additional layer of complexity in tumor biology and have been further validated as regulators of processes fundamental to glioma. This field is rapidly changing. Herein, we have reviewed the emerging roles of miRNAs as drivers of glioma formation and progression with a focus on glioma hallmarks. miRNAs may be essential in glioma growth, angiogenesis, invasion, genomic instability, tumor-promoting inflammation, and glioma-specific metabolism. In recent years, functions of miRNAs in gliomagenesis and microenvironment have been considerably elucidated, and we have validated the tumor suppressive or oncogenic functions of miRNAs in glioma. Now, we should move toward a next phase involving clinical trials with miRNAs as glioma therapies. For example, miR-34, a tumor-suppressive miRNA that simultaneously downregulates the expressions of MET, PDGFRA, and CDK6 is currently in clinical trials as a directed therapy for advanced solid tumors. In glioma, the restoration of miR-34a can possibly outperform any single targeted agents tailored to those targets. There remain several problems to use miRNAs in glioma therapy. These include not only accumulation of our knowledge of miRNAs' biological functions in glioma, but also the development of new and safe methods for delivery to glioma cells. Although the clinical application of miRNAs in GBM has yet to be realized, we believe the future of glioma therapy could be bright.

In this review, we have also focused on circulating miRNAs of serum, plasma, and CSF in patients with glioma. The use of miRNAs has several limitations, such as the diversity of methodologies that exist for miRNA detection and the small cohort size for the validation steps reported in current studies. Nonetheless, circulating miRNAs may exhibit diagnostic values, the combination of biomarkers may improve the diagnostic accuracy, and the combination of circulating miRNAs and other screening methods may be particularly useful in glioma detection. However, a standard protocol of sample treatment and suitable internal controls should be further established to make the level of detection comparable to that of other methods before miRNA biomarkers are fully utilized in clinical practice.

Author details

Takashi Sasayama*, Kazuhiro Tanaka and Eiji Kohmura

*Address all correspondence to: takasasa@med.kobepu.ac.jp

Department of Neurosurgery, Kobe University Graduate School of Medicine, Kusunoki-cho, Chuo-ku, Kobe, Japan

References

[1] Stupp R, Mason WP, van den Bent MJ, Weller M, Fisher B, Taphoorn MJ, et al. Radiotherapy plus concomitant and adjuvant temozolomide for glioblastoma. The New England Journal of Medicine. 2005;352(10):987–96.

[2] Gilbert MR, Dignam JJ, Armstrong TS, Wefel JS, Blumenthal DT, Vogelbaum MA, et al. A randomized trial of bevacizumab for newly diagnosed glioblastoma. The New England Journal of Medicine. 2014;370(8):699–708.

[3] Chinot OL, Wick W, Mason W, Henriksson R, Saran F, Nishikawa R, et al. Bevacizumab plus radiotherapy-temozolomide for newly diagnosed glioblastoma. The New England Journal of Medicine. 2014;370(8):709–22.

[4] Bartel DP, Chen CZ. Micromanagers of gene expression: the potentially widespread influence of metazoan microRNAs. Nature Review Genetics. 2004;5(5):396–400.

[5] Ambros V, Lee RC. Identification of microRNAs and other tiny noncoding RNAs by cDNA cloning. Methods in Molecular Biology. 2004;265:131–58.

[6] Lu J, Getz G, Miska EA, Alvarez-Saavedra E, Lamb J, Peck D, et al. MicroRNA expression profiles classify human cancers. Nature. 2005;435(7043):834–8.

[7] Ciafre SA, Galardi S, Mangiola A, Ferracin M, Liu CG, Sabatino G, et al. Extensive modulation of a set of microRNAs in primary glioblastoma. Biochemical and Biophysical Research Communications. 2005;334(4):1351–8.

[8] Chan JA, Krichevsky AM, Kosik KS. MicroRNA-21 is an antiapoptotic factor in human glioblastoma cells. Cancer Research. 2005;65(14):6029–33.

[9] Sasayama T, Nishihara M, Kondoh T, Hosoda K, Kohmura E. MicroRNA-10b is overexpressed in malignant glioma and associated with tumor invasive factors, uPAR and RhoC. International Journal of Cancer Journal International du Cancer. 2009;125(6):1407–13.

[10] Tanaka H, Sasayama T, Tanaka K, Nakamizo S, Nishihara M, Mizukawa K, et al. MicroRNA-183 upregulates HIF-1alpha by targeting isocitrate dehydrogenase 2 (IDH2) in glioma cells. Journal of Neuro-oncology. 2013;111(3):273–83.

[11] Silber J, Lim DA, Petritsch C, Persson AI, Maunakea AK, Yu M, et al. miR-124 and miR-137 inhibit proliferation of glioblastoma multiforme cells and induce differentiation of brain tumor stem cells. BMC Medicine. 2008;6:14.

[12] Godlewski J, Nowicki MO, Bronisz A, Williams S, Otsuki A, Nuovo G, et al. Targeting of the Bmi-1 oncogene/stem cell renewal factor by microRNA-128 inhibits glioma proliferation and self-renewal. Cancer Research. 2008;68(22):9125–30.

[13] Rao SA, Santosh V, Somasundaram K. Genome-wide expression profiling identifies deregulated miRNAs in malignant astrocytoma. Modern Pathology: An Official Journal of the United States and Canadian Academy of Pathology, Inc. 2010;23(10):1404–17.

[14] Lemmon MA, Schlessinger J. Cell signaling by receptor tyrosine kinases. Cell. 2010;141(7):1117–34.

[15] Cancer Genome Atlas Research N. Comprehensive genomic characterization defines human glioblastoma genes and core pathways. Nature. 2008;455(7216):1061–8.

[16] Furnari FB, Fenton T, Bachoo RM, Mukasa A, Stommel JM, Stegh A, et al. Malignant astrocytic glioma: genetics, biology, and paths to treatment. Genes & Development. 2007;21(21):2683–710.

[17] Liu Z, Jiang Z, Huang J, Huang S, Li Y, Yu S, et al. miR-7 inhibits glioblastoma growth by simultaneously interfering with the PI3K/ATK and Raf/MEK/ERK pathways. International Journal of Oncology. 2014;44(5):1571–80.

[18] Webster RJ, Giles KM, Price KJ, Zhang PM, Mattick JS, Leedman PJ. Regulation of epidermal growth factor receptor signaling in human cancer cells by microRNA-7. The Journal of Biological Chemistry. 2009;284(9):5731–41.

[19] Papagiannakopoulos T, Friedmann-Morvinski D, Neveu P, Dugas JC, Gill RM, Huillard E, et al. Pro-neural miR-128 is a glioma tumor suppressor that targets mitogenic kinases. Oncogene. 2012;31(15):1884–95.

[20] Mathew LK, Skuli N, Mucaj V, Lee SS, Zinn PO, Sathyan P, et al. miR-218 opposes a critical RTK-HIF pathway in mesenchymal glioblastoma. Proceedings of the National Academy of Sciences of the United States of America. 2014;111(1):291–6.

[21] Rao SA, Arimappamagan A, Pandey P, Santosh V, Hegde AS, Chandramouli BA, et al. miR-219-5p inhibits receptor tyrosine kinase pathway by targeting EGFR in glioblastoma. PloS One. 2013;8(5):e63164.

[22] Xu F, Li F, Zhang W, Jia P. Growth of glioblastoma is inhibited by miR-133-mediated EGFR suppression. Tumour biology: The Journal of the International Society for Oncodevelopmental Biology and Medicine. 2015;36(12):9553–8.

[23] Huang D, Qiu S, Ge R, He L, Li M, Li Y, et al. miR-340 suppresses glioblastoma multiforme. Oncotarget. 2015;6(11):9257–70.

[24] Li X, Liu Y, Granberg KJ, Wang Q, Moore LM, Ji P, et al. Two mature products of MIR-491 coordinate to suppress key cancer hallmarks in glioblastoma. Oncogene. 2015;34(13):1619–28.

[25] Kim J, Zhang Y, Skalski M, Hayes J, Kefas B, Schiff D, et al. microRNA-148a is a prognostic oncomiR that targets MIG6 and BIM to regulate EGFR and apoptosis in glioblastoma. Cancer Research. 2014;74(5):1541–53.

[26] Yin D, Ogawa S, Kawamata N, Leiter A, Ham M, Li D, et al. miR-34a functions as a tumor suppressor modulating EGFR in glioblastoma multiforme. Oncogene. 2013;32(9):1155–63.

[27] Genovese G, Ergun A, Shukla SA, Campos B, Hanna J, Ghosh P, et al. microRNA regulatory network inference identifies miR-34a as a novel regulator of TGF-beta signaling in glioblastoma. Cancer Discovery. 2012;2(8):736–49.

[28] Silber J, Jacobsen A, Ozawa T, Harinath G, Pedraza A, Sander C, et al. miR-34a repression in proneural malignant gliomas upregulates expression of its target PDGFRA and promotes tumorigenesis. PloS One. 2012;7(3):e33844.

[29] Brennan CW, Verhaak RG, McKenna A, Campos B, Noushmehr H, Salama SR, et al. The somatic genomic landscape of glioblastoma. Cell. 2013;155(2):462–77.

[30] Li Y, Guessous F, Zhang Y, Dipierro C, Kefas B, Johnson E, et al. MicroRNA-34a inhibits glioblastoma growth by targeting multiple oncogenes. Cancer Research. 2009;69(19): 7569–76.

[31] Verhaak RG, Hoadley KA, Purdom E, Wang V, Qi Y, Wilkerson MD, et al. Integrated genomic analysis identifies clinically relevant subtypes of glioblastoma characterized by abnormalities in PDGFRA, IDH1, EGFR, and NF1. Cancer cell. 2010;17(1):98–110.

[32] Kouri FM, Ritner C, Stegh AH. miRNA-182 and the regulation of the glioblastoma phenotype—toward miRNA-based precision therapeutics. Cell Cycle. 2015;14(24): 3794–800.

[33] Lan F, Yu H, Hu M, Xia T, Yue X. miR-144-3p exerts anti-tumor effects in glioblastoma by targeting c-Met. Journal of Neurochemistry. 2015;135(2):274–86.

[34] Wang L, Shi ZM, Jiang CF, Liu X, Chen QD, Qian X, et al. MiR-143 acts as a tumor suppressor by targeting N-RAS and enhances temozolomide-induced apoptosis in glioma. Oncotarget. 2014;5(14):5416–27.

[35] Wang XR, Luo H, Li HL, Cao L, Wang XF, Yan W, et al. Overexpressed let-7a inhibits glioma cell malignancy by directly targeting K-ras, independently of PTEN. Neuro-oncology. 2013;15(11):1491–501.

[36] Shi Z, Chen Q, Li C, Wang L, Qian X, Jiang C, et al. MiR-124 governs glioma growth and angiogenesis and enhances chemosensitivity by targeting R-Ras and N-Ras. Neuro-oncology. 2014;16(10):1341–53.

[37] Lv Z, Yang L. MiR-124 inhibits the growth of glioblastoma through the downregulation of SOS1. Molecular Medicine Reports. 2013;8(2):345–9.

[38] Tan X, Wang S, Yang B, Zhu L, Yin B, Chao T, et al. The CREB-miR-9 negative feedback minicircuitry coordinates the migration and proliferation of glioma cells. PloS One. 2012;7(11):e49570.

[39] Malzkorn B, Wolter M, Liesenberg F, Grzendowski M, Stuhler K, Meyer HE, et al. Identification and functional characterization of microRNAs involved in the malignant progression of gliomas. Brain Pathology. 2010;20(3):539–50.

[40] Stark MS, Bonazzi VF, Boyle GM, Palmer JM, Symmons J, Lanagan CM, et al. miR-514a regulates the tumour suppressor NF1 and modulates BRAFi sensitivity in melanoma. Oncotarget. 2015;6(19):17753–63.

[41] Huse JT, Brennan C, Hambardzumyan D, Wee B, Pena J, Rouhanifard SH, et al. The PTEN-regulating microRNA miR-26a is amplified in high-grade glioma and facilitates gliomagenesis in vivo. Genes & Development. 2009;23(11):1327–37.

[42] Kim H, Huang W, Jiang X, Pennicooke B, Park PJ, Johnson MD. Integrative genome analysis reveals an oncomir/oncogene cluster regulating glioblastoma survivorship. Proceedings of the National Academy of Sciences of the United States of America. 2010;107(5):2183–8.

[43] Guo P, Nie Q, Lan J, Ge J, Qiu Y, Mao Q. C-Myc negatively controls the tumor suppressor PTEN by upregulating miR-26a in glioblastoma multiforme cells. Biochemical and Biophysical Research Communications. 2013;441(1):186–90.

[44] Tan X, Wang S, Zhu L, Wu C, Yin B, Zhao J, et al. cAMP response element-binding protein promotes gliomagenesis by modulating the expression of oncogenic micro-

RNA-23a. Proceedings of the National Academy of Sciences of the United States of America. 2012;109(39):15805–10.

[45] Tian K, Di R, Wang L. MicroRNA-23a enhances migration and invasion through PTEN in osteosarcoma. Cancer Gene Therapy. 2015;22(7):351–9.

[46] Li H, Yang BB. Stress response of glioblastoma cells mediated by miR-17-5p targeting PTEN and the passenger strand miR-17-3p targeting MDM2. Oncotarget. 2012;3(12): 1653–68.

[47] Xia X, Li Y, Wang W, Tang F, Tan J, Sun L, et al. MicroRNA-1908 functions as a glioblastoma oncogene by suppressing PTEN tumor suppressor pathway. Molecular Cancer. 2015;14:154.

[48] Tokudome T, Sasaki A, Tsuji M, Udaka Y, Oyamada H, Tsuchiya H, et al. Reduced PTEN expression and overexpression of miR-17-5p, -19a-3p, -19b-3p, -21-5p, -130b-3p, -221-3p and -222-3p by glioblastoma stem-like cells following irradiation. Oncology Letters. 2015;10(4):2269–72.

[49] Kleihues P, Burger PC, Scheithauer BW. The new WHO classification of brain tumours. Brain Pathology. 1993;3(3):255–68.

[50] Plate KH, Risau W. Angiogenesis in malignant gliomas. Glia. 1995;15(3):339–47.

[51] Yue X, Wang P, Xu J, Zhu Y, Sun G, Pang Q, et al. MicroRNA-205 functions as a tumor suppressor in human glioblastoma cells by targeting VEGF-A. Oncology Reports. 2012;27(4):1200–6.

[52] Harris AL. Hypoxia—a key regulatory factor in tumour growth. Nature Reviews Cancer. 2002;2(1):38–47.

[53] Zhang KL, Han L, Chen LY, Shi ZD, Yang M, Ren Y, et al. Blockage of a miR-21/EGFR regulatory feedback loop augments anti-EGFR therapy in glioblastomas. Cancer Letters. 2014;342(1):139–49.

[54] Hermansen SK, Nielsen BS, Aaberg-Jessen C, Kristensen BW. miR-21 is linked to glioma angiogenesis: a co-localization study. The Journal of Histochemistry and Cytochemistry: Official Journal of the Histochemistry Society. 2016;64(2):138–48.

[55] Chen L, Han L, Zhang K, Shi Z, Zhang J, Zhang A, et al. VHL regulates the effects of miR-23b on glioma survival and invasion via suppression of HIF-1alpha/VEGF and beta-catenin/Tcf-4 signaling. Neuro-oncology. 2012;14(8):1026–36.

[56] Xiao B, Zhou X, Ye M, Lv S, Wu M, Liao C, et al. MicroRNA566 modulates vascular endothelial growth factor by targeting Von HippelLandau in human glioblastoma in vitro and in vivo. Molecular Medicine Reports. 2016;13(1):379–85.

[57] Babae N, Bourajjaj M, Liu Y, Van Beijnum JR, Cerisoli F, Scaria PV, et al. Systemic miRNA-7 delivery inhibits tumor angiogenesis and growth in murine xenograft glioblastoma. Oncotarget. 2014;5(16):6687–700.

[58] Smits M, Nilsson J, Mir SE, van der Stoop PM, Hulleman E, Niers JM, et al. miR-101 is down-regulated in glioblastoma resulting in EZH2-induced proliferation, migration, and angiogenesis. Oncotarget. 2010;1(8):710–20.

[59] Sun J, Zheng G, Gu Z, Guo Z. MiR-137 inhibits proliferation and angiogenesis of human glioblastoma cells by targeting EZH2. Journal of Neuro-oncology. 2015;122(3):481–9.

[60] Wurdinger T, Tannous BA, Saydam O, Skog J, Grau S, Soutschek J, et al. miR-296 regulates growth factor receptor overexpression in angiogenic endothelial cells. Cancer Cell. 2008;14(5):382–93.

[61] Fang L, Deng Z, Shatseva T, Yang J, Peng C, Du WW, et al. MicroRNA miR-93 promotes tumor growth and angiogenesis by targeting integrin-beta8. Oncogene. 2011;30(7):806–21.

[62] Dews M, Fox JL, Hultine S, Sundaram P, Wang W, Liu YY, et al. The myc-miR-17~92 axis blunts TGF{beta} signaling and production of multiple TGF{beta}-dependent antiangiogenic factors. Cancer Research. 2010;70(20):8233–46.

[63] Kruiswijk F, Labuschagne CF, Vousden KH. p53 in survival, death and metabolic health: a lifeguard with a licence to kill. Nature Reviews Molecular Cell Biology. 2015;16(7):393–405.

[64] Lin J, Teo S, Lam DH, Jeyaseelan K, Wang S. MicroRNA-10b pleiotropically regulates invasion, angiogenicity and apoptosis of tumor cells resembling mesenchymal subtype of glioblastoma multiforme. Cell Death & Disease. 2012;3:e398.

[65] Gabriely G, Yi M, Narayan RS, Niers JM, Wurdinger T, Imitola J, et al. Human glioma growth is controlled by microRNA-10b. Cancer Research. 2011;71(10):3563–72.

[66] Brown CJ, Lain S, Verma CS, Fersht AR, Lane DP. Awakening guardian angels: drugging the p53 pathway. Nature Reviews Cancer. 2009;9(12):862–73.

[67] Suh SS, Yoo JY, Nuovo GJ, Jeon YJ, Kim S, Lee TJ, et al. MicroRNAs/TP53 feedback circuitry in glioblastoma multiforme. Proceedings of the National Academy of Sciences of the United States of America. 2012;109(14):5316–21.

[68] Sun YC, Wang J, Guo CC, Sai K, Wang J, Chen FR, et al. MiR-181b sensitizes glioma cells to teniposide by targeting MDM2. BMC Cancer. 2014;14:611.

[69] Skalsky RL, Cullen BR. Reduced expression of brain-enriched microRNAs in glioblastomas permits targeted regulation of a cell death gene. PloS One. 2011;6(9):e24248.

[70] Burkhart DL, Sage J. Cellular mechanisms of tumour suppression by the retinoblastoma gene. Nature Reviews Cancer. 2008;8(9):671–82.

[71] Serrano M, Hannon GJ, Beach D. A new regulatory motif in cell-cycle control causing specific inhibition of cyclin D/CDK4. Nature. 1993;366(6456):704–7.

[72] Lundberg AS, Weinberg RA. Functional inactivation of the retinoblastoma protein requires sequential modification by at least two distinct cyclin-cdk complexes. Molecular and Cellular Biology. 1998;18(2):753–61.

[73] Deng X, Ma L, Wu M, Zhang G, Jin C, Guo Y, et al. miR-124 radiosensitizes human glioma cells by targeting CDK4. Journal of Neuro-oncology. 2013;114(3):263–74.

[74] Qiu S, Huang D, Yin D, Li F, Li X, Kung HF, et al. Suppression of tumorigenicity by microRNA-138 through inhibition of EZH2-CDK4/6-pRb-E2F1 signal loop in glioblastoma multiforme. Biochim Biophys Acta. 2013;1832(10):1697–707.

[75] Hui W, Yuntao L, Lun L, WenSheng L, ChaoFeng L, HaiYong H, et al. MicroRNA-195 inhibits the proliferation of human glioma cells by directly targeting cyclin D1 and cyclin E1. PloS One. 2013;8(1):e54932.

[76] Nakada M, Nakada S, Demuth T, Tran NL, Hoelzinger DB, Berens ME. Molecular targets of glioma invasion. Cellular and Molecular Life Sciences. 2007;64(4):458–78.

[77] Liu Y, Yan W, Zhang W, Chen L, You G, Bao Z, et al. MiR-218 reverses high invasiveness of glioblastoma cells by targeting the oncogenic transcription factor LEF1. Oncology Reports. 2012;28(3):1013–21.

[78] Song L, Huang Q, Chen K, Liu L, Lin C, Dai T, et al. miR-218 inhibits the invasive ability of glioma cells by direct downregulation of IKK-beta. Biochemical and Biophysical Research Communications. 2010;402(1):135–40.

[79] Li Y, Xu J, Chen H, Bai J, Li S, Zhao Z, et al. Comprehensive analysis of the functional microRNA-mRNA regulatory network identifies miRNA signatures associated with glioma malignant progression. Nucleic Acids Research. 2013;41(22):e203.

[80] Yan W, Zhang W, Sun L, Liu Y, You G, Wang Y, et al. Identification of MMP-9 specific microRNA expression profile as potential targets of anti-invasion therapy in glioblastoma multiforme. Brain Research. 2011;1411:108–15.

[81] Asuthkar S, Velpula KK, Chetty C, Gorantla B, Rao JS. Epigenetic regulation of miRNA-211 by MMP-9 governs glioma cell apoptosis, chemosensitivity and radiosensitivity. Oncotarget. 2012;3(11):1439–54.

[82] Zheng X, Chopp M, Lu Y, Buller B, Jiang F. MiR-15b and miR-152 reduce glioma cell invasion and angiogenesis via NRP-2 and MMP-3. Cancer Letters. 2013;329(2):146–54.

[83] Lu Y, Chopp M, Zheng X, Katakowski M, Buller B, Jiang F. MiR-145 reduces ADAM17 expression and inhibits in vitro migration and invasion of glioma cells. Oncology Reports. 2013;29(1):67–72.

[84] Gabriely G, Wurdinger T, Kesari S, Esau CC, Burchard J, Linsley PS, et al. MicroRNA 21 promotes glioma invasion by targeting matrix metalloproteinase regulators. Molecular and Cellular Biology. 2008;28(17):5369–80.

[85] Fowler A, Thomson D, Giles K, Maleki S, Mreich E, Wheeler H, et al. miR-124a is frequently down–regulated in glioblastoma and is involved in migration and invasion. European Journal of Cancer. 2011;47(6):953–63.

[86] Zhao WH, Wu SQ, Zhang YD. Downregulation of miR-124 promotes the growth and invasiveness of glioblastoma cells involving upregulation of PPP1R13L. International Journal of Molecular Medicine. 2013;32(1):101–7.

[87] Cai J, Zhao J, Zhang N, Xu X, Li R, Yi Y, et al. MicroRNA-542-3p suppresses tumor cell invasion via targeting AKT pathway in human astrocytoma. The Journal of Biological Chemistry. 2015;290(41):24678–88.

[88] Wang H, Tao T, Yan W, Feng Y, Wang Y, Cai J, et al. Upregulation of miR-181s reverses mesenchymal transition by targeting KPNA4 in glioblastoma. Scientific Reports. 2015;5:13072.

[89] Yin F, Zhang JN, Wang SW, Zhou CH, Zhao MM, Fan WH, et al. MiR-125a-3p regulates glioma apoptosis and invasion by regulating Nrg1. PloS One. 2015;10(1):e0116759.

[90] Dontula R, Dinasarapu A, Chetty C, Pannuru P, Herbert E, Ozer H, et al. MicroRNA 203 modulates glioma cell migration via Robo1/ERK/MMP-9 signaling. Genes & Cancer. 2013;4(7–8):285–96.

[91] Chen Z, Li D, Cheng Q, Ma Z, Jiang B, Peng R, et al. MicroRNA-203 inhibits the proliferation and invasion of U251 glioblastoma cells by directly targeting PLD2. Molecular Medicine Reports. 2014;9(2):503–8.

[92] Chung HJ, Choi YE, Kim ES, Han YH, Park MJ, Bae IH. miR-29b attenuates tumorigenicity and stemness maintenance in human glioblastoma multiforme by directly targeting BCL2L2. Oncotarget. 2015;6(21):18429–44.

[93] Sun L, Yan W, Wang Y, Sun G, Luo H, Zhang J, et al. MicroRNA-10b induces glioma cell invasion by modulating MMP-14 and uPAR expression via HOXD10. Brain Research. 2011;1389:9–18.

[94] Liu Q, Zou R, Zhou R, Gong C, Wang Z, Cai T, et al. miR-155 regulates glioma cells invasion and chemosensitivity by p38 isforms in vitro. Journal of Cellular Biochemistry. 2015;116(7):1213–21.

[95] Corsten MF, Miranda R, Kasmieh R, Krichevsky AM, Weissleder R, Shah K. MicroRNA-21 knockdown disrupts glioma growth in vivo and displays synergistic cytotoxicity with neural precursor cell delivered S-TRAIL in human gliomas. Cancer Research. 2007;67(19):8994–9000.

[96] Gaur AB, Holbeck SL, Colburn NH, Israel MA. Downregulation of Pdcd4 by mir-21 facilitates glioblastoma proliferation in vivo. Neuro-oncology. 2011;13(6):580–90.

[97] Papagiannakopoulos T, Shapiro A, Kosik KS. MicroRNA-21 targets a network of key tumor-suppressive pathways in glioblastoma cells. Cancer Research. 2008;68(19):8164–72.

[98] Niu H, Wang K, Zhang A, Yang S, Song Z, Wang W, et al. miR-92a is a critical regulator of the apoptosis pathway in glioblastoma with inverse expression of BCL2L11. Oncology Reports. 2012;28(5):1771–7.

[99] Wang K, Wang X, Zou J, Zhang A, Wan Y, Pu P, et al. miR-92b controls glioma proliferation and invasion through regulating Wnt/beta-catenin signaling via Nemo-like kinase. Neuro-oncology. 2013;15(5):578–88.

[100] Medina R, Zaidi SK, Liu CG, Stein JL, van Wijnen AJ, Croce CM, et al. MicroRNAs 221 and 222 bypass quiescence and compromise cell survival. Cancer Research. 2008;68(8): 2773–80.

[101] Liu F, Gong J, Huang W, Wang Z, Wang M, Yang J, et al. MicroRNA-106b-5p boosts glioma tumorigensis by targeting multiple tumor suppressor genes. Oncogene. 2014;33(40):4813–22.

[102] Polyak K, Lee MH, Erdjument-Bromage H, Koff A, Roberts JM, Tempst P, et al. Cloning of p27Kip1, a cyclin-dependent kinase inhibitor and a potential mediator of extracellular antimitogenic signals. Cell. 1994;78(1):59–66.

[103] Gillies JK, Lorimer IA. Regulation of p27Kip1 by miRNA 221/222 in glioblastoma. Cell Cycle. 2007;6(16):2005–9.

[104] Wan Y, Fei XF, Wang ZM, Jiang DY, Chen HC, Yang J, et al. Expression of miR-125b in the new, highly invasive glioma stem cell and progenitor cell line SU3. Chinese Journal of Cancer. 2012;31(4):207–14.

[105] Le MT, Teh C, Shyh-Chang N, Xie H, Zhou B, Korzh V, et al. MicroRNA-125b is a novel negative regulator of p53. Genes & Development. 2009;23(7):862–76.

[106] Park SY, Lee JH, Ha M, Nam JW, Kim VN. miR-29 miRNAs activate p53 by targeting p85 alpha and CDC42. Nature Structural & Molecular Biology. 2009;16(1):23–9.

[107] He L, He X, Lim LP, de Stanchina E, Xuan Z, Liang Y, et al. A microRNA component of the p53 tumour suppressor network. Nature. 2007;447(7148):1130–4.

[108] Kato M, Paranjape T, Muller RU, Nallur S, Gillespie E, Keane K, et al. The mir-34 microRNA is required for the DNA damage response in vivo in C. elegans and in vitro in human breast cancer cells. Oncogene. 2009;28(25):2419–24.

[109] Yan D, Ng WL, Zhang X, Wang P, Zhang Z, Mo YY, et al. Targeting DNA-PKcs and ATM with miR-101 sensitizes tumors to radiation. PloS One. 2010;5(7):e11397.

[110] Nogueira L, Ruiz-Ontanon P, Vazquez-Barquero A, Moris F, Fernandez-Luna JL. The NFkappaB pathway: a therapeutic target in glioblastoma. Oncotarget. 2011;2(8):646–53.

[111] Li Y, Li W, Yang Y, Lu Y, He C, Hu G, et al. MicroRNA-21 targets LRRFIP1 and contributes to VM-26 resistance in glioblastoma multiforme. Brain Research. 2009;1286:13–8.

[112] Taganov KD, Boldin MP, Chang KJ, Baltimore D. NF-kappaB-dependent induction of microRNA miR-146, an inhibitor targeted to signaling proteins of innate immune responses. Proceedings of the National Academy of Sciences of the United States of America. 2006;103(33):12481–6.

[113] Park H, Huang X, Lu C, Cairo MS, Zhou X. MicroRNA-146a and microRNA-146b regulate human dendritic cell apoptosis and cytokine production by targeting TRAF6 and IRAK1 proteins. The Journal of Biological Chemistry. 2015;290(5):2831–41.

[114] Wu H, Liu Q, Cai T, Chen YD, Wang ZF. Induction of microRNA-146a is involved in curcumin-mediated enhancement of temozolomide cytotoxicity against human glioblastoma. Molecular Medicine Reports. 2015;12(4):5461–6.

[115] Iyer A, Zurolo E, Prabowo A, Fluiter K, Spliet WG, van Rijen PC, et al. MicroRNA-146a: a key regulator of astrocyte-mediated inflammatory response. PloS One. 2012;7(9):e44789.

[116] Yu H, Pardoll D, Jove R. STATs in cancer inflammation and immunity: a leading role for STAT3. Nature Reviews Cancer. 2009;9(11):798–809.

[117] Wei J, Wang F, Kong LY, Xu S, Doucette T, Ferguson SD, et al. miR-124 inhibits STAT3 signaling to enhance T cell-mediated immune clearance of glioma. Cancer Research. 2013;73(13):3913–26.

[118] Tarassishin L, Lee SC. Interferon regulatory factor 3 alters glioma inflammatory and invasive properties. Journal of Neuro-oncology. 2013;113(2):185–94.

[119] Vander Heiden MG, Cantley LC, Thompson CB. Understanding the Warburg effect: the metabolic requirements of cell proliferation. Science. 2009;324(5930):1029–33.

[120] Colavolpe C, Metellus P, Mancini J, Barrie M, Bequet-Boucard C, Figarella-Branger D, et al. Independent prognostic value of pre-treatment 18-FDG-PET in high-grade gliomas. Journal of Neuro-oncology. 2012;107(3):527–35.

[121] Hardie DG. AMP-activated/SNF1 protein kinases: conserved guardians of cellular energy. Nature Reviews Molecular Cell Biology. 2007;8(10):774–85.

[122] Sanders MJ, Ali ZS, Hegarty BD, Heath R, Snowden MA, Carling D. Defining the mechanism of activation of AMP-activated protein kinase by the small molecule A-769662, a member of the thienopyridone family. The Journal of Biological Chemistry. 2007;282(45):32539–48.

[123] Hawley SA, Boudeau J, Reid JL, Mustard KJ, Udd L, Makela TP, et al. Complexes between the LKB1 tumor suppressor, STRAD alpha/beta and MO25 alpha/beta are

upstream kinases in the AMP-activated protein kinase cascade. Journal of Biology. 2003;2(4):28.

[124] Godlewski J, Nowicki MO, Bronisz A, Nuovo G, Palatini J, De Lay M, et al. MicroRNA-451 regulates LKB1/AMPK signaling and allows adaptation to metabolic stress in glioma cells. Molecular Cell. 2010;37(5):620–32.

[125] Guo QM, Malek RL, Kim S, Chiao C, He M, Ruffy M, et al. Identification of c-myc responsive genes using rat cDNA microarray. Cancer Research. 2000;60(21):5922–8.

[126] Zamorano A, Lamas M, Vergara P, Naranjo JR, Segovia J. Transcriptionally mediated gene targeting of gas1 to glioma cells elicits growth arrest and apoptosis. Journal of Neuroscience Research. 2003;71(2):256–63.

[127] Barr LF, Campbell SE, Diette GB, Gabrielson EW, Kim S, Shim H, et al. c-Myc suppresses the tumorigenicity of lung cancer cells and down-regulates vascular endothelial growth factor expression. Cancer Research. 2000;60(1):143–9.

[128] Wang G, Wang J, Zhao H, Wang J, Tony To SS. The role of Myc and let-7a in glioblastoma, glucose metabolism and response to therapy. Archives of Biochemistry and Biophysics. 2015;580:84–92.

[129] Chang TC, Zeitels LR, Hwang HW, Chivukula RR, Wentzel EA, Dews M, et al. Lin-28B transactivation is necessary for Myc-mediated let-7 repression and proliferation. Proceedings of the National Academy of Sciences of the United States of America. 2009;106(9):3384–9.

[130] Rani SB, Rathod SS, Karthik S, Kaur N, Muzumdar D, Shiras AS. MiR-145 functions as a tumor-suppressive RNA by targeting Sox9 and adducin 3 in human glioma cells. Neuro-oncology. 2013;15(10):1302–16.

[131] Dang CV. MYC on the path to cancer. Cell. 2012;149(1):22–35.

[132] Gan B, Lim C, Chu G, Hua S, Ding Z, Collins M, et al. FoxOs enforce a progression checkpoint to constrain mTORC1-activated renal tumorigenesis. Cancer Cell. 2010;18(5):472–84.

[133] Kress TR, Cannell IG, Brenkman AB, Samans B, Gaestel M, Roepman P, et al. The MK5/PRAK kinase and Myc form a negative feedback loop that is disrupted during colorectal tumorigenesis. Molecular Cell. 2011;41(4):445–57.

[134] Masui K, Tanaka K, Akhavan D, Babic I, Gini B, Matsutani T, et al. mTOR complex 2 controls glycolytic metabolism in glioblastoma through FoxO acetylation and upregulation of c-Myc. Cell Metabolism. 2013;18(5):726–39.

[135] Boyerinas B, Park SM, Shomron N, Hedegaard MM, Vinther J, Andersen JS, et al. Identification of let-7-regulated oncofetal genes. Cancer Research. 2008;68(8):2587–91.

[136] Kefas B, Comeau L, Erdle N, Montgomery E, Amos S, Purow B. Pyruvate kinase M2 is a target of the tumor-suppressive microRNA-326 and regulates the survival of glioma cells. Neuro-oncology. 2010;12(11):1102–12.

[137] Zhou J, Xu T, Yan Y, Qin R, Wang H, Zhang X, et al. MicroRNA-326 functions as a tumor suppressor in glioma by targeting the Nin one binding protein (NOB1). PloS One. 2013;8(7):e68469.

[138] de Visser KE, Eichten A, Coussens LM. Paradoxical roles of the immune system during cancer development. Nature Reviews Cancer. 2006;6(1):24–37.

[139] Mantovani A, Sozzani S, Locati M, Allavena P, Sica A. Macrophage polarization: tumor-associated macrophages as a paradigm for polarized M2 mononuclear phagocytes. Trends in Immunology. 2002;23(11):549–55.

[140] Graff JW, Dickson AM, Clay G, McCaffrey AP, Wilson ME. Identifying functional microRNAs in macrophages with polarized phenotypes. The Journal of Biological Chemistry. 2012;287(26):21816–25.

[141] Cai X, Yin Y, Li N, Zhu D, Zhang J, Zhang CY, et al. Re-polarization of tumor-associated macrophages to pro-inflammatory M1 macrophages by microRNA-155. Journal of Molecular Cell Biology. 2012;4(5):341–3.

[142] Tanikawa T, Wilke CM, Kryczek I, Chen GY, Kao J, Nunez G, et al. Interleukin-10 ablation promotes tumor development, growth, and metastasis. Cancer Research. 2012;72(2):420–9.

[143] Zhang C, Han L, Zhang A, Yang W, Zhou X, Pu P, et al. Global changes of mRNA expression reveals an increased activity of the interferon-induced signal transducer and activator of transcription (STAT) pathway by repression of miR-221/222 in glioblastoma U251 cells. International Journal of Oncology. 2010;36(6):1503–12.

[144] Raulet DH, Gasser S, Gowen BG, Deng W, Jung H. Regulation of ligands for the NKG2D activating receptor. Annual Review of Immunology. 2013;31:413–41.

[145] Friese MA, Platten M, Lutz SZ, Naumann U, Aulwurm S, Bischof F, et al. MICA/NKG2D-mediated immunogene therapy of experimental gliomas. Cancer Research. 2003;63(24):8996–9006.

[146] Codo P, Weller M, Meister G, Szabo E, Steinle A, Wolter M, et al. MicroRNA-mediated down-regulation of NKG2D ligands contributes to glioma immune escape. Oncotarget. 2014;5(17):7651–62.

[147] Wei J, Nduom EK, Kong LY, Hashimoto Y, Xu S, Gabrusiewicz K, et al. MiR-138 exerts anti-glioma efficacy by targeting immune checkpoints. Neuro-oncology. 2015.

[148] Ohno M, Natsume A, Kondo Y, Iwamizu H, Motomura K, Toda H, et al. The modulation of microRNAs by type I IFN through the activation of signal transducers and activators

of transcription 3 in human glioma. Molecular Cancer Research: MCR. 2009;7(12):2022–30.

[149] Aleckovic M, Kang Y. Regulation of cancer metastasis by cell-free miRNAs. Biochimica et Biophysica Acta. 2015;1855(1):24–42.

[150] Wang K, Yuan Y, Cho JH, McClarty S, Baxter D, Galas DJ. Comparing the MicroRNA spectrum between serum and plasma. PloS One. 2012;7(7):e41561.

[151] Cheng HH, Yi HS, Kim Y, Kroh EM, Chien JW, Eaton KD, et al. Plasma processing conditions substantially influence circulating microRNA biomarker levels. PloS One. 2013;8(6):e64795.

[152] Sasayama T, Nakamizo S, Nishihara M, Kawamura A, Tanaka H, Mizukawa K, et al. Cerebrospinal fluid interleukin-10 is a potentially useful biomarker in immunocompetent primary central nervous system lymphoma (PCNSL). Neuro-oncology. 2012;14(3):368–80.

[153] Skog J, Wurdinger T, van Rijn S, Meijer DH, Gainche L, Sena-Esteves M, et al. Glioblastoma microvesicles transport RNA and proteins that promote tumour growth and provide diagnostic biomarkers. Nature Cell Biology. 2008;10(12):1470–6.

[154] Roth P, Wischhusen J, Happold C, Chandran PA, Hofer S, Eisele G, et al. A specific miRNA signature in the peripheral blood of glioblastoma patients. Journal of Neurochemistry. 2011;118(3):449–57.

[155] Wang Q, Li P, Li A, Jiang W, Wang H, Wang J, et al. Plasma specific miRNAs as predictive biomarkers for diagnosis and prognosis of glioma. Journal of Experimental & Clinical Cancer Research: CR. 2012;31:97.

[156] Zhao Q, Yin T, Peng J, Zou Y, Yang J, Shen A, et al. Noninvasive metabolomic profiling of human embryo culture media using a simple spectroscopy adjunct to morphology for embryo assessment in in vitro fertilization (IVF). International Journal of Molecular Sciences. 2013;14(4):6556–70.

[157] Dong L, Li Y, Han C, Wang X, She L, Zhang H. miRNA microarray reveals specific expression in the peripheral blood of glioblastoma patients. International journal of oncology. 2014;45(2):746–56.

[158] Manterola L, Guruceaga E, Gallego Perez-Larraya J, Gonzalez-Huarriz M, Jauregui P, Tejada S, et al. A small noncoding RNA signature found in exosomes of GBM patient serum as a diagnostic tool. Neuro-oncology. 2014;16(4):520–7.

[159] Shao N, Wang L, Xue L, Wang R, Lan Q. Plasma miR-454-3p as a potential prognostic indicator in human glioma. Neurological Science. 2015;36(2):309–13.

[160] Wu J, Li L, Jiang C. Identification and Evaluation of Serum MicroRNA-29 Family for Glioma Screening. Molecular Neurobiology. 2015;52(3):1540–6.

[161] Liu Q, Liao F, Wu H, Cai T, Yang L, Fang J. Different expression of miR-29b and VEGFA in glioma. Artificial Cells, Nanomedicine, and Biotechnology. 2015:1–6.

[162] Wei X, Chen D, Lv T, Li G, Qu S. Serum microRNA-125b as a potential biomarker for glioma diagnosis. Molecular neurobiology. 2016;53(1):163–70.

[163] Lai NS, Wu DG, Fang XG, Lin YC, Chen SS, Li ZB, et al. Serum microRNA-210 as a potential noninvasive biomarker for the diagnosis and prognosis of glioma. British Journal of Cancer. 2015;112(7):1241–6.

[164] Ivan M, Huang X. miR-210: fine-tuning the hypoxic response. Advances in experimental medicine and biology. 2014;772:205–27.

[165] Zeng L, He X, Wang Y, Tang Y, Zheng C, Cai H, et al. MicroRNA-210 overexpression induces angiogenesis and neurogenesis in the normal adult mouse brain. Gene Therapy. 2014;21(1):37–43.

[166] Chio CC, Lin JW, Cheng HA, Chiu WT, Wang YH, Wang JJ, et al. MicroRNA-210 targets antiapoptotic Bcl-2 expression and mediates hypoxia-induced apoptosis of neuroblastoma cells. Archives of Toxicology. 2013;87(3):459–68.

[167] Cui H, Seubert B, Stahl E, Dietz H, Reuning U, Moreno-Leon L, et al. Tissue inhibitor of metalloproteinases-1 induces a pro-tumourigenic increase of miR-210 in lung adenocarcinoma cells and their exosomes. Oncogene. 2015;34(28):3640–50.

[168] Sun J, Liao K, Wu X, Huang J, Zhang S, Lu X. Serum microRNA-128 as a biomarker for diagnosis of glioma. International Journal of Clinical and Experimental Medicine. 2015;8(1):456–63.

[169] Yue X, Lan F, Hu M, Pan Q, Wang Q, Wang J. Downregulation of serum microRNA-205 as a potential diagnostic and prognostic biomarker for human glioma. Journal of Neurosurgery. 2016;124(1):122–8.

[170] Baraniskin A, Kuhnhenn J, Schlegel U, Maghnouj A, Zollner H, Schmiegel W, et al. Identification of microRNAs in the cerebrospinal fluid as biomarker for the diagnosis of glioma. Neuro-oncology. 2012;14(1):29–33.

[171] Teplyuk NM, Mollenhauer B, Gabriely G, Giese A, Kim E, Smolsky M, et al. MicroRNAs in cerebrospinal fluid identify glioblastoma and metastatic brain cancers and reflect disease activity. Neuro-oncology. 2012;14(6):689–700.

[172] Akers JC, Ramakrishnan V, Kim R, Skog J, Nakano I, Pingle S, et al. MiR-21 in the extracellular vesicles (EVs) of cerebrospinal fluid (CSF): a platform for glioblastoma biomarker development. PloS One. 2013;8(10):e78115.

[173] Shi R, Wang PY, Li XY, Chen JX, Li Y, Zhang XZ, et al. Exosomal levels of miRNA-21 from cerebrospinal fluids associated with poor prognosis and tumor recurrence of glioma patients. Oncotarget. 2015;6(29):26971–81.

Chapter 3

Novel Endocrine Targets for GBM Therapy

Judith Marcela Dueñas-Jiménez,
Irene Aguilar-García,
María de la Luz Galván-Ramírez,
Sergio Horacio Dueñas-Jiménez,
Jorge David Rivas-Carrillo, Anne Santerre and
Erika Priscilla Domínguez-Rangel

Additional information is available at the end of the chapter

http://dx.doi.org/10.5772/62878

Abstract

Astrocytomas are brain tumors from glial cells, and they are classified by the World Health Organization (WHO) as astrocytoma, grade I or benign; astrocytoma, grade II or malignant; anaplastic astrocytoma, grade III; and glioblastoma multiforme or grade IV. The high-grade gliomas have an incidence of 6.03/100,000. The frequency of GBM is higher in men than in woman by a 50%. The survival of patients with GBM varied between 14 and 18 months, and less than 10% patients survive for 5 years. The main treatments for GBM consist of surgical tumor resection, radiotherapy, and chemotherapy. These tumors present different endocrine characteristics, such as expression of aromatase enzyme, estrogen, progesterone, as well as testosterone receptors. In addition, patients with GBM produce estradiol in high concentrations when compared to those with low-grade astrocytomas. The highest mRNA expression of ERα and aromatase in GBM patients had been postulated as prognostic biomarkers. The aromatase inhibitors had been used in the treatment of breast cancer in postmenopausal women with satisfactory results. At present time, several research groups are interested in testing these inhibitors for treating GBM.

Keywords: glioblastoma, endocrine characteristics, estradiol receptor, aromatase, aromatase inhibitors

1. Introduction

Glioblastoma multiforme (GBM) tumor occurs either as a primary tumor when it is formed de novo or a secondary tumor when the tumor progresses from grade II or III to grade IV. GBM is a diffuse and infiltrative tumor with a high mitotic activity, nuclear atypia, pleomorphism, and necrosis. GBM is the most frequently occurring brain tumor (12–15%) and represents 50–60% of all astrocytomas. There are two variants of glioblastoma: Glioblastoma of giant cells and gliosarcoma. GBM affects the cerebral hemispheres, mostly the white substance of the cerebral hemispheres. GBM primary has a bad prognostic due to its molecular heterogeneity. On the basis of its transcriptional subtype, GBM primary is also classified as neural, classical, and mesenchymal as well as proneural for GBM secondary. In GBM primary occurs the amplification of epidermal growth factor (EGF), and the *PTEN* gene is mutated in 45% of GBM primary cases, whereas in GBM secondary, the EGF amplification does not occur. The chromosome alteration in GBM involves a loss of the chromosome 10. The treatment for this kind of tumor after a safe surgical process also involves radiotherapy (RT) and the pharmacological treatment using the alkylating agent Temozolamide (TMZ), and different combinations of this agent with antitumor drugs such as the Bevacizumab. In spite of these treatments, there is a short survival period for GBM patients (14–18 months), which promotes the development of different clinical trials (II or III) to provide the patient a treatment with a better outcome. These new approaches are based on the molecular aspects of GBM to make the treatments more individualized.. This chapter describes the main GBM endocrine and molecular characteristics now known and makes a proposal on future treatments for GBM patients on the basis of these molecular characteristics.

2. Epidemiology

The incidence can change by age; in adults, for example, gliomas are the most frequent primary central nervous system tumors recurring in 70% of the patients. The average age of patients with GBM primary is 62 years, while for secondary GBM patients, it is approximately 45 years. The ethnicity and geographical localization are also of great importance in their epidemiology [1]. These tumors represent about 31% of newly diagnosed tumors in the United States and 81% of malignant tumors of the brain. The incidence of brain cancer in Europe is of 5.5/100,000 individuals, and the minor incidence is in sub-Saharan Africa with 0.8/100,000 individuals [2]. High-grade gliomas, anaplastic astrocytoma (AA) and GBM, have an incidence of 6.03/100,000 [3,4]. It has been shown that the incidence of GBM with respect to gender and ethnicity was different. The white people had the highest incidence of 2.5/100,000, Latin white people 1.8/100,000, and black people 1.5/100,000 [5].

3. Molecular characteristics of GBM

The current molecular characterization of GBM has allowed different classifications of the tumor subtypes and revealed intracellular pathways that might contribute to the development of new and effective therapeutic targets. The new molecular classification can distinguish individual somatic mutations within the same tumor grade, since tumors are highly variable from patient to patient [6,7]. Thus, using molecular markers facilitate study of heterogeneity of glioma, and subsequently its diagnosis and treatment.

Intensive molecular analyses have revealed a variety of deregulated genetic pathways involved in the DNA damage and repair, apoptosis, cell migration, angiogenesis, and in the cell cycle. Molecular analyses show that they arise from different genomic alterations, which may influence the response to therapy. The Cancer Genome Atlas (TCGA) Research Network (2008) has established a comprehensive catalog of genomic abnormalities driving tumor genesis, thus subclassifying glioblastoma into at least four molecular subtypes, featuring distinct genetic, epigenetic, and transcriptional alterations [6,8]. Tumor variants are classified based on somatic mutations as: isocitrate dehydrogenase (IDH) and Tumor Protein (TP53). Glioblastoma is also classified based on it´s transcriptional signature as: classical, mesenchymal, neural or proneural. Classification is also given by variations in the number of gene copies, by mutations in Epidermal Growth Factor Receptor (EGFR) or by DNA hypermethylation of promotor-associated CpG islands [9].

The majority of glioblastoma cases are primary brain tumors that grow rapidly without major clinical or histological evidence of a less malignant precursor lesion. These tumors mainly affect the elderly and are genetically characterized by loss of heterozygosity (LOH) on 10q, EGFR amplification, p16INK4a deletion, and fosfatidilinositol-3,4,5-trisfosfato 3-fosfatasa (*PTEN*) mutations [10,11]. Secondary glioblastoma tumors develop through progression from low-grade diffuse astrocytoma or AA and are pronounced in younger patients [12]. The disruption of tumor-suppressor gene *TP53* is implicated in the progression of many types of human malignancies; adult glioblastoma patients with *TP53* mutation may have a more severe consequence than those without *TP53* mutations [10]. It has also been shown that *TP53* mutations, but not *p53* expression, correlate with a more aggressive form of the disease. Studies have also reported that glioblastoma with *TP53* mutations are more frequent in women than in men, and may occur in younger patients [13]. In addition, some studies suggest that *TP53* mutations may occur in patients of any age group. In contrast, EGFR amplification preferentially occurs in older patients. Thus, multiple genes are involved in the initiation of the disease, and variability occurs in different age and sex groups in the progression of GBM. It is of interest that after careful analysis of age and disease progression, no significant difference in survival was observed in patients with primary and secondary glioblastoma. During the progression of glioblastoma, additional mutations and genetic alterations accumulate, which may alter disease severity and patient survival.

GBM primary and secondary can also differ significantly, depending on their pattern of promoter methylation and in the expression of profiles at the RNA and protein levels. LOH on 10q is shown to be most frequent in both primary and secondary glioblastomas [14]. *TP53* mutations are detected early in the pathway, and frequent genetic alterations can lead to secondary glioblastoma. In 77 Japanese patients with GBM primary, 22% had *TP53* mutations, 21% *PTEN* mutations, 32% *EGFR* amplification, 42% *p16 INK4a* homozygous deletion, and 69% LOH on chromosome 10q in those patients [15]. The frequencies of these genetic alterations at the population level were similar to those reported in Europe. This study noted a positive association between *EGFR* amplification and *p16 INK4a* deletion.

4. Glioblastoma multiforme risk factors

GBM is the most aggressive form of malignant glioma. Several syndromes are associated with the increased incidence of GBM, such as Lynch syndrome, Li–Fraumeni syndrome, melanoma–neural system tumor syndrome, Ollier disease, and Maffucci syndrome [16]. A small proportion (5–10%) of patients has a family history of glioma. Genes too exist that are involved in gliomagenesis and participate in glioma growth, such as telomerase reverse transcriptase (TERT) [17], *EGFR* [18,19], coiled-coil domain containing protein 26 (*CCDC26*) [20],Cyclin-dependent Kinase inhibitor 2B [17], *TP53* [21,22,23], and the regulator of telomere elongation helicase 1 (*RTEL1*) [24,25].

5. Endocrine characteristics of GBM

5.1. Estrogen receptors

GBM exhibits different endocrine characteristics. GBM expresses high levels of estrogen receptor alpha (mRNA ERα) and low levels of estrogen receptor beta (ERß); expression of mRNA ERα is positively correlated to the survival of GBM patients and could be used as a prognostic factor [26]. In contrast, the low expression of ERß in GBM has been related to a worse prognosis for survival and could be used as a biomarker for prognosis too [27,28]. Furthermore, activation of the signaling pathways induced by ERβ suppresses glioma growth in a model in vivo [29].

The coactivator family of estrogen receptors (SRC) is composed of three members, SRC-1, SRC-2, and SRC-3 [30,31]. SRC-1 increases the transcriptional activity of ER [32,33]; it also participates in the tumor progression and survival of several lines of human cancer [34,35]. SRC-2 is localized in different regions of the brain and mediates a variety of steroids-dependent functions [36,37]. SRC-3 is overexpressed in different types of cancer (breast, ovary, prostate, stomach, endometrium, esophagus, and pancreas) [38,39,40,41]. In astrocytoma cell lines, SRC1 and SRC-3 have been detected [42]. 17-/i> estradiol induces the growth of several cell lines of human astrocytoma through the ERα, and its interaction with SRC-1 and SRC3 suggests that ERα has an important role in the growth of astrocytoma [43].

5.2. Progesterone receptors in GBM

Progesterone receptors (PRs) are expressed in 100% of high-grade astrocytomas. The predominant isoform expression of PR in GBM is PRB. In astrocytomas, the molecular mechanisms involved in the differential expression of PR isoforms are unknown. It is important to know what PR isoform is expressed in the brain tumor, because progesterone can exert different cell functions depending on the expression pattern of PR isoforms [44,45].

In several cell contexts, human PRB functions as a transcriptional activator of progesterone-responsive genes, whereas PRA acts a repressor of transcriptional steroid hormone receptors inclusive PRB [46]; PR expression assessed by immunohistochemistry directly correlates with the histological grades of astrocytomas; these results suggest that PR-positive tumors possess a high proliferative potential [47]. However, no conclusive data exists about the PR as a marker of prognosis.

Progesterone significantly decreases GBM tumor growth and promotes the survival time in approximately 60% of mice. Synergistic effects of progesterone and Temozolomide (TMZ) have been observed in the glioblastoma cell lines U87MG and U118MG. A significant decrease in PCNA (a marker of cell proliferation) expression in both U87MG and U118 cell lines was observed by the effect of progesterone alone (80 μM) or by the combination of 80 μM progesterone and 100 μM TMZ, when compared to control, and this has a significantly statistic outcome than that with TMZ alone. Cell survival was reduced in 58%, with the combined treatment of progesterone and TMZ (P 80 μM + TMZ 100 μM after) when compared to that with MTZ alone. Further, progesterone inhibited O-6-methylguanine-DNA-methyltransferase (MGMT) expression as well as the EGFR/PI3K/AkT/mTOR signaling pathway, which is highly active in GBM. Progesterone + TMZ also inhibited the cell migration, suggesting that the combination therapy could contain the spread of tumor in vivo [48].

5.3. Androgen receptor in GBM

The androgen receptor (AR) is present in astrocytomas of low and high grades, with a higher expression in AA compared to astrocytomas grade I, II, and GBM. AR expression no affect the survival time of GBM patients [49,50] described a higher expression of AR in GBM tumors in women and men compared to periphery normal brain tissue.

5.4. Aromatase

Aromatase is an enzyme encoded by *CYP19* gene localized in chromosome 15q 21.2. It converts androgens in estrogens; this enzyme is expressed mainly in ovary, testis, placenta, brain, lung, stomach, and adipose tissue [51]. Aromatase is composed of 503 amino acids and is the major source for estrogen production in postmenopausal women. The aromatase works in three steps; first, the C19 methyl group of androgenic substrate is oxidized to formic acid in concomitant aromatization of ring A to the characteristic phenolic ring A of estrogen [52].

Aromatase expression in GBM tumor is negatively correlated to the survival of GBM patients and has been proposed as a possible prognosis biomarker for astrocytomas [29].

17–ß estradiol levels in GBM tumor are highest, compared to low-grade astrocytomas (I, II) or astrocytoma anaplastic (grade III). The concentration of 17–ß estradiol in GBM seems to be directly involved in the tumor growth.

6. GBM treatment

GBM tumors show a large number of aberrations with a pronounced mitotic activity, neoangiogenesis, and necrosis. Its proliferative rate is three to five times more than the proliferative rate in AA [53].

On the basis of a recent GBM classification as proneural, neural, classical, and mesenchymal, diverse types of treatments must be created to make a molecular personalized therapy [6] (**Table 1**). Performing molecular assays is complex, as their cost may be an obstacle for a routine use.

Treatment	Overall survival (OS)	Progression-free survival (PFS)	Side effects	Author
TMZ/RT	14.6 months	6.9 months	Myelosuppression	Stupp (2005)
RT	12.1 months	5.0 months	Skin reactions, cardiac complications	Stupp (2005)
Bev/TMZ /RT	20.5 months	10.7 months	Myelosuppression, arterial thromboembolism, gastrointestinal perforation	Gilbert (2014) Chinot (2014)
Bev	15.7	10.6	Arterial thromboembolism, arterial gastrointestinal perforation	
Cilengitide/RT	26.3 months	13.5 months		Stupp (2014)
Nimotuz umab/RT	22.3 months	7.7 months	Headache, nausea, vomiting, anemia, myalgia	Westphal (2015)
Nimustine	28.4 months	18.9 months	Chest pain and cianosis peribucal	Kim (2011)
Enzastaurin	17.1 months	9 months	Lymphopenia	Wick (2013)
Tipifarnib	80.3 weeks	18.1 weeks	Headache, nausea, vomiting	Ducassou (2013)
Everolimus	13.9 months	11.3 months	Anemia, higher levels of cholesterol in the blood, low phosphorus	Hainsworth (2012)

Table 1. Effects on survival of different treatments for GBM patients and their side effects.

The standard treatment for GBM patients includes brain radiation, a maximal surgery and .chemotherapy with the alkylating agent TMZ.

A larger number of new drugs and virus-based therapy are being evaluated in phase II and III trials as well.

In a phase III trial including recently diagnosed GBM patients, the median overall survival (OS) for GBM patients was 14.6 months with chemotherapy and RT, and 12.1 months with RT alone with a median follow-up of 28 months [63].

In phase III of another study, 978 patients received standard radiation and TMZ with or without Bevacizumab, an angiogenesis inhibitor used at 10 mg/kg, every 2 weeks with a median follow-up of 20.5 months. The OS between bevacizumab group and placebo group was no different, and side effects such as hypertension, thromboembolic events, intestinal perforation, and neutropenia were more common in the bevacizumab group. The progression-free survival (PFS) was significantly improved in the experimental arm (10.7 vs 7.3 months, $P = 0.007$) [64]. In another phase (III) trial with 458 patients, newly diagnosed GBM received radiation and TMZ with or without bevacizumab (10 mg/kg each for 2 weeks and TMZ for six cycles). With bevacizumab monotherapy (15 mg/kg), the median of PFS was of 10.6 months in the bevacizumab group as compared to 6.2 months in the placebo group.

6.1. Aromatase inhibitors (AIs)

The conversion of androstenedione and testosterone to estrogens can be blocked by the aromatase inhibitors; these pharmacological agents have a high specific activity to reduce, importantly, estrogen production. The AIs are classified in two types: I.—steroid inhibitors and II.—nonsteroid inhibitors; they are reactive species that bind covalently and irreversibly or noncovalently and reversibly to aromatase, respectively. The latter class interacts with the heme cofactor by employing its azole moiety. Third generation inhibitors are composed of triazole derivatives: anastrozole, letrozole, and the steroidal examestane. These inhibitors provided greater clinical benefits with a robust aromatase inhibition of 98% or more. The aromatase inhibitors have been successfully used for the treatment of estrogen receptor-positive breast cancer in postmenopausal women [65]. Letrozole has a more potent inhibitory effect on estrogen synthesis than anastrozole [66]. Letrozole has been tested in a GBM model using Sprague–Dawley rats orthotopically implanted with C6 cells. Imaging analysis employing μPET/CT showed an important reduction in the volume of tumor (>75%) after 8 days of letrozole treatment (4 mg/kg/day) [67].

The AIs, namely 3b-hydroxyandrost-4-en-17-one (1), androst-4-en-17-one (12), 4a,5a-epoxy androstan-17-one (13a), and 5a-androst-2-en-17-one (16), induced an antiproliferative effect on MCF7 breast cancer cells, and this effect was due to a cell cycle arrest and cell death by apoptosis [68]. Table 1 shows different treatments for GBM and their effect on OS. It also exhibits the progression-free survival, with the side effects observed in these studies.

6.2. Hormone release growth hormone (GHRH) inhibitors

GHRH inhibitors had been used for the treatment of various cancers or disorders that express growth hormone (GH) or GHRH production. GHRH antagonists suppress GH or insulin-like growth factor (IGF-1) in transgenic mice overexpressing the *GHRH* gene; GHRH antagonists can inhibit the rat pituitary tumor cells overexpressing the GHRH receptors (p-GHRH-R). These antagonists also inhibit GH secretion [70]. There is evidence that GHRH antagonists are well tolerated in humans; however, more phase I–III clinical trials are necessary to probe the efficiency of these antagonists [71]. GHRH antagonists inhibit cancers that depend on IGF-1 as a growth factor [72–74]. GHRH antagonists can also inhibit various autocrine factors such as GHRH, GH, or VEGF by binding to the tumoral GHRH receptors, resulting in a tumor growth suppression [75,76]. In addition, GHRH antagonists could provoke tumor cell death by active cell pathways producing apoptosis [77,78].

The presence of the GHRH-R variant SV1 differs from the pGHRH by a short segment of the extracellular ligand-binding domain of the receptor protein in normal tissue and in various neoplastic tumors, lymphomas, small-cell lung carcinomas, pancreatic cancer, glioblastomas, and prostate cancer [79–81]. In several experimentally formed tumors, GHRH antagonist inhibits the growth and metastasis of cells expressing these receptor types. This inhibition occurs by binding to the full length of the GHRH-R or SV1 [79,80,82]. Kovácks et al., 2010 observed a strong GH release inhibition by the JV-1-63, reducing tumor growth (46%) of DBTRG-05 glioblastomas. Their experiments were conducted on nude mice. JV-1-63 antagonists caused an upregulation of mRNA expression of pGHRHR and downregulation of SV1 expression in vitro [82].

The use of aromatase and GHRH inhibitors could have a clinical use in patients with GBM once adequate phase II or III clinical trials are made.

Author details

Judith Marcela Dueñas-Jiménez[1*], Irene Aguilar-García[1], María de la Luz Galván-Ramírez[1], Sergio Horacio Dueñas-Jiménez[1], Jorge David Rivas-Carrillo[1], Anne Santerre[2] and Erika Priscilla Domínguez-Rangel[1]

*Address all correspondence to: judithmarceladuenas@gmail.com

1 University Center for Health Sciences, University of Guadalajara, Guadalajara, Jalisco, México

2 University Center for Biological and Agricultural Sciences, University of Guadalajara, Guadalajara, Jalisco, México

References

[1] Hou LC, Veeravagu A, Hsu AR. Tse VC recurrent glioblastoma multiforme: a review of natural history and management options. Neurosurg Focus 2006; 20(4):E5.

[2] Rosen ST. Cancer Treatment and Research, vol. 163. Duarte, CA, 2015; pp. 1–14. DOI: 10.1007/978-3-319-12048-5

[3] Dolececk TA, Propp J, Stroup N, Kruch C. CBTRUS statistical report: primary brain and central nervous system tumors diagnosed in the United States in 2005–2009. Neuro Oncol 2009; 15(Suppl 5): 1–49. DOI: 10.1093/neuonc/nos218

[4] Wen P, Kesari S. Malignant gliomas in adults. N Engl J Med 2008; 359: 492–507. DOI: 10.1056/NEJMra0708126

[5] Chakrabarti I, Cockburn M, Cozen W, Wang Y-P, Preston-Martin S. A. population-based description of glioblastoma multiforme in Los Angeles County, 1974–1999. Cancer 2008; 104(12): 2798–2806. DOI: 10.1002/cncr.21539

[6] Verhaak RG, Hoadley KA, Purdom E, Wang V, Qi Y, Wilkerson MD, et al. Integrated genomic analysis identifies clinically relevant subtypes of glioblastoma characterized by abnormalities in PDGFRA, IDH1, EGFR, and NF1. Cancer Cell 2010; 17(1): 98–110. DOI: 10.1016/j.ccr.2009.12.020

[7] Dunn G, Rinne M, Wykosky J, Genovese G, Quayle S, Dunn I, et al. Emerging insights into the molecular and cellular basis of glioblastoma. Genes Dev 2012; 26(8): 756–784. DOI: 10.1101/gad.187922.112

[8] Noushmehr H, Weisenberger DJ, Diefes K, Phillips HS, Pujara K, Berman BP, et al. Identification of a CpG island methylator phenotype that defines a distinct subgroup of glioma. Cancer Cell 2010; 17(5): 510–522. DOI: 10.1016/j.ccr.2010.03.017

[9] Brennan CW, Verhaak RGW, McKenna A, Campos B, Noushmehr H, Salama SR, et al. The somatic genomic landscape of glioblastoma. Cell 2013; 155(2): 462–477. DOI: 10.1016/j.cell.2013.09.034.

[10] Huang PH, Mukasa A, Bonavia R, Flynn RA, Brewer ZE, Cavenee WK, Furnari FB, White FM. Quantitative analysis of EGFRvIII cellular signalling networks reveals a combinatorial therapeutic strategy for glioblastoma. Proc Natl Acad Sci U S A 2007; 104: 12867–12872. DOI: 10.1073/pnas.0705158104

[11] Khasraw M, Lassman AB Advances in the treatment of malignant gliomas. Curr Oncol Rep 2010; 12(1): 26–33. DOI: 10.1007/s11912-009-0077-4.

[12] Ohgaki H, Kleihues P. Genetic pathways to primary and secondary glioblastoma. Am J Pathol 2007; 170(5): 1145–1453. DOI: 10.2353/ajpath.2007.070011

[13] Zawlik I, Kita D, Vaccaella S, Mittelbronn M, Franceschi S, Ohgaki H. Common polymorphisms in the MDM and TP53 genes and the relationship outcomes in glioblastomas. Brain Pathol 2009; 19(2): 188–194. DOI: 10.1111/j.1750-3639.2008.00170.x.

[14] Nagajaran R, Costello J. Molecular epigenetics and genetics in neuro–oncology. Neurotherapeutics 200; 6(3): 436–446. DOI: 10.1016/j.nurt.2009.04.002.

[15] Fukushima T, Favereaux A, Huang H, Shimizu T, Yonekawa Y, Nakazato Y, Ohagki H. Genetic alterations in primary glioblastomas in Japan. J Neuropathol Exp Neurol 2006; 65(1):12–18. DOI: http://dx.doi.org/10.1097/01.jnen.0000196132.66464.96

[16] Temel JS, Greer JA, Muzikansky A et al. Early palliative care for patients with metastatic non-small-cell lung cancer. N Engl J Med 2010; 363(8):733–742. DOI: 10.1056/NEJMoa1000678.

[17] Rajaraman P, Melin BS, Wang Z, McKean–Cowdin R, Michaud DS, Wang SS, et al. Genome – wide association study of glioma and meta – analysis. Hum Genet 2010; 131(12): 1877–1888. DOI: 10.1007/s00439-012-1212-0

[18] Walsh KM, Anderson E, Hansen HM, Decker PA, Kosel ML, Kollmeyer T, et al. Analysis of 60 reported glioma risk SNPs replicates published GWAS findings but fails to replicate associations from published candidate–gene studies. Genet Epidemiol 2013; 37(2): 222–228. DOI: 10.1002/gepi.21707

[19] Sanson M, Hosking FJ, Shete S, Zelenika D, Dobbins SE, Ma Y et al. Chromosome 7p11.2 (EGFR) variation influences glioma risk. Hum Mol Genet 2011; 20(14): 2897–2904. DOI: 10.1093/hmg/ddr192

[20] Jenkins RB, Wresnch MR, Johnson D, Fridley BL, Decker PA, Xiao Y, et al. Cancer genetics. Cancer Genet 2011; 204(1): 13–18. DOI: 10.1016/j.cancergencyto.2010.10.002

[21] Enciso–Mora V; Hosking FJ, Di Stefano AL, Zelenika D, Shete S, Broderick P, et al. Low penetrance susceptibility to glioma is caused by the variant rs 783782222. Br J Cancer 2013; 108(10): 2178–2185. DOI: 10.1038/bjc.2013.155

[22] Stacey SN, Sulem P, Jonasdottir A, Masson G, Gudmunson J, Gudbartsson DF et al. A germiline in the TP53 polyadenylation signal confers susceptibility. Nat Genet 2011; 43(11): 1098–1103. DOI: 10.1038/ng.926.

[23] Egan KM, Nabors LB, Olson JJ, Monteiro AN, Browning JE, Madden MH, et al. Rre TP53 genetic variant associated with glioma risk and outcome. J Med Genet 2012; 49(7): 420–421. DOI: 10.1136/jmedgenet-2012-100941

[24] Shete S, Hosking FJ, Robertson LB, Sanson M, Malmer B, et al. Genome - wide association study indentifies five susceptibility loci for glioma. Nat Genet 2009; 41(8): 899–904. DOI: 10.1038/ng.407

[25] Wrensch M, Kenkins RB, Chang JS, Yeh RF, Xiao Y, Decker PA, et al. Variants in the CDKN2B and RTEL1 regions are associated with high grade glioma susceptibility. Nat Genet 2009; 41(8): 905–908. DOI: 10.1038/ng.408.

[26] Dueñas JM, Candanedo A, Santerre A, Orozco S, Sandoval H, Feria R, et al. Aromatase and estrogen receptor alpha mRNA expression as prognostic biomarkers in patients with astrocytomas. J Neurooncol 2014; 119(2): 275–284. DOI: 10.1007/s11060-014-1509-z.

[27] Batistatou A, Kyzas PA, Goussia A, Arkoumani E, Voulgaris S, Polyzoidis K, et al. Estrogen receptor beta (ER – β), protein expression correlates with BAG – 1, and prognosis in brain glial tumors. J Neurooncol 2006; 77(1): 17–23. DOI: 10.1007/s11060-005-9005-0

[28] Batistaou A, Stefanou D, Goussia A, Arkoumani E, Papavassiliou AG, Agnatis N. Estrogen receptor beta (ERβ) is expressed in brain astrocytic tumors and declines with

differentiation of the neoplasm. J Cancer Res Clin Oncol 2004; 130(7): 405–410. DOI: 10.1007/s00432-004-0548-9

[29] Sareddy GR, Nair BC, Gonugunta VK, Zhang QG, Brener A, Brann DW, et al. Therapeutic Significance of estrogen receptor β agonists in gliomas. Mol Cancer Ther 2012; 11(5): 1174–1182. DOI: 10.1158/1535-7163.MCT-11-0960

[30] Oñate SA, Tsai SY, Tsai MJ, O'Malley BW. Sequence and characterization of a coactivator for the steroid hormone receptor superfamily. Science 1995; 270(5240): 1354–1357. DOI: 10.1126/science.270.5240.1354

[31] Anzick SL, Kononen J, Walker RL, Azorsa DO, Tanner MM, Guan XY, et al. ALB1, a steroid receptor coactivator amplified in breast and ovarian cancer. Science. 1997; 277(5328): 965–968. DOI: 10.1126/science.277.5328.965

[32] Tetel MJ, Auger AP, Charlier TD. Who´s in charge? Nuclear receptor coactivator and corepressor function in brain and behavior. Front Neuroendocrinol 2009; 30(3): 328–342. DOI: 10.1016/j.yfrne.2009.04.008

[33] Molenda-Figueira HA, Murphy SD, Shea K, SIegal NK, Zhao Y, Chadwick JG. Steroid receptor coactivator – 1 from brain physically interacts differentially with steroid receptor subtypes. Endocrinology 2008; 149(10): 5272–5279. DOI: 10.1210/en.2008-0048

[34] Vienonen A, Miettinen S, Mannien T, Altuci L, Willhelm E, Ylikomi T. Regulation of nuclear receptor and cofactor expression in breast cancer cell lines. Eur J Endocrinol 2003; 148(4): 469–479. DOI: 10.1530/eje.0.1480469

[35] Weldon CB, Elliott S, Zhu Y, Clayton JL, Curiel TJ, Jaffe BM, Burow ME. Regulation of estrogen-mediated cell survival and proliferation by p160 coactivators. Surgery 2004;136(2): 346–354. DOI: 10.1016/j.surg.2004.05.010

[36] Apostolakis ED, Ramamurphy M, Zhou D, Oñate S, O´Malley BW. Acute disruption of select steroid receptor coactivators prevents reproductive behavior in rats and unmasks genetic adaptation in knockout mice. Mol Endocrinol 2002; 16(7): 1511–1523. DOI: 10.1210/mend.16.7.0877

[37] Nishihara E, Yoshida H, Chan C-S, Liao L, Davis RL, O'Malley BW, et al. SRC–1 null mice exhibit moderate motor dysfunction and delayed development of cerebellar Purkinje cells. J Neurosci 2003; 23(1): 213–222.

[38] Tognoni CM, Chadwick JG, Ackeifi CA, Tetel MJ. Nuclear receptor coactivators are coexpressed with steroid receptors and regulated by estradiol in mouse brain. Neuroendocrinology. 2011; 94: 49–57. DOI: 10.1159/000323780

[39] Lonard DM, Lanz RB, O´Malley BW. Nuclear receptor coregulators and human disease. Endocr Rev. 2007; 28(5): 575–587. DOI: 10.1210/er.2007-0012

[40] Sakaguchi H, Fujimoto J, Sun W-S, Tamaya T. Clinical implications of steroid receptor coactivator (SRC – 3) in uterine endometrial cancers. J Steroid Biochem Mol Biol 2007; 104(3–5): 237–240. DOI: 10.1016/j.jsbmb.2007.03.007

[41] Sakakura C, Hagiwara A, Yasuoka R, Fujita Y, Nakanishi M, Masuda K, et al. Amplification and over expression of the AIB1 nuclear receptor coactivator gene in primary gastric cancers. Int J Cancer 2000; 89(3): 217–223. DOI: 10.1002/1097-0215(20000520)89:3<2

[42] Hernández O, Rodríguez M, González A, Camacho I. Progesterone and estradiol effects on SRC–1 and SRC–3 expression in human astrocitoma cell lines. Endocrine 2010; 37(1): 194–200. DOI: 10.1007/s12020-009-9288-6

[43] González A, Hansberg V, Hernández O, González T, Henderson J, Lemus D, et al. Estradiol increases cell growth in human astrocitoma cell lines through ERα activation and its interaction with SCR–1, SCR–3, coactivators. Biochim Biophys Acta. 2002; 1823(2): 379–386. DOI: 10.1016/j.bbamcr.2011.11.004

[44] Giangrande P, McDonnel DP. The A and B isoforms of the human progesterone receptor: two functionally different transcription factors encoded by a single gene. Recent Prog Horm Res 1999; 54: 291–313.

[45] Tora L, Gronemeyer H, Turcotte B, Gaub MP, Chambon P. The N-terminal region of the chicken progesterone receptor specifies target gene activation. Nature 1988; 333(6169): 185–188. DOI: 10.1038/333185a0

[46] Vegeto E, Shahbaz MM, Wen DX, Goldman ME, O´Malley BW, McDonnell DP. Human Progesterone receptor A for is a cell – and promoter – specific repressor of human progesterone receptor B function. Mol Endocinol 2013; 7(10): 1244–1255. DOI: org/ 10.1210/mend.7.10.8264658#sthash.FjZjmlYb.dpuf

[47] Khalid H, Shibata S, Kishikawa M, Yasunaga A, Iseki M, Hiura T. Inmunohistochemical analysis of progesterone receptor and Ki – 67 labelling index in astrocytic tumors. Cancer. 1997; 80(11): 2133–2140. DOI: 10.1002/(SICI)1097-0142(19971201)80:11<2133::AID-CNCR13>3.

[48] Atif F, Patel N, Yosuf S, Stein D. The synergistic effect of combination progesterone and temozolamide on human glioblastoma cells. Plos One 2015; 10(6): e0131441. DOI: 10.1371/journal.pone.0131441

[49] Yong GC, Kim HK, Kap Lee H, Chan Lee K. Expression of androgen receptors in astrocytoma. J Korean Med Sci 1996; 11(6): 517–521. DOI: 10.3346/jkms.1996.11.6.517

[50] Yu X, Jiang Y, Wei W, Cong P, et al. Androgen receptor signalling regulates growth of glioblastoma multiforme in men. Tumor Biol 2015; 36(2): 967–972. DOI: 10.1007/ s13277-014-2709-z

[51] Miller W, Larionov A. Aromatase 2004, Edinburgh, UK, 6–8 September 2004. Breast Cancer Res 2004; 7: E2. DOI: 10.1186/bcr964

[52] Simpson E, Clyne C, Rubin G, Boon W, Robertson K, Britt K, et al. Aromatase—a brief overview. Annu Rev Physiol 2002; 64: 93–127. DOI: 10.1146/annurev.physiol.64.081601.142703

[53] Kleihues P, Luois D, Scheithauer B, Rorke L, Reifenberger G, Burger P, et al. The WHO classification of tumors of the nervous system. J Neuropathol Exp Neurol. 2002; 61(3): 215–225. DOI: org/10.1093/jnen/61.3.215

[54] Stupp R, Weber D. The role of radio and chemotherapy in glioblastoma. Onkologie. 2005; 28(6–7): 315–317. DOI: 10.1159/000085575

[55] Gilbert M, Dignam J, Armstrong T, Wefel J, Blumenthal D, Vogelbaum M, et al. A randomized trial of bevacizumab for newly diagnosed glioblastoma. N Engl Med. 2014; 370(8): 699–708. DOI: 10.1056/NEJMoa1308573

[56] Chinot O, Reardon D. The future of antiangiogenic treatment in glioblastoma. Curr Opin Neurol 2014; 26(6): 675–682. DOI: 10.1097/WCO.0000000000000142.

[57] Stupp R, Picard M, Weller M. Does cilentigide deserve another chance? – Authors reply. Lancel Oncol 2014; 15(13): 585–586. DOI: 10.1016/S1470-2045(14)71121-0

[58] Westphal M, Heese O, Steinbach J, Schnell O, Schackert G, Mehdorn M, et al. A randomised, open label phase III trial with nimotuzumab, an anti epidermal growth factor receptor monoclonal antibody in the treatment of newly diagnosed adult glioblastoma. Eur J Cancer 2015; 51(4): 522–532. DOI: 10.1016/j.ejca.2014.12.019.

[59] Kim I, Park C, Heo D, Kim C, Rhee C, Nam D, et al. Radiotherapy followed by adjuvant temozolomide with or without neoadjuvant ACNU—CDDP chemotherapy in newly diagnosed glioblastomas: a prospective randomized controlled multicenter phase III trial. J Neurooncol 2011; 103(3): 595–602. DOI: 10.1007/s11060-010-0427

[60] Wick W, Steinbach J, Platten M, Hartmann C, Wenz F, von Deimiling, et al. Enzastaurin before and concomitant with radiation therapy, followed by enzastaurin maintenance therapy, in patients with newly diagnosed glioblastoma without MGMT promoter hypermethylation. Neuro Oncol 2013; 15(10): 1405–1412. DOI: 10.1093/neuonc/not100.

[61] Ducassou A, Uro-Coste E, Verelle P, Filleron T, Benouaich A, Lubrano V, et al. $\alpha v\beta 3$ integrin and Fibroblast growth factor receptor (FGFR1): pronostic factors in a phase I-II clinical trial associating continuous administration of tipifarnib with radiotherapy for patients with newly diagnosed glioblastoma. Eur J Cancer 2013; 49(9): 2161–2169. DOI: 10.1016/j.ejca.2013.02.033

[62] Hainswoth J, Shih K, Shepard G, Tillinghast G, Brinker B, Spigel D. Phase II study of concurrent radiation therapy, temozolamide, and bevacizumab followed by bevacizumab /everolimus as first line treatment for patients with glioblastoma. Cin Adv Hematol Oncol. 2012; 10(4): 240–246.

[63] Burtsein H, Prestud A, Seidenfeld J, Anderson H, Bucholz T, Davidson N, et al. American Society of Clinical Oncology Clinical Practice guideline: update on adjuvant

endocrine therapy for women with hormone receptor –positive breast cancer. J Clin Oncol. 2010; 34(7): 3784–3796.

[64] Geisler J, Haynes B, Anker G, Dowselt M, Lonning E. Influence of letrozole and anastrozole estrogen levels in postmenopausal breast cancer patients evaluated in a randomized, cross – over Study. J Clin Oncol. 2002; 3: 751–757.DOI:10.1038/bjc.2011.58

[65] Amaral C, Varela C, Borges M, Tavares da Silva E, Roleira F, Correia da Silva G, et al. Steroidal aromatase inhibitors inhibit growth of hormone–dependent breast cancer cells by inducing cell cycle arrest and apoptosis. Apoptosis 2013; 18(11): 1426–1436. DOI: 10.1007/s10495-013-0879-6

[66] Kovacs M, Kineman R, Schally A, Zarandi M, Groot K, Frohman L. Effects of antagonist of growth hormone—releasing hormone (GHRH) on GH and insulin—like growth factor 1 levels in transgenic mice overexpression the human GHRH, an animal model of acromegaly. Endocrinology 1997; 138(11): 4536–4542. DOI: org/10.1210/endo. 138.11.5498

[67] Kovacs M, Schally A, Lee E, Busto R, Armatis P, Groot K, Varga J. Inhibitory effects of antagonistic analogues of GHRH on GH3 pituitary cells overexpressing the human GHRH receptor. J Endocrinol. 2002; 175(2): 425–434. DOI: 10.1677/joe.0.1750425

[68] Jenkins PJ, Bustin SA Evidence for a link between IGF-I and cancer. Eur J Endocrinol. 2004; 151:S17–S22. DOI: 10.1530/eje.0.151S017

[69] Kahan Z, Gardi J, Nyari T, Foldesi I, Ormandi K, Lazar G, et al. Elevated levels of circulating insulin-like growth factor-I, IGF-binding globulin-3 and testosterone predict hormone-dependent breast cancer in postmenopausal women a case–control study. Int J Oncol 2006; 29(1):193–200. DOI: 10.3892/ijo.29.1.193

[70] Le Roith D. The insulin - like growth factor system. Experimental Diab Res. 2003; 4(4): 205–212. DOI: 10.1155/EDR.2003.205

[71] Kovacs M, Schally A, Varga J, Zaradi M. Endocrine and antineoplasic actions of growth actions of hormone – releasing hormone antagonists. Curr Med Chem 2008; 15(4): 314–321. DOI: 10.2174/092986708783497355

[72] Schally A, Varga J, Engel J. Antagonists of growth – hormone – releasing hormone: an emerging new therapy for cancer. Nat Clin Pract Endocrinol Metab. 2008; 4(1): 33–43. DOI:10.1038/ncpendmet0677

[73] Hohla F, Buchholz S, Schally A, Rick F, Szalontay L, Varga J, et al. GHRH antagonist causes DNA damage leading to pcell c21 mediated cell cycle arrest and apoptosis in human colon cancer cells. Cell Cycle 2009; 8(19): 3149–3156.

[74] Kanashiro C, Schally A, Zaradi M, Hammann B, Varga J. Alterations of EGFR/HER, angiogenesis and apoptosis pathways after therapy with antagonists of growth hormone releasing and bombesin in non – small cell lung cancer. Int J Oncol 2007; 30(4): 1019–1028. DOI: 10.3892/ijo.30.4.1019

[75] Havt A, Schally A, Halmos G, Varga J, Toller G, Hovarh J, et al. The expression of the pituitary growth hormone – releasing hormone receptor and its splice variants in normal and neoplastic human tissues. PNAS 2005; 102(48): 17424–17429. 18. DOI: 10.1073/pnas.

[76] Heinrih E, Schally A, Bulchholz S, Rock F, Halmos G, Mile M, et al. Dose dependent growth inhibition in vivo of PC – 3 prostate cancer with a reduction in tumoral growth factors after therapy with GHRH antagonist MZ – J – 7 – 138. Prostate 2008; 68(16): 1763–1772.

[77] Resaki Z, Czompoly T, Shally A, Halmos G. Isolation and sequencing of CDNA for splice variants of growth hormone—releasing hormone receptors from human cancers. PNAS 2000; 97(19): 10561–10566. DOI: 10.1073/pnas.

[78] Kovacs M, Schally A, Hohla F, Rick F, Pozsagai E, Szalontay L. A correlation of endocrine and anticancer effects of some antagonists of GHRH. Peptides 2010; 31(10): 1839–1846. DOI: 10.1016/j.peptides.2010.07.006

[79] Chiot O, Reardon D. The future of antiangiogenic treatment in glioblastoma. Curr Opin Neurol. 2014; 27(6): 675–682. DOI: 10.1097/WCO.

[80] Kim I, Park C, Heo D, Kim C, Rhee C, Nam D, et al. Radiotherapy followed by adjuvant temozolomide with or without neoadjuvant ACNU—CDDP chemotherapy in newly diagnosed glioblastomas: a prospective randomized controlled multicenter phase III trial. J Neurooncol 2011; 103(3): 595–602. DOI: 10.1007/s11060-010-0427.

Chapter 4

Genetic Alterations of Glioblastoma

Romana Richterová and Branislav Kolarovszki

Additional information is available at the end of the chapter

http://dx.doi.org/10.5772/63127

Abstract

The current research in oncology is focused on genetics and molecular oncology in order to obtain better understanding of the etiology of tumor disease. Detailed knowledge of oncogenesis mechanisms could lead to invention of effective therapeutic tools against cancer. Under healthy conditions, cell cycle is regulated by oncogenes and tumor suppressor genes, which should be in strict balance. Genesis of tumor is a consequence of the accumulation of genetic alterations, which help the cell to escape normal cellular regulatory mechanisms and destruction by immune system. Glioblastoma (GBM) is a highly malignant primary brain tumor occurring mostly in population of adults. Patients suffering from GBM have very poor prognosis. Despite development in radiology methods promising earlier diagnosis and development of clinical and radiation oncology with newer treatment regimes, the effect of therapy remains limited and prognosis of patients has not improved as expected. Target of GBM research are genes involved in response to oxidative stress and DNA damage, genes regulating cell cycle, genes determining immune response, growth factors, and others. Genetic alterations are studied in connection to their possible relationship to susceptibility of brain tissue for tumor formation, to sensitivity of brain tissue for various environmental etiology factors, to effect of anticancer treatment or resistance of tumor tissue to therapy, to overall survival, and progression-free interval.

Keywords: glioblastoma, genes, alteration, mutations, genetic pathways

1. Introduction

Glioblastoma (GBM) is a brain tumor of neuroectodermal origin. It is a second most common primary brain neoplasm and the most common from malignant brain tumors. This tumor arises from neural stem cells (NSCs), progenitor cells, dedifferentiated mature neural cells or neuroepithelial stem cells that transform into cancer stem cells (CSCs) or glioblastoma stem (GSC) or stem-like cells [1]. Stem cells have a high potential of self-renewal and differentiation. GBM is a tumor with highest degree of anaplasia within gliomas. It is classified as grade IV according to the WHO classification of brain tumors from 2007. This lesion has a rapid growth, is unbounded, infiltrates surrounding brain tissue, but rarely metastasizes. When metastases occur, it is usually within the central nervous system. Typical histopathological features of this tumor are cells of recognizably astrocyte origin, but displaying cellular pleomorphism with multinucleation, frequent mitoses, and areas of necrosis surrounded by palisading nuclei (increased tumor cell density) and endothelial proliferation as a manifestation of cellular hyperplasia with numerous clusters of blood vessels forming so-called glomeruloid formations. GBM cells spread along tracts in white matter infiltrate cerebrospinal fluid and vessels between meningeal layers. Invasion of GBM cells begins with the degradation of surrounding matrix proteins by proteases and proteinases. Movement of tumor cells through surrounding brain tissue requires receptor turnover, formation and degradation of focal adhesion molecules and rearrangement of cytoskeleton components. These changes are consequences of genetic alterations, such as overexpression, amplification, deletion or mutation in focal adhesion kinase and phosphatidylinositol 3-kinase (PI3K) pathways [2] and mainly caused by activation of growth factors and their receptors (integrins and protein deleted in colorectal cancer (DCC), hyaluron receptors CD44, RHAMM, BEHAB, ontogenetic protein SPARC, receptors for platelet-derived growth factor (PDGF), transforming growth factor (TGF)-α, epidermal growth factor (EGF), and basic fibroblast growth factor (bFGF)). Some components of extracellular matrix such as laminin or fibronectin are overexpressed in GBM and their silencing reduces invasiveness of GBM cells [3]. Besides microscopic characteristics, GBM is connected with a huge amount of genetic alterations causing higher proliferation, migration, and invasiveness of tumor cells. The intrinsic ability of GBM cells to invade normal brain tissue impedes complete surgical resection and predictably results in early local recurrence and mortality. Thoroughgoing explanation of GBM genetic pathways with their gene alterations is necessary for choosing of more suitable therapy and in predicting patient prognosis. This chapter offers an overview of the most common genetic alterations occurring in GBM.

2. Classification of GBM

According to the WHO classification of brain tumors based on histopathological origin, GBM is a primary brain tumor of neuroepithelial, glial origin. Ranking of GBM in clinical and prognostic significance is within the highest grade IV. GBM could also be classified according to mode of occurrence, as it could be a result of progression from less malignant glial tumor (so-called secondary type) or it could occur de novo (primary type). Another specific type is pediatric GBM. The most common is primary type. Primary, secondary, and pediatric GBMs have their own specific genetic and epigenetic alterations occurring in their gliomagenesis (see **Figure 1**). As diagnosis of GBM presents with heterogeneity of altered genetic pathways evidenced by The Cancer Genome Atlas Research Network's study, classification based on gene expression profile distinguishes a classical, mesenchymal, proneural, and neural type of GBM. Classical type typically harbors no TP53 mutations, but very high rate of epidermal growth factor receptor (EGFR) mutations. This type has a slightly better survival. Mesenchy-

http://dx.doi.org/10.5772/63127

mal type displays frequent mutations of neurofibromatosis gene 1 (NF1), TP53, and PTEN genes and aggressive anticancer therapy brings a significant increase in survival of these patients. Third, proneural subtype presents with highest mutation rate of TP53, PDGFRA, and isocitrate dehydrogenase (IDH) and usually affects younger adults. Last, neural type occurs more often in older population and contains several gene mutations at an average rate [4]. These classifications show high heterogeneity of genetic profile, aggressiveness, clinical characteristics, and expected prognosis of GBM patients with a strong need of definite uniform classification of subtypes leading to more specific treatment for each GBM subtype.

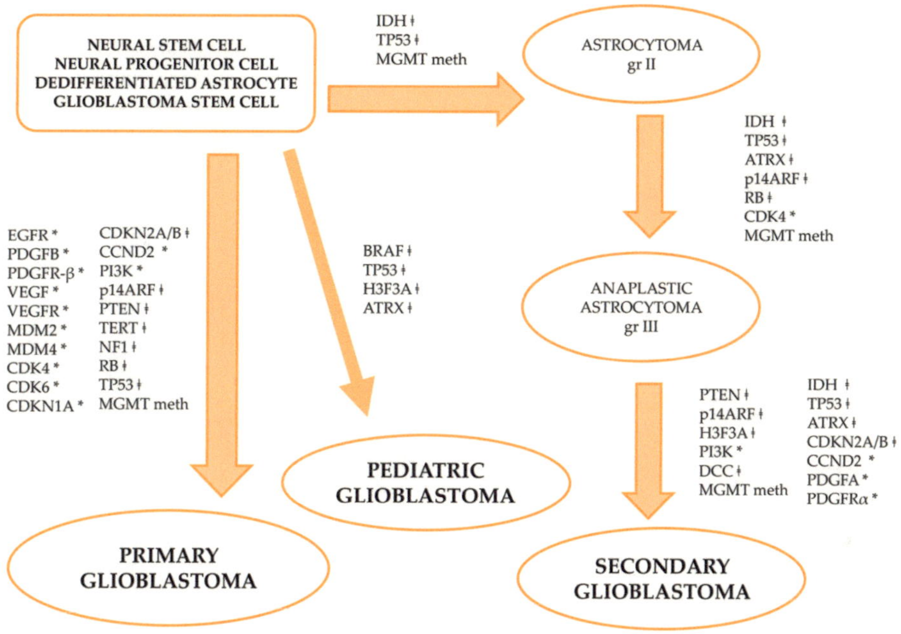

Figure 1. Genes involved in genesis of primary, secondary, and pediatric glioblastoma. *Gain of function through amplification or mutation; ǂhomozygous deletion or mutation.

3. Most frequent genetic alterations of GBM

As mentioned above, alterations of oncogenes and tumor suppressor genes could deflect cell from normal cell cycle. Accumulation of genetic alterations of these genes initiates oncogenesis. In oncogenes, lesion of one allele is sufficient to cause mutation. Activation of oncogene causes avoidance of apoptosis and cell further proliferates. Amplification and activating mutation are the most common genetic alteration of oncogenes. On the other hand, lesion of both alleles is required to evoke mutation in tumor suppressor genes. These genes and their protein products when activated inhibit cell proliferation. Frequently observed alterations are deletion and inhibitory mutation.

During years of genetic research, there have been established three critical genetic pathways whose alterations lead to the formation of GBM: inactivation of p53 and retinoblastoma (RB) pathways (see **Figure 2**), activation of the PI3K pathway, and deregulation of growth factor (receptor tyrosine kinase—RTK) signaling (see **Figure 3**). TP53 signaling pathway is altered in 87% of GBMs, mostly affecting p53, murine double minute-2 (MDM2), MDM4, and cyclin-dependent kinase (CDK)N2A genes. Approximately 78% of GBMs harbor RB signaling disruption with most frequently altered genes: RB1, CDK4, CDK6, CCND2, and cyclin-dependent kinase inhibitor 2 (CDKN2) family. Finally, RTK/RAS/PI3K activation was found in 88% of tumors, affecting usually NF1, PIK3R1, and PIK3CA genes.

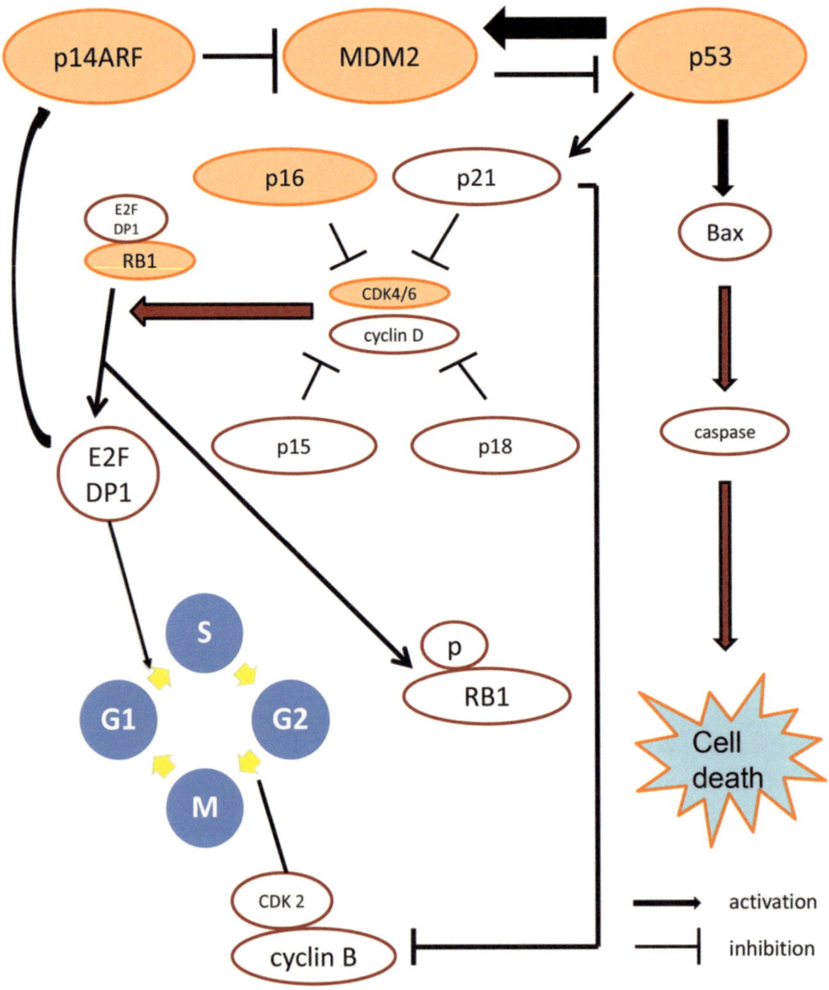

Figure 2. p53 and RB cell cycle and cell death signaling pathway. Proteins marked with full color are most frequently altered in glioblastoma.

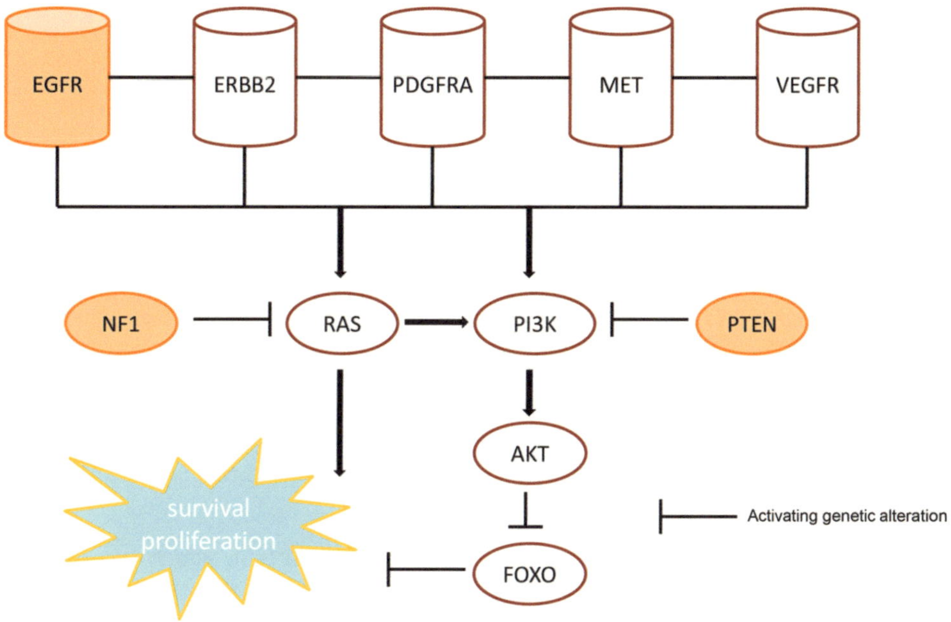

Figure 3. RTK/RAS/PI3K pathway. Proteins marked with full color are most frequently altered in glioblastoma.

GBM is classified as primary or secondary according to altered genes. Primary GBM is a tumor with de novo formation. On the other hand, GBM as a result of malignant transformation of lower-grade glial tumor is called secondary [1]. Also, clinical manifestation and age of diagnosis vary within these two types. Typical for primary GBM is very short anamnesis and age over 50. On the contrary, patients with secondary GBM usually have previous anamnesis of lower grade glioma and younger age depending on the age at the time of diagnosis of preexisting lower grade glioma. Both – primary and secondary GBM – have their own specific gene alterations occurring in their gliomagenesis (see **Figure 1**). Typical alterations for primary GBM are homozygous deletion or mutation of *EGFR, PDGFRα, MDM2, CDK4,* and *PI3K* genes, and amplification or mutation of *CDKN2A/B, PTEN, NF1,* and *RB* genes. Secondary GBM also has some typical alterations, which are mutation of *IDH* and *TP53* genes and 9p deletion. The best-known prognostic factor of GBM, hypermethylation of methylguanin-O-methyltransferase *(MGMT)* gene promoter, occurs in both primary and secondary GBM.

Gene **TP53** is a crucial tumor suppressor gene located on 17p13.1. It is one of the most frequently mutated genes in human tumor cells [5]. Protein p53 restricts cell proliferation and growth, modulates cell reaction to DNA damage, activates DNA repair, causes cell arrest in G1/S regulation point, and induces apoptosis, senescence, and autophagy. TP53 also regulates neovascularization and cell differentiation [6]. Suppression of pluripotency and inhibition of self-renewal of stem cells belong to the most recently discovered functions of TP53 [7]. TP53-mediated apoptosis is almost not present in glioma cells. Dysfunction of TP53 disrupts the p14ARF pathway, what delays apoptosis and that further promotes genome instability. [8]. High incidence of alterations is in p53-binding domain, mainly codons 175, 248, and 273.

Polymorphism Arg72Pro is under suspicion of higher susceptibility to GBM, but this relationship is not yet definitely confirmed. Mutation or deletion of TP53 is found in 35% of GBM cases, but is more frequent in astrocytomas grade II [6, 9] and plays a role in their progression to secondary GBM. On the other hand, it is present in only about 10% of primary GBM [10].

Oncogene **MDM2** is located on 12q14.3-q15. Protein product of this oncogene is E3 ubiquitin ligase which acts like transcriptional factor. This ligase has five forms and two of them have the ability to interact with p53. The function of this protein is suppression of cell cycle arrest and apoptosis by negative effect on p53 and promotion of cell growth and renewal [11]. The effect of MDM2 is repression of transcriptional activity of p53 and amplification or overexpression of this oncogene completely excludes p53 from having an effect on cell cycle. MDM2 overexpression plays an important role in genesis of glioma, but it seems that they are not involved in glioma progression into higher grade [12]. This overexpression is present in about 10–14% of GBM and is always connected with the presence of wild type TP53. It is an alternative mechanism to disrupt p53 pathway in tumor genesis [6]. This alteration is typical for primary GBM [12].

MDM4 is located on 1q32. MDM4 encodes mdm2-related protein, which has p53-binding domain and RING finger domain. MDM4 binds p53 protein and so inhibits p53-mediated transcriptional transactivation. It also binds MDM2 protein via RING finger domain. Overexpression and amplification of MDM4 occur in GBM, though it is not common (7%). MDM4 alterations do not occur together with p53 or MDM2 alteration. It is an alternative mechanism by which a small part of GBMs escapes p53-regulated growth control. This oncoprotein may inhibit oncogenesis. Ubiquitin-specific protease 2a (USP2A) binds to MDM4, stabilizes it and protects against degradation. USP2–MDM4 interaction could be a determinant of malignant potential. MDM4 and USP2a are highly expressed in GBMs from patients with longer survival [13].

RB gene located on 13q14.2 has a protein product RB, which controls cell cycle, and acts as a gatekeeper to S-phase entry. RB protein is an end point of kinase activities of CDK4/6-cyclin D complexes. Transcription factor E2F binds to RB protein, which is normally not phosphorylated. Complex RB–E2F is a silencing complex restricting access to transcription factors. Phosphorylation of RB leads to release of E2F and such conformation allows CDK2 to access cell cycle during S-phase and this promotes another phosphorylation and that further inhibits the binding of E2F to RB protein [14]. Mutation of this gene has the same effect on cell cycle as the amplification of CDK4/CDK6 or mutation of CDKN2A/CDKN2B, but these alterations are never present together. This means that gliomagenesis proceeds by only one of these alternative genetic pathways. RB pathway is frequently altered in GBM and has a huge role in gliomagenesis [15]. Alterations of RB pathway are present almost universally in human cancers. It is very common in primary GBM, and is present in about 80% [4, 16]. Impaired RB1 expression is associated with increased tumor proliferation and decreased survival; however, more direct correlation with prognosis is in astrocytomas grade II and III than in GBM [17]. Mutation or deletion of RB1 is present in 11% of GBM [16].

CDKN1A gene encodes protein p21 and is located on chromosome 6p. Protein p21 is a member of kinase inhibitor protein family (KIP). Level of p53 protein regulates transcription of p21.

Apoptosis and cell cycle arrest mediated by p53 induce transcription of p21. This protein controls cell proliferation by regulatory binding to complexes of CDK. It negatively effects complexes of cyclin E/CDK2 and cyclin A/CDK2 and activates cyclin D/CDK. CDKN1A amplification is frequent in GBM [18].

Gene **CDKN1B** is localized on 12p13.1-p12. Its protein product is p27, which is also a member of KIP family. This protein also binds to CDK complexes, inhibits cyclin E/CDK2 and cyclin A/CDK2, and it activates cyclin D/CDK. In proliferating cells, p27 was found in complex with cyclin D/CDK and in G_1 – arrested cells, p27 was bound to cyclin E/CDK2. Very low levels of expression [19] are typical of GBM.

On 9p21 are located genes **CDKN2A** (protein product p16) and **CDKN2B** (product p15). These proteins are inhibitors of CDK and they inhibit phosphorylation of RB1 protein by binding to cyclin D, what prevents their interaction with CDK4/6. Regulation of p16/p14ARF pathway is determining the susceptibility to the only proved environmental risk factor of gliomagenesis – ionizing radiation [20]. Higher risk of glioma formation was observed in patients with CDKN2A and CDKN2B mutations [21, 22]. Homozygous deletion of CDKN2A is present in almost 50% of gliomas and is connected with poor prognosis [14]. But polymorphisms of *CDKN2A/CDKN2B* genes are not proved to be connected with tumor grade and prognosis [23].

Protein **p14ARF** is an alternate reading frame product of CDKN2A locus on 9p21. This protein has tumor suppressor activity, regulates cell cycle, initiates p53-dependent cell cycle arrest and apoptosis [20] and is induced by mitogenic stimulation. It inhibits MDM2 and so promotes p53. The finding of p14ARF loss in conjunction with p53 gene loss suggests that the protein may have other p53-independent tumor suppressor functions. P14ARF mediates antiangiogenic effects by upregulating expressions of tissue inhibitor of metalloproteinase-3 in p53-independent fashion. About 60–80% of high-grade gliomas show loss of tumor suppressor p14ARF activity by homozygous mutation [24].

CDKN2C gene has locus on 1p32, encodes protein p18, interacts with CDK4 and CDK6 and prevents their activation. It functions as a cell growth regulator that controls G1 cell cycle progression and also suppresses tumorigenesis. Homozygous deletion is a most common cause of CDKN2C inactivation. This deletion occurs in tumors harboring also CDKN2A deletions. Expression of CDKN2C is almost absent in 43% of GBMs. It is suggested that p16 deletion occurs as an early event in tumorigenesis and p18 inactivation should happen later in tumor formation [25].

Genes **CDK4** (12q14) and **CDK6** (7q21-22) have protein products CDK4 and CDK6 with catalytic kinase activity. Their inhibitors are proteins p15 and p16. CDK4 and CDK6 proteins make complexes with cyclin D. Gene CDK6 is an oncogene, which is required for proliferation of tumor cells and its viability [16]. Overexpression of CDK proteins inhibits the function of their inhibitors – proteins p15 and p16. Amplification of CDK4 is observed in 18% and CDK6 in 1% of GBMs [16].

CCND2 gene (cyclin D2), locus 12p13, encodes a protein of cyclin family that function as regulators of CDK kinases. Cyclin D2 makes a complex with CDK4 and CDK6 and works as a regulatory subunit of this complex, which is required for G1/S cell cycle transition. Association of cyclin D2 and CDK4/6 leads to phosphorylation of RB and RB-related proteins that allows cell to enter S phase of cell cycle. Deregulation of this cell cycle transition often causes formation of tumor and is frequently seen in GBM. Amplification of CCND2 occurs in 2% of GBM cases. Study on *in vitro* GSC showed high expression levels of cyclin D2 and suppression of its expression led in experimental model to G1 arrest. This suggests an important role of cyclin D2 in cell cycle progression and in tumorigenicity of GSC [26].

PIK3CA gene (phosphatidylinositol-4, 5-bisphosphate 3-kinase catalytic subunit alpha) located on 3q26.3 encodes ATP-dependent IA PI3K alpha catalytic subunit of phosphatidylinositol 3-kinase. This gene is a part of PI3K pathway, which plays a role in proliferation, cellular metabolism, apoptosis, differentiation, migration, and survival [27]. Binding of RTK to its receptor activates regulatory units of PI3K pathway, this activates catalytic subunits, which phosphorylates phosphatidylinositol 4, 5-bisphosphate (PIP2), converts it to phosphatidylinositol 3, 4, 5-triphosphate (PIP3). PIP3 activates downstream signaling cascades as the AKT and mTOR pathways, which are involved in proliferation and cell survival [28]. Hyperactivation of these pathways contributes to tumor progression. Mutations of this gene constitutively activate the PI3K catalytic activity and drive the GBM formation and progression [29]. Treatment of GBM with PI3K-targeted agents is promising [28]. PIK3CB gene (phosphatidylinositol-4, 5-bisphosphate 3-kinase catalytic subunit beta) located on 3q22.3 encodes IA PI3K beta catalytic subunit of phosphatidylinositol 3-kinase. This gene was identified as a marker predicting recurrence and prognosis of GBM [30].

PIK3R1 gene (phosphatidylinositol-3-kinase regulatory subunit 1) located on 5q13.1 is also part of PI3K pathway. Mutations and amplifications of these genes also occur in GBM [29]. PIK3R1 mutations act through the catalytic subunit by binding to it and inhibiting its activity [31]. Result of such PIK3R1 mutation is no inhibition of catalytic subunit and so constant activity of whole pathway leading to invasion and migration of tumor cells. Experimental knockdown of PIK3CA and PIK3R1 leads to decrease in proliferation, migration, and invasion of GBM cell lines [32].

Gene phosphatase and tensin homology – **PTEN** located on 10q23.3 is a tumor suppressor gene. PTEN protein, product of this gene, is a lipid phosphatase counteracting the effect of PI3K signaling. PTEN regulates this pathway by converting PIP3 to PIP2. After exposure to ionizing radiation, PTEN acts as a critical determinant of cell fate between the senescence and apoptosis [33]. Germ line mutations of PTEN were described in some autosomal hereditary diseases, such as Cowden disease, Bannayan-Zonana syndrome, etc. Monosomy of chromosome 10 is frequently present in GBM and rarely in low-grade astrocytoma. Inactivation of this tumor suppressor gene is present in both primary and secondary GBM [6]. PTEN gene is mutated or lost in 60–70% of GBM and this condition is associated with poor prognosis [18].

Signal transducer and activator of transcription 3 – **STAT3** gene (locus 17q21.31) encodes a protein member of STAT family. In response to growth factors or cytokines, this protein becomes phosphorylated and acts as a transcription factor. STAT3 regulates cell growth, nervous system development, stem cell differentiation, apoptosis, and is commonly activated in tumors. It also regulates growth and self-renewal of GBM stem cells. STAT3 has an antiapoptotic role, is activated in high percentage of GBM, and is required for maintaining of multipotency of tumor cells [34].

Oncogene **AKT3** (v-akt murine thymoma viral oncogene homolog 3) located on 1q44 codes a protein, member of serine/threonine protein kinase family (AKT). These AKT kinases are regulators of processes such as cell proliferation, differentiation, apoptosis, tumorigenesis, glycogen synthesis, and glucose uptake and their overexpression induces cell survival and malignant transformation. Enhanced DNA repair can allow damaged or mutated cells to survive, contributing to resistance and tumor recurrence [35]. Inhibition of AKT kinases activity leads to apoptosis. AKTs have three isoforms AKT1, AKT2, AKT3, being one of the major downstream effectors of PI3K. AKT pathway is activated in 70% of gliomas and is usually associated with PTEN mutations [36]. AKT3 is also essential for normal brain development [37] and is stimulated by PDGF, insulin, and insulin-like growth factor (IGF)1. AKT1 protein does not seem to be overexpressed in GBM, level of AKT2 increases with the malignancy grade and AKT3 expression decreases. It seems that AKT3 protein is affected by the negative feedback caused by AKT2 overexpression. Even though ATK3 is downregulated, it exhibits high kinase activity and retained the functional capacity as an oncoprotein and so may inhibit the growth of malignant cells. AKT3 is often amplified in GBM [35]. AKT2 and AKT3 isoform-specific knockdown inhibits cell growth and induces apoptosis [38] and thus is a potential target for therapy of AKT pathway-altered GBM.

NF1 (locus 17q11.2) codes tumor suppressor protein neurofibromin 1, Ras GTPase-activating protein, which was first found to be mutated in a genetic neurodevelopmental disease neurofibromatosis. Neurofibromin negatively regulates Ras and m-TOR signaling in astrocytes. Approximately 23% of GBM harbor inactivating mutation of NF1, typically mesenchymal subtype. NF1 inactivation could be due to genetic loss or mutation or to extensive proteasomal degradation [39].

MYC oncogene (v-myc avian myelocytomatosis viral oncogene homolog) has locus on 8q24.21. Its protein product is a nuclear phosphoprotein and transcriptional factor with various functions in cell cycle progression, cellular transformation, and apoptosis. Oncogenic activation is achieved by mutation, amplification, overexpression, and chromosomal translocation. This gene is an important target for the cooperative actions of p53 and PTEN in the regulation of normal and malignant cell differentiation, self-renewal, and tumorigenic potential. Overexpression of MYC is present in up to 70% of GBM [40] and surprisingly is highly correlated with better overall survival, what could be a result of enhancement of the proapoptotic effect of upregulated MYC [41]. Moreover, a direct relationship was found between MYC overexpression and MGMT methylation, so that MYC overexpression can be considered a good indicator of response to temozolomide treatment [42].

BMI1 – polycomb ring finger oncogene (10p11.23) is a transcriptional epigenetic repressor of genes governing self-renewal, differentiation, and proliferation, which is directly regulated by MYC. It plays a role in the development of the cerebellum and is required for self-renewal of stem cells in the hematopoietic, epithelial, and nervous system [43]. Overexpression of BMI1 is frequently present in GBM and is concurrent with MYC activation and MYC directly induces upregulation of BMI1 [41, 44].

Isocitrate dehydrogenase system comprises two genes: IDH1 located on 2q33.3 and IDH2 located on 15q26.1. Their products are enzymes (IDH1, IDH2, and IDH3) involved in citric acid cycle. The function of IDHs in this basic metabolic pathway is to catalyze oxidative decarboxylation of isocitrate to α-ketoglutarate and reducing NADP+ to NADPH (NAD+ to NADH in case of IDH3). Crucial effect on interaction of an enzyme with a substrate has arginine 132 (R132) in IDH1 and R172 in IDH2. Mutations of these important areas lead to significant reduction of enzyme activity [45, 46]. Mutations of IDH genes are common in patients with secondary GBM, but rare in primary and pediatric (11%) GBM [47, 48]. The fact that IDH mutations are found in a wide spectrum of histologic tumor types indicates that they occur as an early alteration in tumorigenesis [49]. Only 3–7% of primary GBM shows IDH mutations, but is often found in astrocytoma grade II and III and secondary GBM [50]. Though IDH mutations in primary GBM are rare, they create a prognostically favorable subgroup [21]. Also, IDH2 mutation, which is much less frequent than IDH1 mutation, occurs in gliomas [51], but only in about 6% of secondary GBMs [52]. There is also a possible association between the presence of IDH1 mutation and longer overall survival in patients with GBM [53, 54]. Furthermore, IDH mutation appears to be a significant marker of positive chemosensitivity in secondary GBM. Patients with this mutation show a higher response rate to temozolomide, which is widely used in chemotherapy of malignant gliomas. This makes IDH mutation an independent favorable prognostic factor for overall survival with comparable importance to hypermethylation of MGMT promotor [52]. Patients having both IDH mutation and MGMT promoter methylation seem to have best response to therapy and progression-free survival. Mechanism leading to increased effect of chemotherapy is not clearly known, it is possible that IDH mutation promotes treatment-induced apoptosis by inhibiting the cell-protective mechanisms against oxidative stress [55]. Prolonged survival of secondary GBM patients with IDH mutation was proved in patients with tumors of astrocytic, but not oligodendroglial origin [56]. Tumors with IDH mutation often show also the presence of TP53 mutation; on the other hand, tumors with wild type IDH often have alteration typical for primary GBM (*PTEN, EGFR, CDKN2A*, or *CDKN2B*). This fact confirms the existence of separate genetic pathways for primary and secondary GBM [50]. IDH mutations are novel and very important and useful prognostic factor of gliomas [21]. An inhibitor of IDH1 significantly retards GBM growth through inducing differentiation [57].

DCC gene with locus on 18q21.3 has product DCC protein. This protein is highly expressed in the nervous system. DCC is a transmembrane protein and creates part of the receptor for netrin 1. Netrins play a role in direct cell and axon migration during neural development. Their expression is also detectable in adult tissue, but their function is not yet clear [58]. DCC induces apoptosis and cell cycle arrest in G2 phase. Also plays a role in chemo-attraction to netrin-1 slowing the rate of spontaneous cell migration. DCC has probably anti-oncogenic function, although if disruption of netrin signaling contributes to tumorigenesis is not yet understood [59]. According to immunohistochemical examination, expression of DCC decreases in many malignancies including GBM and also decreases during progression from low-grade astrocytomas to GBM. This points out the connection of DCC with the formation of secondary, but not with primary GBM [59].

Paternally expressed gene 3 – **PEG3**, located on 19.chromosome, is an imprinted gene expressed mainly during embryogenesis, but also in some adult tissues – ovary, testis, muscle, and brain [60]. Overexpression is frequent in oligodendrogliomas, for GBM very low expression is typical. Deregulation of PEG3 induces the formation of gliomas [61].

GST genes – glutathione S-transferases genes: GSTP1 (location 11q13), GSTM1 (1p13.3), GSTT1 (22q11.23), and GSTO1 (10q25.1). Proteins of these genes are phase II biotransformation enzymes, which detoxify a wide range of exogenous agents including carcinogens. GSTs are responsible for glutathion conjugation of alkylators and scavenging of free radicals generated by radiation [62]. These enzymes provide enzymatic and nonenzymatic functions. GSTs also have important roles in cellular processes as cell proliferation, apoptosis, oncogenesis, tumor progression, drug resistance, and cell response to stress [63]. Genetic variations of GST genes determine the response to carcinogens. Polymorphisms of these genes result in absent or altered enzyme activity and are associated with survival rate in cancer patients. The relationship between these polymorphisms and brain tumor risk is not clear, although there have been some results referring to possible association between GSTM1 null genotype and brain tumor incidence [64]. Patients with brain tumors and GST polymorphisms have higher risk of adverse effects of chemotherapy with nitrosourea alkylating agents.

EGF gene is located on 4q25. EGF is a ligand for its receptor (EGFR), inducing a dimerization of one or several members of the EGFR family (ErbB1-4). This activates several tyrosine kinases and other downstream signal molecules promoting transcription in the cell nucleus [65]. These molecules are important for cell proliferation, survival, migration, and differentiation. EGF polymorphism 61G/A on the promoter part of this gene is associated with glioma susceptibility and with the degree of malignancy [66]; however, results of studies are controversial, probably due to diverse distribution of EGF gene frequencies among the different ethnic groups. EGF 61G/A polymorphism is also probably associated with the survival time of glioma patients [67].

EGFR gene, located on 7p12, encodes EGFR protein, which is a transmembrane receptor responsible for communication with its extracellular ligands – EGF and TGF-α and for transmission of their signalization within the cell. EGFR has an effect on cell apoptosis, angiogenesis, tumor proliferation, and ability to metastasize and is connected to sensitivity to therapy and drug resistance. EGFR is the most frequently amplified gene in astrocytomas, mainly in GBM. Expression of EGFR is higher in high-grade and poorly differentiated GBMs. Both overexpression and amplification of EGFR are correlated with tumor progression. Over 50% of GBM have mutations of EGFR. Presence of EGFR mutation is associated with early relapses and poor prognosis [68]. These mutations exist in three variations: EGFRvIII, δEGFR, and de2-7EGFR (deletion, loss of exons 2-7 of mRNA strand). δEGFR promotes tumorigenesis of GBM by increasing cellular proliferation, decreasing apoptosis, and promoting tumor cell invasiveness. Amplification and de2-7EGFR-specific mutation is typical for primary GBM, in which monosomy of chromosome 10 is also simultaneously present. Amplification of EGFR is mostly associated with CDKN2A deletion, but usually occurs without homozygote deletion or mutation of PTEN. Alteration of EGFR alone is probably not sufficient to cause tumorigenesis, but another alteration in RB1 pathway is required.

PDGF exists in five types of dimers consisting of four types of polypeptides, each encoded by a different gene – A, B, C, and D. PDGFA (7p22), PDGFB (22q13.1), PDGFC (4q32), and PDGFD (8q11). This system comprises two receptors: PDGFR-α (gene PDGFRA, 4q11-q13) and PDGFR-β (gene PDGFRB, 5q31-q32). PDGF system is involved in cell cycle regulation, cell migration, and chemotaxis and has also developmental functions – also in glial development [69]. PDGFR-α is expressed only in subset of GBMs. PDGFR-β is more commonly expressed in GBM by self-renewing GBM stem cells. PDGF pathway aberrations are mostly associated proneural and mesenchymal subtypes of GBM [70]. Overexpression of PDGF and its receptors is often found also in low-grade gliomas, suggesting this alteration as an early oncogenic event and if often found in secondary GBM [71].

IGF system is composed of two ligands: IGF1 (gene IGF1, 12q23.2), IGF2 (also called somatomedin A, gene IGF2, 11p15.5), their receptors: IGF1R (15q26.3) and IGF2R (6q26), six binding proteins (IGFBP 1-6), and various IGFBP-related peptides. IGF has a role in regulation of cell processes. IGF1 is a major physiological mediator of the growth hormone and has a huge influence on cell proliferation and differentiation. It inhibits apoptosis by blocking the initiation of the apoptotic pathway. IGF1R is involved in malignant transformation processes. IGF-binding proteins modulate interactions between IGF and IGFR. IGFBP3 (located on 7p13-p12) acts as an apoptotic agent and inhibits the activity of IGF1 and has growth-promoting effects [72]. Amplification of IGF1, IGF2, and IGF1R genes occurs in gliomas and other cancers. No association between IGF polymorphism and GBM risk has been found.

FGF system is a family of factors involved in various cellular processes, such as developmental, mitogen, cytoprotective, and angiogenic functions. System comprises 18 ligands and four FGF receptors and FGF-binding protein, which increases FGF2-dependent proliferation of fibroblast cells and may have an important role in oncogenesis. FGF2 (bFGF, 4q27-q25), known as a pro-angiogenic factor for vessel formation and wound repair, is a potential oncoprotein in GBM. Upregulated FGF2–FGFR1 signaling is implicated in the pathogenesis of GBM. Overexpression of FGF2 promotes GBM cell proliferation and also exerts an anti-apoptotic function by upregulating of anti-apoptotic genes BCL-2 and BCL-X and thus making tumor resistant to chemotherapy [73]. FGF2 also modulates apoptosis and thus promotes survival via resistance to radiation-induced cell death [74].

Vascular endothelial growth factor – **VEGF** system is the most potent angiogenesis- and vasculogenesis-promoting system. There are known six VEGF ligands and three receptors (VEGFR1, locus 13q12, VEGFR2, locus 4q11-q12, VEGFR3, locus 5q34-q35). VEGF system stimulates endothelial cell migration, growth, proliferation, and survival, also acts as microvascular permeability factor and increases extravasation of plasma proteins [75]. Activation of endothelial nitric oxide (NO) synthase leads to generation of NO and thus further activates angiogenesis. The main angiogenic effect of this system is mediated by interaction of VEGF (VEGFA) with VEGFR2. Angiogenesis is crucial for tumor formation, growth, and maintenance of blood supply. As the tumor develops, it may activate secondary angiogenic pathways, such as bFGF, TGF, and PDGF. GBMs exhibit high levels of VEGF [76]. Higher vascular permeability leads also to radiologic postcontrast enhancement. GBMs with high levels of VEGF are more likely to exhibit ring-like enhancement, what makes relatively clear border on postcontrast imaging. In such tumors, the gross total resection is easier to obtain. High expression of VEGF is associated with poor prognosis, but there are other factors determining prognosis, such as the extent of resection [76].

TGFβ superfamily is involved in morphogenesis, embryonic development, adult stem cell differentiation, immune reaction, wound healing, and inflammation [77]. This superfamily comprises over 30 proteins divided into two branches: TGFβ subfamily and the bone morphogenetic protein-like (BMP-like) group. The TGFβ subfamily contributes to carcinogenesis and makes tumors more aggressive and BMP-like group has a tumor suppression effect [78]. TGFβ subfamily is composed of three isoforms coded by three different genes – TGFBI (19q13), TGFBII (1q41), and TGFBIII (14q24). This subfamily regulates cell proliferation, differentiation, and extracellular matrix production [79]. All three isoforms are widely expressed in GBM, but TGFβ expression is increased in mesenchymal GBM [80].

Proto-oncogene **MET** (7q31) codes hepatocyte growth factor receptor with tyrosine kinase activity and belongs to RTK family. This receptor is usually expressed in epithelial cells. MET after binding with its ligand hepatocyte growth factor (HGF) plays a role in various cellular signaling pathways involved in proliferation, motility, migration, invasion, and tissue homeostasis by activating the RAS, PI3K, STAT, beta-catenin, and NOTCH signal transduction pathways [81]. It is aberrantly activated in many cancers (lung, pancreas, ovary, salivary gland, and breast cancers) as well as in GBM via mutation, amplification, or overexpression. Mutation of MET in GBM is rare [4]. Amplification is present in 5% and overexpression in 13% of GBM [82]. Overexpression and amplification of MET are not perfectly concordant. This abnormal activation of MET promotes malignancy and is partially associated with the aggressiveness as it was found only in grade IV, not in grade II or III gliomas, but relationship to prognosis is not clear [82, 83]. Amplification of EGFR could be associated with aberrant MET expression [4]. Under research are MET inhibitors in GBM treatment. Moreover, targeting the MET pathway potentiates the responsiveness of GBM to γ-radiation [82].

HGF gene (7q21.1) codes for HGF protein, a pleiotropic factor and cytokine, promoting cell proliferation, survival, motility, scattering, differentiation, and morphogenesis [84]. It is usually expressed by mesenchymal cells, but could be secreted also by tumor cells. In addition, HGF has a protective function in several diseases, including liver cirrhosis and promotes tissue regeneration. It also stimulates mobility and invasiveness of tumor cells and induces angiogenesis [81]. GBM with autocrine activation of HGF has also activated MET signaling and that predicts sensitivity to MET inhibitors in treatment [85]. HGF serum levels serve as biomarkers of responsiveness to such therapy. HGF levels in serum and cerebrospinal fluid correlate with prognosis, and are associated with higher mortality and recurrence rates [86].

Gene **ATRX** (α-thalassemia/mental-retardation-syndrome-X-linked), located at Xq21.1, was discovered as a gene responsible for rare developmental disorder characterized by α-thalassemia and intellectual impairment. It also has a role in the regulation of transcription, heterochromatin structure, and genome stability and is frequently deregulated in human cancer [87]. ATRX alterations are commonly present together with IDH and TP53 mutations. They are detected in 80% of secondary GBMs, but only in 7% of primary [88]. Mutations of ATRX gene are frequent also in pediatric GBM [89].

The B-Raf proto-oncogene serine/threonine kinase – **BRAF** gene, located on 7q34, is a member of Raf kinase family and serves as a strong activator of the extracellular signal-regulated kinase/ mitogen-activated protein kinase 1 and 2 (Erk 1/2) signal transduction cascade which modulates cell growth, proliferation, migration, differentiation, and apoptosis. Mutations of BRAF gene usually occur at codon 600, which is a site of activation loop of the kinase domain. Consequence of this BRAF V600E mutation is a protein with increased kinase activity. This mutation is usually present in lower-grade gliomas, but was found in 54% of epithelioid GBM [90], in 7% of giant cell GBM [91]. Within classical GBM types, BRAF mutation was present in 8% of adult and in 12% of pediatric GBM cases. These GBMs were all classified as primary. In adults, they create a group of tumors that are present in younger age (mean age of 39 years), none of these tumors harbored IDH mutation and seem to have slightly longer survival [92]. GBMs with BRAF V600E mutation may represent a small, but more favorable subgroup. In such patients, BRAF/MEK inhibitor treatment may be beneficial in combination with other therapies [93].

H3 histone, family 3A – **H3F3A** gene, located on 1q42.12, encodes replication-independent histone H3.3. Histones are basic nuclear proteins responsible for the nucleosome structure of the chromosomal fiber. ATRX and DAXX genes are encoding subunits of a chromatin remodeling complex required for H3.3 incorporation at pericentric heterochromatin and telomeres [94]. The histone H3.3 mutations result in amino acid substitution at K27 or G34 – two critical positions within the histone tail involved in key regulatory posttranslational modifications. H3F3A mutations are often seen in tumors with somatic TP53 mutation, within histological grades are specific for GBM and are highly prevalent in children and young adults, and they are present in one-third of pediatric GBMs [95]. Interestingly, K27-mutated tumors were predominantly seen in midline structures – thalamus, pons (diffuse intrinsic pontine gliomas), and spinal cord and have potentially poor prognosis. G34-mutated GBMs have better overall survival [96].

Telomerase reverse transcriptase –**TERT** gene is located on 5p15.33. This gene encodes the enzymatic core of telomerase. Telomeres are repeated sequences of DNA at the ends of chromosomes. Under physiological conditions, as the cell divides, telomeres become progressively shorter. Telomerase counteracts the shortening of telomeres by adding small segments of DNA at the end of chromosome after each cell division. Enhanced telomerase activity facilitates cellular immortality and promotes oncogenesis. Mutations of TERT promoter unmask binding sites for transcription factors, upregulate TERT expression and cellular telomerase activity [97]. TERT mutations are much more common in primary GBM and are inversely correlated with IDH mutations. Primary GBMs with TERT mutation exhibit significantly shorter overall survival than TERT-wild type tumors [98]. This unfavorable prognosis was absent after gross total resection and temozolomide therapy, what may indicate that TERT mutation makes tumor more susceptible to chemotherapy.

Tumor suppressor **PARK2** gene (parkin RBR E3 ubiquitin protein ligase) has locus on 6q25.2-q27. The exact function of this gene is still to be explored. It codes an E3 ubiquitin ligase mediating the targeting of substrate proteins for proteasome degradation. Germ line mutations of this gene cause Parkinson's disease, somatic mutations contribute to cancer. PARK2 is one of the most commonly inactivated tumor suppressor genes in GBM [99]. Deletion or inactivating mutation of this gene causes inability of PARK2 to promote ubiquitination and results in cyclin E deregulation, which can promote tumor cell growth. Low expression of PARK2 is associated with poor survival [100].

MGMT gene encodes a protein with alkyltransferase activity. MGMT is a DNA repair enzyme, which is responsible for tumor resistance to alkylating and methylating agents. Activity of this enzyme is regulated by this promoter area. This promoter, when methylated, causes inactivation of MGMT. Approximately 44% of GBM has MGMT promoter methylation [21]. Methylation status of MGMT is clinically the most relevant molecular parameter to predict sensitivity of gliomas do DNA alkylating chemotherapeutics [101]. This methylation is associated with prolonged progression-free survival and overall survival in patients with GBM treated with alkylating agents, such as temozolomide. [102]. Expression of MGMT is not associated with tumor grade [68].

4. Conclusion

GBM is the most aggressive and devastating primary brain tumor with very grim prognosis. The patient's survival rarely exceeds a year and a half with all accessible therapy used. Only 3% of GBM patients have survival over 5 years. This fact makes this tumor a very severe diagnosis directly affecting life expectancy of the patient and quality of his/her life. Explanation of its genesis could bring us closer to invention of effective treatment and genetic profile of concrete GBM tissue would help to design the individualized therapy management for each patient. Understanding the genetic and epigenetic characterization could help to distinguish various GBM subgroups, indistinguishable by histological appearance, but classified according to molecular and genetic alterations. This could lead to establishment of GBM classification with clinical impact, subgroup-specific treatment, and better design of future trials. The aim was to achieve prolonged progression-free interval and overall survival with maintaining satisfactory quality of life. It is very important if concrete genetic alteration is connected to tumor formation or if it is prognostic factor. Other factors influencing prognosis are histological type and tumor grade, age of patient, Karnofsky performance score at the time of diagnosis, extend of surgical resection, tumor localization, and appropriate therapeutic management. Tumor localization and extend of its surgical resection influence progression-free interval as well as overall survival. Detailed and complete explanation and discovery of altered genes and whole genetic pathways of GBM is the basis for new distinctive GBM classification. Such a new tumor division could bring us closer to routine genetic examination of frequently altered genetic pathways from tumor sample and aiming of therapy directly against specific genetic and epigenetic targets. Such individualized therapy could decrease the number of adverse effects, but first of all, hopefully, would finally ameliorate survival and life quality of patients, suffering from this severe disease.

Acknowledgements

This work was supported by projects: Competence Center for Research and Development in the diagnosis and therapy of oncological diseases, ITMS 26220220153 and The application of PACS (Picture Archiving and Communication System) in the reasearch and development, ITMS 26210120004.

Author details

Romana Richterová* and Branislav Kolarovszki

*Address all correspondence to: romana.richterova@gmail.com

Department of Neurosurgery, Jessenius Faculty of Medicine in Martin, Comenius University in Bratislava, Martin, Slovakia

References

[1] Ricard D, Idbaih A, Ducray F, Lahutte M, Hoang-Xuan K, Delattre JY: Primary brain tumours in adults. Lancet. 2012;379:1984–1996. DOI: 10.1016/S0140-6736(11)61346-9

[2] Michael KE, Dumbauld DW, Burns KL, Hanks SK, Garcia AJ: Focal adhesion kinase modulates cell adhesion strengthening via integrin activation. Mol Biol Cell. 2009;20:2508–2519. DOI: 10.1091/mbc.E08-01-0076

[3] Sengupta SNS, Hindi ES, Wainwright DA, Han Y, Lesniak MS: Short hairpin RNA-mediated fibronectin knockdown delays tumor growth in a mouse glioma model. Neoplasia. 2010;12:837–847.

[4] Cancer Genome Atlas Research Network: Comprehensive genomic characterization defines human GBM genes and core pathways. Nature. 2008;455:1061–1068. DOI: 10.1038/nature07385

[5] Iacob G, Dinca EB: Current data and strategy in GBM multiforme. J Med Life. 2009;2:386–393.

[6] Hede SM, Nazarenko I, Nistér M, Lindström MS: Novel perspectives on p53 function in neural stem cells and brain tumors. J Oncol. 2011;2011:852970. DOI: 10.1155/2011/852970

[7] Zhao Z, Xu Y: p53 and stem cells: new developments and new concerns. Trends Cell Biol. 2010;20:170–175. DOI: 10.1016/j.tcb.2009.12.004

[8] Krakstad C, Chekenya M: Survival signaling and apoptosis resistance in GBMs: opportunities for targeted therapeutics. Mol Cancer. 2010;9:135–149. DOI: 10.1186/1476-4598-9-135

[9] Wade M, Wang YV, Wahl GM: The p53 orchestra: Mdm2 and Mdmx set the tone. Trends Cell Biol. 2010;20:299–309. DOI: 10.1016/j.tcb.2010.01.009

[10] Furnari FB, Fenton T, Bachoo RM, Mukasa A, Stommel JM, Stegh A, Hahn WC, Ligon KL, Louis DN, Brennan C, Chin L, DePinho RA, Cavenee WK: Malignant astrocytic glioma: genetics, biology, and paths to treatment. Genes Dev. 2007;21:2683–2710. DOI: 10.1101/gad.1596707

[11] Thomasova D, Mulay SR, Bruns H, Anders HJ: p53-independent roles of MDM2 in NF-κB signaling: implications for cancer therapy, wound healing, and autoimmune diseases. Neoplasia. 2012;14:1097–1101.

[12] Wang AL, Liu ZX, Li G, Zhang LW: Expression and significance of P53 protein and MDM-2 protein in human gliomas. Chin Med J (Engl). 2011;124:2530–2533.

[13] Wang CL, Wang JY, Liu ZY, Ma XM, Wang XW, Jin H, Zhang XP, Fu D, Hou LJ, Lu YC: Ubiquitin-specific protease 2a stabilizes MDM4 and facilitates the p53-mediated intrinsic apoptotic pathway in GBM. Carcinogenesis. 2014;35:1500–1509. DOI: 10.1093/carcin/bgu015

[14] Goldhoff P, Clarke J, Smirnov I, Berger MS, Prados MD, James CD, Perry A, Phillips JJ: Clinical stratification of GBM based on alterations in retinoblastoma tumor suppressor protein (RB1) and association with the proneural subtype. J Neuropathol Exp Neurol. 2012;71:83–89. DOI: 10.1097/NEN.0b013e31823fe8f1

[15] Chow LM, Endersby R, Zhu X, Rankin S, Qu C, Zhang J, Broniscer A, Ellison DW, Baker SJ: Cooperativity within and among Pten, p53, and Rb pathways induces high-grade astrocytoma in adult brain. Cancer Cell. 2011;19:305–316. DOI: 10.1016/j.ccr.2011.01.039

[16] Wiedemeyer WR, Dunn IF, Quayle SN, Zhang J, Chheda MG, Dunn GP, Zhuang L, Rosenbluh J, Chen S, Xiao Y, Shapiro GI, Hahn WC, Chin L: Pattern of retinoblastoma pathway inactivation dictates response to CDK4/6 inhibition in GBM. Proc Natl Acad Sci USA. 2010;107:11501–11506. DOI: 10.1073/pnas.1001613107

[17] Kim CS, Jung S, Jung TY, Jang WY, Sun HS, Ryu HH: Characterization of invading glioma cells using molecular analysis of leading-edge tissue. J Korean Neurosurg Soc. 2011;50:157–165. DOI: 10.3340/jkns.2011.50.3.157

[18] Walker C, Baborie A, Crooks D, Wilkins S, Jenkinson MD: Biology, genetics and imaging of glial cell tumours. Br J Radiol. 2011;84:90–106. DOI: 10.1259/bjr/23430927

[19] Yue WY, Sai K, Wu QL, Xia YF, Yu SH, Chen ZP: Long-term molecular changes in WHO grade II astrocytomas following radiotherapy. Chin J Cancer. 2012;31:159–165. DOI: 10.5732/cjc.011.10149

[20] Liu Y, Shete S, Hosking FJ, Robertson LB, Bondy ML, Houlston RS: New insights into susceptibility to glioma. Arch Neurol. 2010;67:275–278. DOI: 10.1001/archneurol.2010.4

[21] Weller M, Felsberg J, Hartmann C, Berger H, Steinbach JP, Schramm J, Westphal M, Schackert G, Simon M, Tonn JC, Heese O, Krex D, Nikkhah G, Pietsch T, Wiestler O, Reifenberger G, von Deimling A, Loeffler M: Molecular predictors of progression-free and overall. Survival in patients with newly diagnosed GBM: a prospective translational study of the German glioma network. J Clin Oncol. 2009;27:5743–5750. DOI: 10.1200/JCO.2009.23.0805

[22] Shete S, Hosking FJ, Robertson LB, Dobbins SE, Sanson M, Malmer B, Simon M, Marie Y, Boisselier B, Delattre JY, Hoang-Xuan K, El Hallani S, Idbaih A, Zelenika D, Andersson U, Henriksson R, Bergenheim AT, Feychting M, Lönn S, Ahlbom A, Schramm J, Linnebank M, Hemminki K, Kumar R, Hepworth SJ, Price A, Armstrong G, Liu Y, Gu X, Yu R, Lau C, Schoemaker M, Muir K, Swerdlow A, Lathrop M, Bondy M, Houlston RS: Genome-wide association study identifies five susceptibility loci for glioma. Nat Genet. 2009;41:899–904. DOI: 10.1038/ng.407

[23] Simon M, Hosking FJ, Marie Y, Gousias K, Boisselier B, Carpentier C, Schramm J, Mokhtari K, Hoang-Xuan K, Idbaih A, Delattre JY, Lathrop M, Robertson LB, Houlston RS, Sanson M: Genetic risk profiles identify different molecular etiologies for glioma. Clin Cancer Res. 2010;16:5252–5259. DOI: 10.1158/1078-0432.CCR-10-1502

[24] Zerrouqi A, Pyrzynska B, Febbraio M, Brat DJ, Van Meir EG: P14ARF inhibits human GBM-induced angiogenesis by upregulating the expression of TIMP3. J Clin Invest. 2012;122:1283–1295. DOI: 10.1172/JCI38596

[25] Solomon DA, Kim JS, Jenkins S, Ressom H, Huang M, Coppa N, Mabanta L, Bigner D, Yan H, Jean W, Waldman T: Identification of p18 INK4c as a tumor suppressor gene in GBM multiforme. Cancer Res. 2008;68:2564–2569. DOI: 10.1158/0008-5472.CAN-07-6388

[26] Koyama-Nasu R, Nasu-Nishimura Y, Todo T, Ino Y, Saito N, Aburatani H, Funato K, Echizen K, Sugano H, Haruta R, Matsui M, Takahashi R, Manabe E, Oda T, Akiyama T: The critical role of cyclin D2 in cell cycle progression and tumorigenicity of GBM stem cells. Oncogene. 2013;32:3840–3845. DOI: 10.1038/onc.2012.399

[27] Courtney KD, Corcoran RB, Engelman JA: The PI3K pathway as drug target in human cancer. J Clin Oncol. 2010;28:1075–1083. DOI: 10.1200/JCO.2009.25.3641

[28] Wen PY, Lee EQ, Reardon DA, Ligon KL, Alfred Yung WK: Current clinical development of PI3K pathway inhibitors in GBM. Neuro Oncol. 2012;14:819–829. DOI: 10.1093/neuonc/nos117.

[29] Parsons DW, Jones S, Zhang X, Lin JC, Leary RJ, Angenendt P, Mankoo P, Carter H, Siu IM, Gallia GL, Olivi A, McLendon R, Rasheed BA, Keir S, Nikolskaya T, Nikolsky Y, Busam DA, Tekleab H, Diaz LA Jr, Hartigan J, Smith DR, Strausberg RL, Marie SK, Shinjo SM, Yan H, Riggins GJ, Bigner DD, Karchin R, Papadopoulos N, Parmigiani G,

Vogelstein B, Velculescu VE, Kinzler KW: An integrated genomic analysis of human GBM multiforme. Science. 2008;321:1807–1812. DOI: 10.1126/science.1164382

[30] Varghese RT, Liang Y, Guan T, Franck CT, Kelly DF, Sheng Z: Survival kinase genes present prognostic significance in glioblastoma. Oncotarget. 2016;7:20140-20151. DOI: 10.18632/oncotarget.7917

[31] Sun MHP, Hofmann BT, Hart JR, Vogt PK: Cancer derived mutations in the regulatory subunit p85alpha of phosphoinositide 3-kinase function through the catalytic subunit p110alpha. Proc Natl Acad Sci USA. 2010;107:15,547–15,552. DOI: 10.1073/pnas.1009652107

[32] Weber GL, Parat MO, Binder ZA, Gallia GL, Riggins GJ: Abrogation of PIK3CA or PIK3R1 reduces proliferation, migration, and invasion in GBM multiforme cells. Oncotarget. 201;2:833–849.

[33] Lee JJ, Kim BC, Park MJ, Lee YS, Kim YN, Lee BL, Lee JS: PTEN status switches cell fate between premature senescence and apoptosis in glioma exposed to ionizing radiation. Cell Death Differ. 2011;18:666–677. DOI: 10.1038/cdd.2010.139

[34] Sherry MM, Reeves A, Wu JK, Cochran BH: STAT3 is required for proliferation and maintenance of multipotency in GBM stem cells. Stem Cells. 2009;27:2383–2392. DOI: 10.1002/stem.185

[35] Turner KM, Sun Y, Ji P, Granberg KJ, Bernard B, Hu L, Cogdell DE, Zhou X, Yli-Harja O, Nykter M, Shmulevich I, Yung WK, Fuller GN, Zhang W: Genomically amplified Akt3 activates DNA repair pathway and promotes glioma progression. Proc Natl Acad Sci USA. 2015;112:3421–3426. DOI: 10.1073/pnas.1414573112

[36] Omuro AM, Faivre S, Raymond E: Lessons learned in the development of targeted therapy for malignant gliomas. Mol Cancer Ther. 2007;6:1909–1919.

[37] Easton RM, Cho H, Roovers K, Shineman DW, Mizrahi M, Forman MS, Lee VM, Szabolcs M, de Jong R, Oltersdorf T, Ludwig T, Efstratiadis A, Birnbaum MJ: Role for Akt3/protein kinase Bgamma in attainment of normal brain size. Mol Cell Biol. 2005;25:1869–1878.

[38] Mure H, Matsuzaki K, Kitazato KT, Mizobuchi Y, Kuwayama K, Kageji T, Nagahiro S: Akt2 and Akt3 play a pivotal role in malignant gliomas. Neuro Oncol. 2010;12:221–232. DOI: 10.1093/neuonc/nop026

[39] Verhaak RG, Hoadley KA, Purdom E, Wang V, Qi Y, Wilkerson MD, Miller CR, Ding L, Golub T, Mesirov JP, Alexe G, Lawrence M, O'Kelly M, Tamayo P, Weir BA, Gabriel S, Winckler W, Gupta S, Jakkula L, Feiler HS, Hodgson JG, James CD, Sarkaria JN, Brennan C, Kahn A, Spellman PT, Wilson RK, Speed TP, Gray JW, Meyerson M, Getz G, Perou CM, Hayes DN; Cancer Genome Atlas Research Network: Integrated genomic analysis identifies clinically relevant subtypes of GBM characterized by abnormalities

in PDGFRA, IDH1, EGFR and NF1. Cancer Cell. 2010;17:98–110. DOI: 10.1016/j.ccr.2009.12.020

[40] Faria MH, Gonçalves BP, do Patrocínio RM, de Moraes-Filho MO, Rabenhorst SH: Expression of Ki-67, topoisomerase II alpha and c-MYC in astrocytic tumors: correlation with the histopathological grade and proliferative status. Neuropathology. 2006;26:519–527.

[41] Cenci T, Martini M, Montano N, D'Alessandris QG, Falchetti ML, Annibali D, Savino M, Bianchi F, Pierconti F, Nasi S, Pallini R, Larocca LM: Prognostic relevance of c-Myc and BMI1 expression in patients with glioblastoma. Am J Clin Pathol. 2012;138:390–396. DOI: 10.1309/AJCPRXHNJQLO09QA

[42] De Salvo M, Maresca G, D'agnano I, Marchese R, Stigliano A, Gagliassi R, Brunetti E, Raza GH, De Paula U, Bucci B: Temozolomide induced c-Myc-mediated apoptosis via Akt signaling in MGMT expressing glioblastoma cells. Int J Radiat Biol. 2011;87:518–533. DOI: 10.3109/09553002.2011.556173

[43] Shakhova O, Leung C, Marino S: Bmi1 in development and tumorigenesis of the central nervous system. J Mol Med. 2005;83:596–600.

[44] Guo WJ, Datta S, Band V, Dimri GP: Mel-18, a polycomb group protein, regulates cell proliferation and senescence via transcriptional repression of Bmi-1 and c-Myc oncoproteins. Mol Biol Cell. 2007;18:536–546.

[45] Pusch S, Sahm F, Meyer J, Mittelbronn M, Hartmann C, von Deimling A: Glioma IDH1 mutation patterns off the beaten track. Neuropathol Appl Neurobiol. 2011;37:428–430. DOI: 10.1111/j.1365-2990.2010.01127.x

[46] Zhao S, Lin Y, Xu W, Jiang W, Zha Z, Wang P, Yu W, Li Z, Gong L, Peng Y, Ding J, Lei Q, Guan KL, Xiong Y: Glioma-derived mutations in IDH1 dominantly inhibit IDH1 catalytic activity and induce HIF-1alpha. Science. 2009;324:261–265. DOI: 10.1126/science.1170944

[47] Toedt G, Barbus S, Wolter M, Felsberg J, Tews B, Blond F, Sabel MC, Hofmann S, Becker N, Hartmann C, Ohgaki H, von Deimling A, Wiestler OD, Hahn M, Lichter P, Reifenberger G, Radlwimmer B: Molecular signatures classify astrocytic gliomas by IDH1 mutation status. Int J Cancer. 2011;128:1095–1103. DOI: 10.1002/ijc.25448

[48] Kim W, Liau LM: IDH mutations in human glioma. Neurosurg Clin N Am. 2012;23:471–480. DOI: 10.1016/j.nec.2012.04.009

[49] Yan H, Parsons DW, Jin G, McLendon R, Rasheed A, Yuan W, Kos I, Batinic-Haberle I, Jones S, Riggins GJ, Friedman H, Friedman A, Reardon D, Herndon J, Kinzler KW, Velculescu VE, Vogelstein B, Bigner DD: IDH1 and IDH2 mutations in gliomas. N Engl J Med. 2009;360:765–773. DOI: 10.1056/NEJMoa0808710

[50] Ichimura K, Pearson DM, Kocialkowski S, Bäcklund LM, Chan R, Jones DT, Collins VP: IDH1 mutations are present in the majority of common adult gliomas but rare in primary GBMs. Neuro Oncol. 2009;11:341–347. DOI: 10.1215/15228517-2009-025

[51] Reitman ZJ, Yan H: Isocitrate dehydrogenase 1 and 2 mutations in cancer: alterations at a crossroads of cellular metabolism. J Natl Cancer Inst. 2010;102:932–941. DOI: 10.1093/jnci/djq187

[52] SongTao Q, Lei Y, Si G, YanQing D, HuiXia H, XueLin Z, LanXiao W, Fei Y: IDH mutations predict longer survival and response to temozolomide in secondary GBM. Cancer Sci. 2012;103:269–273. DOI: 10.1111/j.1349-7006.2011.02134.x

[53] Nobusawa S, Watanabe T, Kleihues P, Ohgaki H: IDH1 mutations as molecular signature and predictive factor of secondary GBMs. Clin Cancer Res. 2009;15:6002–6007. DOI: 10.1158/1078-0432.CCR-09-0715

[54] Beiko J, Suki D, Hess KR, Fox BD, Cheung V, Cabral M, Shonka N, Gilbert MR, Sawaya R, Prabhu SS, Weinberg J, Lang FF, Aldape KD, Sulman EP, Rao G, McCutcheon IE, Cahill DP: IDH1 mutant malignant astrocytomas are more amenable to surgical resection and have a survival benefit associated with maximal surgical resection. Neuro-Oncology. 2014;16:81–91. DOI: 10.1093/neuonc/not159

[55] Reitman ZJ, Yan H: Isocitrate dehydrogenase 1 and 2 mutations in cancer: alterations at a crossroads of cellular metabolism. J Natl Cancer Inst. 2010;102:932–941. DOI: 10.1093/jnci/djq187

[56] Takahashi Y, Nakamura H, Makino K, Hide T, Muta D, Kamada H, Kuratsu J: Prognostic value of isocitrate dehydrogenase 1, O6-methylguanine-DNA methyltransferase promoter methylation, and 1p19q co-deletion in Japanese malignant glioma patients. World J Surg Oncol. 2013;11:284. DOI: 10.1186/1477-7819-11-284

[57] Rohle D, Popovici-Muller J, Palaskas N, Turcan S, Grommes C, Campos C, Tsoi J, Clark O, Oldrini B, Komisopoulou E, Kunii K, Pedraza A, Schalm S, Silverman L, Miller A, Wang F, Yang H, Chen Y, Kernytsky A, Rosenblum MK, Liu W, Biller SA, Su SM, Brennan CW, Chan TA, Graeber TG, Yen KE, Mellinghoff IK: An inhibitor of mutant IDH1 delays growth and promotes differentiation of glioma cells. Science. 2013;340:626–630. DOI: 10.1126/science.1236062

[58] Rajasekharan S, Kennedy TE: The netrin protein family. Genome Biol. 2009;10:239. DOI: 10.1186/GBM-2009-10-9-239

[59] Jarjour AA, Durko M, Luk TL, Marçal N, Shekarabi M, Kennedy TE: Autocrine netrin function inhibits glioma cell motility and promotes focal adhesion formation. PLoS One. 2011;6:e25408. DOI:10.1371/journal.pone.0025408

[60] Jiang X, Yu Y, Yang HW, Agar NY, Frado L, Johnson MD: The imprinted gene PEG3 inhibits Wnt signaling and regulates glioma growth. J Biol Chem. 2010;285:8472–8480. DOI: 10.1074/jbc.M109.069450

[61] Otsuka S, Maegawa S, Takamura A, Kamitani H, Watanabe T, Oshimura M, Nanba E: Aberrant promoter methylation and expression of the imprinted PEG3 gene in glioma. Proc Jpn Acad Ser B. 2009;85:157–165. DOI: 10.2183/pjab.85.157

[62] Kilburn L, Okcu F, Wang T, Cao Y, Renfro-Spelman A, Aldape KD, Gilbert MR, Bondy M: Glutathione S-transferase polymorphism are associated with survival in anaplastic glioma patients. Cancer. 2010;116:2242–2249. DOI: 10.1002/cncr.25006

[63] Lo H, Ali-Osman F: Genetic polymorphism and function of glutathione S-transferases in tumor drug resistance. Curr Opin Pharmacol. 2007;7:367–374. DOI: 10.1016/j.coph. 2007.06.009

[64] Schwartzbaum JA, Ahlbom A, Lönn S, Warholm M, Rannug A, Auvinen A, Christensen HC, Henriksson R, Johansen C, Lindholm C, Malmer B, Salminen T, Schoemaker MJ, Swerdlow AJ, Feychting M: An international casecontrol study of glutathione transferase and functionally related polymorphisms and risk of primary adult brain tumors. Cancer Epidemiol Biomarkers Prev. 2007;16:559–565. DOI: 10.1158/1055-9965.EPI-06-0918

[65] Sjöström S, Anderson U, Liu Y, Brännström T, Broholm H, Johansen C, Collatz-Laier H, Henriksson R, Bondy M, Melin B: Genetic variation in EGF and EGFR and GBM outcome. Neuro-Oncol. 2010;12:815–821. DOI: 10.1093/neuonc/noq018

[66] Chen X, Yang G, Zhang D, Zhang W, Zou H, Zhao H, Zhang X, Zhao S: Association between the epidermal growth factor +61 G/A polymorphism and glioma risk: a meta-analysis. PLoS One. 2014;9:e95139. DOI: 10.1371/journal.pone.0095139

[67] Pinto GR, Yoshioka FK, Clara CA, Santos MJ, Almeida JR, Burbano RR, Rey JA, Casartelli C: Association study of an epidermal growth factor gene functional polymorphism with the risk and prognosis of gliomas in Brazil. Int J Biol Markers. 2009;24:277–281.

[68] Hu X, Miao W, Zou Y, Zhang W, Zhang Y, Liu H: Expression of p53, epidermal growth factor receptor, Ki-67 and O6-methylguanine-DNA methyltransferase in human gliomas. Oncol Lett. 2013;6:130–134.

[69] Ozawa T, Brennan CW, Wang L, Squatrito M, Sasayama T, Nakada M, Huse JT, Pedraza A, Utsuki S, Yasui Y, Tandon A, Fomchenko EI, Oka H, Levine RL, Fujii K, Ladanyi M, Holland EC: PDGFRA gene rearrangements are frequent genetic events in PDGFRA-amplified GBMs. Genes Dev. 2010;24:2205–2218. DOI: 10.1101/gad.1972310

[70] Kim Y, Kim E, Wu Q, Guryanova O, Hitomi M, Lathia JD, Serwanski D, Sloan AE, Weil RJ, Lee J, Nishiyama A, Bao S, Hjelmeland AB, Rich JN: Platelet-derived growth factor receptors differentially inform intertumoral and intratumoral heterogeneity. Genes Dev. 2012;26:1247–1262. DOI: 10.1101/gad.193565.112

[71] Westermark B: Platelet-derived growth factor in GBM-driver or biomarker? Ups J Med Sci. 2014;119:298–305. DOI: 10.3109/03009734.2014.970304

[72] Lönn S, Rothman N, Shapiro WR, Fine HA, Selker RG, Black PM, Loeffler JS, Hutchinson AA, Inskip PD: Genetic variation in insulin-like growth factors and brain tumor risk. Neuro-Oncol. 2008;10:553–559. DOI: 10.1215/15228517-2008-026

[73] Pardo OE, Wellbrock C, Khanzada UK, Aubert M, Arozarena I, Davidson S, Bowen F, Parker PJ, Filonenko VV, Gout IT, Sebire N, Marais R, Downward J, Seckl MJ: FGF-2 protects small cell lung cancer cells from apoptosis through a complex involving PKCepsilon, B-Raf and S6K2. The EMBO Journal. 2006;25:3078–3088.

[74] Haley EM, Kim Y: The role of basic fibroblast growth factor in GBM multiforme and GBM stem cells and in their in vitro culture. Cancer Lett. 2014;346:1–5. DOI: 10.1016/j.canlet.2013.12.003

[75] Desjardins A, Friedman HS: Bevacizumab therapy for GBM: a passionate discussion. CNS Oncol. 2014;3:1–3. DOI: 10.2217/cns.13.53

[76] Wang K, Wang YY, Wang JF, Ma J, Jiang T, Dai JP: Radiologic features and expression of vascular endothelial growth factor stratify survival outcomes in patients with GBM. AJNR Am J Neuroradiol. 2016;37:629-635. DOI:10.3174/ajnr.A4567

[77] Santibanez JF, Quintanilla M, Bernabeu C: TGF-beta/ TGF-beta receptor system and its role in physiological and pathological conditions. Clin Sci (Lond). 2011;121:233–251. DOI: 10.1042/CS20110086

[78] Weiss A, Attisano L: The TGFbeta superfamily signaling pathway. Wiley Interdisciplinary Reviews. Developmental Biol. 2013;2:47–63. DOI: 10.1002/wdev.86

[79] Kaminska B, Kocyk M, Kijewska M: TGF beta signaling and its role in glioma pathogenesis. Adv Exp Med Biol. 2013;986:171–187. DOI: 10.1007/978-94-007-4719-7_9

[80] Frei K, Gramatzki D, Tritschler I, Schroeder JJ, Espinoza L, Rushing EJ, Weller M: Transforming growth factor-β pathway activity in GBM. Oncotarget. 2015;6:5963–5977.

[81] Organ SL, Tsao MS: An overview of the c-MET signaling pathway. Ther Adv Med Oncol. 2011;3:7–19. DOI: 10.1177/1758834011422556

[82] Kwak Y, Kim SI, Park CK, Paek SH, Lee ST, Park SH: C-MET overexpression and amplification in gliomas. Int J Clin Exp Pathol. 2015;8:14932–14938.

[83] Kong DS, Song SY, Kim DH, Joo KM, Yoo JS, Koh JS, Dong SM, Suh YL, Lee JI, Park K, Kim JH, Nam DH: Prognostic significance of c-Met expression in GBMs. Cancer. 2009;115:140–148. DOI: 10.1002/cncr.23972

[84] Basilico C, Arnesano A, Galluzzo M, Comoglio PM, Michieli P: A high affinity hepatocyte growth factor-binding site in the immunoglobulin-like region of Met. J Biol Chem. 2008;283:21,267–21,277. DOI: 10.1074/jbc.M800727200

[85] Xie Q, Bradley R, Kang L, Koeman J, Ascierto ML, Worschech A, De Giorgi V, Wang E, Kefene L, Su Y, Essenburg C, Kaufman DW, DeKoning T, Enter MA, O'Rourke TJ, Marincola FM, Vande Woude GF: Hepatocyte growth factor (HGF) autocrine activation

predicts sensitivity to MET inhibition in GBM. Proc Natl Acad Sci USA. 2012;109:570–575. DOI: 10.1073/pnas.1119059109

[86] Garcia-Navarrete R, Garcia E, Arrieta O, Sotelo J: Hepatocyte growth factor in cerebrospinal fluid is associated with mortality and recurrence of GBM, and could be of prognostic value. J Neurooncol. 2010;97:347–351. DOI: 10.1007/s11060-009-0037-8

[87] Watson LA, Goldberg H, Bérubé NG: Emerging roles of ATRX in cancer. Epigenomics. 2015;7:1365–13678. DOI: 10.2217/epi.15.82

[88] Liu XY, Gerges N, Korshunov A, Sabha N, Khuong-Quang DA, Fontebasso AM, Fleming A, Hadjadj D, Schwartzentruber J, Majewski J, Dong Z, Siegel P, Albrecht S, Croul S, Jones DT, Kool M, Tonjes M, Reifenberger G, Faury D, Zadeh G, Pfister S, Jabado N: Frequent ATRX mutations and loss of expression in adult diffuse astrocytic tumors carrying IDH1/IDH2 and TP53 mutations. Acta Neuropathol. 2012;124:615–625. DOI: 10.1007/s00401-012-1031-3

[89] Appin CL, Brat DJ: Molecular pathways in gliomagenesis and their relevance to neuropathologic diagnosis. Adv Anat Pathol. 2015;22:50–58. DOI: 10.1097/PAP.0000000000000048

[90] Kleinschmidt-DeMasters BK, Aisner DL, Birks DK, Foreman NK: Epithelioid GBMs show a high percentage of BRAF V600E mutation. Am J Surg Pathol. 2013;37:685–698. DOI: 10.1097/PAS.0b013e31827f9c5e

[91] Schindler G, Capper D, Meyer J, Janzarik W, Omran H, Herold-Mende C, Schmieder K, Wesseling P, Mawrin C, Hasselblatt M, Louis DN, Korshunov A, Pfister S, Hartmann C, Paulus W, Reifenberger G, von Deimling A: Analysis of BRAF V600E mutation in 1320 nervous system tumors reveals high mutation frequencies in pleomorphic xanthoastrocytoma, ganglioglioma and extra-cerebellar pilocytic astrocytoma. Acta Neuropathol. 2011;121:397–405. DOI: 10.1007/s00401-011-0802-6

[92] Gutmann DH: BRAF-V600E mutation in pediatric and adult GBM. Neuro-Oncology. 2014;16:318–319. DOI: 10.1093/neuonc/not146

[93] Takahashi Y, Akahane T, Sawada T, Ikeda H, Tempaku A, Yamauchi S, Nishihara H, Tanaka S, Nitta K, Ide W, Hashimoto I, Kamada H: Adult classical GBM with a BRAFV600E mutation. World J Surg Oncol. 2015;13:100. DOI: 10.1186/s12957-015-0521-x

[94] Lewis PW, Elsaesser SJ, Noh KM, Stadler SC, Allis CD: Daxx is an H3.3-specific histone chaperone and cooperates with ATRX in replication-independent chromatin assembly at telomeres. Proc Natl Acad Sci USA. 2010;107:14,075–14,080. DOI: 10.1073/pnas.1008850107

[95] Schwartzentruber J, Korshunov A, Liu XY, Jones DTW, Pfaff E, Jacob K, Sturm D, Fontebasso AM, Quang DA, Tonjes M, Hovestadt V, Albrecht S, Kool M, Nantel A, Konermann C, Lindroth A, Jäger N, Rausch T, Ryzhova M, Korbel JO, Hielscher T, Hauser P, Garami M, Klekner A, Bognar L, Ebinger M, Schuhmann MU, Scheurlen W,

Pekrun A, Frühwald MC, Roggendorf W, Kramm C, Dürken M, Atkinson J, Lepage P, Montpetit A, Zakrzewska M, Zakrzewski K, Liberski PP, Dong Z, Siegel P, Kulozik AE, Zapatka M, Guha A, Malkin D, Felsberg J, Reifenberger G, von Deimling A, Ichimura K, Collins VP, Witt H, Milde T, Witt O, Zhang C, Castelo-Branco P, Lichter P, Faury D, Tabori U, Plass C, Majewski J, Pfister SM, Jabado N: Driver mutations in histone H3.3 and chromatin remodelling genes in paediatric GBM. Nature. 2012;482:226–231. DOI: 10.1038/nature10833

[96] Sturm D, Witt H, Hovestadt V, Khuong-Quang DA, Jones DT, Konermann C, Pfaff E, Tönjes M, Sill M, Bender S, Kool M, Zapatka M, Becker N, Zucknick M, Hielscher T, Liu XY, Fontebasso AM, Ryzhova M, Albrecht S, Jacob K, Wolter M, Ebinger M, Schuhmann MU, van Meter T, Frühwald MC, Hauch H, Pekrun A, Radlwimmer B, Niehues T, von Komorowski G, Dürken M, Kulozik AE, Madden J, Donson A, Foreman NK, Drissi R, Fouladi M, Scheurlen W, von Deimling A,Monoranu C, Roggendorf W, Herold-Mende C, Unterberg A, Kramm CM, Felsberg J, Hartmann C, Wiestler B, Wick W, Milde T, Witt O, Lindroth AM, Schwartzentruber J, Faury D, Fleming A, Zakrzewska M, Liberski PP, Zakrzewski K, Hauser P, Garami M, Klekner A, Bognar L, Morrissy S, Cavalli F, Taylor MD,van Sluis P, Koster J, Versteeg R, Volckmann R, Mikkelsen T, Aldape K, Reifenberger G, Collins VP, Majewski J, Korshunov A, Lichter P, Plass C, Jabado N, Pfister SM: Hotspot mutations in H3F3A and IDH1 define distinct epigenetic and biological subgroups of GBM. Cancer Cell. 2012;22:425–437. DOI: 10.1016/j.ccr.2012.08.024

[97] Huang FW, Hodis E, Xu MJ, Kryukov GV, Chin L, Garraway LA: Highly recurrent TERT promoter mutations in human melanoma. Science. 2013;339:957–959. DOI: 10.1126/science.1229259

[98] Simon M, Hosen I, Gousias K, Rachakonda S, Heidenreich B, Gessi M, Schramm J, Hemminki K, Waha A, Kumar R: TERT promoter mutations: a novel independent prognostic factor in primary GBMs. Neuro Oncol. 2015;17:45–52. DOI: 10.1093/neuonc/nou158

[99] Veeriah S, Taylor BS, Meng S, Fang F, Yilmaz E, Vivanco I, Janakiraman M, Schultz N, Hanrahan AJ, Pao W, Ladanyi M, Sander C, Heguy A, Holland EC, Paty PB, Mischel PS, Liau L, Cloughesy TF, Mellinghoff IK, Solit DB, Chan TA: Somatic mutations of the Parkinson's disease-associated gene PARK2 in glioblastoma and other human malignancies. Nat Genet. 2010;42:77–82. DOI: 10.1038/ng.491

[100] Lin DC, Xu L, Chen Y, Yan H, Hazawa M, Doan N, Said JW, Ding LW, Liu LZ, Yang H, Yu S, Kahn M, Yin D, Koeffler HP: Genomic and Functional Analysis of the E3 Ligase PARK2 in Glioma. Cancer Res. 2015;75:1815–1827. DOI: 10.1158/0008-5472.CAN-14-1433

[101] Von Deimling A, Korshunov A, Hartmann C: The next generation of glioma biomarkers: MGMT methylation, BRAF fusions and IDH1 mutations. Brain Pathol. 2011;21:74–87. DOI: 10.1111/j.1750-3639.2010.00454.x

[102] Glas M, Happold C, Rieger J, Wiewrodt D, Bähr O, Steinbach JP, Wick W, Kortmann RD, Reifenberger G, Weller M, Herrlinger U: Long-term survival of GBM patients treated with radiotherapy and lomustine plus temozolomide. J Clin Oncol. 2009;27:1257–1261. DOI: 10.1200/JCO.2008.19.2195

Chapter 5

Mechanisms of Glioma Cell Invasion

Scott G. Turner, Maleeha Ahmad and
Steven A. Toms

Additional information is available at the end of the chapter

http://dx.doi.org/10.5772/63126

Abstract

Malignant gliomas are the most aggressive primary brain tumors. Although current treatment includes surgery and chemo/radiation therapy, life expectancy remains on the order of 2 years. One of the features, which make these tumors incurable, is their infiltration into normal brain tissue. This process is incompletely understood at a molecular level and appropriate targets need to be developed. This review discusses (1) the unique structure of the neural extracellular matrix (ECM), (2) the basis of the proliferation to migration transition that initiates the infiltrative process, (3) the remodeling of the ECM by degradation and synthesis of new components, and (4) trophic factors that act as chemoattractants and chemorepellents for migrating cells. Finally we briefly discuss the challenges facing the study of this complex process and future directions in attacking this important problem in neuro-oncology.

Keywords: glioma, migration, invasion, extracellular matrix, protease, signaling

1. Introduction

Malignant gliomas are the most common primary tumors of the central nervous system (CNS) accounting for over 22,000 new cases in the USA each year [1]. Glioblastoma multiforme (GBM) is the most aggressive (WHO grade IV) glioma and is characterized histologically by high mitotic activity leading to hypoxia and necrosis, nuclear atypia and cellular pleomorphism, and microvascular proliferation due to secretion of pro-angiogenic factors. These tumors are uniformly fatal with standard treatment consisting of maximal surgical resection followed by radiation and chemotherapy which targets cell proliferation (Temozolomide or other DNA modifying agents) [2] or angiogenesis (Bevacizumab) [3], as well as other newly developed methods of attacking dividing tumor cells (Optune-TTF) [4].

Gliomas differ from metastatic tumors in their ability to migrate into the surrounding brain parenchyma. While most recurrence occurs within 1–2 cm of the original tumor bed [5], seemingly multifocal disease or so-called "butterfly glioma" can develop at distant sites as a consequence of migration of cells along blood vessels and white matter tracts [6] (**Figure 1**). Although they are highly infiltrative, less than 2% of gliomas spread outside the CNS, suggesting that tumor cells are either not able to cross the basement membrane and enter the vasculature or that they require a specific neural environment containing specific molecules through which they can proliferate and migrate. Tumor cells switch from a proliferative to a migratory or mesenchymal phenotype, resorting to this more primitive state, which mimics the behavior of their migratory progenitors such as the radial glia that traversed white matter pathways and other structures during embryonic development [7]. The molecular mechanisms of this transition are currently poorly understood.

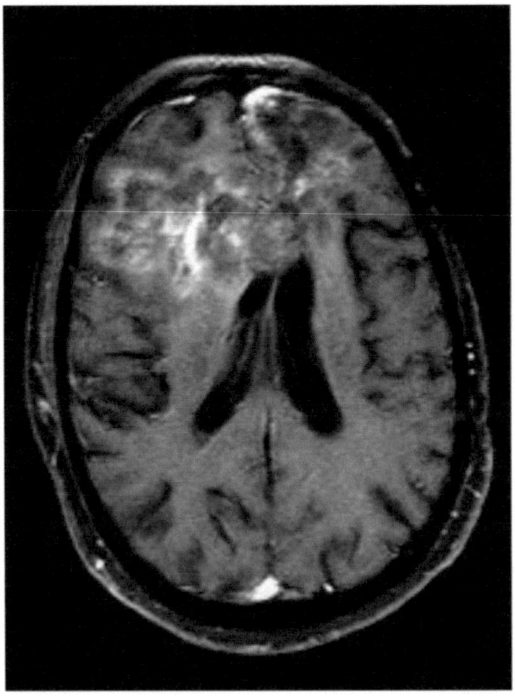

Figure 1. Butterfly glioma in a patient with bihemispheric spread due to involvement of the corpus callosum.

In this chapter, we discuss the composition of the brain's extracellular matrix, as well as the mechanisms by which tumor cells transition to a migratory phenotype and remodel the ECM through degradation by novel proteases and their inhibitors. We discuss the search for ECM molecules expressed by the tumor cells, which then respond to chemoattractants in the environment in order to direct growth. Finally, we discuss potential targets of anti-infiltrative therapy and the obstacles that must yet be overcome to address this important neuro-oncologic problem.

http://dx.doi.org/10.5772/63126

2. The Extracellular Matrix

The ECM consists of three components: (1) perineural nets (PN) which surround neural cells and their processes and provide support and regulate plasticity, (2) a complex interstitial matrix between cells, and (3) basement membranes that surround blood vessels made up primarily of laminin, fibronectin, and collagens. ECM components are secreted by resident cells and serve to provide structural cell support, regulate cell-cell connectivity and communication, and sequester growth factors and chemoattractants to regulate cell motility. The composition of the ECM varies from tissue to tissue and is comprised of proteoglycans such as chondroitin sulfate, heparin sulfate, keratin sulfate, and a lattice of interconnected fibrous proteins [8].

The neural extracellular matrix comprises 10–20% by volume of the brain and spinal cord and is structurally and functionally distinct from the ECM in other tissues [9] (**Figure 2**). The most abundant component of the neural ECM is hyaluronan (HA) and its associated glycoproteins. HA is a large hygroscopic glycosaminoglycan composed of alternating D-glucuronic acid and N-acetylglucosamine which is synthesized by hyaluronan synthase anchored to cell membranes [10]. In the developing brain, HA is organized into fiber-like structures along which neural precursors migrate. HA is anchored to astrocytes through its receptor, CD44, a transmembrane glycoprotein that couples the ECM to the actin cytoskeleton [11] and to hyaluronan synthase on neurons. Overexpression of CD44 was shown to increase the length of filopodia of neuroblastoma cells *in vitro* and promote invasion into a HA-rich matrix, demonstrating how overexpression of this single gene can affect the complex sequence of events for an invading cell to detach from its substrate, adhere to and degrade the surrounding matrix, and migrate through it [12].

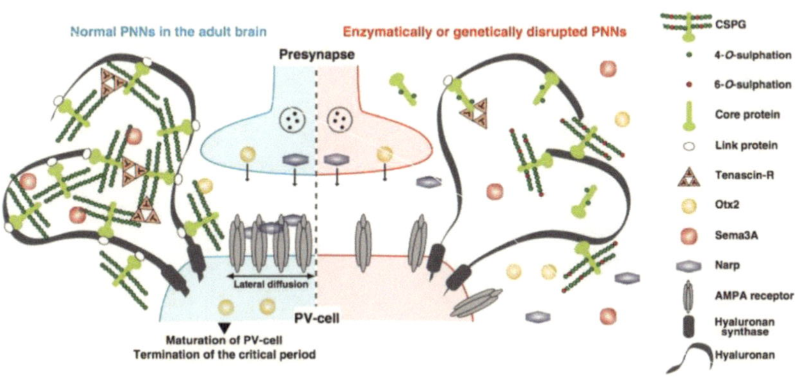

Figure 2. Structure of neural extracellular matrix (ECM). Reproduced with permission from Miyata et al. [14].

HA is associated with a number of proteins that are organized into a scaffold within the ECM. The major group is chondroitin sulfate proteoglycans (CSPGs) whose structure consists of a core protein covalently linked to chondroitin sulfate glycosaminoglycan (CS-GAG) through serine residues [13, 14]. Chondroitin sulfate is a disaccharide chain consisting of glucuronic acid and N-acetylgalactosamine linked via a β-glycosidic bond and is polymerized into chains through the activity of chondroitin synthase and polymerizing factor [15]. Variability within CSPG derives from variation within the core protein of CSPGs as well as the number and

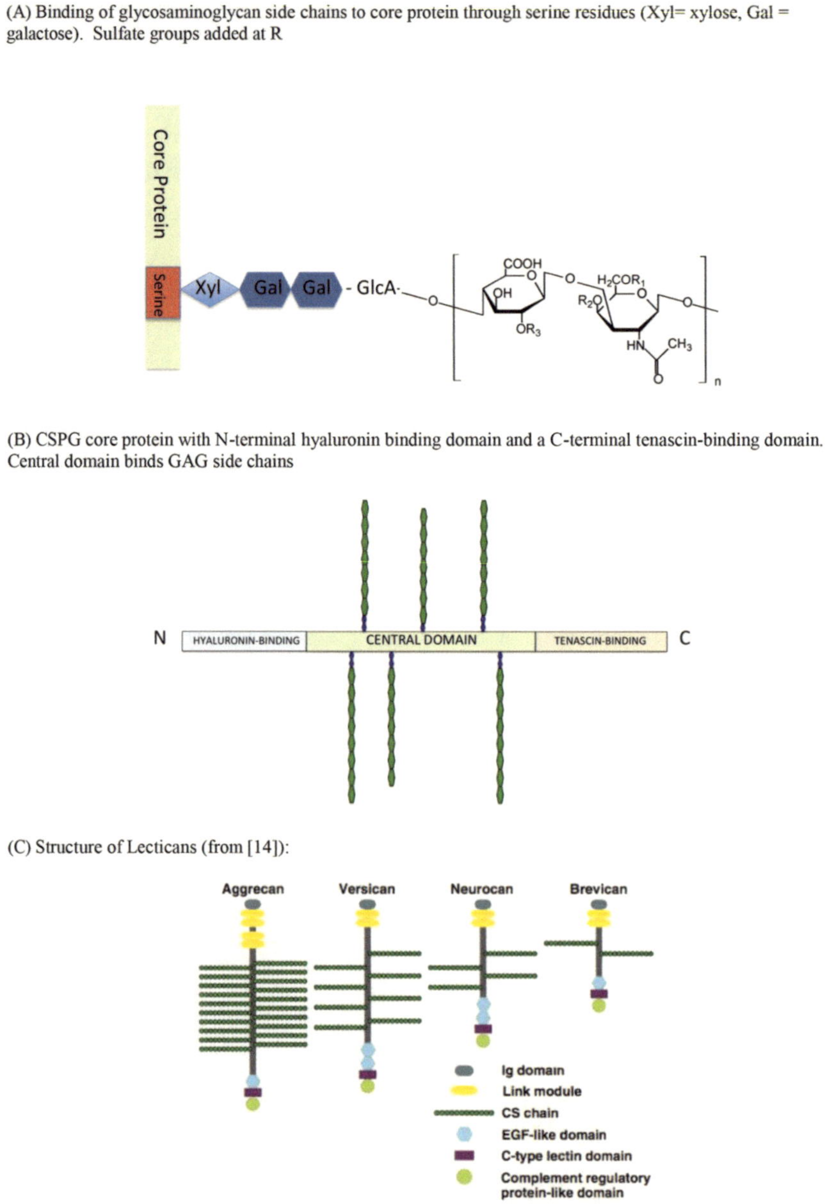

Figure 3. Chondroitin sulfate proteoglycan structure. (A) Binding of glycosaminoglycan side chains to core protein through serine residues (Xyl, xylose; Gal, galactose). Sulfate groups added at R. (B) CSPG core protein with N-terminal hyaluronan binding domain and a C-terminal tenascin-binding domain. Central domain binds GAG side chains. (C) Structure of Lecticans (Reproduced with permission from Miyata et al. [14]).

http://dx.doi.org/10.5772/63126

positions of sulfate groups, which are added via chondroitin sulfotransferases [16, 17]. This variability determines the CSPG binding properties and their function. Link proteins such as Bral-1 and 2, [18], Crtl1 [19], and HAPLN1 [20] stabilize the interaction between HA and CSPG within the PN. Mice lacking Crtl1 have attenuated PN and persistent plasticity in the visual cortex [21].

The classes of CSPG include (1) lecticans such as aggrecan, brevican, neurocan, and versican [22], (2) phosphacan (a tyrosine phosphatase) [23], and (3) small leucine-rich proteoglycans [24]. CSPG can be associated with the plasma membrane through a membrane-spanning domain [25] or a GPI-anchor [26], or can be secreted into the ECM (e.g., lecticans and phosphacan). In the CNS, the chondroitin sulfate side chains act as chemorepellents, and CPSGs are known to inhibit axon projection and cell motility and limit neural plasticity [27]. The lecticans are the principal CSPGs in the CNS, whose core proteins consist of an N-terminal HA-binding domain and a C-terminal domain that binds tenascin-R [28] and tenascin-C [29] (**Figure 3**).

The tenascin family of glycoproteins has four members, tenascin-R, -C, -X, and -W, which are encoded by four genes with a number of splice variants [30] and are believed to modulate cell adhesion and migration. Tenascin-R (formerly called restrictin) is found exclusively in the adult CNS and forms trimers which crosslink CSPGs. Tenascin-R inhibits adhesion of neural cells to fibronectin [31]. Tenascin-C is expressed during embryonic development by migrating neural crest cells, is re-expressed during wound healing and in gliomas, and is thought to be involved with increasing glioma cell proliferation and migration [32]. In tenascin-C knockout mice, CSPGs aggregate and fewer PN form [33]. Tenasacin-X is not found in the nervous system. Tenascin-W is expressed in blood vessels within gliomas and may be involved in angiogenesis [34].

The interstitial ECM forms a highly compressible network of HA and CSPG filaments that is resistant to cell migration by virtue of the inhibitory actions of CPSG, especially their CS components, paucity of anchorage points in the water-rich environment, and the presence of sequestered inhibitory molecules such as slits [35], semaphorins [36], and netrins [37].

In contrast to the hydrated PN that surrounds neurons and the loose interstitial matrix of the brain parenchyma, the ECM around the brain's vasculature and subpial surfaces forms a more rigid basal lamina that contains laminin, fibronectin, and type IV and VI collagens and is similar to the ECM in other tissues [35]. This substrate is more likely to allow adhesion of migrating cells and for this reason, gliomas tend to follow blood vessels and subpial surfaces as they invade into the surrounding tissue [36]. They do not, however, degrade the basal lamina and thus do not generally intravasate and spread hematogenously to distant sites.

3. Migration vs. proliferation

One of the characteristics of malignant gliomas that makes them universally fatal is their ability to infiltrate normal brain parenchyma. This diffuse spread makes surgical cure impossible and makes treatment with radiation and chemotherapy difficult and inefficient. The rapid proliferation of cells in malignant gliomas changes the tumor microenvironment, which becomes hypoxic, acidic, and devoid of glucose and other nutrients. Tumor cells must adapt to these changes to survive and thus change from a proliferative to a migratory phenotype in order to reach a more favorable environment. The mechanism by which tumor cells transition to this migratory state and the factors which trigger this process are therefore important to understand as it serves as an excellent target for therapy. This complex metabolic change, sometimes called the "epithelial-mesenchymal transition," is poorly understood, however, and involves multiple signal transduction pathways with many molecules needed to effect the changes in gene expression needed to bring about this transition.

One of the key molecules involved with sensing stress in a cell's microenvironment is the AMP-activated serine/threonine protein kinase (AMPK) [37]. AMPK is activated by a high AMP/ATP ratio and other conditions of metabolic stress and causes cells to conserve energy, thus regulating their cellular homeostasis in response to environmental cues. AMPK is activated in response to environmental stress through phosphorylation by three known protein kinases: liver kinase-B1 (LKB1) and the two calmodulin-dependent protein kinases, CaMKKα and CaMKKβ, that phosphorylate AMPK in response to high intracellular calcium levels [38]. Once activated, AMPK exerts its effects on cellular metabolism through many downstream molecules, one of which is cyclooxygenase-2 (COX2), whose inhibition by AMPK leads to more aggressive tumor growth and invasion [39]. Overexpression of COX2 has been seen in many types of cancer including colon, breast, and lung [40].

LKB1, a tumor suppressor gene, is constitutively active and is the primary AMPK kinase. Its phosphorylation of AMPK sets off a cascade that results in liberation of intracellular ATP and conservation of energy through regulation of biosynthetic pathways [41]. Mutations in LKB1 are found in Peutz-Jeghers syndrome [42] as well as melanoma [43], lung [44], and pancreatic cancers [45]. LKB1 signaling pathways also are involved in cell migration by virtue of their control of cytoskeletal proteins involved in cell polarization and migration. LKB1 deficiency leads to alterations in cell polarity and impaired migration of neural progenitor cells *in vivo* [46], while LKB1 activation is known to inhibit cell proliferation and can affect cellular polarity, which is essential for cell migration [47]. The latter effect is thought to be mediated, in part, through phosphorylation of MAP/microtubule affinity regulating kinase-3 (MARK-3), which regulates phosphorylation of microtubule-associated proteins [48] and phosphorylation of myosin light chain-2 directly by AMPK [49].

While the activation of AMPK leads to energy conservation in nutrient-poor environments, the mammalian target of rapamycin complex-1 (mTORC1) is a serine/threonine kinase, which promotes cell growth and proliferation. Inhibition of apoptosis [50] by mTOR overactivity has been observed in several types of cancers [51]. The balance between AMPK and mTOR is maintained in part by the tuberous sclerosis complex-2 gene (TSC-2), which is activated by AMPK and which, in turn, inactivates mTOR [50] (**Figure 4**). In addition, AMPK directly phosphorylates Raptor, a scaffold protein in the mTOR1 complex, resulting in direct inactivation of mTORC1 [52]. Mammalian target of rapamycin complex-2 (mTORC2) is considered resistant to rapamycin and is not sensitive to nutrients in the cellular microenvironment. It activates PKC-α and AKT to regulate the structure of the actin cytoskeleton [53].

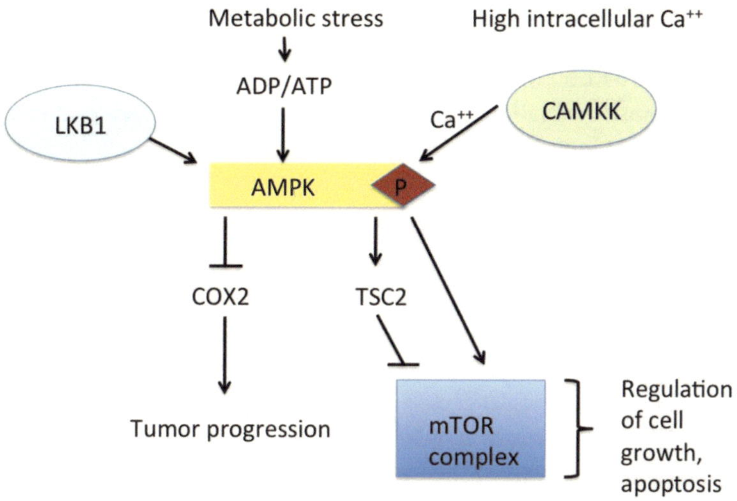

Figure 4. The AMPK/mTOR system. AMPK, AMP-activated serine/threonine protein kinase; CAMKK, Ca(2+)/calmodulin-dependent protein kinase kinase; COX2, cyclooxygenase-2; LKB1, liver kinase B1, mTOR, mammalian target of rapamycin; TSC2, tuberous sclerosis-2.

In addition to intracellular energy levels, hypoxia and acidity are triggers for cells to regulate their gene expression to adapt to a hostile environment. In tumors, hypoxia occurs due to rapid cell proliferation and inadequate blood supply from aberrant blood vessels. It leads to resistance to radiation and chemotherapy and is associated with a more aggressive disease and a poorer outcome. Oxygen homeostasis is mediated by the hypoxia-inducible factor (HIF) family of basic helix-loop-helix transcription factors, which consist of heterodimer of a constitutively expressed beta-subunit and an alpha-subunit which, when translated, is only stabilized under hypoxic conditions and is degraded once hypoxia has been corrected [54–56]. HIF-1 induces expression of dozens of target genes involved in the regulation of angiogenesis, cellular metabolism, and cell migration by binding to hypoxia-responsive elements (HREs) in their promoters. HIF-1α directly activates transcription of vascular endothelial growth factor (VEGF) [57, 58], which is the major regulator of angiogenesis and directs new blood vessel growth into hypoxic areas. HIF-2α knockdown leads to reduced levels of VEGF and poorly vascularized, highly necrotic tumors in neuroblastoma [59]. In order to adapt to hypoxia, cells switch from aerobic to anaerobic metabolism, and this shift is regulated, in part, by HIF-1. Glycolytic enzymes such as pyruvate kinase M2, phosphoglycerate kinase, and aldolase are induced by HIF-1 [60, 61] as are the glucose transporters, GLUT-1 and GLUT-3 [62]. Additionally, pyruvate dehydrogenase kinase-1 is activated, reducing mitochondrial oxygen consumption by preventing pyruvate from entering the citric acid cycle [63]. Finally,

HIF-1 is essential in the epithelial-mesenchymal transition by directly regulating the expression of Twist, which is essential for cancer metastasis [64]. Twist is a basic helix-loop-helix transcription factor whose expression is regulated through a number of signal transduction pathways including Akt, Ras, and Wnt and whose expression correlates with higher tumor grade [65]. It inhibits the E-cadherin-mediated adhesion between cells, which enables tumor cells to adopt a more motile phenotype [66]. Twist also serves as a survival factor by inhibiting p53-induced apoptosis by counteracting the effects of c-MYC in neuroblastoma [67]. HIF-1 regulates expression of a number of adhesion molecules, such as alpha- and beta-integrins and E-cadherin [68–70], matrix metalloproteinase-2 and -9 [71, 72] as well as a number of chemokines and their receptors including c-Met and CXCR4 [73–75], suggesting how hypoxia may play a role in triggering cell migration and digestion of the ECM.

Much remains to be elucidated regarding the molecular cascades through which cells transition to a migratory phenotype. Rapid proliferation creates a toxic microenvironment that, when sensed by the cell, sends a signal through the AMPK-mTORC axis or by HIF-1 and others to effect the changes in transcription needed to bring about the transformation to a migratory phenotype so the cell may escape to a more favorable environment. As they leave the main tumor mass and move into the brain parenchyma which limits and inhibits their migration, glioma cells remodel their environment by secreting degradative enzymes and novel ECM components which attempt to recapitulate the more permissive, primitive structure of the developing brain.

4. ECM Remodeling

4.1. Degradation

In 1946, Fisher [76] proposed that metastatic spread of tumors may be mediated by proteolytic degradation of the ECM. Since then, several classes of intracellular and extracellular proteases, both secreted and membrane-bound, have been identified which play roles in tumorigenesis including cell proliferation, adhesion, migration, angiogenesis, and apoptosis. The coordination between ECM degradation and subsequent cell adhesion to ECM components through integrin and other receptors followed by migration is the basis of glioma infiltration into brain parenchyma.

Lysosomal cathepsins are proteases, which are critical in removing other proteases which are in turn critical in removing unwanted cellular and extracellular components such as collagens, fibronectin, and laminin [77], and secreted cathepsins also mediate the activity of matrix metalloproteases (MMPs) by degrading their inhibitors TIMP-1 and TIMP-2 [78]. Cathepsin B promoter activity and protein levels are higher in high grade gliomas than in low-grade gliomas, and the protein is maximally expressed at the leading infiltrating edge of enlarging tumors [79]. Additionally, upregulation of cathepsins B and D has been shown to correlate with glioma tumor grade and invasiveness [80, 81], while inhibition inhibits glioma cell invasion *in vitro* [82]. Another class of intracellular proteases is the caspases, a family of intracellular cysteine proteases essential for apoptosis that are synthesized as inactive pro-caspases and activated by pro-apoptotic signals [83]. Malignant cells have the ability to escape apoptosis and, in neuroblastoma cells, the caspase 8 gene (CASP8) has been shown to be either deleted or silenced [84]. Loss of CASP8 correlates with increased risk of metastasis in patients with neuroblastoma. Other caspases, including CASP10, 3, 5, 6, and 7, have also found to be mutated in various tumor types [85–89].

Extracellular proteases are secreted by migrating tumor cells in order to degrade ECM components and to release chemoattractant and chemorepellent molecules to direct further tumor cell migration [90]. MMPs are a class of 28 zinc-dependent endopeptidases whose expression by tumor cells has been linked to increased invasion, proliferation, angiogenesis, and morbidity [91]. There are both membrane-bound MMPs and secreted forms which are released as inactive zymogens in response to growth factors such as platelet-derived growth factor (PDGF), epidermal growth factor (EGF), and transforming growth factor beta (TGF-β) [92], as well as in response to cell–cell and cell–ECM interactions and signaling [93]. These inactive proenzymes contain a pro-peptide residue at the N-terminus, which masks the zinc ion within the catalytic region. Proteolytic cleavage of this region exposes the catalytic domain and activates the enzyme [94]. MMP2 and MMP9 are both expressed in human glioma cells *in vitro* [95, 96] and overexpression in gliomas correlates with higher tumor grade and poorer prognosis [97]. The MMPs localize to the leading edges of migrating cells, and many components of the neural ECM have been identified as substrates for MMP2 and MMP9 including the lecticans-aggrecan [98], versican [99], brevican [100], and neurocan, as well as link protein and tenascin [101] and components of the vascular basement membrane such as laminin, fibronectin, and collagen [102]. Although these substrates have been demonstrated *in vitro*, the exact role of MMP *in vivo* is unclear. Versican, for example, appears not be a major MMP substrate *in vivo*, and glioma cells do not degrade the basal laminae of blood vessels to enter the bloodstream. MMP activity is tightly regulated at the level of transcription, activation of the zymogen, and by activity of tissue inhibitors of metalloproteases (TIMS) [103]; the degree of ECM digestion during migration is clearly a complex and carefully regulated process. MMPs are also involved in the "pro-angiogenic switch" that stimulates the production of new blood vessels into the growing tumor mass [104], a process mediated, in large part, by the VEGF signaling pathway [105]. The transmembrane metalloprotease, MT1-MMP, can directly degrade the ECM and also activate pro-MMP2 and upregulate VEGF expression [106], suggesting that this MMP may play a major role in tumor invasiveness and angiogenesis and may serve as a potential target for therapy.

Another class of zinc-dependent metalloproteases is the ADAMS (a disintegrin and metalloproteinase) and the related ADAMTS (a disintegrin and metalloproteinase with thrombospondin motifs). ADAMS are membrane-bound, zinc-dependent metalloproteases that contain a pro-domain which is cleaved to activate the metalloprotease, a disintegrin domain which can bind to integrin receptors, a cysteine-rich domain, an EGF-like domain, and a transmembrane domain at the C terminus [107] (**Figure 5**). ADAMTS are extracellular proteases similar in structure but lack the EGF and transmembrane domains and contain an additional thrombospondin type I motif at the C terminus which may bind them to the ECM [108]. ADAM-8 and ADAM-19 are expressed at high levels in gliomas, and its expression correlates with invasiveness [109]. ADAM-17 activates the EGF/phosphoinositide-3 kinase/serine/threonine kinase signal transduction pathway under hypoxic conditions and leads to increased tumor cell invasion [110]. ADAM-22 normally inhibits astrocyte proliferation in normal brain via interactions between its disintegrin domain and cell surface integrins. It is downregulated in high-grade gliomas leading to elimination of this growth inhibition [111]. ADAMTS-4 and ADAMTS-5 degrade the lectican and small leucine-rich repeat families of proteoglycans, and their expression also correlates with glioma invasiveness [112].

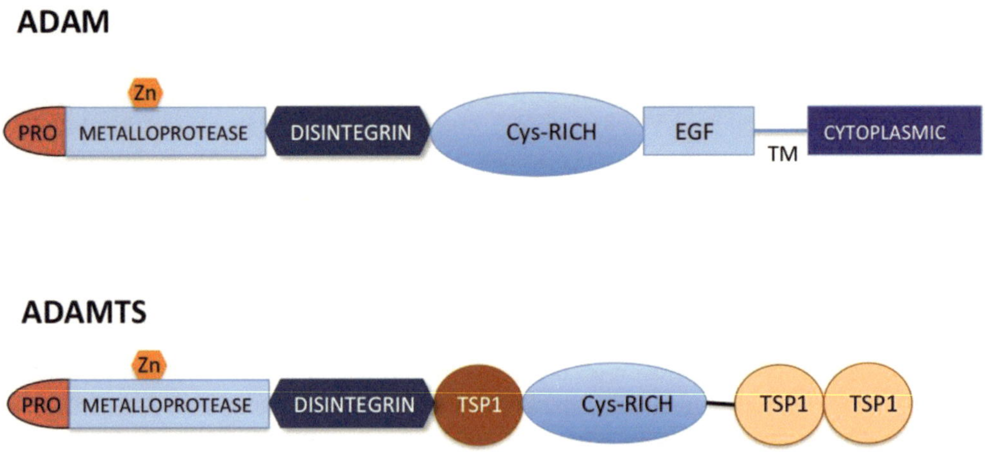

Figure 5. ADAM/ADAMT structure. ADAM and ADAMT members contain a propeptide domain (Pro) followed by the enzymatic metalloprotease domain containing the Zn-binding site followed by the disintegrin- and cystein-rich domains. ADAM members contain an EGF-like domain and ADAMTS contain additional thrombospondin type 1 motifs (TSP1) transmembrane (TM).

Finally, plasmin degrades ECM components and activates several MMPs, and the plasminogen activators, urokinase-type PA (uPA), expressed by glioma cells, and tissue-type PA (tPA) transmembrane (TM) expressed in the endothelium of blood vessels, both play an important role in tumor cell invasion and angiogenesis [113, 114]. There is a higher level of expression of uPA in higher-grade gliomas than in lower-grade gliomas [115] and its binding to its receptor (uPAR) causes it to form a heteromeric complex with integrin receptors, which are also highly expressed on glioma cells. These then initiate signal transduction cascades that result in the upregulation of uPA, MMP, and other molecules that promote cell migration through the ECM [116].

4.2. Synthesis

It is evident that intracellular and extracellular proteases play important roles in the complex process of glioma cell-cell adhesion and attachment and detachment to ECM components during migration. This process is mediated by a well-regulated cascade of signal transduction pathways that also lead to the production of novel ECM components to create a new scaffold on which tumor cells can migrate. As migrating cells degrade the ECM, they further change their microenvironment by secreting novel proteins and liberating peptides on which to migrate and generating chemoattractants and chemorepellents for guidance. In many ways, this new environment is reminiscent of that of the primitive CNS in which cell migration was abundant in setting up the organization of the brain.

One of the earliest events in glioma formation is the loss of the p53 tumor suppressor gene and upregulation of secreted protein acidic and rich in cysteine (SPARC), an ECM-associated glycoprotein that has an anti-adhesive role and leads to cell rounding and detachment from the ECM [117]. This is thought to be accomplished through the activation of P38 mitogen-activated protein kinase (MAPK)-heat shock protein (HSP)-27, Akt, and Shc-Raf-extracellular signal-regulated kinase (ERK) signaling pathways [118]. SPARC is secreted at the leading edge of the invading cells [119] and has been shown to increase invasion *in vitro* [120] and *in vivo* [121]. Additionally, the combination of SPARC overexpression and loss of p53 may play a role in promoting cell survival by escaping immune surveillance [122]. SPARC is highly expressed in gliomas, and increased levels are associated with poorer prognosis [123]. Interestingly, SPARC levels are higher in developing brain, where cell migration is necessary for setting up the architecture of the developing brain, so it is not surprising that invading glioma cells try to recapitulate this more permissive environment.

The Receptor-type protein tyrosine phosphatase mu (PTPμ) is a cell adhesion molecule normally found in neurons and glia but is absent in higher-grade, infiltrative gliomas. It is hypothesized to be involved with cell-cell adhesion and contact inhibition and that its loss allows for cell migration [124]. PTPμ is cleaved in human GBM tumor tissue and cell lines by a number of proteases including ADAMS, calpain, and serine proteases to generate protein fragments with unique biologic functions affecting cell adhesion and migration [125]. In addition to the degradation of the protein component of the ECM, glioma cells secrete hyaluronidases, which break down HA in the ECM, generating soluble HA, which activates MMP and promotes invasion [126]. Increased levels of HA and hyaluronectin are found in peripherally invasive regions of certain tumors [127] creating a more disorganized matrix through which cells can migrate. Receptor-type protein tyrosine phosphatase zeta (RPTP-ζ) is a membrane-bound proteoglycan expressed in developing and adult brains as well as in migrating glioma cells [128]. The soluble factor pleiotrophin is overexpressed in gliomas and, through binding to RPTP-ζ, promotes cytoskeletal changes through modification of beta-catenin, beta-adducin, and Fyn [129]. RPTP-ζ undergoes differential splicing and one splice variant, phosphacan, is a soluble factor lacking the cytoplasmic phosphatase domain. Phosphacan is also highly expressed during embryogenesis and in migrating glioma cells and may regulate glioma migration through interactions with tenascin in the ECM [130] and axonin [131].

Two members of the lectican family, which are normally inhibitory to cell migration, versican and brevican, have unique isoforms that are present at different times of development, and these tumor-specific isoforms have been shown to promote invasion. Versican undergoes differential splicing to generate four different isoforms (V0, V1, V2, and V3), which vary in their GAG-binding domains. The V2 isoform is predominant in the adult CNS and is a potent inhibitor of axonal growth into the ECM [132]. The V0/V1 isoform, however, is found in the primitive developing brain and is upregulated by TGF-β in malignant glioma [133], where it acts as a pro-migratory factor by upregulating membrane type 1 matrix metalloprotease (MT1-MMP) through the activation of microglial Toll-like receptor 2 (TLR2) [134]. Brevican, on the other hand, undergoes differential glycosylation and there are novel glycoforms in gliomas in developing and mature brain [135]. It is overexpressed in malignant gliomas, and its brevican knockdown inhibits proliferation, invasion, and spread of brevican-expressing glioma cells *in vitro* [136]. Not only is brevican overexpressed in gliomas, it is also proteolytically cleaved by metalloproteases of the ADAMTS family including ADAMTS-4 and -5, which are also overexpressed in gliomas [137]. If this posttranslational cleavage is blocked, brevican does not enhance glioma cell invasion *in vitro* or tumor progression *in vivo* [138].

Because the basal lamina of blood vessels presents a more favorable substrate for migration, it is not surprising that migrating glioma cells secrete basal lamina components to travel on. For example, certain laminin isoforms are secreted by glioma cells, and these cells interact with these isoforms and others on the tumor vasculature through the alpha3beta1 integrin during migration [139]. As tumor cells proliferate, the tumor mass becomes denser, and this mechanical stress induces secretion of collagens, their crosslinker LOX, and the angiogenic factor VEGF [140]. Collagens bind to integrins via integrin-binding domains at the cell surface and can thus activate signal transduction pathways that control proliferation, angiogenesis, and migration [141]. Integrins are associated with the actin cytoskeleton through the interaction with talin and with the microtubule network via paxillin and binding to components of the cytoskeleton modulates the affinity of integrins for the ECM [142]. Glioma cells can migrate along fibronectin in the vascular ECM, and both versican and brevican can increase synthesis of fibronectin through an EGFR-dependent mechanism by binding to β-1 integrin and β-3 integrin, respectively [143–145]. These newly synthesized fibronectin fibrils accumulate at the migrating cell surface and serve to reorganize the ECM and promote cell attachment [146, 147].

4.3. Transcriptional control

The regulation of the expression of novel proteins in gliomas is poorly understood but is surely a complex process involving many signal transduction pathways and transcription factors, and some candidates have emerged that may regulate cell migration. The Oct-3/4 transcription factor is involved in regulating self-renewal in stem cells and was recently found to be overexpressed in malignant gliomas. Oct-3/4 expressing-glioblastoma cells exhibited increased migration and invasion *in vitro* and resulted in upregulated FAK and c-Src expression, which mediate integrin signals as well as increased MMP-13 expression [148]. ATF2, another transcription factor expressed in malignant glioma, is thought to be involved in the regulation of cell invasion as its level of expression is correlated with cell invasion *in vitro* [149]. Finally, suppressor of fused (Sufu) is a tumor suppressor which downregulates hedgehog, WNT, and other signaling pathways to prevent tumorigenesis [150, 151]. Overexpression suppresses glioma cell proliferation and invasiveness, angiogenesis, and *in vivo* tumor growth, while knockdown of Sufu promoted these effects, possibly by directly affecting Gli1, a transcription factor in the hedgehog signaling pathway [152].

http://dx.doi.org/10.5772/63126

4.4. Chemotaxis

Once glial cells switch to a migratory phenotype, they degrade the ECM surrounding them, detach from the matrix and extend "invadopodia", actin-rich protrusions with ECM proteolytic activity that bind to and digest ECM components as a result of complex signal transduction pathways linking the extracellular microenvironment to the actin cytoskeleton [153]. Cells respond to soluble molecules in this environment and use these cues to direct migration through various signal transduction pathways. These include growth factors, soluble peptides generated by proteolysis of cell surface adhesion molecules [118], and small chemotactic cytokines.

The EGF family of growth factors is known to stimulate cell proliferation and migration [154], and overexpression of EGF receptor (EGFR) is an important feature distinguishing high-grade from low-grade gliomas [155], and the highest level of expression is found at the invasive border of the expanding tumor [156]. EGFR is amplified in 40% of GBM and of these, half have a mutant form of the receptor (EGFRvIII) lacking the ligand-binding domain leading to constitutive activation [157]. Ligand binding induces dimerization and activation of EGFR, a receptor tyrosine kinase (RTK), whose signaling results in cell proliferation, angiogenesis as well as metastatic spread through the activation of PI3K-AKT-GSK3b-Rac1 and Ras-Raf-MEK-ERK signal transduction pathways [158]. However, the activation of wild-type EGFR promotes invasion independent of angiogenesis, whereas loss of its activity results in angiogenic tumor growth. EGFRvIII might only be involved in stimulating angiogenic tumor growth when wild-type EGFR expression is lost [159,160]. Formylpeptide receptor (FPR) is a G-protein-coupled receptor that has been shown to be expressed in highly malignant gliomas [161]. Necrotic GBM cells release a number of potential ligands for FPR, and the activation of this pathway promotes chemotaxis as well as the production of VEGF [162, 163]. In addition, FPR has been shown to transactivate EGFR leading to increased chemotaxis and proliferation [164].

Scatter factor/hepatocyte growth factor (SF/HGF) as well as its receptor which is encoded by the c-MET proto-oncogene are both are upregulated in malignant gliomas. MET is a transmembrane RTK whose signal transduction cascade leads to increased gliomas motility *in vitro* as well as survival and angiogenesis [165]. Fibroblast growth factor (FGF) may act synergistically with upregulated VEGF and SF/HGF in GBM cells to enhance malignancy [166].

Serine-threonine kinases also play a role in tumorigenesis. TGF-β is an important growth factor whose signaling is involved in invasion as well as proliferation and survival of glioma cells [167]. Its receptor is a serine-threonine kinase that, on ligand binding, oligomerizes and activates a signal transduction cascade that results in the translocation of activated Smads to the nucleus where they interact with other transcription factors to regulate expression of genes involved in cell motility and proliferation [168]. TGF-β signaling upregulates MMP expression and suppresses tissue inhibitors of metalloproteinase (TIMP), thus promoting invasion [169] and inhibition of TGF-β1 or knockdown of its receptor reduces invasiveness *in vitro* [170].

Chemotactic cytokines are a group of small molecules that have been found to regulate the migration of leukocytes in the immune system and have been found to be involved in metastatic behavior of certain cancers [171]. Chemokine receptors are G-protein-coupled transmembrane receptors whose signaling pathways regulate many cellular activities including motility. Chemokines and their receptors are expressed throughout the CNS by neurons and glia and are overexpressed in high-grade gliomas [172]. Stromal-derived factor 1 (SDF-1) also called CXCL2 is a chemotactic cytokine, which, along with its receptor CXCR4, is overexpressed in gliomas as well as within the vascular endothelium along the hypoxic rim of the tumor [173, 174]. SDF-1 has been shown to promote the migration of glioma cells *in vitro* [175] by upregulating the expression of membrane type-2 matrix metalloproteinase (MT2-MMP) [176]. CXCL1 is another small chemokine known to be involved in the metastatic spread in melanoma [177] and has been shown to be highly expressed in glioma samples and promotes migration *in vitro* by upregulating MMP-2 and β1-integrin [178]. TGF-β signaling promotes invasion by reducing expression of neurotactin, a chemokine also known as CX3CL1 whose pro-adhesive properties must be overcome to allow cells to detach and migrate. The treatment of glioma cells with recombinant TGF-β1 reduced CX3CL1, expression and facilitated glioma cell detachment and dispersion [179].

Both positive and negative signals exist within the microenvironment of glioma cells, and hypoxia is an important chemorepellent as described previously which induces cell migration away from the tumor mass. HIF-1α is stabilized at the leading tumor edge and mediates cell invasion and angiogenesis through integrin and RTK signaling pathways [180]. Slit glycoproteins are secreted into the ECM and normally serve as chemorepulsive factors but whose expression is diminished in invasive gliomas through promoter methylation. They normally bind to members of the Roundabout (Robo) family of transmembrane receptors and lead to depolymerization of the actin cytoskeleton within the invadopodia to promote cell adhesion [181, 182]. This may be accomplished through the inactivation of Cdc42, a Rho GTPase known to be involved in cell motility [183].

Semaphorins and their receptors (plexins and neuropilins) have been found to be involved in cell migration and metastasis as well as proliferation and angiogenesis in several types of cancers [184–188], and different members of the family have different functions depending on the type of tumor involved. For example, Sema 3A inhibits migration in GBM and has anti-angiogenic properties in meningioma [189, 190]. Secreted semaphorins contain an N-terminal sema domain followed by variable numbers of PSI (plexins, semaphorins, and integrins) and immunoglobulin-like domains in their extracellular regions [191]. Sema 3A binds to the Neuropilin-1 receptor that recruits the PlexinA1 receptor to transduce a chemorepulsive signal. Sema3A also binds Neuropilin-2 but at a lower affinity than Neuropilin-1, and the binding of Neuropilin-2 acts to modulate cell signaling and converts the repulsive signal into an attractive one. Blocking Neuropilin-1 or Plexin A1 switches the Sema3A response from repulsion to attraction, while blockade of Neuropilin-2 suppresses Sema3A's typical chemorepulsive effect [192]. Similarly, Sema 4D which binds to PlexinB1 and acts through Rho [193], and Sema5A which binds to PlexinB3 and acts through Rac1, both act as chemorepellents by ultimately affecting the actin cytoskeleton and altering cell morphology [194].

Finally, Netrins are secreted laminin-associated chemotactic molecules that regulate embryonic axon migration [195] which have also been shown to be involved in glioma cell migra-

http://dx.doi.org/10.5772/63126

tion, mediated by binding to their receptors, deleted in colorectal cancer (DCC), neogenin, and uncoordinated-5 (UNC5) [196–198]. Netrins have been shown to localize to cell surfaces and interact with laminins in the basement membrane of blood vessels. Netrin-1 binding to DCC receptors on migrating glia promotes the formation of focal adhesions, limiting migration. GBMs have been shown to downregulate Netrins, thus releasing the inhibition and promoting loss of cell-cell interaction, promoting migration along basement membranes [199]. Though Netrin-1 binding to the DCC receptor tends to promote adhesion, limiting migration, UNC5 binding transforms this to repulsion [200]. This switch from attachment to motility is reminiscent of that described earlier with the semaphorins.

5. Future Directions

Current therapy for malignant gliomas is aimed at reducing tumor burden and targeting dividing cells with cytotoxic chemotherapy, anti-angiogenic agents, or tumor-treating fields. New agents targeting new pathways are desperately needed as survival still remains extremely poor and glioma cells become resistant over time to current therapies. Delivering therapy to normal brain parenchyma containing infiltrating tumor cells is also difficult as the blood-brain barrier remains largely intact, though several strategies have been attempted to overcome this [201]. Limiting the invasiveness of these aggressive tumors is desirable; however, the molecular pathways involved in this complex process remain incompletely understood and new targets and therapies are lacking. Additionally, because tumor cells seem to adopt either a proliferative or migratory phenotype, preventing migration may impose a selective advantage for cells to proliferate rather than migrate leading to more rapid local recurrences. There is also no way to visualize invading cells until they stop migrating and proliferate to create a radiographically evident tumor mass. Two-dimensional *in vitro* assays have been used to study this process using glass or plastic substrates and more recently, assays using hydrogels or nanofiber scaffolds have been developed to better simulate the three-dimensional microenvironment encountered by migrating tumor cells [202–204].

Identifying molecular targets has been a priority in developing new therapies for GBM, and the complex process of cell migration offers many potential targets including ECM components, proteases, and members of signal transduction pathways. The neural ECM has many unique components that are potential targets for therapy. Because tenascin is upregulated in malignant gliomas and may be a stem cell marker [205], it is an attractive target and phase I trials are underway exploring the use of radiolabeled monoclonal antibodies to tenascin-C or tenascin-R to deliver a radiation boost to the resection cavity. Since many signal transduction pathways involved in glioma invasion often involve RTKs, and since various RTKs are mutated or overexpressed in GBM, RTK inhibitors are an obvious choice of targeted therapy. The results, however, have been disappointing, and no clear RTK inhibitor or combination has demonstrated a significant survival benefit [206]. Similarly, several inhibitors of MMPs have been investigated and, though some have shown efficacy *in vitro*, no clear clinical benefit has yet been demonstrated [207–209]. Cilengitide is an arginine-glycine-aspartic acid containing peptide that targets integrins and, though it was promising in preclinical studies, it failed to show improvement in progression-free survival or overall survival in both the CENTRIC [210] and CORE [211] trials investigating the addition of cilengitide to standard therapy in patients with newly diagnosed GBM with or without MGMT promoter methylation.

Many molecules involved in regulating cell migration in malignant gliomas are also involved in angiogenesis, cell proliferation, and avoidance of apoptosis; so agents targeting these molecules would be expected to have multiple antitumor effects. However, results have been mixed and, though *in vitro* data are encouraging for many agents, none has proven successful in showing clinical improvement in survival. There is apparently much redundancy in these signaling pathways, requiring a more complete understanding of these molecular events as well as more accurate modeling with which to study the complex processes involved in tumor spread. The earliest events leading to a migratory phenotype would be ideal candidates for therapy, though inhibiting migration could select for a proliferating phenotype leading to faster local recurrence. Hopefully, as we achieve a better understanding of the genetics and molecular alterations leading to glioma invasion, new therapies will arise to limit this aggressive, deadly disease.

Author details

Scott G. Turner*, Maleeha Ahmad and Steven A. Toms

*Address all correspondence to: sgturner@geisinger.edu

Departments of Neurology and Neurosurgery, Geisinger Medical Center, Danville, PA, USA

References

[1] Dolecek TA, Propp JM, Stroup NE, Kruchko C. CBTRUS statistical report: primary brain and central nervous system tumors diagnosed in the United States in 2005–2009. Neuro Oncol. 2012; 14 Suppl 5:v1-49.

[2] Stupp R, Mason WP, van den Bent MJ, et al. Radiotherapy plus Concomitant and Adjuvant Temozolomide for Glioblastoma. N Engl J Med. 2005; 352:987–996.

[3] Vredenburgh JJ, Desjardins A, Herndon JE, Marcello J, Reardon DA, Quinn JA, Rich JN, Sathornsumetee S, Gururangan S, Sampson J, Wagner M, Bailey L, Bigner DD, Friedman AH, Friedman HS. Bevacizumab plus irinotecan in recurrent glioblastoma multiforme. J Clin Oncol. 2007; 25(30):4722–9.

[4] Stupp R, Taillibert S, Kanner AA, et al. Maintenance Therapy With Tumor-Treating Fields Plus Temozolomide vs Temozolomide Alone for Glioblastoma: A Randomized Clinical Trial. JAMA. 2015; 314(23):2535–2543.

[5] Hou LC, Veeravagu A, Hsu AR, Tse VCK. Recurrent Glioblastoma Multiforme: A Review of Natural History and Management Options. Neurosurg Focus. 2006; 20(4):E5.

[6] Giese A, Westphal M. Glioma invasion in the central nervous system. Neurosurgery. 1996;39(2):235–250.

[7] Wolf K, Mazo I, Leung H, Engelke K , von Andrian UH., Deryugina EI, Strongin AY, Bröcker EB, Friedl P. Compensation mechanism in tumor cell migration/mesenchymal–amoeboid transition after blocking of pericellular proteolysis. JCB. 2003; 160(2): 267–277.

[8] Lau LW, Cua R, Keough MB, Haylock-Jacobs S, Yong VW. Pathophysiology of the Brian Extracellular Matrix: a new target of remyelination. Natire Reviews. 2013; 14:722–729.

[9] Bignami A, Hosley M, Dahl D. Hyaluronic Acid and Hyaluronic Acid-Binding Proteins in Brain Extracellular Matrix. Anat. Embryol. 1993; 188:419–433.

[10] Delpech B, Maingonnat C, Girard N, Chauzy C, Maunoury R, Olivier A, Tayot J, Creissard P. Hyaluronan and hyaluronectin in the extracellular matrix of human brain tumour stroma. Eur J Cancer. 1993; 29A(7):1012–7.

[11] Misra S, Heldin P, Hascall VC, Karamanos NK, Skandalis SS, Markwald RR, Ghatak S. Hyaluronan-CD44 interactions as potential targets for cancer therapy. FEBS J. 2011; 278(9):1429–43.

[12] Pusch A, Boeckenhoff A, Glaser T, Kaminski T, Kirfel G, Hans M, Steinfarz B, Swandulla D, Kubitscheck U, Gieselmann V, Brüstle O, Kappler J. CD44 and hyaluronan promote invasive growth of B35 neuroblastoma cells into the brain. Biochimica et Biophysica Acta (BBA) - Molecular Cell Research. 2010; 1803(2): 261–274.

[13] Mikami T, Kitagawa H. Biosynthesis and function of chondroitin sulfate. Biochim. Biophys Acta. 2013; 1830: 4719–4733.

[14] Sugahara K, Mikami T. Chondroitin/der- matan sulfate in the central nervous system. Curr. Opin. Struct. Biol. 2007; 17:536–545.

[15] Mikami T, Kitagawa H. Biosynthesis and function of chondroitin sulfate. Biochim. Biophys. Acta. 2013; 1830:4719–4733.

[16] Ohtake S, Ito Y, Fukuta M, Habuchi O. Human N-acetylgalactosamine 4-sulfate 6-O-sulfotrans- ferase cDNA is related to human B cell recombination activating gene-associated gene. J. Biol. Chem. 2001; 276: 43894–43900.

[17] Kobayashi M, Sugumaran G, Liu J, Shworak NW, Silbert JE, Rosenberg RD. Molecular cloning and characterization of a human uronyl 2-sulfo- transferase that sulfates iduronyl and glucuronyl residues in dermatan/chondroitin sulfate. J. Biol. Chem. 1999; 274:10474–10480.

[18] Oohashi T, Hirakawa S, Bekku Y, Rauch U, Zimmermann DR, Su WD, Ohtsuka A, Murakami T, Ninomiya Y. Bral1, a brain-specific link protein, colocalizing with the

versican V2 isoform at the nodes of Ranvier in developing and adult mouse central nervous systems. Mol. Cell. Neurosci. 2002; 19:43–57.

[19] Carulli D, Pizzorusso T, Kwok JCF, Putignano E, Poli A, Forostyak S, Andrews MR, Deepa SS, Glant TT, Fawcett JW. Animals lacking link protein have attenuated perineuronal nets and persistent plasticity. Brain 2010; 133:2331–2347.

[20] Sim H, Hu B, Viapiano MS. Reduced Expression of the Hyaluronan and Proteoglycan Link Proteins in Malignant Gliomas. J Biol Chem. 2009; 284(39):26547–26556.

[21] Carulli D, Pizzorusso T, Kwok JCF, Putignano E, Poli A, Forostyak S, Andrews MR, Deepa SS, Glant TT, Fawcett JW. Animals lacking link protein have attenuated perineuronal nets and persistent plasticity. Brain 2010; 133:2331–2347.

[22] Yamaguchi Y. Lecticans: organizers of the brain extracellular matrix. Cell. Mol. Life Sci. 2000; 57:276–289.

[23] Levy JB, Canoll PD, Silvennoinen O, Barnea G, Morse B, Honegger AM, Huang JT, Cannizzaro LA, Park SH, Druck T. The cloning of a receptor-type protein tyrosine phosphatase expressed in the central nervous system. J Biol Chem. 1993; 268(14):10573–10581.

[24] Dellett M, Hu W, Papadaki V, Ohnuma S. Small leucine rich proteoglycan family regulates multiple signalling pathways in neural development and maintenance. Dev Growth Differ. 2012; 54(3):327–340.

[25] Kinugasa Y, Ishiguro H, Tokita Y, Oohira A, Ohmoto H, Higashiyama S. Neuroglycan C, a novel member of the neuregulin family. Biochem Biophys Res Commun. 2004; 321(4):1045–9.

[26] Seidenbecher CI, Smalla KH, Fischer N, Gundelfinger ED, Kreutz MR. Brevican isoforms associate with neural membranes. Journal of Neurochemistry. 2002; 83(3):738–746.

[27] Niederost BP, Zimmermann DR, Schwab ME, Bandtlow CE. Bovine CNS myelin contains neurite growth-inhibitory activity associated with chondroitin sulfate proteoglycans. J. Neurosci. 1999; 19:8979–8989.

[28] Yamaguchi Y. Lecticans: organizers of the brain extracellular matrix. Cell. Mol. Life Sci. 2000; 57:276–289.

[29] Day JM, Olin AI, Murdoch AD, Canfield A, Sasaki T, Timpl R, Hardingham TE, Aspberg A. Alternative splicing in the aggrecan G3 domain influences binding interactions with Tenascin-C and other extracellular matrix proteins. J. Biol. Chem. 2004; 279:12511–12518.

[30] Hsia H, Schwarzbauer J. Meet the tenascins: multifunctional and mysterious. J Biol Chem. 2005; 280 (29): 26641–26644.

[31] Pesheva P, Probstmeier R, Skubitz AP, McCarthy JB, Furcht LT, Schachner M. Tenascin-R (J1 160/180) inhibits fibronectin-mediated cell adhesion–functional relatedness to tenascin-C. J Cell Sci. 1994; 107: 2323–2333.

[32] Herold-Mende C, Mueller MM, Bonsanto MM, Schmitt HP, Kunze S, Steiner HH. Clinical impact and functional aspects of tenascin-C expression during glioma progression. Int. J. Cancer. March 2002; 98(3): 362–369.

[33] Garcion E, Faissner A, Ffrench-Constant C. Knockout mice reveal a contribution of the extracellular matrix molecule tenascin-C to neural precursor proliferation and migration. Development. 2001; 128(13):2485–2496.

[34] Martina E, Degen M, Rüegg C, Merlo A, Lino MM, Chiquet-Ehrismann R, Brellier F. Tenascin-W is a specific marker of glioma-associated blood vessels and stimulates angiogenesis in vitro. FASEB J. 2010; 24(3):778–787.

[35] Gladson CL. The extracellular matrix of gliomas: modulation of cell function. J Neuropathol Exp Neurol. 1999; 58(10):1029–1040.

[36] Cuddapah VA, Robel S, Watkins S, Sontheimer HA. Neurocentric perspective on glioma invasion. Nature Reviews. 2014; 15: 455–465.

[37] Hue L, Rider MH. The AMP-activated protein kinase: more than an energy sensor. Essays Biochem. 2007; 43:121–137.

[38] Woods A, Dickerson K, Heath R, Hong SP, Momcilovic M, Johnstone SR, Carlson M, Carling D. Ca2+/calmodulin-dependent protein kinase kinase-beta acts upstream of AMP-activated protein kinase in mammalian cells. Cell Metab. 2005; 2(1):21–33.

[39] Lee YK, Park SY, Kim YM, Lee WS, Park OJ. AMP kinase/cyclooxygenase-2 pathway regulates proliferation and apoptosis of cancer cells treated with quercetin. Experimental & Molecular Medicine. 2009; 41:201–207.

[40] Sobolewski C, Cerella C, Dicato M, Ghibelli L, Diederich M. The Role of Cyclooxygenase-2 in Cell Proliferation and Cell Death in Human Malignancies. International Journal of Cell Biology. 2009; 2010:1–21.

[41] Woods A, Johnstone SR, Dickerson K, Leiper FC, Fryer LG, Neumann D, Schlattner U, Wallimann T, Carlson M, Carling D. LKB1 is the upstream kinase in the AMP-activated protein kinase cascade. Curr Biol. 2003; 13(22):2004–2008.

[42] Hemminki A, Avizienyte E, Roth S, Loukola A, Aaltonen LA, Jarvinen H, de la Chapelle A. A serine/ threonine kinase gene defective in Peutz–Jeghers syndrome. Duodecim 1998; 114:667–668.

[43] Guldberg P, thor Straten P, Ahrenkiel V, Seremet T, Kirkin AF, Zeuthen J. Somatic mutation of the Peutz–Jeghers syndrome gene, LKB1/STK11, in malignant melanoma. Oncogene 1999; 18:1777–1780.

[44] Hearle N, Schumacher V, Menko FH, Olschwang S, Boardman LA, Gille JJ, Keller JJ, Westerman AM, Scott RJ, Lim W, et al. Frequency and spectrum of cancers in the Peutz–Jeghers syndrome. Clin Cancer Res. 2006; 12:3209–3215.

[45] Su GH, Hruban RH, Bansal RK, Bova GS, Tang DJ, Shekher MC, Westerman AM, Entius MM, Goggins M, Yeo CJ, Kern SE. Germline and somatic mutations of the STK11/LKB1 Peutz–Jeghers gene in pancreatic and biliary cancers. Am J Pathol 1999; 154:1835–1840.

[46] Asada N, Sanada K, Fukada Y. LKB1 regulates neuronal migration and neuronal differentiation in the developing neocortex through centrosomal positioning. J Neurosci. 2007; 27(43):11769–11775.

[47] Alessi DR, Sakamoto K, Bayascas JR. LKB1-dependent signaling pathways. Annu Rev Biochem. 2006; 75:137–163.

[48] Sapir T, Sapoznik S, Levy T, Finkelshtein D, Shmueli A, Timm T, Mandelkow EM, Reiner O. Accurate balance of the polarity kinase MARK2/Par-1 is required for proper cortical neuronal migration. J Neurosci. 2008; 28(22):5710–5720.

[49] Lee JH, Koh H, Kim M, Kim Y, Lee SY, Karess RE, Lee SH, Shong M, Kim JM, Kim J, Chung J. Energy-dependent regulation of cell structure by AMP-activated protein kinase. Nature. 2007; 447(7147):1017–1020.

[50] Shaw RJ. LKB1 and AMPK control of mTOR signalling and growth Acta Physiol (Oxf). 2009; 196(1): 65–80.

[51] Hardt M, Chantaravisoot N, Tamanoi F. Activating mutations of TOR (target of rapamycin). Genes Cells. 2011; 16(2):141–151.

[52] Gwinn DM, Shackelford DB, Egan DF, Mihaylova MM, Mery A, Vasquez DS, Turk BE, Shaw RJ. AMPK phosphorylation of raptor mediates a metabolic checkpoint. Mol Cell. 2008; 30(2):214–26.

[53] Jacinto E, Loewith R, Schmidt A, Lin S, Rüegg MA, Hall A, Hall MN. Mammalian TOR complex 2 controls the actin cytoskeleton and is rapamycin insensitive. Nat Cell Biol. 2004 ;6(11):1122–1128.

[54] Wang GL, Jiang B, Rue EA, Semenza GL. Hypoxia-inducible factor 1 is a basic-helix-loop-helix-PAS heterodimer regulated by cel- lular O2 tension. Proc Natl Acad Sci USA. 1995; 92:5510–5514.

[55] Yang J, Zhang L, Erbel PJ, Gardner KH, Ding K, Garcia JA, Bruick RK. Functions of the Per/ARNT/Sim domains of the hypoxia-in- ducible factor. J Biol Chem. 2005; 280:36047–36054 .

[56] Chapman-Smith A, Lutwyche JK, Whitelaw ML. Contribution of the Per/Arnt/Sim (PAS) domains to DNA binding by the basic helix-loop-helix PAS transcriptional regulators. J Biol Chem. 2004; 279:5353- 5362.

[57] Dery MA, Michaud MD, Richard DE. Hypoxia-inducible factor 1: regulation by hypoxic and non-hypoxic activators. Int J Biochem Cell Bio. 2004; 37:535–540.

[58] Vaupel P. The Role of Hypoxia-Induced Factors in Tumor Progression. Oncologist. 2004; 9:10–17.

[59] Pietras A, Johnsson AS, Påhlman S. The HIF-2α-driven pseudo-hypoxic phenotype in tumor aggressiveness, differentiation, and vascularization. Curr Top Microbiol Immunol. 2010; 345:1–20.

[60] Luo W, Hu H, Chang R, Zhong J, Knabel M, O'Meally R, Cole RN, Pandey A, Semenza GL. Pyruvate kinase M2 is a PHD3-stimulated coactivator for hypoxia-inducible factor 1. Cell. 2011; 145(5):732–744.

[61] Kress S, Stein A, Maurer P, Weber B, Reichert J, Buchmann A, Huppert P, Schwarz M. Expression of hypoxia-inducible genes in tumor cells. J Cancer Res Clin Oncol. 1998; 124(6):315–320.

[62] Mobasheri A, Richardson S, Mobasheri R, Shakibaei M, Hoyland JA. Hypoxia inducible factor-1 and facilitative glucose transporters GLUT1 and GLUT3: putative molecular components of the oxygen and glucose sensing apparatus in articular chondrocytes. Histol Histopathol. 2005; 20(4):1327–1338.

[63] Papandreou I, Cairns RA, Fontana L, Lim AL, Denko NC. HIF-1 mediates adaptation to hypoxia by actively downregulating mito- chondrial oxygen consumption. Cell Metab. 2006; 3:150–151.

[64] Yang MH, Wu MZ, Chiou SH, Chen PM, Chang SY, Liu CJ, Teng SC, Wu KJ. Direct regulation of TWIST by HIF-1alpha promotes metastasis. Nat Cell Biol. 2008; 10(3):295–305.

[65] Je EC, Lca BS, Ga GA. The Role of Transcription Factor TWIST in Cancer Cells. Je et al. J Genet Syndr Gene Ther 2013; 4:1.

[66] Martin A, Cano A. Tumorigenesis: Twist1 links EMT to self-renewal. Nat Cell Biol. 2010; 12(10):924–925.

[67] Valsesia-Wittmann S, Magdeleine M, Dupasquier S, Garin E, Jallas AC, Combaret V, Krause A, Leissner P, Puisieux A. Oncogenic cooperation between H-Twist and N-Myc overrides failsafe programs in cancer cells. Cancer Cell. 2004; 6(6):625–630.

[68] Lee SH, Lee YJ, Han HJ. Role of hypoxia- induced fibronectin-integrin beta1 expression in embryonic stem cell proliferation and migra- tion: Involvement of PI3K/Akt and FAK. J Cell Physiol 2011; 226:484–493.

[69] Ryu MH, Park HM, Chung J, Lee CH and Park HR. Hypoxia-inducible factor-1alpha mediates oral squamous cell carcinoma invasion via upregulation of alpha5 integrin and fibronectin. Biochem Biophys Res Commun 2010; 393:11–15.

[70] Krishnamachary B, Zagzag D, Nagasawa H, Rainey K, Okuyama H, Baek JH, Semenza GL. Hypoxia-inducible factor-1-dependent re- pression of E-cadherin in von Hippel-

Lindau tumor suppressor-null renal cell carcinoma mediated by TCF3, ZFHX1A, and ZFHX1B. Can- cer Res. 2006; 66:2725–2731.

[71] LuoY, He DL, Ning L, Shen SL, Li L, Li X, Zhau HE, Chung LW. Over-expression of hypoxia- inducible factor-1alpha increases the invasive potency of LNCaP cells in vitro. BJU Int. 2006; 98:1315–1319.

[72] O'Toole EA, van Koningsveld R, Chen M, Woodley DT. Hypoxia induces epidermal kerati- nocyte matrix metalloproteinase-9 secretion via the protein kinase C pathway. J Cell Physiol. 2008; 214:47–55.

[73] Pennacchietti S, Michieli P, Galluzzo M, Mazzone M, Giordano S, Comoglio PM. Hypoxia promotes invasive growth by transcriptional activation of the met protooncogene. Cancer Cell. 2003; 3:347–361.

[74] Ishikawa T, Nakashiro K, Klosek SK, Goda H, Hara S, Uchida D, Hamakawa H. Hypoxia enhances CXCR4 expression by activating HIF-1 in oral squamous cell carcinoma. Oncol Rep. 2009; 21:707–712.

[75] Li Y, Qiu X, Zhang S, Zhang Q, Wang E. Hypoxia induced CCR7 expression via HIF-1alpha and HIF-2alpha correlates with migration and invasion in lung cancer cells. Cancer Biol Ther. 2009; 8:322–330.

[76] Fisher, A. Mechanism of the proteolytic activity of malignant tissue cells. Nature 1946;157:442.

[77] Buck MR, Karustis DG, Day NA, Honn KV, and Sloane BF. Degradation of extracellular-matrix proteins by human cathepsin B from normal and tumour tissues. Biochem J. 1992; 282(Pt 1):273–278.

[78] Kostoulas G, Lang A, Nagase H, Baici A. Stimulation of angiogenesis through cathepsin B inactivation of the tissue inhibitors of matrix metalloproteinases. FEBS Lett. 1999; 455:286–290.

[79] Mikkelsen T, et al. Immunolocalization of cathepsin B in human glioma: implications for tumor invasion and angiogenesis. J. Neurosurg. 1995; 83:285–290.

[80] Demchik LL, Sameni M, Nelson K, Mikkelsen T, Sloane BF. Cathepsin B and glioma invasion. Int J Dev Neurosci. 1999;17(5–6):483–94.

[81] Rempel SA, Rosenblum ML, Mikkelsen T, Yan PS, Ellis KD, Golembieski WA, Sameni M, Rozhin J, Ziegler G, Sloane BF. Cathepsin B expression and localization in glioma progression and invasion. Cancer Res. 1994; 54:6027–6031.

[82] Liu Y, Zhou Y, Zhu K. Inhibition of glioma cell lysosome exocytosis inhibits glioma invasion. PLoS One. 2012;7(9):e45910.

[83] López-Otín C, Lynn M. Matrisian Emerging roles of proteases in tumour suppression. Nature Reviews Cancer. 2007; 7:800–808.

[84] Teitz T, Wei T, Valentine MB, Vanin EF, Grenet J, Valentine VA, Behm FG, Look AT, Lahti JM, Kidd VJ. Caspase 8 is deleted or silenced preferentially in childhood neuroblastomas with amplification of MYCN. Nature Med. 2000; 6:529–535.

[85] Harada K, Toyooka S, et al. Deregulation of caspase 8 and 10 expression in pediatric tumors and cell lines. Cancer Res. 2002; 62:5897–5901.

[86] Soung YH, Lee JW, Kim SY, Park WS, Nam SW, Lee JY, Yoo NJ, Lee SH. Somatic mutations of CASP3 gene in human cancers. Hum. Genet. 2004; 115:112–115.

[87] Offman J, Gascolgne K, et al. Repeated sequences in CASPASE-5 and FANCD2 but not NF1 are targets for mutation in microsatellite-unstable acute leukemia/ myelodysplastic syndrome. Mol. Cancer Res. 2005; 3: 251–260.

[88] Lee JW, Kim MR, Soung YH, Nam SW, Kim SH, Lee JY, Yoo NJ, Lee SH. Mutational analysis of the CASP6 gene in colorectal and gastric carcinomas. APMIS. 2006; 114:646–650.

[89] Soung YH, Lee JW, et al. Inactivating mutations of CASPASE-7 gene in human cancers. Oncogene. 2003; 22:8048–8052.

[90] McCawley LJ , and Matrisian LM. Matrix metalloproteinases: they're not just for matrix anymore! Curr. Opin. Cell Biol. 2001; 13:534–540.

[91] Hagemann C, Anacker J, Ernestus R, Vince GH. A complete compilation of matrix metalloproteinase expression in human malignant gliomas. World J Clin Oncol. 2012; 3(5):67–79.

[92] Borden P, Heller RA. Transcriptional control of matrix me- talloproteinases and the tissue inhibitors of matrix metallo- proteinases. Crit Rev Eukaryot Gene Expr. 1997; 7:159–178.

[93] Nagase H, Woessner JF. Matrix metalloproteinases. J Biol Chem 1999; 274:21491–21494.

[94] Van Wart HE, Birkedal-Hansen H. The cysteine switch: a principle of regulation of metalloproteinase activity with potential applicability to the entire matrix metalloproteinase gene family. Proc Natl Acad Sci USA 1990; 87:5578–5582.

[95] Rao JS, Go Y, Kyritisis AP, Uhm J, Venkaiah B, Mohanam S, Gokaslan ZL, Rao JS. Elevated levels of Mr 92,000 type IV collagenase in human brain tumors. Cancer Res. 1993; 53:2208–2211.

[96] Forsyth PA, Wong H, Laing TD, Rewcastle NB, Morris DG, Muzik H, Leco KJ, Johnston RN, Brasher PM, Sutherland G, Edwards DR. Gelatinase-A (MMP-2), gelatinase-B (MMP-9) and membrane type matrix metalloproteinase-1 (MT1-MMP) are involved in different aspects of the pathophysiology of malignant gliomas. Br. J. Cancer 1999; 79:1828–1835.

[97] Rao JS. Molecular mechanisms of glioma invasiveness: the role of proteases. Nat Rev Cancer. 2003; 3(7):489–501.

[98] Struglics A, Hansson M. MMP proteolysis of the human extracellular matrix protein aggrecan is mainly a process of normal turnover. Biochem J. 2012; 446(2):213–223.

[99] Barascuk NF, Genovese F, et al. A MMP derived versican neo-epitope is elevated in plasma from patients with atherosclerotic heart disease. Int. J. Clin. Exp. Med (2013); 6:174–184.

[100] Nakamura H, Fujii Y, et al. Brevican Is Degraded by Matrix Metalloproteinases and Aggrecanase-1 (ADAMTS4) at Different Sites. The Journal of Biological Chemistry. 2000; 275(49):38885–38890.

[101] Hagemann C, Anacker J, Ernestus RI, Vince GH. A complete compilation of matrix metalloproteinase expression in human malignant gliomas. World J Clin Oncol. 2012; 3(5):67–79.

[102] Wang M, Wang T, Liu S, Yoshida D, Teramoto A.The expression of matrix metalloproteinase-2 and -9 in human gliomas of different pathological grades. Brain Tumor Pathol. 2003;20(2):65–72.

[103] Bergers G, Brekken R, McMahon G, Vu TH, Itoh T, Tamaki K, Tanzawa K, Thorpe P, Itohara S, Werb Z, Hanahan D. Matrix metalloproteinase-9 triggers the angiogenic switch during carcinogenesis. Nat Cell Biol. 2000; 2(10):737–744.

[104] Plate KH, Breier G, Weich HA, Risau W. Vascular endothelial growth factor is a potential tumour angiogenesis factor in human gliomas in vivo. Nature 1992; 359:845–848.

[105] Sounni NE, Devy L, Hajitou A, Frankenne F, Munaut C, Gilles C, Deroanne C, Thompson EW, Foidart JM, Noel A. MT1-MMP expression promotes tumor growth and angiogenesis through an up-regulation of vascular endothelial growth factor expression. FASEB J. 2002; 16(6):555–64.

[106] Viapiano MS, Hockfield S, Matthews RT. BEHAB/brevican requires ADAMTS-mediated proteolytic cleavage to promote glioma invasion. J Neurooncol. 2008; 88(3): 261–272.

[107] Wolfsberg TG, Straight PD, Gerena RL, et al. ADAM, a widely distributed and developmentally regulated gene family encoding membrane proteins with a disintegrin and metalloprotease domain. Dev. Biol. 1995; 169(1):378–383.

[108] Porter S, Clark IM, Kevorkian L, Edwards DR. The ADAMTS metalloproteinases. Biochemical Journal 2005; 386 (1): 15–27.

[109] Wildeboer D, Naus S, Amy Sang QX, Bartsch JW, Pagenstecher A. Metalloproteinase disintegrins ADAM8 and ADAM19 are highly regulated in human primary brain tumors and their expression levels and activities are associated with invasiveness. J Neuropathol Exp Neurol. 2006; 65(5):516–527.

[110] Zheng X, Jiang F, Katakowski M, Kalkanis SN, Hong X, Zhang X, Zhang ZG, Yang H, Chopp M. Inhibition of ADAM17 reduces hypoxia-induced brain tumor cell invasiveness. Cancer Sci. 2007; 98(5):674–684.

[111] D'Abaco GM, Ng K, Paradiso L, Godde NJ, Kaye A, Novak U. ADAM22, expressed in normal brain but not in high-grade gliomas, inhibits cellular proliferation via the disintegrin domain. Neurosurgery. 2006; 58(1):179–186.

[112] Stanton H, Melrose J, Little CB, Fosang AF. Proteoglycan degradation by the ADAMTS family of proteinases. Biochimica et Biophysica Acta (BBA) - Molecular Basis of Disease. 2011; 1812(12):1616–1629.

[113] Akai T, Niiya K, Sakuragawa N, Iizuka H, Endo S. Modulation of tissue-type plasminogen activator expression by platelet activating factor in human glioma cells. J Neurooncol. 2002; 59(3):193–198.

[114] Rustamzadeh E, Li C, Doumbia S, Hall WA, Vallera DA. Targeting the over-expressed urokinase-type plasminogen activator receptor on glioblastoma multiforme. J Neurooncol. 2003; 65(1):63–75.

[115] Yamamoto M, Sawaya R, Mohanam S, Rao VH, Bruner JM, Nicolson GL, et al. Expression and localization of urokinase-type plasminogen activator receptor in human gliomas. Cancer Res. 1994; 54:5016–5020.

[116] Lakka SS, Gondi CS, Yanamandra N, Dinh DH, Olivero WC, Gujrati M, Rao JS. Synergistic down-regulation of urokinase plasminogen activator receptor and matrix metalloproteinase-9 in SNB19 glioblastoma cells efficiently inhibits glioma cell invasion, angiogenesis, and tumor growth. Cancer Res. 2003; 63(10):2454–24561.

[117] Sage EH, Bornstein P. Extracellular proteins that modulate cell-matrix interactions. SPARC, tenascin and thrombospondin. J Biol Chem. 1991; 266:14831–14834.

[118] Alam R, Schultz CR, Golembieski WA, Poisson LM, Rempel SA. PTEN suppresses SPARC-induced pMAPKAPK2 and inhibits SPARC-induced Ser78 HSP27 phosphorylation in glioma. Neuro Oncol. 2013; 15(4):451–461.

[119] Rempel SA, Golembieski WA, Ge S, Lemke N, Elisevich K, Mikkelsen T, Gutiérrez JA: SPARC: a signal of astrocytic neoplastic transformation and reactive response in human primary and xenograft gliomas. J Neuropathol Exp Neurol. 1998; 57:1112–1121.

[120] Rempel SA, Golembieski WA, Fisher JL, Maile M, Nakeff A. SPARC modulates cell growth, attachment and migration of U87 glioma cells on brain extracellular matrix proteins. J Neurooncol. 2001; 53:149–160.

[121] Schultz C, Lemke N, Ge S, Golembieski WA, Rempel SA. Secreted protein acidic and rich in cysteine promotes glioma invasion and delays tumor growth in vivo. Cancer Res 2002; 62:6270–6277.

[122] Rich JN, Hans C, Jones B, et al. Gene expression profiling and genetic markers in glioblastoma survival. Cancer Res. 2005; 65:4051–4058.

[123] Thomas SL, Schultz CR, Mouzon E, Golembieski WA, El Naili R, Radakrishnan A, Lemke N, Poisson LM, Gutiérrez JA, Cottingham S, Rempel SA. Loss of Sparc in p53-null Astrocytes Promotes Macrophage Activation and Phagocytosis Resulting in Decreased Tumor Size and Tumor Cell Survival . Brain Pathology. 2015; 25:391–400.

[124] Burgoyne AM, Palomo JM, Phillips-Mason PJ, Burden-Gulley SM, Major DL, Zaremba A, Robinson S, Sloan AE, Vogelbaum MA, Miller RH, Brady-Kalnay SM. PTPμ suppresses glioma cell migration and dispersal. Neuro Oncol. 2009; 11(6):767–778.

[125] Phillips-Mason PJ, Craig SE, Brady-Kalnay SM. A protease storm cleaves a cell-cell adhesion molecule in cancer: multiple proteases converge to regulate PTPmu in glioma cells. J Cell Biochem. 2014; 115(9):1609–1623.

[126] Isnard N, Legeais JM, Renard G, Robert L. Effect of hyaluronan on MMP expression and activation. Cell Biol Int. 2001; 25(8):735–739.

[127] Bertrand P, Girard N, Delpech B, Duval C, d'Anjou J, Dauce JP. Hyaluronan (hyaluronic acid) and hyaluronectin in the extracellular matrix of human breast carcinomas: comparison between invasive and non-invasive areas. Int J Cancer. 1992; 52(1):1–6.

[128] Sakurai T, Friedlander DR, Grumet M. Expression of polypeptide variants of receptor- type protein tyrosine phosphatase beta: the secreted form, phosphacan, increases dramatically during embryonic development and modulates glial cell behavior in vitro. J Neurosci Res. 1996; 43(6):694–706.

[129] Pariser H, Ezquerra L, Herradon G, Perez-Pinera P, Deuel TF. Fyn is a downstream target of the pleiotrophin/receptor protein tyrosine phosphatase beta/zeta-signaling pathway: regulation of tyrosine phosphorylation of Fyn by pleiotrophin. Biochem Biophys Res Commun. 2005; 332:664–669.

[130] Grumet M, Milev P, Sakurai T, Karthikeyan L, Bourdon M, Margolis RK, Margolis RU. Interactions with tenascin and differential effects on cell adhesion of neurocan and phosphacan, two major chondroitin sulfate proteoglycans of nervous tissue. The Journal of Biological Chemistry. 1994; 269:12142–12146.

[131] Milev P, Maurel P, Häring M, Margolis RK, Margolis RU. TAG-1/Axonin-1 Is a High-affinity Ligand of Neurocan, Phosphacan/Protein-tyrosine Phosphatase-ζ/β, and N-CAM. The Journal of Biological Chemistry.1996; 27:15716–15723.

[132] Schmalfeldt M, Bandtlow CE, Dours-Zimmermann MT, Winterhalter KH, Zimmermann DR. Brain derived versican V2 is a potent inhibitor of axonal growth. J Cell Sci. 2000; 113(Pt 5):807–816.

[133] Arslan F, Bosserhoff AK, Nickl-Jockschat T, Doerfelt A, Bogdahn U, Hau P. The role of versican isoforms V0/V1 in glioma migration mediated by transforming growth factor-β2. British Journal of Cancer. 2007; 96, 1560–1568.

[134] Hu F, a Dzaye OD, Hahn A, Yu Y, Scavetta RJ, Dittmar G, Kaczmarek AK1, Dunning KR, Ricciardelli C, Rinnenthal JL, Heppner FL, Lehnardt S, Synowitz M, Wolf SA, Kettenmann H. Glioma-derived versican promotes tumor expansion via glioma-associated microglial/macrophages Toll-like receptor 2 signaling. Neuro-Oncology. 2015; 17(2), 200–210.

[135] Viapiano MS, Bi WL, Piepmeier J, Hockfield S, Matthews RT. Novel tumor-specific isoforms of BEHAB/brevican identified in human malignant gliomas. Cancer Res. 2005; 65(15):6726–6733.

[136] Lu R, Wu C, et al. The role of brevican in glioma: promoting tumor cell motility in vitro and in vivo. BMC Cancer. 2012; 12:607–616.

[137] Held-Feindt J, Paredes EB, Blömer U, Seidenbecher C, Stark AM, Mehdorn HM, Mentlein R. Matrix-degrading proteases ADAMTS4 and ADAMTS5 (disintegrins and metalloproteinases with thrombospondin motifs 4 and 5) are expressed in human glioblastomas. Int J Cancer. 2006; 118(1):55–61.

[138] Viapiano MS, Hockfield S, Matthews RT. BEHAB/brevican requires ADAMTS-mediated proteolytic cleavage to promote glioma invasion. J Neurooncol. 2008; 88(3): 261–272.

[139] Kawataki T, Yamane T, Naganuma H, Rousselle P, Andurén I, Tryggvason K, Patarroyo M. Laminin isoforms and their integrin receptors in glioma cell migration and invasiveness: Evidence for a role of alpha5-laminin(s) and alpha3beta1 integrin. Exp Cell Res. 2007; 313(18):3819–3831.

[140] Mammoto T, Jiang A, Jiang E, Panigrahy D, Kieran M W, Mammoto A. Role of Collagen Matrix in Tumor Angiogenesis and Glioblastoma Multiforme Progression. Am J Pathol. 2013; 183(4):1293–1305.

[141] Leitinger B. Transmembrane collagen receptors. Annu Rev Cell Dev Biol. 2011; 27:265–290.

[142] Tanentzapf G, Brown NH. An interaction between integrin and the talin FERM domain mediates integrin activation but not linkage to the cytoskeleton. Nat Cell Biol. 2006; 8:601–606.

[143] Xiang YY, Dong H, Wan Y, Li J, Yee A, Yang BB, Lu WY. Versican G3 domain regulates neurite growth and synaptic transmission of hippocampal neurons by activation of epidermal growth factor receptor. J Biol Chem. 2006; 281(28):19358–19368.

[144] Wu Y, Sheng W, Chen L, Dong H, Lee V, Lu F, Wong CS, Lu WY, Yang BB. Versican V1 isoform induces neuronal differentiation and promotes neurite outgrowth. Mol Biol Cell. 2004; 15(5):2093–2104.

[145] Hu B, Kong LL, Matthews RT, Viapiano M S. The Proteoglycan Brevican Binds to Fibronectin after Proteolytic Cleavage and Promotes Glioma Cell Motility. J Biol Chem. 2008; 283(36): 24848–24859.

[146] Schwarzbauer JE, Sechler JL. Fibronectin fibrillogenesis: a paradigm for extracellular matrix assembly. Curr Opin Cell Biol. 1999; 11(5):622–627.

[147] Larsen M, Artym VV, Green JA, Yamada KM. The matrix reorganized: extracellular matrix remodeling and integrin signaling. Curr Opin Cell Biol. 2006; 18(5):463–471.

[148] Kobayashi K, Takahashi H, Inoue A, Harada H, Toshimori S, Kobayashi Y, Goto K, Sugimoto K, Yano H, Ohnishi T, Tanaka J. Oct-3/4 promotes migration and invasion of glioblastoma cells. J Cell Biochem. 2012; 113(2):508–517.

[149] Zhang R, Luo H, Wang S, Chen Z, Hua L, Wang HW, Chen W, Yuan Y, Zhou X, Li D, Shen S, Jiang T, You Y, Liu N, Wang H. MiR-622 suppresses proliferation, invasion and migration by directly targeting activating transcription factor 2 in glioma cells. J Neurooncol. 2015; 121(1):63–72.

[150] Lee Y, Kawagoe R, Sasai K, Li Y, Russell HR, Curran T, McKinnon PJ. Loss of suppressor-of-fused function promotes tumorigenesis. Oncogene. 2007; 26:6442–6447.

[151] Jenkins D. Hedgehog signalling: emerging evidence for non-canonical pathways. Cellular signalling. 2009; 21:1023–1034.

[152] Liu X, Wang X, et al. Suppressor of fused (Sufu) represses Gli1 transcription and nuclear accumulation, inhibits glioma cell proliferation, invasion and vasculogenic mimicry, improving glioma chemo-sensitivity and prognosis. Oncotarget. 2014; 5(22):11681–11694.

[153] Stylli SS, Kaye AH, Lock P. Invadopodia: at the cutting edge of tumour invasion. J Clin Neurosci. 2008; 15(7):725–737.

[154] Herbst RS. Review of epidermal growth factor receptor biology. International Journal of Radiation Oncology, Biology, Physics. 2004; 59(2 Suppl):21–26.

[155] Huang PH, Xu AM, White FM. Oncogenic EGFR signaling networks in glioma. Sci Signal. 2009; 2(87):re6.

[156] Okada Y, Hurwitz EE, Esposito JM, Brower MA, Nutt CL, Louis DN. Selection pressures of TP53 mutation and microenvironmental location influence epidermal growth factor receptor gene amplification in human glioblastomas. Cancer Res. 2003; 63(2):413–416.

[157] Ekstrand AJ, James CD, Cavenee WK, Seliger B, Pettersson RF, Collins VP. Genes for epidermal growth factor receptor, transforming growth factor α, and epidermal growth factor and their expression in human gliomas in vivo. Cancer Res. 1991; 51, 2164–2172.

[158] Guillamo JS, de Bouard S, Valable S, Marteau L, Leuraud P, Marie Y, Poupon MF, Parienti JJ, Raymond E, Peschanski M. Molecular mechanisms underlying effects of epidermal growth factor receptor inhibition on invasion, proliferation, and angiogenesis in experimental glioma. Clin Cancer Res. 2009; 15:3697–3704.

[159] Talasila KM, Soentgerath A, et al. EGFR wild-type amplification and activation promote invasion and development of glioblastoma independent of angiogenesis. Acta Neuropathol. 2013; 125(5):683–698.

[160] Huang J, Hu J, et al. Transactivation of the Epidermal Growth Factor Receptor by Formylpeptide Receptor Exacerbates the Malignant Behavior of Human Glioblastoma Cells. Cancer Res. 2007; 67(12):5906–5913.

[161] Zhou Y, Bian X, Le Y, et al. Formylpeptide receptor FPR and the rapid growth of malignant human gliomas. J Natl Cancer Inst. 2005; 97:823–835.

[162] Le Y, Gong W, Li B, et al. Utilization of two seven-transmembrane, G protein-coupled receptors, formyl peptide receptor-like 1 and formyl peptide receptor, by the synthetic hexapeptide WKYMVm for human phagocyte activation. J Immunol. 1999; 163:6777–6784.

[163] Zhou Y, Bian X, Le Y, et al. Formylpeptide receptor FPR and the rapid growth of malignant human gliomas. J Natl Cancer Inst. 2005; 97:823–835.

[164] Huang J, et al. Receptor "hijacking" by malignant glioma cells: a tactic for tumor progression. Cancer Lett. 2008; 267(2):254–261.

[165] Brockmann MA, Papadimitriou A, Brandt M, Fillbrandt R, Westphal M, Lamszus K. Inhibition of intracerebral glioblastoma growth by local treatment with the scatter factor/hepatocyte growth factor-antagonist NK4. Clin Cancer Res. 2003; 9(12):4578–4585.

[166] Lamszus K, Laterra J, Westphal M, Rosen EM. Scatter factor/hepatocyte growth factor (SF/HGF) content and function in human gliomas. Int J Dev Neurosci. 1999; 17(5–6):517–530.

[167] Kaminska B, Kocyk M, Kijewska M. TGF beta signaling and its role in glioma pathogenesis. Adv Exp Med Biol. 2013; 986:171–87.

[168] Derynck R, Zhang Y, Feng XH. SMADS: transcriptional activators of TGF beta responses. Cell. 1998; 95 (6): 737–40.

[169] Wick W, Platten M, Weller M. Glioma cell invasion: regulation of metalloproteinase activity by TGF-beta. J Neurooncol. 2001; 53:177–185.

[170] Ye XZ, Xu SL, Xin YH, Yu SC, Ping YF, Chen L, Xiao HL, Wang B, Yi L, Wang QL, Jiang XF, Yang L, Zhang P, Qian C, Cui YH, Zhang X, Bian XW. Tumor-associated microglia/macrophages enhance the invasion of glioma stem-like cells via TGF-beta1 signaling pathway. J Immunol. 2012; 189:444–453.

[171] Balkwill F. Cancer and the chemokine network. Nature Reviews Cancer. 2004; 4:540–550.

[172] Ambrosini E, Aloisi F. Chemokines and glial cells: a complex network in the central nervous system. Neurochem Res. 2004; 29(5):1017–1038.

[173] Rempel SA, Dudas S, Ge S, Gutiérrez JA. Identification and localization of the cytokine SDF1 and its receptor, CXC chemokine receptor 4, to regions of necrosis and angiogenesis in human glioblastoma. Clin Cancer Res. 2000; 6(1):102–111.

[174] Ehtesham M, Winston JA, Kabos P, Thompson RC.. CXCR4 expression mediates glioma cell invasiveness. Oncogene. 2006; 25(19):2801–2806.

[175] Barbieri F, Bajetto A, Porcile C, Pattarozzi A, Massa A, Lunardi G, Zona G, Dorcaratto A, Ravetti JL, Spaziante R, Schettini G, Florio T. CXC receptor and chemokine expression in human meningioma: SDF1/CXCR4 signaling activates ERK1/2 and stimulates meningioma cell proliferation. Ann N Y Acad Sci. 2006; 1090:332–343.

[176] Zhang J, Sarkar S, Yong VW. The chemokine stromal cell derived factor-1 (CXCL12) promotes glioma invasiveness through MT2-matrix metalloproteinase. Carcinogenesis. 2005; 26(12):2069–2077.

[177] Zhou Y, Zhang J, Liu Q, Bell R, Muruve DA, Forsyth P, Arcellana-Panlilio M, Robbins S, Yong VW. The chemokine GRO-alpha (CXCL1) confers increased tumorigenicity to glioma cells. Carcinogenesis. 2005; 26(12):2058–2068.

[178] Richmond A, Thomas HG. Melanoma growth stimulatory activity: isolation from human melanoma tumors and characterization of tissue distribution. J. Cell. Biochem. 2008; 36(2):185–198.

[179] Sciumé G, Soriani A, Piccoli M, Frati L, Santoni A, Bernardini G. CX3CR1/CX3CL1 axis negatively controls glioma cell invasion and is modulated by transforming growth factor-beta. Neuro-Oncology. 2010; (7)701–710.

[180] Kaur B, Khwaja FW, Severson EA, Matheny SL, Brat DJ, Van Meir EG. Hypoxia and the hypoxia-inducible-factor pathway in glioma growth and angiogenesis. Neuro Oncol. 2005; 7(2):134–153.

[181] Spitzweck B, Brankatschk M, Dickson BJ. Distinct protein domains and expression patterns confer divergent axon guidance functions for Drosophila Robo receptors. Cell. 2010; 140(3):409–420.

[182] Evans TA, Bashaw GJ. Functional diversity of Robo receptor immunoglobulin domains promotes distinct axon guidance decisions. Curr. Biol. 2010; 20(6):567–572.

[183] Wong K, Ren XR, Huang YZ, Xie Y, Liu G, Saito H, Tang H, Wen L, Brady-Kalnay SM, Mei L, Wu JY, Xiong WC, Rao Y. Signal transduction in neuronal migration: roles of GTPase activating proteins and the small GTPase Cdc42 in the Slit-Robo pathway. Cell. 2001; 107(2):209–221.

[184] Xiang RH, Hensel CH, Garciaeta DK. Isolationofthe human semaphorin III/F Gene (SEM A3F) at chromosome 3p21, a region deleted in lung cancer. Genomics. 1996; 32(1): 39–48.

[185] Tomizawa Y, Sekido Y, and Kondo Y, et al., Inhibition of lung cancer cell growth and induction of apoptosis after reexpres- sion of 3p21.3 candidate tumor suppressor gene

SEMA3B, Proceedings of the National Academy of Sciences of the United States of America. 2001; 98(24):13954–13959.

[186] Castro-Rivera E, Ran S, Thorpe P, Minna JD. Semaphorin 3B (SEMA3B) induces apoptosis in lung and breast cancer, whereas VEGF165 antagonizes this effect. Proceedings of the National Academy of Sciences of the United States of America. 2004; 101(31):11432–11437.

[187] De Ponnat C, Buffard V, Leroy K, et al. Antiproliferative effect of semaphorin 3F on human melanoma cell lines. Journal of Investigative Dermatology. 2006; 126(10):2343–2345.

[188] Wu F, Zhou Q, Yang J, et al. Endogenous axon guiding chemorepulsant semaphorin-3F inhibits the growth and metastasis of colorectal carcinoma. Clinical Cancer Research 2011; 17(9):2702–2711.

[189] Tamagnone L, Artigiani S, Chen H, et al. Plexins are a large family of receptors for transmembrane, secreted, and GPI- anchored semaphorins in vertebrates. Cell. 1999; 99(1):71–80.

[190] Bagci T, Wu JK, Pfannl R, Ilag LL, Jay DG. Autocrine semaphorin 3A signaling promotes glioblastoma dispersal. Oncogene. 2009; 28(40):3537–3550.

[191] Barresi V, Vitarelli E, Cerasoli S. Semaphorin3A immunohistochemical expression in human meningiomas: cor- relation with the microvessel density. Virchows Archiv. 2009; 454(5):563–571.

[192] Nasarre C, Concina E, et al. Neuropilin-2 acts as a modulator of Sema3A-dependent glioma cell migration. Cell Adh Migr. 2009; 3(4):383–389.

[193] Swiercz JM, Kuner R, Behrens K, and Offermanns S. Plexin-B1 directly interacts with PDZ-RhoGEF/LARG to regulate RhoA and growth cone morphology. Neuron. 2002; 35(1):51–63.

[194] Li X, Lee, AYW. Semaphorin 5A and plexin-B3 inhibit human glioma cell motility through RhoGDIα-mediated inactivation of Rac1 GTPase. The Journal of Biological Chemistry. 2010; 285(42):32436–32445.

[195] Rajasekharan S, Kennedy TE. The netrin protein family. Genome Biol. 2009; 10:239.1–239.8.

[196] Meyerhardt JA, Look AT, Bigner SH, Fearon ER. Identification and characterization of neogenin, a DCC-related gene. Oncogene1997; 14:1129–1136.

[197] Meyerhardt JA, Caca K, et al. Netrin- 1: interaction with deleted in colorectal cancer (DCC) and alterations in brain tumors and neuroblastomas. Cell Growth Differ. 1999; 10:35–42.

[198] Thiebault K, Mazelin L, et al. The netrin-1 receptors UNC5H are putative tumor suppressors controlling cell death commitment. Proceedings of the National Academy of Sciences of the United States of America. 2003; 100:4173–4178.

[199] Jarjour AA, Durko M, Luk TL, Marçal N, Shekarabi M, Kennedy TE. Autocrine netrin function inhibits glioma cell motility and promotes focal adhesion formation. PLoS One. 2011; 6(9):e25408.

[200] Hong K, Hinck L, Nishiyama M, Poo MM, Tessier-Lavigne M, Stein E. A Ligand-Gated Association between Cytoplasmic Domains of UNC5 and DCC Family Receptors Converts Netrin-Induced Growth Cone Attraction to Repulsion. Cell. 1999; 97(7):927–941.

[201] van Tellingen O, Yetkin-Arik B, de Gooijer MC, Wesseling P, Wurdinger T, de Vries HE. Overcoming the blood-brain tumor barrier for effective glioblastoma treatment. Drug Resist Updat. 2015; 19:1–12.

[202] Agudelo-Garcia PA, De Jesus JK, et al. Glioma Cell Migration on Three-dimensional Nanofiber Scaffolds Is Regulated by Substrate Topography and Abolished by Inhibition of STAT3 Signaling. Neoplasia. 2011; 13(9):831–840.

[203] Viapiano MS, Lawler SE. Glioma invasion: mechanisms and therapeutic challenges. In: Van Meir, E.G., ed. CNS Cancer: Models, Markers, Prognostic Factors, Targets, and Therapeutic Approaches. 1st ed. New York: Humana Press (Springer), 2009. pp. 1219.

[204] Valster A, Tran NL, Nakada M, Berens ME, Chan AY, Symons M. Cell migration and invasion assays. Methods. 2005; 37(2):208–15.

[205] Nie S, Gurrea M, Zhu J, Thakolwiboon S, Heth JA, Muraszko KM, Fan X, Lubman DM. Tenascin-C: a novel candidate marker for cancer stem cells in glioblastoma identified by tissue microarrays. J Proteome Res. 2015; 14(2):814–822.

[206] Joshi AD, Loilome W, Siu IM, Tyler B, Gallia GL, Riggins GJ. Evaluation of tyrosine kinase inhibitor combinations for glioblastoma therapy. PLoS One. 2012; 7(10):e44372.

[207] Wang M, Yoshida D, Liu S, Teramoto A. Inhibition of cell invasion by indomethacin on glioma cell lines: in vitro study. J Neurooncol. 2005; 72(1):1–9.

[208] Blázquez C, Salazar M, Carracedo A, Lorente M, Egia A, González-Feria L, Haro A, Velasco G, Guzmán M. Cannabinoids Inhibit Glioma Cell Invasion by Down-regulating Matrix Metalloproteinase-2 Expression. Cancer Res. 2008; 68:1945–1952.

[209] Gabelloni P, Da Pozzo E, Bendinelli S, Costa B, Nuti E, Casalini F, Orlandini E, Da Settimo F, Rossello A, Martini C. Inhibition of metalloproteinases derived from tumours: new insights in the treatment of human glioblastoma. Neuroscience. 2010; 168(2):514–522.

[210] Stupp R, Hegi ME, et al. Cilengitide combined with standard treatment for patients with newly diagnosed glioblastoma with methylated MGMT promoter (CENTRIC

EORTC 26071–22072 study): a multicentre, randomised, open-label, phase 3 trial. Lancet Oncol. 2014; 15(10):1100–108.

[211] Nabors LB, Fink KL, et al. Two cilengitide regimens in combination with standard treatment for patients with newly diagnosed glioblastoma and unmethylated MGMT gene promoter: results of the open-label, controlled, randomized phase II CORE study. Neuro Oncol. 2015; 17(5):708–717.

Section 2

Investigations

Chapter 6

Critical Molecular and Genetic Markers in Primary Brain Tumors with Their Clinical Importance

Ilhan Yaylim, Sumeyya Azam,
Ammad Ahmad Farooqi, Özlem Küçükhüseyin,
Muhammad Ismail and Ali Metin Kafadar

Additional information is available at the end of the chapter

http://dx.doi.org/10.5772/63550

Abstract

Classification of primary brain tumors is based mainly on histopathological characteristics. Due to the peculiarity of the central nervous system (CNS), the location of the tumor is also used in the naming of the CNS tumors. These features, histopathology, and location determine the main prognostic factors in these tumors. Updated molecular and genetic findings in the last two decades accumulated vast amount of knowledge about the biological behavior, response to the treatment, and consequently the prognosis of CNS tumors. After the clinical use of these data, a recent classification is proposed by the International Society of Neuropathology named as "integrated diagnosis."

This classification considers the histopathological classification, World Health Organization (WHO) grade along with the molecular information. The emerging molecular-genetic data about the CNS tumors will allow the translational researchers to deliberately understand the oncogenic mechanisms involved in the evolution of these tumors and judge the optional treatment strategies.

Evaluating the check points of cell cycle and apoptosis provides valuable information about the tumor biology (tumorigenesis). These mechanisms (pathways) also play an exclusive role in CNS tumors. Knowledge concerning the gene repressors and gene activators or some epigenetic changes in proliferative and antiproliferative pathways that regarded gliomas may yield new individualized treatment options.

In this chapter, we will review the basic and translational research molecular-genetic data of gliomas with special interest on proliferative and antiproliferative pathways. Further emerging treatment options and treatment responses in gliomas will be critically evaluated with regard to their histopathology, anatomical location, and molecular-genetic fingerprints.

Keywords: gliomas, proliferation, apoptosis, cell cycle, gene

1. Introduction

Primary brain tumors are a distinct group of pathologies due to their location, low incidence compared to other human tumors, histopathologic diversities, and unexpected response to treatment methods mainly caused by their peculiar genetic and molecular characteristics. Evaluating new important biomarkers which affect the etiopathogenesis of brain tumors may also help clinicians in consulting patients about prognosis, potential clinical studies, and following response to the treatment strategies [1]. Nowadays, the value of early detection of various types of cancer before metastasis has become a very significant issue. This approach may increase life expectancy and the quality of life in these patients [2]. It is known that one of the best management strategies of cancer is to predict its prognosis and response to the updated therapeutic procedures. In order to achieve this, it is significant to consider the blood, serum, plasma, or tissue biomarkers. Although the value of liquid biopsy in different human tumors is established, there is a lack of data regarding primary brain tumors [3]. Confluence of information suggested that genetic, epigenetic, functional or compositional heterogeneity of diseased and healthy tissues presented a major challenge to strategies to improve clinical outcome. [4]. Many molecules found in various fluids, tissues, and cell lines are produced either by the tumor itself, other tissues, or tumor microenvironment, in response to the presence of cancer or other associated conditions including inflammation. The scientists study on cancer search for proper candidate tumor markers and for identifying patients who face different diagnosis or clinical stages of cancer. This type of biomarkers must have some characteristics which can be used to estimate tumor volume, determine response to treatment, and assess disease recurrence through monitoring. Recent advancements have shown that amplifications/translocations, genetic mutations and changes in microarray-generated profiles (genetic signatures) are contributory in cancer development, metastasis and development of resistance against different therapeutics. These genetic signatures are referred according to the type of tumor marker or profile and may be associated with clinical outcomes or good prognosis or enhanced quality of life [3,4]. An ideal tumor marker is described as easily measurable, reliable, and cost-effective by use of an assay with high analytical sensitivity and specificity. Although we have developed a deeper understanding of the underlying mechanisms, there are only a few markers which have been used in routine applications and only a limited number of them can be used to identify patients or monitor progression of cancer types and clinical staging.

Gene overexpression is described as increase in copy number of genes or chromosomes (i.e., gene amplification) through increased transcriptional activity. It is known that imbalance between the gene repressors and gene activators or some epigenetic changes as DNA methylation or chromosomal translocations can alter transcriptional activity of the gene [3,4].

http://dx.doi.org/10.5772/63550

2. Defined molecular markers which changed our clinical attitude

The use of biomarkers in glioblastoma (GBM) has been evaluated in a recent survey by neuro-oncologists [5]. Current evidences indicate that MGMT, EGFR, 1p/19q, EGFR, p53, phosphatase and tensin homolog (PTEN) mutation or deletion, EGFRvIII, IDH1/2, PDGFR, and PIK3CA are the most commonly used markers. But, use of these biomarkers claimed to be prognostic in GBM cases is still debated. There exist significantly varying clinical representations and cases of GBM, and the structure of the signaling molecules is highly complex, and therefore, use of these markers is not very common as of now. In addition, glioblastoma, still a heterogeneous disease, also possesses additional difficulties such as having limited biomarkers to diagnosis and monitoring and therapeutic options, having poorly understood pathogenesis, and requiring individualized treatments. On the other hand, the discovery of new biomarkers together with currently used markers can enable us to better stratify patients regarding treatment paradigms and clinical trials (**Figure 1**) [6,7].

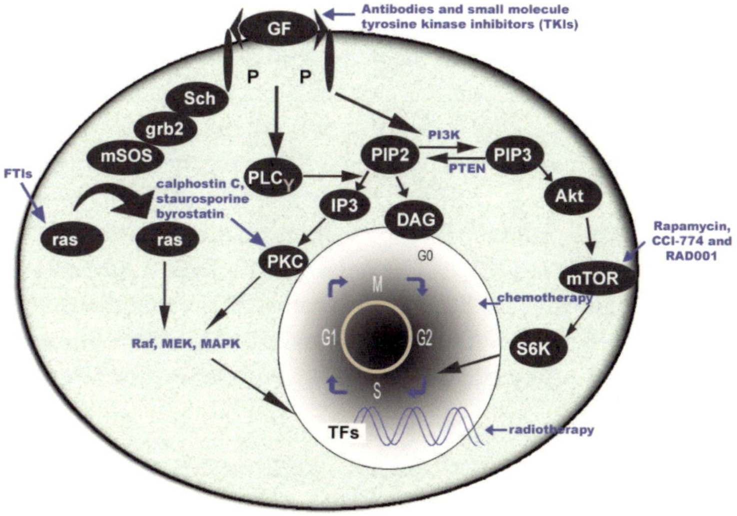

Figure 1. Some signaling pathways with therapeutic implications in gliomas [7]. Some abbreviations are shown below. EGF: epidermal growth factor; PIP2, phosphatidylinositol phosphate-2; PIP3, phosphatidylinositol phosphate-2; PKC, protein kinase C; Grb2, growth factor receptor-bound protein-2; VEGF, vascular endothelial growth factor; S6K, p70 S6 kinase; mTOR, mammalian target of rapamycin; TF, transcription factors; SOS, son of sevenless molecule.

3. Proliferative and antiproliferative pathways and their roles in gliomas

As more and more detailed studies into intracellular signaling cascades and modulators that regulate these pathways are published, intricacy of the fine-balance between celluar survival and death is revealed. A revolution in the signaling cascades has provided near complete resolution of how physiologically important signaling proteins interact with extracellular cues to trigger proliferation. More detailed understanding of the regulatory and activation processes of uncontrolled cellular proliferation is proving to be a key in identification of newer approaches to improve the efficacy of existing therapeutics. The homeostasis of mitogenic signaling is tactfully controlled by multiple mechanisms. The past several years have seen a dramatic leap in our understanding of how Receptor tyrosine kinase (RTK) mediated signaling is rewired during tumorigenesis to support the transformed phenotype. Activation of RTK results in receptor dimerization and autophosphorylation. More importantly, docking sites are created for different adaptor protein complexes such as Grb2/SOS. Mutant Ras is reportedly involved in 50% of all human tumors. There are direct pieces of evidence emphasizing on role of mutant Ras in gliomas. High Ras-GTP levels in advanced astrocytomas have been reported [8, 9].

Epidermal growth factor receptor (EGFR), coded as a cell-surface-bound receptor, is another important molecule involved in cell proliferation with potential effects on clinical prognosis of GBM. It is known that approximately <10% of secondary GBMs and 50% of primary GBMs have EGFR mutations [10]. The presence of EGFR variant III mutation (EGFRvIII) is known to upregulate mitogenic signaling pathways. There is a deletion of the regulator N-terminal domain (▪ 6–273) of EGFR in this pattern of EGFR. About 10–60% of the patients with GBM have EGFRvIII which can be detected in the peripheral blood of brain tumors. The detection of this mutation in brain cancer patients has great importance for anti-EGFRvIII therapies and patients can be monitored to track their response to these therapies [11,12]. Better and deeper knowledge of mechanistic insights that cause EGFR heterogeneity in GBM will prove to be helpful in identification of drugs with maximum efficacy. *EGFRvIII* mutation to identify patients for treatments such as erlotinib therapy for non-small cell lung cancer or RNA-directed treatments and vaccine therapies [13]. As of now, we still have a limited knowledge about downstream signaling pathways for EGFR and whether *EGFR* mutations affect these downstream signaling pathways, such as AKT, MAPK, and STAT3. On the other hand, it has been suggested that the clinical utility of this biomarker and its use for targeted treatment are complicated [1].

Platelet-derived growth factor receptor (PDGFR), a cell-surface tyrosine kinase, plays role in GBM proliferation and stem cell renewal. There are multiple isoforms of PDGFR, mutated in up to 30% of GBMs. One of them, the most significant one regarding GBM, is PDGFRA. The other isoform is also PDGFRAD (with a deletion of exons 8 and 9), seen in 40% of GBMs, and leads to constitutive activation [14,15]. According to the Cancer Genome Atlas, PDGFRA has a crucial role in the proneural subtype of GBM; however, no changes were observed in prognosis of the evaluated patients [16].

The phosphatidylinositol 3-kinase (PI3K)/AKT (PI3K/AKT) pathway is known as a crucial intracellular signaling pathway, taking role in regulating cell proliferation, migration, quiescence, proliferation, cancer, and longevity [17]. PI3K is an enzyme which phosphorylates phosphatidylinositol-4,5-bisphosphate (PIP2) to phosphatidylinositol-3,4,5-trisphosphate (PIP3) at the cell inner membrane. This activation process leads to recruit and upregulate various downstream pathways including AKT, a molecule localized in the plasma membrane [18].

Phosphatase and tensin homolog (PTEN) is known as a natural inhibitor of PI3K/AKT pathway. It has been shown to inhibit transduction of signals to downstream effectors via dephosphorylation of PIP_3 to PIP_2 [19]. It has been reported that an increased PI3K/Akt/mTOR signaling is seen in ~88% of all glioblastomas [20,21]. All of these biological pathways has been related to genetic alterations of key regulatory molecules involved in mitogenic signaling in RTKs and also in the PI3K-PTEN-Akt signaling axis.

Some regulatory and effector molecules play important role in classical cell death networks of both extrinsic (death receptor-mediated) and intrinsic (mitochondria-dependent) apoptosis signaling pathways [22]. Since the discovery of TNF (Tumor Necrosis Factor) family members, a new milestone in apoptosis-inducing cancer therapies has emerged. TRAIL (tumor necrosis factor-related apoptosis-inducing ligand) is a protein reportedly involved in selective killing of cancer cells while leaving normal cells intact. The major biological role of this 281-amino acid-type II transmembrane protein is apoptosis induction after interacting with its receptors to trigger extrinsically and intrinsically controlled pathways. Four different homologous human TRAIL receptors have been categorized into TRAIL-R1/DR4, TRAIL-R2/DR5 also known as Killer, TRAIL-R3 or DcR1, and TRAIL-R4 or DcR2. Substantial fraction of information has been added into the existing pool of knowledge related to TRAIL biology and known that different cancers are resistant to TRAIL-based therapeutics. Mechanistically it has been shown that downregulation of death receptors considerably impaired TRAIL-induced apoptosis in cancer cells. In the upcoming section, we briefly summarize advancements in our understanding related to the underlying mechanisms of resistance against TRAIL-induced apoptosis. We also discuss how TRAIL has shown as a potent anticancer agent in xenografted mice. Natural products have also added more options in the armory against brain tumor. Detailed mechanistic insights have provided a near complete resolution of protein network TRAIL-resistant glioblastoma and increasingly it is being realized that imbalance of stoichiometric ratios of proapoptotic and antiapoptotic proteins modulates response of cancer cells to TRAIL. Previously, it has been convincingly revealed that Znf domain of A20 E3 ligase ubiquitinated RIP1 through a K63-linked polyUB chain that structurally interacted with p18 domain of caspase-8 and blocked its dimerization and cleavage. Functionally inactive caspase-8 was unable to proteolytically process downstream effectors that resulted in impairment of TRAIL-induced apoptosis in glioblastoma [23]. Adeno-associated virus (AAV) vectors are being used to efficiently deliver secreted, soluble TRAIL in different preclinical studies. Additionally, these are also used in combination with TRAIL-sensitizing cardiac glycoside, lanatoside C (lan C). Tumor growth was considerably reduced in intracranial U87 tumor-bearing mice treated with AAV-sTRAIL and lanatoside C [24]. Mesenchymal stem cells (MSCs) have the ability to migrate toward intracranial glioma xenografts. Experimentally verified data indicated that MSCs expressing firefly luciferase (fluc) injected into the left hemisphere migrated rapidly toward right, tumor-bearing region of the brain. Results revealed that 11% of implanted MSCs were noted to be localized in right hemisphere within 2 hours after MSC inoculation. Coculture of GBM43 and U87 glioma cells with MSCs-TRAIL displayed notable rise in caspase-3 activity. Survival rate of tumor-bearing mice was enhanced intranasally delivered with MSCs-TRAIL [25]. Carbenoxolone (CBX), a derivative of 18-glycyrrhetinic acid, has been shown to effectively enhance killing activity of TRAIL-expressing MSCs. CBX considerably upregulated cell-surface expression of DR5 in CBX-treated ΔGli36 and U87MG cells. CBX also inhibited gap junction (GJ) communication via modulation of connexin (Cx43). CBX remarkably reduced expression levels of Cx43 in U87MG and ΔGli36 cells after 72 hours. Results revealed that TRAIL-induced apoptosis was markedly higher in cells transfected with Cx43-siRNA [26] .

Antibody-based anticancer therapies have attracted considerable attention and different structural variations are being tested for efficacies which involve smaller antibody fragments such as ScFvs, Fabs, and nanobodies. Single-chain Fv fragment (scFv) consists of a variable light-chain (VL) and variable heavy-chain (VH) domains, which contains whole antigen-binding site.

Multidrug resistance protein 3 (MRP3) is frequently overexpressed in glioblastoma multiforme cells. scFvM58-sTRAIL is an engineered protein formed by fusion of MRP3-specific scFv antibody M58 with N-terminus of soluble TRAIL. scFvM58-sTRAIL was effective against MRP3-positive GBM cells. Expectedly, scFvM58-sTRAIL did not show significant activity against MRP3-negative Jurkat cells. These results indicated that scFvM58-sTRAIL was effective against MRP3-positive cancer cells [27].

Various bivalent EGFR-targeting nanobodies (ENbs) have been designed and noted to be effective. Neural stem cells (NSC) are potent agents to deliver ENbs. Preclinical study revealed that tumor regression was significantly higher in xenografted mice treated with NSC-ENb2-TRAIL. Xenografted mice survived for 51 days upon treatment with control NSC-ENb2 and 80% of mice survived for 80 days after treatment with NSC-ENb2-TRAIL. These findings indicated that tumoritropic NSC-releasing ENb2 inhibited growth of glioblastoma and effectiveness of ENb2-based therapy was markedly improved by NSC-releasing ENb2-TRAIL [28].

Diethylamino-curcumin mimics with substituted triazolyl groups have previously been synthesized and reported to effectively sensitize resistant CRT-MG astroglioma cells to TRAIL [29].

Gingerol, a major bioactive component of ginger, has been shown to trigger expression of DR5 in a p53-dependent manner in U87 glioblastoma cells. Digitoxin (DT), a clinically approved cardiac glycoside, has been observed to overcome resistance against TRAIL in resistant U87MG glioblastoma cells. Digitoxin effectively enhanced DR5 expression on cell surface of resistant cancer cells [30].

4. Natural products mediated targeting of proliferative protein network in glioblastoma

Crude hydromethanolic extracts produced by maceration of *Spartium junceum* flowers and *Onopordum acanthium* leaves were tested for anticancer activity against glioblastoma U-373 cancer cells. *O. acanthium* was effective against glioblastoma cells and induced apoptosis [31] .

Aqueous extract of *Ruta graveolens* L. notably enhanced phosphorylated ERK1/2 and Akt levels in glioma cells. The results indicated that *Ruta graveolens* exerted inhibitory effects via activation of ERK1/2 and Akt-induced signaling pathways [32].

Triterpenoid saponins from *Albizia lebbeck* (L.) showed activity against TG1 and U-87 MG cancer cells with IC_{50} values of 2.10 and 2.24 μM for compound 2 and 3.46 and 1.36 μM for compound 1 [33].

Isocitrate Dehydrogenase 1 and 2 (IDH1/2) are two important enzymes involved in the Krebs cycle and oxidatively decarboxylate isocitrate to produce a-ketoglutarate and CO_2. IDH1 is a cytosolically located protein. IDH2 encodes a mitochondrial protein. Parsons et al. reported that IDH1/2 was mutated in approximately 60–80% of secondary gliomas and 5% of primary gliomas [34]. There are two common IDH mutation (IDH1R132H and IDH2172 mutations) types. It has been reported that these mutations are seen in GBM (>90% samples with IDH1/2 mutation). These mutations lead to increased production of the oncometabolite D-2-hydroxyglutarate. This metabolite has previously been noted to modify DNA methylation patterns in GBM and transcriptional activity of different target genes [35]. *IDH1* mutation may be correlated with several clinical factors such as younger patient age and frontal location. It has also been reported that additional survival benefit (median survival 9.75 years) was achieved from greater tumor resection (<5 cm^3 residual) in *IDH1* mutants, except for wild-type *IDH1*. It has also been suggested that the presence of *IDH1/2* mutation supports increased therapeutic efficacy with chemoradiotherapy and greater resection [1]. When IDH mutations occur, enzymatic activities of some important molecules can be altered. While alpha-ketoglutarate (α-KG) is decreased, produced 2-hydroxyglutarate (2-HG) can inhibit the activity of some enzymes. These enzymes play a significant role in regulating DNA and histone methylation (α-KG-dependent dioxygenase), including histone demethylases and the TET family of 5mC hydroxylases [36–38].

TET proteins are described as a new class of enzymes which can alter the methylation status of the DNA by converting 5-methylcytosine (5mC) to 5-hydroxymethylcytosine (5hmC). The biological function of 5hmC is not clear. It has been suggested that it is an intermediate in DNA demethylation process. 5hmC offers remarkable reduction in human gliomas as compared to normal brain. An inverse relationship has been reported between 5hmC levels and cell proliferation [39,40].

p53 is a very important protein involved in many physiological and pathological process in the regulation of cell viability in terms of cell cycle, apoptosis, cell differentiation, and other mechanisms of cell regulation during exposure to DNA-damaging agents (e.g., ultraviolet radiation, toxins, chemotherapeutic agents) [1]. It has been reported that P53 gene is mutated in 28% of primary GBMs [41]. There are three patterns regarding p53 dysfunction. One is called loss of function. This pattern may describe a lot of endogenous growth inhibitor effects of wild-type p53. The other is gain of function. This means that mutant p53 upregulates a distinct subset of genes from wild-type p53. The last one is dominant-negative effects of p53. It is associated with a tetramer pattern of mutant p53/wild-type p53 and leads to downregulate activity [42]. It is known that some other mechanisms of p53 inactivation include mutations of its modulators including MDM2 inhibitor or deletion of p14ARF [43,44]. Whether there is a correlation between p53 and GBM prognosis is still unclear due to the complexity of the p53 signaling pathway. P53 pathway includes many important regulators and the heterogeneity of p53 mutation types can also affect the p53 molecule. Because of those mentioned, therapies targeting P53 have been limited in this field [42].

The deletion of 1p and 19q, occurring early in tumorigenesis, is known as an important genetic signature. The deletion is seen in 50–70% of patients with low-grade oligodendrogliomas. This can be predictive for the tumor's chemosensitivity to some agents [46,47]. It has been reported that *P190RhoGAP*, localized on 19q13.3, can be one of the candidate genes as a tumor suppressor [48]. A large-scale genomic analysis by array CGH has reported two different patterns about 1p deletion for prognostic factors. One of them is the whole 1p (associated with the deletion of the whole 19q). This may be associated with a good prognosis for oligodendrogliomas. Another is 1p deletion (not associated with 19q loss). This deletion has a negative prognostic value and improves progression-free survival (PFS) and overall survival (OS). It is mostly associated with astrocytomas [49]. It is also related to the response to chemotherapy and radiation in oligodendroglioma. Data obtained from EORTC 26951 and RTOG 9402 trials showed an improvement in OS with the addition of radiation to procarbazine/lomustine/vincristine chemotherapy in anaplastic oligodendroglioma with 1p/19q mutation [50]. There are some studies correlated with these similar findings, In GBM, similar findings have been demonstrated in some studies [51,52], but not in others [53,54]. It has also been reported that codeletion of 1p and 19q is related with *IDH1* mutation and *MGMT* hypermethylation [47,55].

O-6-Methylguanine-DNA-methyltransferase (MGMT) is involved in removal of alkylation at the O6 position of guanine. Hypermethylation of *MGMT* transcriptionally down-regulated its expression. This situation results in impaired repair capability response to chemotherapeutic agents and radiation. Some clinical trials have confirmed the prognostic and predictive roles of *MGMTm* [56]. It has been suggested that patients with *MGMTm* are responsive to chemotherapy. However, *MGMT* status was not distinguished between patients with glioblastoma (GBM) and those with anaplastic astrocytoma (AA) and this restricts interpretation of the study. The European Organisation for Research and Treatment of Cancer (EORTC) 26981/22981 and National Cancer Institute of Canada (NCIC) trials also indicates increased responsiveness to temozolomide for patients with MGMTm [57]. It has been suggested that a standard marker both following prognosis and identifying patients for clinical trials, in which alkylation therapies and/or radiation therapy are applied, may be used for MGMTm [1].

5. Epigenetics in human gliomas with some details

Acetylation of lysine residues is a post-tranlational modification controlled by the opposing action of histone deacetylases (HDACs) and histone acetyl transferases (HATs) [58–60]. Histone methylation may generally occur on the side chains of lysines and arginines, which can alter the activity of effector proteins of the transcriptional machinery [58–60]. It has been reported that some mutations in some regulatory genes such as HDACs (HDAC2 and HDAC9), histone demethylases (JMJD1A and JMJD1B), and histone methyltransferases (SET7, SETD7, MLL, MLL3, and MLL4) have been detected to a large extent in genomic analysis of GBM samples [34]. However, it is still unclear whether histone modifications play significant roles in gliomas and their potential can serve as biomarkers and/or therapeutic targets. Noncoding RNAs are known to play an important role in the epigenetic regulation of gene expression [61,62].

One group of RNAs are described as microRNAs (miRNAs). miRNAs are important regulators for gene expression. miRNAs post-transcriptionally regulate expression of target genes. miRNAs are double-stranded RNA molecules of approximately 22 nucleotides (nt) in length. miRNA binds to specific recognition sequences within the 3′-untranslated region (3′-UTR) of target mRNAs [61–63]. miRNAs are characterized functionally into tumor suppressors and oncogenic miRNAs. Tumor suppressor miRNAs are frequently down-regulated in gliomas as compared to normal brain [64–67]. In contrast, some miRNAs are defined as oncogenes with enhanced expression in glioma such as miR-21, targeting regulators, miR-10b and miR-221, targeting cell cycle inhibitors, miR-30e, and targeting IjBa [68–71]. It has been suggested that there is a link between miRNAs and well-known stem cell-regulating proteins [72]. It has also been reported that miR-17-92 plays a critical role in regulation of glioma stem cell (GSC) differentiation, apoptosis, and proliferation [73]. miR-451 expression reduced notably in cancer cells kept in low glucose conditions. Results revealed that cancer cells kept in low glucose conditions had reduced cell proliferation but an enhanced rate of cell migration and survival in glioblastomas. Glucose sufficiency induced upregulation of miR-451 notably inhibited LKB1/AMPK pathway activation [74]. miR-128, downregulated in glioblastoma tissue, has a tumor-suppressive function. Both in vitro and in vivo, miR-128 expression significantly reduces glioma cell proliferation via downregulation of *Bmi-1 oncogene*, a component of the polycomb repressor complex (PRC). In addition, miR-128 inhibits GSC self-renewal [75]. The PRC has been shown to induce normal and cancer stem cell self-renewal and plays role in GSC regulation [76]. When miR-124 has overexpression, it can inhibit the CD133+ cell subpopulation of the neurosphere and downregulate stem cell markers, such as *BMI1*, *Nanog*, and *Nestin* [77]. Both miR-124 and miR-137 are up-regulated during adult neural stem cell differentiation and down-regulated in high-grade gliomas [78]. Although there are comprehensive studies about miRNa in gliomas, it should not be forgotten that one miRNA can affect the expression of various target genes. It must be reconsidered in terms of several important aspects before miRNAs may be used therapeutically [79].

LncRNAs which have more than 200 nucleotides and are up to 100 kb in length are described as an important RNA molecule that plays role in some biological cellular actions such as stemness, development, and cell survival [80–82]. Maternally expressed gene 3 (*MEG3*) is a maternally expressed imprinted gene that can also act as an lncRNA. Its expression in glioma tissues is lower than that in normal adjacent tissues [83]. The tumor-suppressive role of *MEG3* is confirmed by the fact that it can associate with p53. It is known that this association is needed for p53 activation [84].

6. Possible relationships between location and genetic signature in primary brain tumors

A unique finding is that the location of certain primary brain tumors determines their genetic characteristics. Cranial base meningiomas are less malignant compared to the non-cranial base meningiomas [85]. The frequencies of grade II and III cranial base and non-cranial base meningiomas are 3.5 and 12.1%, respectively. These findings origin from a clinical-pathological observation. The biological, molecular, and genetic basis of this fact requires further explanation. A simple answer would be the diverse embryological origins of the dura mater in various locations of human skull [86]. A recently published paper showed (utmost) intriguing data about meningioma biology, which is going to help our understanding of this tumor, of which 85–90% is classified as benign (grade I), but has in certain locations an aggressive course. Meningiomas regarding their genetic origin are divided as NF2 and non-NF2 meningiomas. The non-NF2 meningiomas behave clinically different and are generally always benign, with chromosomal stability, and originate from the medial skull base. In contrast to these findings, meningiomas with mutant NF2 and/or chromosome 22 loss are more likely to be atypical and demonstrate genomic instability and are localized to the cerebral and cerebellar hemispheres. This group concludes their study: "Collectively, these findings identify distinct meningioma subtypes, suggesting avenues for targeted therapeutics" [87]. There is a mutational profile of a meningioma, which can be predicted based on its anatomical location in human calvarium. This finding may provide a unique treatment strategy for midline tumors, which may have a response to medical treatment like hedgehog inhibitors. There are treatment-resistant meningiomas, which are surgically unresectable, recurrent, or invasive. In these patients one can reserve surgery or irradiation, bearing in mind that there is an independent risk factor for progression of these generally benign considered primary brain tumors. This location-based molecular and genetic data provides an updated information about prognosis and treatment response of meningiomas. This update research, which is collected over 300 meningiomas, is a valuable finding, regarding designing personalized management strategies for meningiomas.

Another fact about meningioma is that there is a subgroup of meningiomas, which are histopathologically classified as grade I meningioma, but recurs during follow-up in a short distance unexpectedly as grade II and later as grade III meningiomas. Although the malignant progression of gliomas is considerably well defined and researched entity, there is lack of scientific data about meningiomas, regarding which one is going to transform malignantly. Al-Mefty et al. explained this clinical observation with their FISH analysis of primary and recurring meningiomas with malignant progression in their series. They studied 175 recurrent meningiomas and found that 11 tumors showed histopathologically verified progression to a higher grade. In this study, the cytogenetic analysis with FISH showed deletions of 22, 1p, and 14q. The interesting finding was that in all but one case, these aberrations have been shown to be also present in the previous specimen despite their lower histopathological grades [88].

The conclusion of this translational paper from 2004 was defined: "Tumors that present with complex genetic alterations, even those with a benign histopathological grade are potentially aggressive and require closer follow-up." After 12 years this sentence is still valid for meningiomas and other primary brain tumors, which are genetically prone to upgrade. The designated malignant progression of primary brain tumors is an important issue for designing molecular-genetic-based therapeutic approaches in the near future. The finding that oligodendrogliomas show allelic deletions on 19q and 1p has been defined in 1994 by Reifenberger et al. [89]. Clinical relevance and its implication in changing management strategies followed this genetic finding. The chemotherapeutic response and survival in patients with anaplastic oligodendrogliomas were explained with the over-mentioned genetic background [90]. Its relationship with better prognosis and response to chemotherapy is today an established fact and will be considered in the update "integrated-layered" classification of central nervous system tumors after Haarlem consensus [91]. The location of oligodendrogliomas and its relationship with 1p19q deletion further changed our direction in a phylogenetic explanation of primary brain tumor development and coexisting molecular-genetic mechanisms. Frontal location of oligodendroglioma was suggested to be a favorable prognostic factor. The accumulated data clearly demonstrated that frontal location was strongly correlated with 1p19q deletion [92]. Prognostic variables in oligodendroglial tumors: a single-institution study of 95 cases. This translational information eased (helped) to predict the prognosis of these peculiar tumors. The embryological developmental basis of oligodendroglioma and its molecular-genetic relationship are other issues, which require further investigation.

Lucius Annaeus Seneca, known as Seneca the Younger (c. 4 BC–AD 65), stated: "No one can wear a mask for very long." We can further apply this wise quote to our update neuro-oncological approach, which requires redefinition in the coming decades: "No tumor can wear a mask for very long." The molecular-genetic data and determining its relationship with primary brain tumors will further relieve "the mask" of the primary brain tumors. The upcoming new WHO classification of central nervous system tumors will consider this issue.

Author details

Ilhan Yaylim[1], Sumeyya Azam[2], Ammad Ahmad Farooqi[3], Özlem Küçükhüseyin[1], Muhammad Ismail[3] and Ali Metin Kafadar[4*]

*Address all correspondence to: ctfkafadar@gmail.com

1 Institute of Experimental Medicine, Department of Molecular Medicine, Istanbul University, Istanbul, Turkey

2 First Affiliated Hospital of Xinjiang Medical University, Xinjiang, Urumqi, PR China

3 Institute of Biomedical and Genetic Engineering (IBGE), Islamabad, Pakistan

4 Department of Neurosurgery, Cerrahpaşa Medical Faculty, Istanbul University, Istanbul, Turkey

References

[1] Karsy M, Neil JA, Guan J, Mahan MA, Colman H, Jensen RL: A practical review of prognostic correlations of molecular biomarkers in glioblastoma. Neurosurg Focus. 2015;38(3):E4. doi: 10.3171/2015.1.FOCUS14755.

[2] Etzioni R, Urban N, Ramsey S, McIntosh M, Schwartz S, Reid B, Radich J, Anderson G, Hartwell L: The case for early detection. Nat Rev Cancer. 2003;3(4):243–252.

[3] Kulasingam V, Diamandis EP: Strategies for discovering novel cancer biomarkers through utilization of emerging technologies. Nat Clin Pract Oncol. 2008;5:588–599.

[4] Hayes DF, Bast RC, Desch CE, Fritsche H Jr, Kemeny NE, Jessup JM, Locker GY, Macdonald JS, Mennel RG, Norton L, Ravdin P, Taube S, Winn RJ: Tumor marker utility grading system: a framework to evaluate clinical utility of tumor markers. J Natl Cancer Inst. 1996;88(20):1456–1466.

[5] Holdhoff M, Ye X, Blakeley JO, Blair L, Burger PC, Grossman SA, et al: Use of personalized molecular biomarkers in the clinical care of adults with glioblastomas. J Neurooncol. 2012;110:279–285.

[6] Westhoff MA, Karpel-Massler G, Brühl O, Enzenmüller S, La Ferla-Brühl K, Siegelin MD, Nonnenmacher L Debatin KM: A critical evaluation of PI3K inhibition in glioblastoma and neuroblastoma therapy. Mol Cell Ther. 2014;2:32.

[7] Rao RD, James CD: Altered molecular pathways in gliomas: an overview of clinically relevant issues. Semin Oncol. 2004;31(5):595–604

[8] Guha A, Feldkamp MM, Lau N, Boss G, Pawson A: Proliferation of human malignant astrocytomas is dependent on Ras activation. Oncogene. 1997;15:2755–2765.

[9] Pandey V, Bhaskara VK, Babu PP: Implications of mitogen-activated protein kinase signaling in glioma. J Neurosci Res. 2016;94:114–127. doi: 10.1002/jnr.23687.

[10] Wong AJ, Ruppert JM, Bigner SH, Grzeschik CH, Humphrey PA, Bigner DS, et al: Structural alterations of the epidermal growth factor receptor gene in human gliomas. Proc Natl Acad Sci U S A. 1992;89:2965–2969.

[11] Frederick L, Wang XY, Eley G, James CD: Diversity and frequency of epidermal growth factor receptor mutations in human glioblastomas. Cancer Res. 2000;60:1383–1387.

[12] Salkeni MA, Zarzour A, Ansay TY, McPherson CM, Warnick RE, Rixe O, et al: Detection of EGFRvIII mutant DNA in the peripheral blood of brain tumor patients. J Neurooncol. 2013;115:27–35

[13] Taylor TE, Furnari FB, Cavenee WK: Targeting EGFR for treatment of glioblastoma: molecular basis to overcome resistance. Curr Cancer Drug Targets. 2012;12:197–209.

[14] Brennan C, Momota H, Hambardzumyan D, Ozawa T, Tandon A, Pedraza A, et al: Glioblastoma subclasses can be defined by activity among signal transduction pathways and associated genomic alterations. PLoS ONE. 2009;4:e7752.

[15] Ozawa T, Brennan CW, Wang L, Squatrito M, Sasayama T, Nakada M, et al: PDGFRA gene rearrangements are frequent genetic events in PDGFRA-amplified glioblastomas. Genes Dev. 2010;24:2205–2218.

[16] Verhaak RGW, Hoadley KA, Purdom E, Wang V, Qi Y, Wilkerson MD, et al: Integrated genomic analysis identifies clinically relevant subtypes of glioblastoma characterized by abnormalities in PDGFRA, IDH1, EGFR, and NF1. Cancer Cell. 2010;17:98–110.

[17] Sami A, Karsy M: Targeting the PI3K/AKT/mTOR signaling pathway in glioblastoma: novel therapeutic agents and advances in understanding. Tumour Biol. 2013;34:1991–2002.

[18] King D, Yeomanson D, Bryant HE: PI3King the lock: targeting the PI3K/Akt/mTOR pathway as a novel therapeutic strategy in neuroblastoma. J Pediatr Hematol Oncol. 2015;37:245–251.

[19] Rafalski VA, Brunet A: Energy metabolism in adult neural stem cell fate. Prog Neurobiol. 2011;93(2):182–203. doi: 10.1016/j.pneurobio.2010.10.007. PMID 21056618.

[20] Network CGAR: Comprehensive genomic characterization defines human glioblastoma genes and core pathways. Nature. 2008;455:1061–1068.

[21] Fan QW, Weiss WA: Targeting the RTK–PI3K–mTOR axis in malignant glioma: overcoming resistance. Curr Top Microbiol Immunol. 2010;347:279–296.

[22] Lavrik IN, Golks A, and Krammer PH: Caspases: pharmacological manipulation of cell death. J Clin Invest. 2005;115:2665–2672.

[23] Bellail AC, Olson JJ, Yang X, Chen ZJ, Hao C: A20 ubiquitin ligase-mediated polyubiquitination of RIP1 inhibits caspase-8 cleavage and TRAIL-induced apoptosis in glioblastoma. Cancer Discov. 2012;2(2):140–155.

[24] Crommentuijn MH, Maguire CA, Niers JM, Vandertop WP, Badr CE, Würdinger T, Tannous BA: Intracranial AAV–sTRAIL combined with lanatoside C prolongs survival in an orthotopic xenograft mouse model of invasive glioblastoma. Mol Oncol. 2015;11. pii: S1574-7891(15)00226-4.

[25] Balyasnikova IV, Prasol MS, Ferguson SD, Han Y, Ahmed AU, Gutova M, Tobias AL, Mustafi D, Rincón E, Zhang L, Aboody KS, Lesniak MS: Intranasal delivery of mesenchymal stem cells significantly extends survival of irradiated mice with experimental brain tumors. Mol Ther. 2014;22(1):140–148.

[26] Yulyana Y, Endaya BB, Ng WH, Guo CM, Hui KM, Lam PY, Ho IA: Carbenoxolone enhances TRAIL-induced apoptosis through the upregulation of death receptor 5 and

inhibition of gap junction intercellular communication in human glioma. Stem Cells Dev. 2013;22(13):1870–1882.

[27] Wang LH, Ni CW, Lin YZ, Yin L, Jiang CB, Lv CT, Le Y, Lang Y, Zhao CY, Yang K, Jiao BH, Yin J: Targeted induction of apoptosis in glioblastoma multiforme cells by an MRP3-specific TRAIL fusion protein in vitro. Tumour Biol. 2014;35(2):1157–1168.

[28] van de Water JA, Bagci-Onder T, Agarwal AS, Wakimoto H, Roovers RC, Zhu Y, Kasmieh R, Bhere D, Van Bergen en Henegouwen PM, Shah K: Therapeutic stem cells expressing variants of EGFR-specific nanobodies have antitumor effects. Proc Natl Acad Sci U S A. 2012;109(41):16642–16647

[29] Ahn Y, Oh S, Lee SJ, Park BG, Park YS, Shin WS, Jang HJ, Park JH, Kwon D, Lee S: Synthesis of diethylamino-curcumin mimics with substituted triazolyl groups and their sensitization effect of TRAIL against brain cancer cells. Bioorg Med Chem Lett. 2014;24(15):3346–3350.

[30] Lee DH, Lee CS, Kim DW, Ae JE, Lee TH: Digitoxin sensitizes glioma cells to TRAIL-mediated apoptosis by upregulation of death receptor 5 and downregulation of survivin. Anticancer Drugs. 2014;25(1):44–52.

[31] Abusamra YA, Scuruchi M, Habibatni S, Maammeri Z, Benayache S, D'Ascola A, Avenoso A, Campo GM, Spina E: Evaluation of putative cytotoxic activity of crude extracts from *Onopordum acanthium* leaves and Spartium junceum flowers against the U-373 glioblastoma cell line. Pak J Pharm Sci. 2015;28(4):1225–1232.

[32] Gentile MT, Ciniglia C, Reccia MG, Volpicelli F, Gatti M, Thellung S, Florio T, Melone MA, Colucci-D'Amato L: *Ruta graveolens* L. induces death of glioblastoma cells and neural progenitors, but not of neurons, via ERK 1/2 and AKT activation. PLoS One. 2015;10(3):e0118864.

[33] Noté OP, Jihu D, Antheaume C, Zeniou M, Pegnyemb DE, Guillaume D, Chneiwess H, Kilhoffer MC, Lobstein A: Triterpenoid saponins from *Albizia lebbeck* (L.) Benth and their inhibitory effect on the survival of high grade human brain tumor cells. Carbohydr Res. 2015;404:26–33.

[34] Parsons DW, Jones S, Zhang X, Lin JC, Leary RJ, Angenendt P, Mankoo P, Carter H, Siu IM, Gallia GL, Olivi A, McLendon R, Rasheed BA, Keir S, Nikolskaya T, Nikolsky Y, Busam DA, Tekleab H, Diaz LA Jr, Hartigan J, Smith DR, Strausberg RL, Marie SK, Shinjo SM, Yan H, Riggins GJ, Bigner DD, Karchin R,Papadopoulos N, Parmigiani G, Vogelstein B, Velculescu VE, Kinzler KW: An integrated genomic analysis of human glioblastoma multiforme. Science. 2008;321:1807–1812. doi: 10.1126/science.1164382.

[35] Noushmehr H, Weisenberger DJ, Diefes K, Phillips HS, Pujara K, Berman BP, et al: Identification of a CpG island methylator phenotype that defines a distinct subgroup of glioma. Cancer Cell. 2010;17:510–522.

[36] Lu C, Ward PS, Kapoor GS, Rohle D, Turcan S, Abdel-Wahab O, Edwards CR, Khanin R, Figueroa ME, Melnick A, Wellen KE, O'Rourke DM, Berger SL, Chan TA, Levine RL,

Mellinghoff IK, Thompson CB: IDH mutation impairs histone demethylation and results in a block to cell differentiation. Nature. 2012;483:474–478.

[37] Dang L, White DW, Gross S, Bennett BD, Bittinger MA, Driggers EM, Fantin VR, Jang HG, Jin S, Keenan MC, Marks KM, Prins RM, Ward PS, Yen KE, Liau LM, Rabinowitz JD, Cantley LC, Thompson CB, Vander Heiden MG, Su SM: Cancer-associated IDH1 mutations produce 2-hydroxyglutarate. Nature. 2010;465:966.

[38] Xu W, Yang H, Liu Y, Yang Y, Wang P, Kim SH, Ito S, Yang C, Wang P, Xiao MT, Liu LX, Jiang WQ, Liu J, Zhang JY, Wang B, Frye S, Zhang Y, Xu YH, Lei QY, Guan KL, Zhao SM, Xiong Y: Oncometabolite 2-hydroxyglutarate is a competitive inhibitor of alpha-ketoglutarate-dependent dioxygenases. Cancer Cell. 2011;19:17–30.

[39] Jin SG, Jiang Y, Qiu R, Rauch RA, Wang Y, Schackert G, Krex D, Lu Q, Pfeifer GP: 5-Hydroxymethylcytosine is strongly depleted in human cancers but its levels do not correlate with IDH1 mutations. Cancer Res. 2011;71:7360–7365.

[40] Kraus TF, Globisch D, Wagner M, Eigenbrod S, Widmann D, Munzel M, Muller M, Pfaffeneder T, Hackner B, Feiden W, Schuller U, Carell T, Kretzschmar HA: Low values of 5-hydroxymethylcytosine (5hmC), the "sixth base," are associated with anaplasia in human brain tumors. Int J Cancer. 2012, http://dx.doi.org/10.1002/ijc.27429.

[41] Ohgaki H, Kleihues P: Genetic profile of astrocytic and oligodendroglial gliomas. Brain Tumor Pathol. 2011;28:177–183.

[42] England B, Huang T, Karsy M: Current understanding of the role and targeting of tumor suppressor p53 in glioblastoma multiforme. Tumour Biol. 2013;34:2063–2074.

[43] Biernat W, Kleihues P, Yonekawa Y, Ohgaki H: Amplification and overexpression of MDM2 in primary (de novo) glioblastomas. J Neuropathol Exp Neurol. 1997;56:180–185.

[44] Nakamura M, Watanabe T, Klangby U, Asker C, Wiman K, Yonekawa Y, et al: p14ARF deletion and methylation in genetic pathways to glioblastomas. Brain Pathol. 2001;11:159–168.

[45] Blough MD, Beauchamp DC, Westgate MR, Kelly JJ, Cairncross JG: Effect of aberrant p53 function on temozolomide sensitivity of glioma cell lines and brain tumor initiating cells from glioblastoma. J Neurooncol. 2011;102:1–7.

[46] Ino Y, Betensky RA, Zlatescu MC, Sasaki H, Macdonald DR, Stemmer-Rachamimov AO, Ramsay DA, Cairncross JG, Louis DN: Molecular subtypes of anaplastic oligodendroglioma: implications for patient management at diagnosis. Clin Cancer Res. 2001;7:839–845.

[47] Jeuken JW, von Deimling A, Wesseling P: Molecular pathogenesis of oligodendroglial tumors. J Neurooncol. 2004;70:161–181.

[48] Wolf RM, Draghi N, Liang X, Dai C, Uhrbom L, Eklof C, Westermark B, Holland EC, Resh MD: p190RhoGAP can act to inhibit PDGF induced gliomas in mice: a putative

tumor suppressor encoded on human chromosome 19q13.3. Genes Dev. 2003;17:476–487.

[49] Idbaih A, Marie Y, Pierron G, Brennetot C, Hoang-Xuan K, Kujas M, Mokhtari K, Sanson M, Lejeune J, Aurias A, Delattre O, Delattre JY: Two types of chromosome 1p losses with opposite significance in gliomas. Ann Neurol. 2005;58:483– 487.

[50] Cairncross G, Wang M, Shaw E, Jenkins R, Brachman D, Buckner J, et al: Phase III trial of chemoradiotherapy for anaplastic oligodendroglioma: long-term results of RTOG 9402. J Clin Oncol. 2013;31:337–343.

[51] Boots-Sprenger SHE, Sijben A, Rijntjes J, Tops BBJ, Idema AJ, Rivera AL, et al: Significance of complete 1p/19q codeletion, IDH1 mutation and MGMT promoter methylation in gliomas: use with caution. Mod Pathol. 2013;26:922–929.

[52] Schmidt MC, Antweiler S, Urban N, Mueller W, Kuklik A, Meyer-Puttlitz B, et al: Impact of genotype and morphology on the prognosis of glioblastoma. J Neuropathol Exp Neurol. 2002;61:321–328.

[53] Hartmann C, Hentschel B, Simon M, Westphal M, Schackert G, Tonn JC, et al: Long-term survival in primary glioblastoma with versus without isocitrate dehydrogenase mutations. Clin Cancer Res. 2013;19:5146–5157.

[54] Laxton RC, Popov S, Doey L, Jury A, Bhangoo R, Gullan R, et al: Primary glioblastoma with oligodendroglial differentiation has better clinical outcome but no difference in common biological markers compared with other types of glioblastoma. Neuro Oncol. 2013;15:1635–1643.

[55] SongTao Q, Lei Y, Si G, YanQing D, HuiXia H, XueLin Z, et al: IDH mutations predict longer survival and response to temozolomide in secondary glioblastoma. Cancer Sci. 2012;103:269–273.

[56] Wick W, Hartmann C, Engel C, Stoffels M, Felsberg J, Stockhammer F, Sabel MC, Koeppen S, Ketter R, Meyermann R, Rapp M, Meisner C, Kortmann RD,Pietsch T, Wiestler OD, Ernemann U, Bamberg M, Reifenberger G, von Deimling A, Weller M: NOA-04 randomized phase III trial of sequential radiochemotherapy of anaplastic glioma with procarbazine, lomustine, and vincristine or temozolomide. J Clin Oncol. 2009;27(35):5874–5880. doi: 10.1200/JCO.2009.23.6497.

[57] Gorlia T, van den Bent MJ, Hegi ME, Mirimanoff RO, Weller M, Cairncross JG, Eisenhauer E, Belanger K, Brandes AA, Allgeier A, Lacombe D, Stupp R.: Nomograms for predicting survival of patients with newly diagnosed glioblastoma: prognostic factor analysis of EORTC and NCIC trial 26981-22981/CE.3. Lancet Oncol. 2008;9:29–38.

[58] Karlic R, Chung HR, Lasserre J, Vlahovicek K, Vingron M: Histone modification levels are predictive for gene expression. Proc Natl Acad Sci U S A. 2010;107:2926–2931.

[59] Bannister AJ, Kouzarides T: Regulation of chromatin by histone modifications. Cell Res. 2011;21:381–395.

[60] Santos-Rosa H, Schneider R, Bannister AJ, Sherriff J, Bernstein BE, Emre NC, Schreiber SL, Mellor J, Kouzarides T: Active genes are tri-methylated at K4 of histone H3. Nature. 2002;419:407–411.

[61] Costa FF: Non-coding RNAs, epigenetics and complexity. Gene. 2008;410:9–17.

[62] Esteller M: Non-coding RNAs in human disease. Nat Rev Genet. 2011;12:861–874.

[63] Mendell JT: MicroRNAs: critical regulators of development, cellular physiology and malignancy. Cell Cycle. 2005;4:1179–1184.

[64] Li Y, Guessous F, Zhang Y, diPierro C, Kefas B, Johnson E, Marcinkiewicz L, Jiang J, Yang Y, Schmittgen TD, Lopes B, Schiff D, Purow B, Abounader R: MicroRNA-34a inhibits glioblastoma growth by targeting multiple oncogenes. Cancer Res. 2009;69:7569–7576.

[65] Mei J, Bachoo R, Zhang CL: MicroRNA-146a inhibits glioma development by targeting Notch1. Mol Cell Biol. 2011;31:3584–3592.

[66] Kefas B, Godlewski J, Comeau L, Li Y, Abounader R, Hawkinson M, Lee J, Fine H, Chiocca EA, Lawler S, Purow B: MicroRNA-7 inhibits the epidermal growth factor receptor and the Akt pathway and is down-regulated in glioblastoma. Cancer Res. 2008;68:3566–3572.

[67] Zhang QQ, Xu H, Huang MB, Ma LM, Huang QJ, Yao Q, Zhou H, Qu LH: MicroRNA-195 plays a tumor-suppressor role in human glioblastoma cells by targeting signaling pathways involved in cellular proliferation and invasion. Neuro Oncol. 2012;14:278–287.

[68] Gabriely G, Yi M, Narayan RS, Niers JM, Wurdinger T, Imitola J, Ligon KL, Kesari S, Esau C, Stephens RM, Tannous BA, Krichevsky AM: Human glioma growth is controlled by microRNA-10b. Cancer Res. 2011;71;3563–3572.

[69] Gabriely G, Wurdinger T, Kesari S, Esau CC, Burchard J, Linsley PS, Krichevsky AM: MicroRNA 21 promotes glioma invasion by targeting matrix metalloproteinase regulators. Mol Cell Biol. 2008;28:5369–5380.

[70] Jiang L, Lin C, Song L, Wu J, Chen B, Ying Z, Fang L, Yan X, He M, Li J, Li M: MicroRNA-30e_ promotes human glioma cell invasiveness in an orthotopic xenotransplantation model by disrupting the NF-kappaB/IkappaBalpha negative feedback loop. J Clin Invest. 2012;122:33–47.

[71] Zhang CZ, Zhang JX, Zhang AL, Shi ZD, Han L, Jia ZF, Yang WD, Wang GX, Jiang T, You YP, Pu PY, Cheng JQ, Kang CS: MiR-221 and miR-222 target PUMA to induce cell survival in glioblastoma. Mol Cancer. 2010;9;229.

[72] Piccirillo SG, Reynolds BA, Zanetti N, Lamorte G, Binda E, Broggi G, et al: Bone morphogenetic proteins inhibit the tumorigenic potential of human brain tumour-initiating cells. Nature. 2006;444:761–765. doi: 10.1038/nature 05349.

[73] Ernst A, Campos B , Meier J, Devens F, Liesenberg F, Wolter M, et al: De-repression of CTGF via the miR-17-92 cluster upon differentiation of human glioblastoma spheroid cultures. Oncogene. 2010;29:3411–3422. doi: 10.1038/onc.2010.83.

[74] Godlewski J, Nowicki MO, Bronisz A,Nuovo G, Palatini J, DeLay M, et al: MicroRNA-451regulates LKB1/AMPKsignalingandallows adaptation to metabolic stress in glioma cells. Mol Cell. 2010;37:620–632. doi: 10.1016/j.molcel.2010.02.018.

[75] Godlewski J, Nowicki MO, Bronisz A, Williams S, Otsuki A, Nuovo G, et al: Targeting of the Bmi-1 oncogene/stemcell renewal factor by microRNA-128 inhibits glioma proliferation and self-renewal. Cancer Res. 2008;68:9125–9130. doi: 10.1158/0008-5472.CAN-08-2629.

[76] Natsume A, Ito M, Katsushima K,Ohka F, Hatanaka A,Shinjo K, et al: Chromatin regulator PRC2Is a key regulator of epigenetic plasticity in glioblastoma. Cancer Res. 2013;73:4559–4570.

[77] Xia H, Cheung WK, Ng SS, Jiang X, Jiang S, Sze J, et al: Loss of brain-enriched miR-124 microRNA enhances stem-like traits and invasiveness of glioma cells. J Biol Chem. 2012. 287:9962–9971. doi: 10.1074/jbc.M111.332627

[78] Silber J, Lim DA,Petritsch C, Persson AI, Maunakea AK, Yu M, et al: miR-124 and miR-137 inhibit proliferation of glioblastoma multiforme cells and induce differentiation of brain tumor stem cells. BMC Med. 2008;6:14. doi: 10.1186/1741-7015-6-14.

[79] Kreth S, Thon N, Kreth FW: Epigenetics in human gliomas. Cancer Lett. 2014;342:185–192

[80] Mercer TR, Dinger ME, Mattick JS: Long non-coding RNAs: insights into functions. Nat Rev Genet. 2009;10:155–159. doi: 10.1038/nrg2521

[81] Koziol MJ, Rinn JL: RNA traffic control of chromatin complexes. Curr Opin Genet Dev. 2010;20:142–148. doi: 10.1016/j.gde.2010.03.003.

[82] Zhang H, Chen Z, Wang X, Huang Z, He Z, Chen Y. Long non-coding RNA:a new player in cancer. J Hematol Oncol. 2013;6:37. doi: 10.1186/1756-8722-6-37.

[83] Wang P, Ren Z, Sun P: Overexpression of the long non-coding RNA MEG3 impairs in vitro glioma cell proliferation. J Cell Biochem. 2012;113:1868–1874. doi: 10.1002/jcb.24055

[84] Lu KH, Li W, Liu XH, Sun M, Zhang ML, Wu WQ, et al: Long non-coding RNA MEG3 inhibits NSCLC cells proliferation and induces apoptosis by affecting p53 expression. BMC Cancer. 2013;13:461. doi: 10.1186/1471-2407-13-461.

[85] Sade B, Chahlavi A, Krishnaney A, Nagel S, Choi E, Lee JH: World Health Organization grades II and III meningiomas are rare in the cranial base and spine. Neurosurgery. 2007;61:1194–1198.

[86] O'Rahilly R, Muller F: The meninges in human development. J Neuropathol Exp Neurol. 1986;45:588–608.

[87] Clark VE, Erson-Omay EZ, Serin A, Jun Yin J, Cotney J, Ozduman K, et al: Genomic analysis of non-NF2 meningiomas reveals mutations in TRAF7, KLF4, AKT1, and SMO. Science. 2013;339(6123)1077–1080.

[88] Al-Mefty O, Kadri P, Pravdenkova S, Sawyer JR, Stangeby C, Husain M: Malignant progression in meningioma: documentation of a series and analysis of cytogenetic findings. J Neurosurg. 2004;101:210–218.

[89] Reifenberger J, Reifenberger G, Liu L, James CD, Wechsler W, Collins VP: Molecular genetic analysis of oligodendroglial tumors shows preferential allelic deletions on 19q and 1p. Am J Pathol. 1994;145(5):1175–1190.

[90] Cairncross JG, Ueki K, Zlatescu MC, Lisle DK, Finkelstein DM, Hammond RR, Silver JS, Stark PC, Macdonald DR, Ino Y, Ramsay DA, Louis DN: Specific genetic predictors of chemotherapeutic response and survival in patients with anaplastic oligodendrogliomas. J Natl Cancer Inst. 1998;90:1473–1479.

[91] Louis DN, Perry A, Burger P, Ellison DW, Reifenberger G, von Deimling A, Aldape K, Brat D, Collins VP, Eberhart C et al.International society of neuropathology-haarlem consensus guidelines for nervous system tumor classification and grading. Brain Pathol. 2014;24:429–435.

[92] Scheie D, Meling TR, Cvancarova M, Skullerud K, Mørk S, Lote K, Eide TJ, Helseth E, Beiske K. Prognostic variables in oligodendroglial tumors: a single-institution study of 95 cases. Neuro Oncol. 2011;13:1225–1233.

Chapter 7

Advanced MR Imaging Techniques in the Diagnosis of Intra-axial Brain Tumors

Anastasia Zikou, George Alexiou and
Maria Argyropoulou

Additional information is available at the end of the chapter

http://dx.doi.org/10.5772/62840

Abstract

Intracranial masses are a significant health problem and present several imaging challenges. The role of imaging is no longer limited to merely providing anatomic details but the advanced MR techniques permit the assessment of the freedom of water molecule movement, the microvascular structure and hemodynamic characteristics, and the chemical makeup of certain metabolites of lesions. In the current chapter, we will discuss the role of the advanced MR imaging techniques, namely perfusion, diffusion-weighted imaging, and MR spectroscopy in the diagnosis and classification of the most frequent brain tumors in adults. We provide a brief description of the advanced MR techniques that are currently used, and we discuss in detail the imaging findings for each lesion. These lesions include gliomas both high and low grade, metastatic lesions, lymphomas, and lesions that may mimic tumors such as tumefactive demyelinating lesions, abscesses, and encephalitis. Our goal is to summarize the diagnostic information that advanced MR imaging techniques offer for establishing a diagnosis and clinical decision making.

Keywords: MRI, brain tumors, perfusion, diffusion tensor imaging, spectroscopy

1. Introduction

Among primary brain and central nervous system tumors in adults, meningiomas are the most common, accounting for 36.4% of all, followed by pituitary tumors (15.5%) and glioblastoma (WHO Grade IV) (15.1%), which is the most malignant primary brain tumor. Other types are nerve sheath tumors (8.1%), all other astrocytomas (5.7%), lymphoma (2%), ependymal tumors

(1.9%), oligodendrogliomas (1.6%), embryonal tumors (1.1%), oligoastrocytic tumors (0.9%), and all other less frequent tumors (11.7%) [1].

Imaging has a fundamental role in intracranial tumor management. Magnetic resonance imaging (MRI) is the imaging modality of choice for establishing diagnosis, classification, surgical planning, and post-treatment follow-up. The latest MRI techniques, namely diffusion, perfusion, and spectroscopy, offer more than the anatomical information that conventional imaging provides. Diffusion allows the assessment of water displacement within tissue. Diffusion tensor imaging permits the mapping of axonal organization. Perfusion MRI is a technique for the assessment of cerebral perfusion. Dynamic susceptibility contrast imaging (DSC-MRI) perfusion technique is currently the most widely used and allows the calculation of relative cerebral blood volume (rCBV) and relative cerebral blood flow (rCBF). MR spectroscopy, with single-voxel or multi-voxel techniques, can detect metabolites within tissue such as N-acetyl aspartate (NAA), choline-containing compounds (Cho), myoinositol (mI), lactate (Lac), creatine (Cr), and other molecules. However, no tumor-specific metabolite has been recognized to date.

Although the discrimination between intra-axial and extra-axial lesions is relatively straightforward, for the accurate discrimination of the variety of intra-axial tumors of several difficulties exist. This is of paramount importance for timely and appropriate patients' management. Herewith, we provide an overview of the latest MR techniques for the differential diagnosis of intra-axial tumors.

2. Primary tumors

Gliomas are the most common primary brain tumors. Glioblastoma accounts for 55% of all cases followed by diffuse astrocytoma (8.6%), ependymal tumors (6.9%), anaplastic astrocytomas (6.1%), oligodenrogliomas (5.7%), pilocytic astrocytomas (5.2%), and other less frequent glioma types [1]. Incidence is higher in males and in whites than in blacks. For glioblastoma, the median age of diagnosis is 64 years but for low-grade gliomas (grades I and II), most often occur between 20 and 40 years. The major diagnostic goal in gliomas is the differentiation of low-grade from high-grade gliomas and from other pathologies that have similar imaging features.

2.1. Diffusion-weighted imaging

Apparent diffusion coefficient (ADC) maps alone cannot differentiate between glioma from another neoplasm or glioma type. Malignancy is usually associated with increased cellular density, resulting in decreased signal intensity on ADC images. High-grade gliomas usually have significant lower ADC values than low-grade gliomas. A lesion-to-normal (L/N) ADC ratio of 1.43 could differentiate low-grade from high-grade gliomas with 100% sensitivity and 94.4% specificity [2]. Evaluation of the perilesion area may aid the diagnosis of a primary tumor due to its infiltrative nature (**Figure 1**).

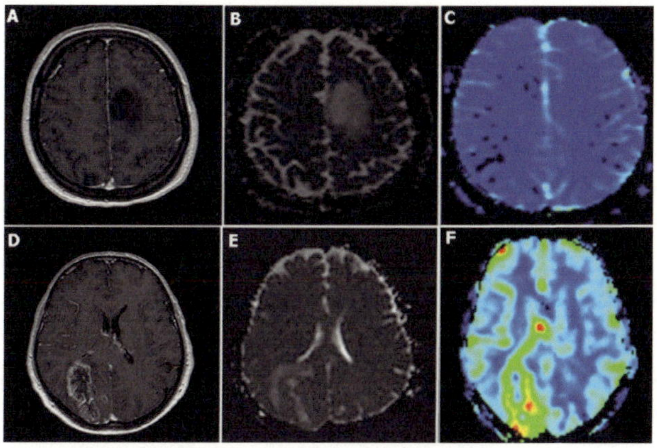

Figure 1. (A) A case of a grade II astrocytoma and of glioblastoma (D). There is a lower ADC value in astrocytoma (B) than glioblastoma (E). The rCBV map shows increased perfusion in glioblastoma (F) contrary to astrocytoma (C).

2.2. Perfusion imaging

Perfusion MRI can be performed using a variety of methods. The most common techniques are as follows: T2-weighted dynamic susceptibility contrast (DSC), T1-weighted dynamic contrast enhanced (DCE), and arterial spine labeling (ASL). The latter do not require contrast administration. The relative cerebral blood volume (rCBV) is the most frequent reported metric. This can be calculated by comparing the cerebral blood volume in a region of interest that is drawn over the tumor to the CBV of a mirror region of interest placed over the normal white matter in the contralateral side.

Gliomas are characterized by increased blood vessels formation for the transport of nutrients and oxygen which are essential for tumor growth. Furthermore, apart from glioma infiltration to parenchyma, malignant cells can also migrate using a perivascular route through microvasculature [3]. Recent reports showed that glioblastoma cells can even differentiate into endothelial cells and pericytes, thus aiding tumor vascularization [4]. High-grade gliomas have a significantly higher rCBV ratio than low-grade gliomas (**Figure 1**). A cut-off ratio of 0.63 has been suggested for the differentiation between them [2]. Furthermore, a significant linear correlation has been reported between rCBV ratio and glioma proliferation potentials as assessed by Ki-67 index and tumor's cell cycle analysis [5, 6]. High-grade tumors had higher Ki-67 index, higher percentage of cells in G2/M phase, and lower percentage of cells in G0/G1 phase.

Oligodendrogliomas contrary to other low-grade gliomas have significant higher rCBV values (mean 3.68 ± 2.39) [7], overlapping even with high-grade gliomas. A possible explanation to this is their increased vascular density and cortical localization [7]. Another important exception is pilocytic astrocytoma, the most common pediatric brain tumor with usually infratentorial localization [8]. The tumor's mural nodule may show increased rCBV ratio in comparison with other low-grade gliomas. Clinicians should also bear in mind that hemangioblastomas may also demonstrate high rCBV ratios.

2.3. MR spectroscopy

Initial studies with MR spectroscopy showed promise for the diagnosis of brain lesions and grading; however, recent evidences are controversial. Several metabolites can be measured that correlate with various pathological alterations within lesions. NAA is the acetylated form of the amino acid, aspartate, which is found in increased concentrations in viable neurons. Given that non-neuronal neoplasms destroy normal neurons there is a reduction in NAA signal. Choline is a marker of cell membrane and can be found elevated in tumors and inflammatory processes. Creatine is a measure of energy stores, whereas lactate increases in cases of ischemia, in which the cell switches to anaerobic glycolysis and lactates accumulates. Thus, lactate is more likely to be present in high-grade than low-grade gliomas. Lipids have been recognized as a marker of myelin breakdown. Several studies have evaluated both single-voxel and multi-voxel spectroscopy. Multi-voxel has the advantage of greater spatial resolution and extent of coverage, thus permits the evaluation of different components of heterogeneous masses. Within tumor, some areas may be more metabolically active than others. In brain tumors, there is usually an increased signal of Cho, whereas NAA and Cr are reduced. Cho/Cr ratio tends to increase as glioma malignancy progresses. In a recent meta-analysis, Cho/NAA ratio showed a sensitivity of 80% and specificity of 76%, higher than Cho/Cr ratio and NAA/Cr ratio for the differentiation of high-grade from low-grade gliomas [9]. However, both sensitivity and specificity do not enable an accurate diagnosis, thus additional imaging modalities may be needed. A CHO/NAA ratio >1, in voxels outside of the enhancement region, suggests tumor infiltration and is indicative of a high-grade glioma (**Figure 2**).

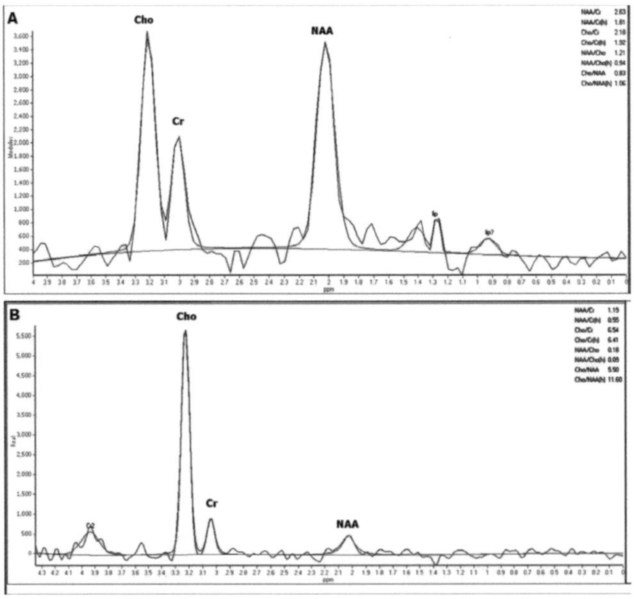

Figure 2. MR proton spectrum of a grade II astrocytoma (A) and of a glioblastoma (B). Contrary to low-grade glioma, glioblastoma exhibits depression of the NAA and creatine (Cr) peaks and elevation of the choline (Cho) peak.

3. Gliomatosis cerebri

Gliomatosis cerebri is a rare diffuse primary neoplastic process of glial origin with dismal prognosis. Based on WHO criteria, this diffusely infiltrating glial neoplasm involves at least three cerebral lobes. There is often bilateral involvement of the cerebral hemispheres and/or deep gray matter (**Figure 3**) [10]. Histopathologically, it is characterized by diffuse infiltration of brain parenchyma by small, immature glial cells that resembles astrocytes, oligodendroglia, or undifferentiated cells [10, 11]. The lesion can contain areas of WHO grades II or III tumors, and less frequent grade IV. Symptomatology is subtle and may involve changes in personality and mental status, headache, hemiparesis, ataxia, and seizures. Although it appears radiologically as extensive disease, clinical symptomatology may be silent. Diagnosis requires brain biopsy and histopathological examination.

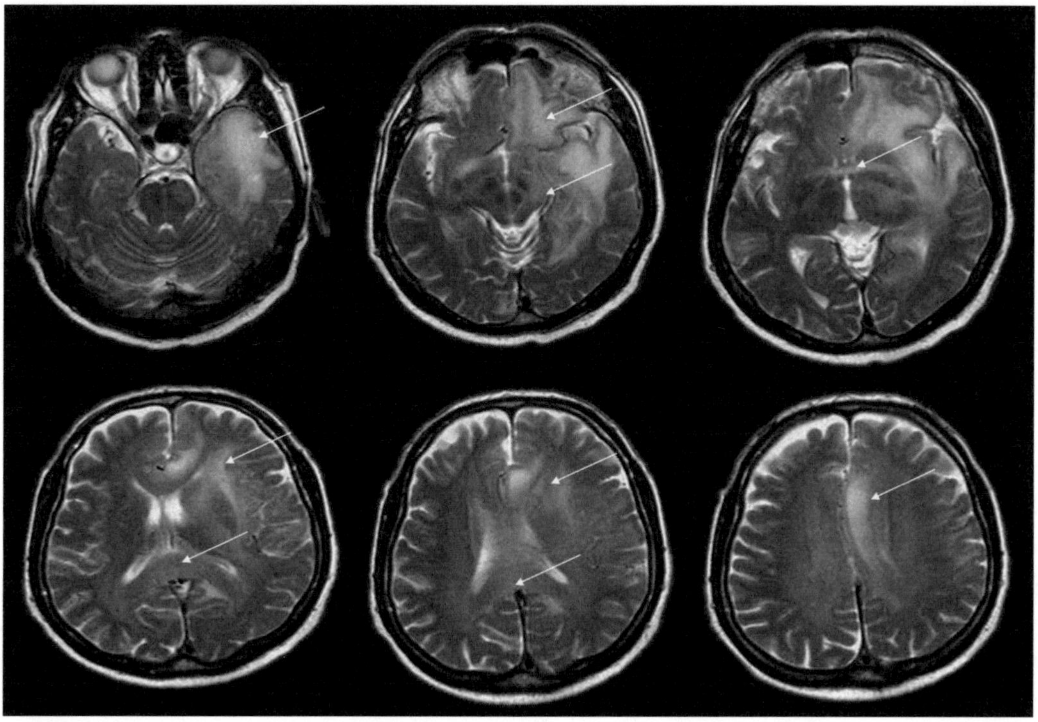

Figure 3. T2-W axial images show diffuse hyperintense lesions with enlargement of the involved structures and little mass effect (arrows).

Two subtypes can be identified radiologically: type 1 with no discrete component and type II with a solid component and diffuse CNS involvement. *IDH1* mutations have been reported more frequent in type II GC [12]. MRI findings are essential for establishing the correct diagnosis. Hypointensity in T1-weighted sequences and hyperintensity in T2-weighted and FLAIR sequences are the classical findings. Another usual MRI finding consists of diffuse infiltration of the cortex with an enlargement of the cortical sulci and the absence of clear delineation between white and gray. Contrast enhancement is absent [13]. In DWI, there is usually no restriction. Perfusion MR shows low or normal rCBV values correlating with the absence of vascular hyperplasia. MR spectroscopy reveals elevated Cho/NAA ratios and marked elevation of myoinositol [14] (**Figure 4**).

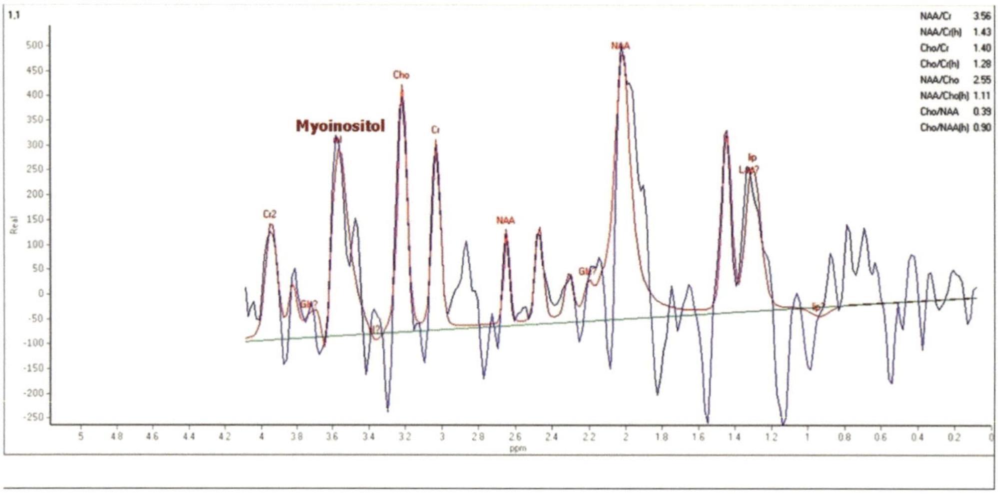

Figure 4. Short-echo MR proton spectrum shows an elevated myoinositol (mI) peak (at 3.55 ppm) in a case of gliomatosis cerebri.

4. Primary central nervous system lymphoma

Primary central nervous system lymphoma (PCNSL) is a rare variant of extranodal non-Hodgkin lymphoma and affects about 1,000 people in the United States each year. Non-invasive diagnosis of PCNSL is of paramount importance given the dramatic benefits of chemotherapy in this tumor. Typical MR imaging features of PCNSLs are frequent periventricular locations, perilesional edema, well-defined margin, and homogeneous and intense nodular enhancement.

4.1. Diffusion-weighted imaging

PCNSLs tend to have a low ADC value because of high cellularity (**Figure 5**). Brain abscess has higher ADC values than lymphomas; thus, this feature can help in differentiating these two entities [15].

http://dx.doi.org/10.5772/62840

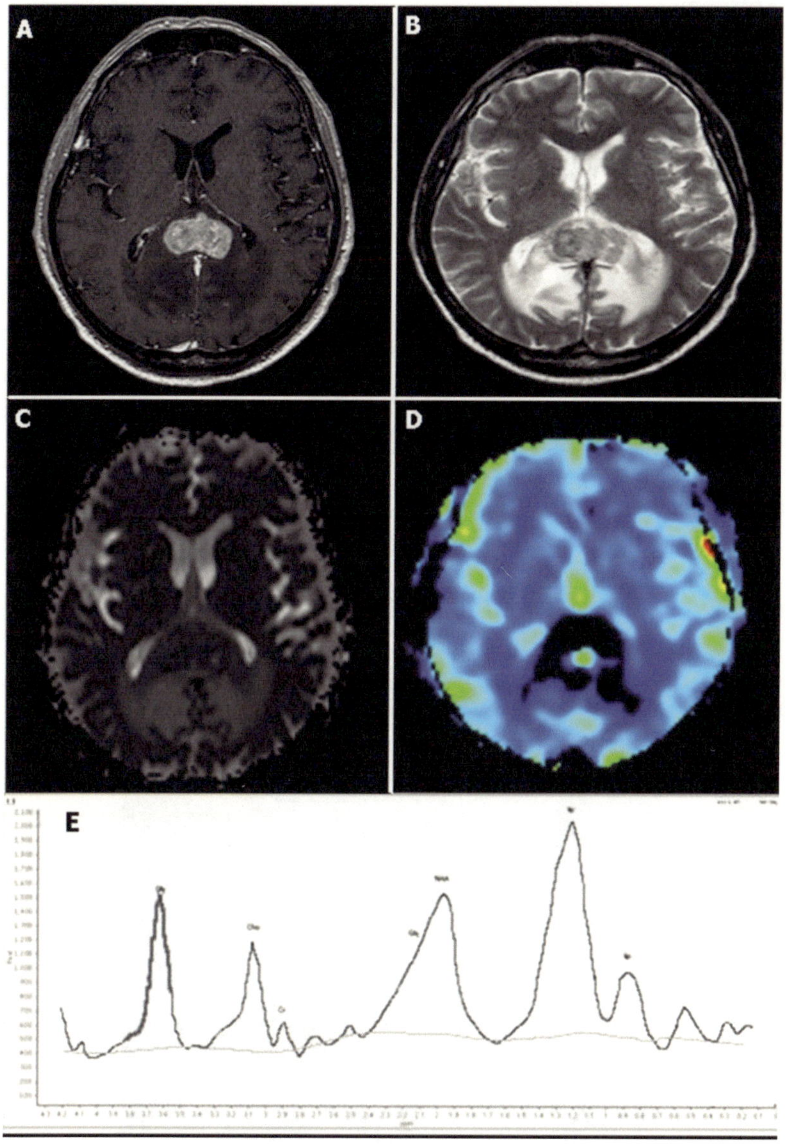

Figure 5. A case of lymphoma (A, B) revealing a low ADC value (C), low perfusion (D), and elevated levels of Lipids (E).

4.2. Perfusion imaging

PCNSL has low rCBV compared with that of high-grade gliomas and metastasis; however, overlapping values may exist (**Figure 5**). An important clue is that PCNSL demonstrates a significant increase in signal intensity above the baseline due to massive leakage of contrast media into the interstitial space contrary to high-grade gliomas [16]. Lymphoma tends to demonstrate higher rCBV compared with toxoplasmosis [15].

4.3. MR spectroscopy

Characteristic spectroscopic findings for PCNSL include elevated signals of lipid, choline, and lactate and reduced NAA signal **(Figure 5**). Large lipid peaks on lesions without central necrosis are also strongly suggestive of PCNSL [17]. High lipid peak may be due to increased turnover of the membrane components in transformed lymphoid cells.

5. Differential diagnosis

5.1. Tumefactive demyelinating lesions

Tumefactive demyelinating lesions (TDLs) can be seen either during a relapse of a known multiple sclerosis or on acute onset. TDL can mimic high-grade gliomas on conventional MRI. In both conditions, there is contrast enhancement, perilesional edema, and central necrosis. Additional histopathology is not always straightforward since abnormal mitotic figures in reactive astrocytes can be present. In TDL, there is usually incomplete rim enhancement on MRI and little mass effect and edema (**Figure 6**).

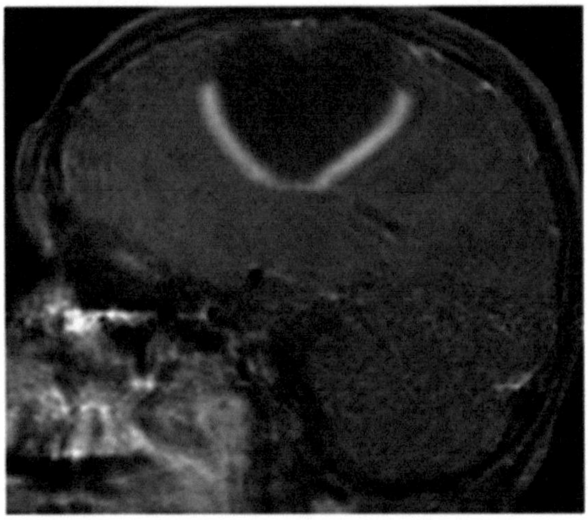

Figure 6. A case of TDL demonstarting incomplete rim enhancement on sagittal T1-weighted images after intravenous contrast administration.

5.1.1 Diffusion-weighted imaging

Min ADC values were higher in TDL than in PCNSLs or high-grade gliomas given that TDL is lesser cellular lesions than both PCNSLs and high-grade gliomas [18]. An important exception might be an acute demyelinating lesion which has areas of low ADC values (**Figure 7**). In acute phase in the TDL rim, there is peripheral restricted diffusion. The abnormal diffusion resolves within 1–3 weeks. Following restricted diffusion on initial MRI, subsequent Gd enhancement can be seen [19].

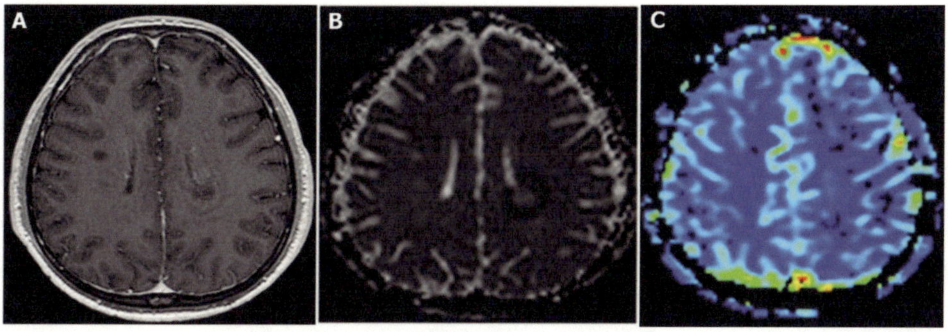

Figure 7. A case of TDL (A) demonstrating moderate ADC values (B). The rCBV maps show no elevation of Blood volume compared with contralateral normal white matter (C).

5.1.2. Perfusion imaging

TDL shows significant lower rCBV values (mean 0.88 ± 0.46) than high-grade gliomas (mean 6.47 ± 6.52), given the increased angiogenesis that the latter have (**Figure 7**). However, PCNSL had a less pronounced difference with a mean value of 2.11 ± 0.53 [20].

5.1.3. MR spectroscopy

TDL findings on spectroscopy are usually involve an elevated choline peak and reduced NAA signal. There may be also increased lactate and increased Cho/NAA that can reach high levels similar to that of high-grade gliomas; thus, differential diagnosis is problematic. The detection of glutamate and glutamine elevations has also been suggestive of TDL [21].

5.2. Brain abscess

Brain abscesses usually result from the extension of inflammation from the sinuses, the orbit, the mastoid cells, or the middle ear. As possible ways of spreading are either direct infection from a penetrating trauma, septic emboli, and contiguous or hematogenous spread. The most common pathogen is *Streptococcus pneumoniae*. Symptomatology is similar to any other mass lesions but tend to progress rapidly. Classical MRI findings of abscess in T2-weighted images are high-signal intensity with a thin rim of low intensity surrounded by edema. Furthermore, satellite lesions are more common in abscesses contrary to neoplastic lesions.

5.2.1. Diffusion-weighted imaging

The characteristic finding of brain abscess in DWI is a core of restricted diffusion due to pus consistency, whereas in neoplasms, there is usually low DWI signal (**Figure 8**). However, some necrotic brain metastasis may also display high signal intensity on DWI [22]. ADC values usually increase as treatment is successful even if cavity remains. Another finding in the rim of neoplastic lesions is a lower ADC value than that of an abscess.

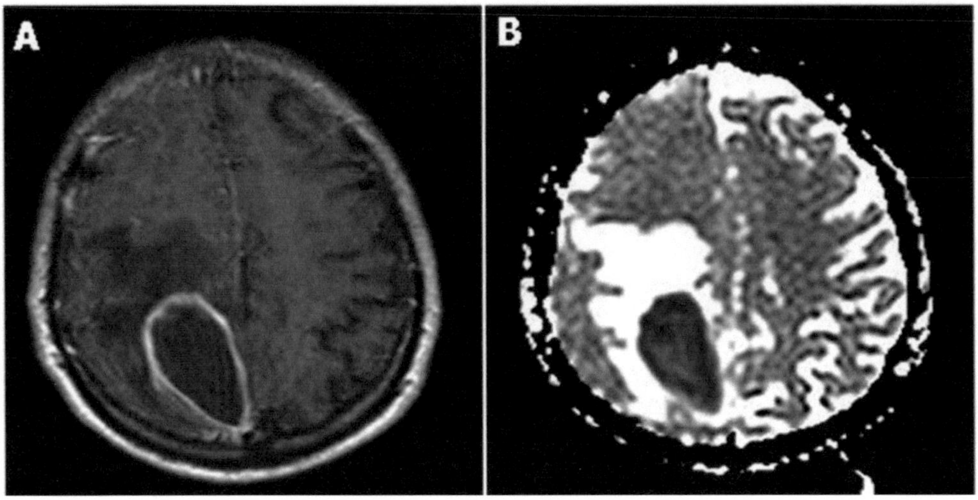

Figure 8. A case of an abscess (A) revealing low ADC values corresponding to the nonenhancing portion of the abscess (B).

5.2.2. Perfusion imaging

Contrary to glioblastomas and metastases, the enhancing rims of abscesses usually demonstrate lower rCBV values. The rCBV ratio of the enhancing portions of abscesses has be reported to be 0.79 ± 0.18, whereas in tumors was 1.40 ± 0.54 [23].

5.2.3. MR spectroscopy

Relative-specific MR spectroscopic feature of brain abscess is a succinate peak; however, it is not present in all cases. Apart from that elevated peaks of lactate, acetate, amino acids, alanine, valine, leucine, and isoleucine can be found. In abscesses reduced peaks of Cho/Crn and NAA are usually present [24]. Tuberculous abscesses typically have high lipid (mostly short-chain fatty acids such as butyric, isobutyric, caproic). Disappearance of metabolites of bacterial origin has been correlated with positive response to therapy [25].

5.3. Encephalitis

Encephalitis is an acute, usually diffuse, inflammatory process affecting the brain and may mimic mass lesions. Herpes simplex (HSV) encephalitis is the most common cause. Biopsy is helpful in some instances. Patients are usually confused and disoriented at the beginning and progress to coma within days. MRI demonstrates edema as high signal on T2, primarily within the temporal lobe, that may extend across sylvian fissure. Enhancement is usually present after the second week. Foci of hemorrhage occasionally can be found on MRI.

5.3.1. Diffusion-weighted imaging

Encephalitis typically demonstrates low ADC values due to cytotoxic edema. However, encephalitis may mimic an infarct that involves the cortical regions of the temporal lobe.

5.3.2. Perfusion imaging

Perfusion MRI has not been widely studied in encephalitis. At an early stage, there is an abnormal increase of blood flow in the affected area, followed by hypoperfusion at a later stage.

5.3.3. MR spectroscopy

On MR spectroscopy, finding encephalitis needs to be differentiated from a low-grade glioma which has similar findings. In general, there is a decrease in NAA peak usually 1–2 weeks after onset. After clinical recovery, there is a corresponding increase in NAA [26, 27]. Frequently, there is an increase in choline and myoinositol peak. An increased Cho/Cr ratio may be attributed to myelin breakdown. Sporadically, the lactate peak may be elevated.

5.4. Metastasis

Although the annual incidence of brain tumors is 17,000, for brain metastasis is 170,000 [28]. Thus, brain metastasis is the most common brain tumor seen clinically. The source of more than 50% of metastatic lesions is lung and breast cancer. When a single-brain lesion is found in a patient with a history of cancer, in 11% of these cases the lesion will not be metastatic. Four out of five of solitary metastases are located in the cerebral hemispheres. The majority tends to occur at the gray/white matter junction and is usually located posterior to the Sylvian fissure.

5.4.1. Diffusion-weighted imaging

The characteristic diffusion-weighted imaging feature for metastatic neoplasms is an elevated ADC. However, there is an overlap of the ADC values of metastatic lesions with those of primary neoplasms (**Figure 9**). Evaluation of ADC values in the non-enhancing T2-hyperintense areas surrounding the lesion may provide clues for the differentiation of high-grade gliomas from metastasis, given the lower ADC values in infiltrated areas of primary neoplasms compared with metastatic lesions. A threshold value of 1.302×10^{-3} mm^2/s for the minimum ADC value in the peritumoral regions had a sensitivity of 82.9% and specificity of 78.9% for distinguishing between glioblastoma and metastasis [29]. Although some studies have not found correlation between restricted diffusion or ADC values and various histologic types of metastases; however, a study reported that well-differentiated adenocarcinomas had lower DWI signal intensity compared with poorly differentiated carcinomas [30, 31].

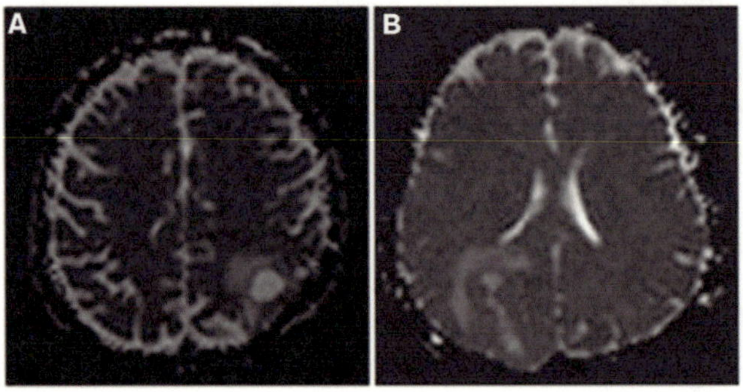

Figure 9. There is overlapping in the ADC values between a metastatic (A) and a primary brain tumor (B).

5.4.2. Perfusion imaging

Angiogenesis is essential for metastatic tumors growth. Thus, these lesions are associated with increased rCBV values compared with contralateral normal white matter. Thus, perfusion metrics tend to overlap between high-grade gliomas and metastatic lesions (**Figure 10**). The peak height and the percentage of signal intensity recovery derived from the T2* relaxivity curve on DSC MR has been reported to provide important clues [32]. Apart from that, metastasis from melanoma and renal cell carcinoma has been reported to have significant higher rCBV values than high-grade gliomas and metastases from lung cancer [33].

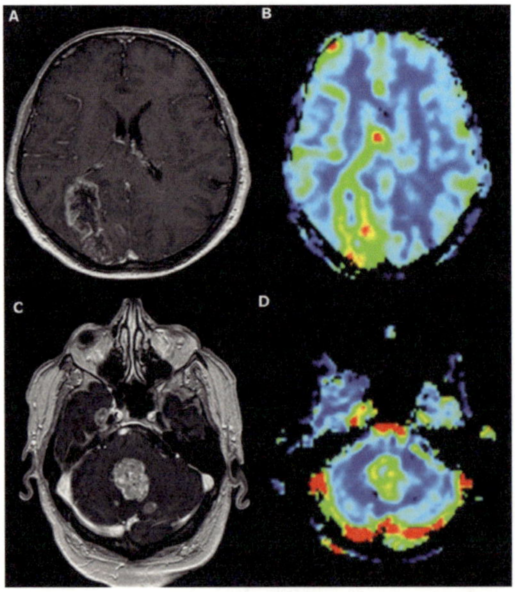

Figure 10. Both glioblastoma (A, B) and metastatic lesions (C, D) exhibits increased rCBV values, not permitting a differentiation based on perfusion imaging.

http://dx.doi.org/10.5772/62840

The rCBV values of perilesional area are usually higher for gliomas than metastatic lesions, due to glioma's infiltrative nature. In a study of 22 high-grade gliomas and 26 metastatic lesions, the rCBV ratios of peritumoural edema were 0.89 ± 0.51 in high-grade gliomas and 0.31 ± 0.12 in metastasis. A threshold rCBV value of 0.46 has been proposed, with a sensitivity of 77.3% and specificity of 96.2% for the differentiation of the two entities [34].

5.4.3. MR spectroscopy

Accurate differentiation between high-grade gliomas and metastatic lesion based on the enhancing part is problematic based on MR spectra. In metastatic lesions, there is no NAA peak, whereas necrosis results in a lipid peak. Lipid and lactate may be also elevated in primary brain tumors due to necrosis. Myoinosital peaks have not been reported to date in brain metastases, contrary to high-grade gliomas which tend to have elevated peaks [35, 36]. Given that primary tumors have a tendency to infiltrate, evaluation of the T2 hyperintense perilesional tissue provide more important information. Thus, although there is an intratumoral choline peak in both primary and metastatic lesions, there is no choline elevation in the peritumoural edema in metastatic lesions [37].

6. Conclusion

Intra-axial brain lesions are a significant health problem and are often a diagnostic imaging challenge. Advanced MRI techniques including proton spectroscopy, perfusion, and DWI have all been evaluated primarily in the context of distinguishing high-grade gliomas from metastases, abscess, and CNS lymphoma. Knowledge of the imaging characteristics of the most common intra-axial masses may allow the non-invasive diagnosis and classification of these masses.

Author details

Anastasia Zikou[1], George Alexiou[2*] and Maria Argyropoulou[1]

*Address all correspondence to: alexiougrg@yahoo.gr

1 Department of Radiology, School of Medicine, University of Ioannina, Ioannina, Greece

2 Department of Neurosurgery, School of Medicine, University of Ioannina, Ioannina, Greece

References

[1] Ostrom QT, Gittleman H, Fulop J, Liu M, Blanda R, Kromer C, Wolinsky Y, Kruchko C, Barnholtz-Sloan JS. CBTRUS statistical report: primary brain and central nervous system tumors diagnosed in the United States in 2008–2012. Neuro Oncol. 2015;14(Suppl 4):iv1–62.

[2] Alexiou GA, Zikou A, Tsiouris S, Goussia A, Kosta P, Papadopoulos A, Voulgaris S, Kyritsis AP, Fotopoulos AD, Argyropoulou MI. Correlation of diffusion tensor, dynamic susceptibility contrast MRI and (99m)Tc-Tetrofosmin brain SPECT with tumour grade and Ki-67 immunohistochemistry in glioma. Clin Neurol Neurosurg. 2014;116:41–5.

[3] Würdinger T, Tannous BA. Glioma angiogenesis: towards novel RNA therapeutics. Cell Adh Migr. 2009;3(2):230–5.

[4] Das S, Marsden PA. Angiogenesis in glioblastoma. N Engl J Med. 2013;369(16):1561–3.

[5] Zikou AK, Alexiou GA, Kosta P, Goussia A, Astrakas L, Tsekeris P, Voulgaris S, Malamou-Mitsi V, Kyritsis AP, Argyropoulou MI. Diffusion tensor and dynamic susceptibility contrast MRI in glioblastoma. Clin Neurol Neurosurg. 2012;114(6):607–12.

[6] Zikou A, Alexiou GA, Vartholomatos G, Goussia A, Xydis VG, Kosta P, Voulgaris S, Kyritsis AP, Argyropoulou MI. Correlation of diffusion tensor and dynamic susceptibility contrast MRI with DNA ploidy and cell cycle analysis of gliomas. Clin Neurol Neurosurg. 2015;139:119–24.

[7] Cha S, Tihan T, Crawford F, Fischbein NJ, Chang S, Bollen A, Nelson SJ, Prados M, Berger MS, Dillon WP. Differentiation of low-grade oligodendrogliomas from low-grade astrocytomas by using quantitative blood-volume measurements derived from dynamic susceptibility contrast-enhanced MR imaging. AJNR Am J Neuroradiol. 2005;26(2):266–73.

[8] Alexiou GA, Moschovi M, Stefanaki K, Sfakianos G, Prodromou N. Epidemiology of pediatric brain tumors in Greece (1991–2008). Experience from the Agia Sofia Children's Hospital. Cent Eur Neurosurg. 2011;72(1):1–4.

[9] Wang Q, Zhang H, Zhang J, Wu C, Zhu W, Li F, Chen X, Xu B. The diagnostic performance of magnetic resonance spectroscopy in differentiating high-from low-grade gliomas: a systematic review and meta-analysis. Eur Radiol. 2015 Oct 15 [Epub ahead of print].

[10] Chen S, Tanaka S, Giannini C, et al. Gliomatosis cerebri: clinical characteristics, management, and outcomes. J Neurooncol. 2013;112(2):267–75.

[11] Fuller GN, Scheithauer BW. The 2007 revised World Health Organization (WHO) classification of tumors of the central nervous system: newly codified entities. Brain Pathol. 2007;17:304–7.

[12] Chen S, Tanaka S, Giannini C et-al. Gliomatosis cerebri: clinical characteristics, management, and outcomes. J Neurooncol. 2013;112(2):267–75.

[13] Desclée P, Rommel D, Hernalsteen D, Godfraind C, de Coene B, Cosnard G. Gliomatosis cerebri, imaging findings of 12 cases. J Neuroradiol. 2010;37(3):148–58.

[14] Bendszus M, Warmuth-metz M, Klein R et-al. MR spectroscopy in gliomatosis cerebri. AJNR Am J Neuroradiol. 2000;21(2):375–80.

[15] Al-Okaili RN, Krejza J, Wang S, Woo JH, Melhem ER. Advanced MR imaging techniques in the diagnosis of intraaxial brain tumors in adults. Radiographics. 2006;26(Suppl 1):S173–89.

[16] Hartmann M, Heiland S, Harting I, Tronnier VM, Sommer C, Ludwig R, Sartor K. Distinguishing of primary cerebral lymphoma from high-grade glioma with perfusion-weighted magnetic resonance imaging. Neurosci Lett. 2003;338(2):119–22.

[17] Yamasaki F, Takayasu T, Nosaka R, Amatya VJ, Doskaliyev A, Akiyama Y, Tominaga A, Takeshima Y, Sugiyama K, Kurisu K. Magnetic resonance spectroscopy detection of high lipid levels in intraaxial tumors without central necrosis: a characteristic of malignant lymphoma. J Neurosurg. 2015;122(6):1370–9.

[18] Mabray MC, Cohen BA, Villanueva-Meyer JE, Valles FE, Barajas RF, Rubenstein JL, Cha S. Performance of apparent diffusion coefficient values and conventional MRI features in differentiating tumefactive demyelinating lesions from primary brain neoplasms. AJR Am J Roentgenol. 2015;205(5):1075–85.

[19] Hyland M, Bermel RA, Cohen JA. Restricted diffusion preceding gadolinium enhancement in large or tumefactive demyelinating lesions. Neurol Clin Pract. 2013;3(1):15–21.

[20] Cha S, Pierce S, Knopp EA, Johnson G, Yang C, Ton A, Litt AW, Zagzag D. Dynamic contrast-enhanced T2*-weighted MR imaging of tumefactive demyelinating lesions. AJNR Am J Neuroradiol. 2001;22(6):1109–16.

[21] Al-Okaili RN, Krejza J, Wang S, Woo JH, Melhem ER. Advanced MR imaging techniques in the diagnosis of intraaxial brain tumors in adults. Radiographics. 2006;26(Suppl 1):S173–89.

[22] Park SH, Chang KH, Song IC, Kim YJ, Kim SH, Han MH. Diffusion-weighted MRI in cystic or necrotic intracranial lesions. Neuroradiology. 2000;42:716–21.

[23] Holmes TM, Petrella JR, Provenzale JM. Distinction between cerebral abscesses and high-grade neoplasms by dynamic susceptibility contrast perfusion MRI. AJR Am J Roentgenol. 2004;183(5):1247–52.

[24] Pal D, Bhattacharyya A, Husain M, Prasad KN, Pandey CM, Gupta RK. In vivo proton MR spectroscopy evaluation of pyogenic brain abscesses: a report of 194 cases. AJNR Am J Neuroradiol. 2010;31(2):360–6.

[25] Lai PH, Weng HH, Chen CY, Hsu SS, Ding S, Ko CW, Fu JH, Liang HL, Chen KH. In vivo differentiation of aerobic brain abscesses and necrotic glioblastomas multiforme using proton MR spectroscopic imaging. AJNR Am J Neuroradiol. 2008;29(8):1511–8.

[26] Sämann PG, Schlegel J, Müller G, Prantl F, Emminger C, Auer DP. Serial proton MR spectroscopy and diffusion imaging findings in HIV-related herpes simplex encephalitis. AJNR Am J Neuroradiol. 2003;24(10):2015–9.

[27] Takanashi J, Sugita K, Ishii M, Aoyagi M, Niimi H. Longitudinal MR imaging and proton MR spectroscopy in herpes simplex encephalitis. J Neurol Sci. 1997;149(1):99–102.

[28] Johnson J D, Young B. Demographics of brain metastasis. Neurosurg Clin N Am. 1996;7(3):337–44.

[29] Lee EJ, terBrugge K, Mikulis D, Choi DS, Bae JM, Lee SK, Moon SY. Diagnostic value of peritumoral minimum apparent diffusion coefficient for differentiation of glioblastoma multiforme from solitary metastatic lesions. AJR Am J Roentgenol. 2011;196(1): 71–6.

[30] Hayashida Y, Hirai T, Morishita S, Kitajima M, Murakami R, Korogi Y, et al. Diffusion-weighted imaging of metastatic brain tumors: comparison with histologic type and tumor cellularity. AJNR Am J Neuroradiol. 2006;27:1419–25.

[31] Duygulu G, Ovali GY, Calli C, Kitis O, Yünten N, Akalin T, et al. Intracerebral metastasis showing restricted diffusion: correlation with histopathologic findings. Eur J Radiol. 2010;74:117–20.

[32] Cha S, Lupo JM, Chen MH, Lamborn KR, McDermott MW, Berger MS, Nelson SJ, Dillon WP. Differentiation of glioblastoma multiforme and single brain metastasis by peak height and percentage of signal intensity recovery derived from dynamic susceptibility-weighted contrast-enhanced perfusion MR imaging. AJNR Am J Neuroradiol. 2007;28(6):1078–84.

[33] Kremer S, Grand S, Berger F, Hoffmann D, Pasquier B, Rémy C, Benabid AL, Bas JF. Dynamic contrast-enhanced MRI: differentiating melanoma and renal carcinoma metastases from high-grade astrocytomas and other metastases. Neuroradiology. 2003;45(1):44–9.

[34] Hakyemez B, Erdogan C, Gokalp G, Dusak A, Parlak M. Solitary metastases and high-grade gliomas: radiological differentiation by morphometric analysis and perfusion-weighted MRI. Clin Radiol. 2010;65(1):15–20.

[35] Bendini M, Marton E, Feletti A, Rossi S, Curtolo S, Inches I, et al. Primary and metastatic intraaxial brain tumors: prospective comparison of multivoxel 2D chemical-shift

imaging (CSI) proton MR spectroscopy, perfusion MRI, and histopathological findings in a group of 159 patients. Acta Neurochir (Wien). 2011;153:403–12.

[36] Fan G, Sun B, Wu Z, Guo Q, Guo Y. In vivo single-voxel proton MR spectroscopy in the differentiation of high-grade gliomas and solitary metastases. Clin Radiol. 2004;59:77–85.

[37] Fink KR, Fink JR. Imaging of brain metastases. Surg Neurol Int. 2013;4(Suppl 4):S209–19.

Chapter 8

Molecular Imaging of Brain Tumours

W. Phillip Law

Additional information is available at the end of the chapter

http://dx.doi.org/10.5772/62823

Abstract

This chapter is a review of the most common radiotracers currently used in clinical brain tumour imaging, and an update of future potentially useful radiotracers for imaging brain tumours with positron emission tomography (PET). It will focus mainly on glioma —the most common type of primary brain tumour—and intracranial metastases, as the cause of the majority of morbidity and mortality in neurooncology. Emerging data support the use of somatostatin analogue PET in the treatment planning and surveillance of meningiomas. There is currently a limited role of PET in other non-glial brain neoplasms including neuronal tumours, pineal and pituitary tumours, germ cell tumours and embryonal tumours (PNET, neuroblastoma). Finally, the newest hybrid imaging modality of PET/MRI and the promise it holds for obtaining state-of-the-art structural and functional imaging data simultaneously, are concisely reviewed.

Keywords: PET, molecular imaging, brain tumour, neurooncology, radiotracer

1. Introduction

Structural imaging using contrast-enhanced computed tomography (CT) and magnetic resonance imaging (MRI) is crucial for the initial detection and diagnosis of brain tumours. However, it has limitations in post-treatment surveillance where tumour- and therapy-related changes can appear similarly. Molecular imaging with positron emission tomography (PET) provides additional information that can better delineate tumour extent and burden, for example fluorodeoxyglucose (FDG) depicts the metabolic activity and fluroethyltyrosine (FET) and fluorodihydroxyphenylalanine (FDOPA) depict the amino acid turnover of otherwise nonspecific soft tissue changes on CT and MRI. This could ultimately improve clinical decision-making and anatomical targeting of tumour for biopsy, radiotherapy or surgery.

2. Brain tumour types

Brain tumours affect approximately 5–10 persons per 100,000 populations. In adults, about half of all brain neoplasms are primary tumours and the other half are metastatic. In childhood, brain neoplasms account for up to 20% of all cancers. Seventy percentage of childhood brain tumours arise from the posterior cranial fossa, whereas in adults, a similar proportion arises above the tentorium [1].

Intracranial tumours may spread directly to adjacent structures, along white matter tracts, or through the cerebrospinal fluid (CSF) spaces. It is rare for brain malignancy to metastasise to other parts of the body.

The most widely accepted system for classifying brain tumours is the World Health Organisation (WHO) classification of tumours of the central nervous system (CNS), which is based on the histological characteristics of the tumour. The latest revision was published in 2007 [2].

2.1. Gliomas

Gliomas are tumours of glial cells and include astrocytomas, oligodendrogliomas and ependymomas. Unlike most neurons, glial cells retain the ability to undergo cell division in the adult CNS. Since carcinogenesis is related to the sequential accumulation of genetic aberrations through cell division, it is not surprising that gliomas are the most common primary brain malignancy and account for about half of all adult brain tumours. The WHO classification of CNS tumours additionally classifies gliomas into Grade I to IV depending on the degree of tumour histological differentiation (**Table 1**).

	I	II	III	IV		I	II	III	IV
Astrocytic tumours									
Subependymal giant cell astrocytoma	•				Central neurocytoma		•		
Pilocytic astrocytoma	•				Extraventricular neurocytoma		•		
Pilomyxoid astrocytoma		•			Cerebellar liponeurocytoma		•		
Diffuse astrocytoma		•			Paraganglioma of the spinal cord	•			
Pleomorphic xanthoastrocytoma		•			Papillary glioneuronal tumour	•			
Anaplastic astrocytoma			•		Rosette-forming glioneuronal tumour of the fourth ventricle	•			
Glioblastoma				•					
Giant cell glioblastoma				•					
Gliosarcoma				•	**Pineal tumours**				
					Pineocytoma	•			
Oligodendroglial tumours					Pineal parenchymal tumour of intermediate differentiation		•	•	
Oligodendroglioma		•			Pineoblastoma				•
Anaplastic oligodendroglioma			•		Papillary tumour of the pineal region		•	•	
Oligoastrocytic tumours									
Oligoastrocytoma		•			**Embryonal tumours**				
Anaplastic oligoastrocytoma			•		Medulloblastoma				•
					CNS primitive neuroectodermal tumour (PNET)				•
Ependymal tumours					Atypical teratoid / rhabdoid tumour				•
Subependymoma	•								
Myxopapillary ependymoma	•				**Tumours of the cranial and paraspinal nerves**				
Ependymoma		•			Schwannoma	•			

http://dx.doi.org/10.5772/62823

	I	II	III	IV		I	II	III	IV
Anaplastic ependymoma			•		Neurofibroma	•			
					Perineurioma	•	•	•	
Choroid plexus tumours					Malignant peripheral nerve sheath tumour (MPNST)		•	•	•
Choroid plexus papilloma	•								
Atypical choroid plexus papilloma		•			**Meningeal tumours**				
Choroid plexus carcinoma			•		Meningioma	•			
					Atypical meningioma		•		
Other neuroepithelial tumours					Anaplastic/malignant meningioma			•	
Angiocentric glioma	•				Haemangiopericytoma		•		
Chordoid glioma of the third ventricle		•			Anaplastic haemangiopericytoma			•	
					Haemangioblastoma	•			
Neuronal and mixed neuronal-glial tumours									
Gangliocytoma	•				**Tumours of the sellar region**				
Ganglioglioma	•				Craniopharyngioma	•			
Anaplastic ganglioglioma			•		Granular cell tumour of the neurohypophysis	•			
Desmoplastic infantile astrocytoma and ganglioglioma	•				Pituicytoma	•			
Dysembryoplastic neuroepithelial tumour	•				Spindle cell oncocytoma of the adenohypophysis	•			

Table 1. WHO grading of tumours of the CNS.

2.2. Brain metastases

The most common primary malignancies that metastasise to the brain are carcinomas of the lung, breast and melanoma [3]. The meninges are also a frequent site of metastatic disease involvement.

The following sections on molecular imaging with PET radiotracers will focus on gliomas and intracranial metastases as the cause of the majority of morbidity and mortality in neurooncology.

3. Fluorodeoxyglucose

3.1. Tumour detection

F-18 FDG is an analogue of glucose (**Figure 1**). Its active transport into the cell is mediated by a group of structurally related glucose transport proteins (GLUT) and once intracellular, FDG

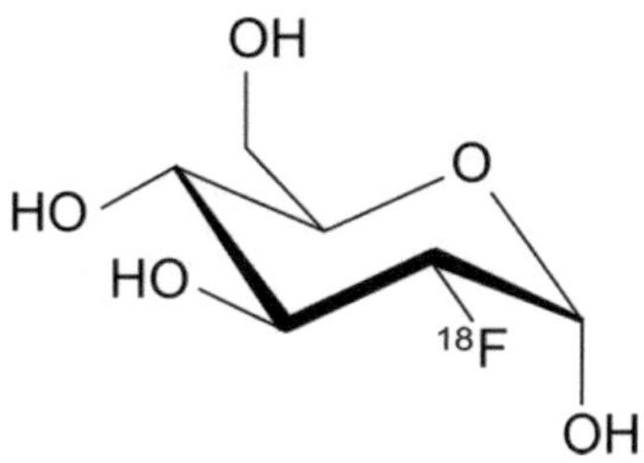

Figure 1. Chemical structure of F-18 fluorodeoxyglucose.

is phosphorylated by the enzyme hexokinase as the first step towards glycolysis. However, unlike glucose, once phosphorylated FDG-6-phosphate cannot continue along the glycolytic pathway and effectively becomes trapped intracellularly. FDG uptake in PET is thus an indication of the metabolic activity of the structure in which it is being taken up. Most malignant cells are metabolically active and demonstrate an increased expression of glucose transport proteins, particularly GLUT-1 and GLUT-3, as well as higher levels of hexokinase.

FDG is the single most important, widely used and explored radiotracer in PET; however, its current role in brain tumour imaging is limited due to the presence of intense physiological FDG uptake in the normal brain resulting in poor tumour-to-background contrast. Thus, an underlying brain tumour, even if FDG-avid, can escape detection on FDG PET (**Figure 2**). In some studies, increased FDG uptake in gliomas was only reported in 21–47% of high-grade tumours and as few as 3–6% of low-grade tumours [4, 5]. Delayed imaging (e.g. 6 h) following FDG administration instead of the usual imaging performed 60–90 min post-radiotracer can improve discrimination between tumour and physiological background uptake as FDG is retained in tumour longer than in normal brain parenchyma [6].

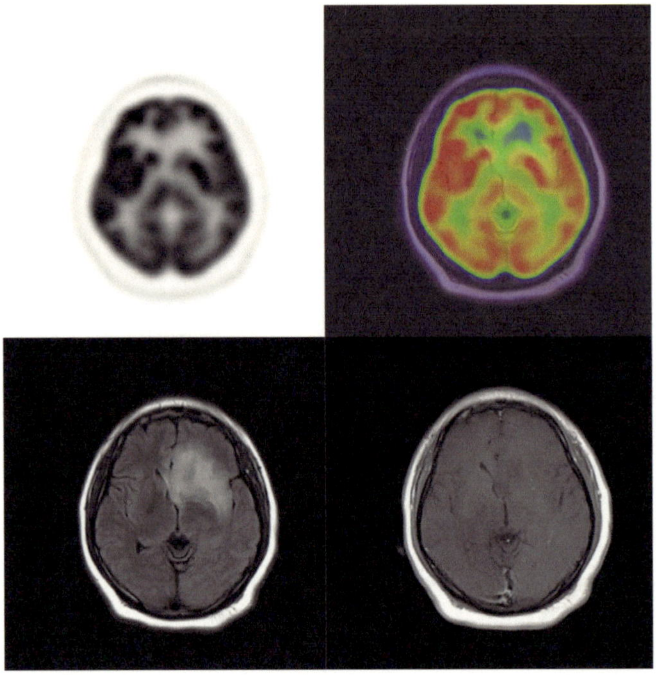

Figure 2. FDG uptake in a left frontal cerebral glioma on PET/CT. *Top row:* The tumour is not readily discernible from intense physiological FDG activity in the adjacent cerebral parenchyma. *Bottom row:* The tumour is much better depicted on MRI FLAIR imaging (*bottom left panel*) and shows no contrast enhancement due to its low grade (*bottom right panel*).

3.2. Tumour grading and prognosis

The uptake of FDG in a neoplasm is a consequence of the increased expression and activity of glucose transporter proteins and of hexokinase, a glucose phosphorylating enzyme. FDG uptake generally correlates with tumour grade [7–9], with low-grade tumours showing similar FDG uptake as white matter, and high-grade tumours similar uptake as grey matter. Tumours can be heterogeneous and contain areas of low- and high-grade dedifferentiation.

FDG uptake in gliomas has also been shown to correlate with survival [10, 11]. Median survival for intracranial metastases is typically less than 1 year, with these metastases generally showing a high-grade pattern of FDG uptake.

3.3. Localisation for biopsy

FDG PET can be useful in selection of a biopsy site where uptake is highest in the tumour, thereby ensuring sampling of the most malignant tissue [12–16].

3.4. Radiotherapy planning

MRI is the current technique of choice for radiotherapy planning. Due to its relatively low tumour-to-background contrast, FDG PET has limited utility for conventional treatment planning. More recently, the addition of PET imaging of some radiotracers—in particular the amino acid analogues—in radiotherapy planning has been shown to be promising in the identification of microscopic residual tumour post-surgery and differentiation of tumour from brain tissue, thereby improving local control and reducing radiation to healthy brain parenchyma (see Section 4).

3.5. Assessment of treatment response

The differentiation of tumour recurrence from radiation necrosis following treatment is one of the most common and important clinical indications for MRI and PET. Both viable tumour and post-radiotherapy necrosis demonstrate contrast enhancement on MRI. Similarly, increased FDG uptake cannot reliably differentiate residual/recurrent tumour from radiation necrosis. Furthermore, false-negative MRI and FDG PET can result from decreased enhancement (due to antiangiogenic therapy) and poor tumour-to-background contrast, respectively.

Whilst the criteria for Response Assessment in Neuro-Oncology have been updated to mitigate these potentially confounding factors in MRI [17–19], advancements in response assessment in PET have focused on other (non-metabolic) radiotracers.

4. Amino acid radiotracers

Amino acids are the building blocks of proteins and critical to nearly every biological process in the human body. They serve as components in metabolic cycles which are upregulated in cancer cells with increased proliferative activity. Because the brain uses glucose almost exclusively for fuel (except during prolonged starvation), PET imaging of brain tumours with amino acid and amino acid analogue radiotracers has a significant advantage of high tumour-to-background contrast (**Figure 3**).

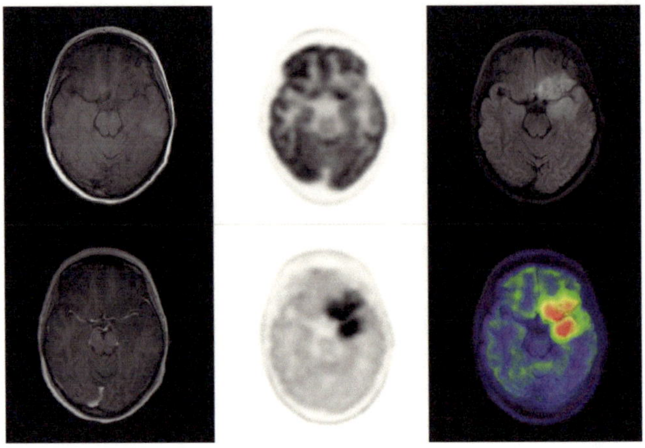

Figure 3. F-18 FDG PET/CT (*top row*) and F-18 FDOPA PET/CT (*bottom row*) of a left frontotemporal low-grade non-enhancing cerebral glioma showing the high tumour-to-background contrast of amino acid imaging compared with metabolic imaging.

4.1. Methionine

Methionine (MET) is a sulphur-containing naturally occurring amino acid (**Figure 4**) whose transport into malignant glioma cells and the supporting vasculature of these tumours is strongly upregulated [20–22].

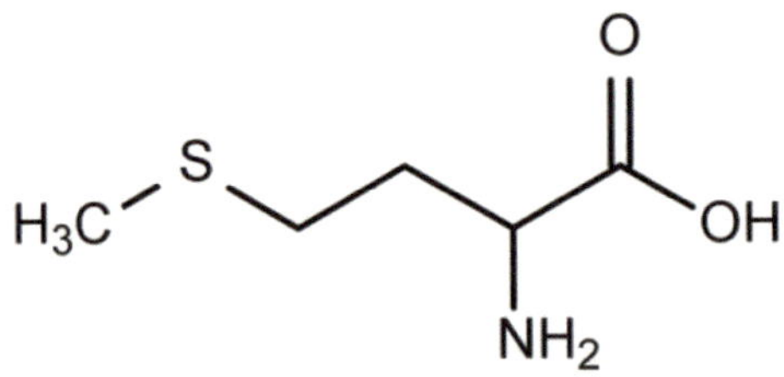

Figure 4. Chemical structure of methionine.

C-11 MET is one of the most widely used amino acid radiotracers for PET imaging in neuro-oncology, mainly due to its relative ease of production that can be performed rapidly with high yield and without the need for complicated purification steps.

The overall sensitivity of MET PET for malignant gliomas ranges from 76 to 95%, with higher rates of detection for higher grade tumours [23]. Increased uptake of MET is also seen in low-grade gliomas—with reported sensitivities of 65–85% [23, 24]—in which there is typically little or absent contrast enhancement on MRI and low uptake on FDG PET [24, 25].

MET is also generally regarded as the reference in prognostication of disease, image-guided biopsy and radiotherapy planning, and the detection of tumour recurrence [26–34], making it the most important radiotracer in the amino acid category.

The main limitation of C-11 MET is its short half-life (20 min), confining its use to centres with a cyclotron on-site or very nearby. It has also been shown to accumulate in brain abscesses and inflammation (cerebritis) [35], important false positives to exclude in the diagnosis of brain tumour.

F-18 has a much longer half-life (110 min) than C-11 and opens up the possibility of radiotracer transport to another centre for diagnostic imaging. F-18 labelled amino acids include F-18-labelled fluoroethyltyrosine (FET) and dihydroxyfluorophenylalanine (FDOPA).

4.2. Fluoroethyltyrosine

FET is an artificial amino acid (**Figure 5**) taken up by upregulated tumour cells but not incorporated into proteins (unlike naturally occurring amino acids such as methionine). As such, its use in the characterisation of brain lesions and the grading of gliomas requires dynamic analysis of activity over time [36]. Its overall accuracy in the diagnosis of gliomas is comparable to MET [37, 38]. It is an excellent tool for differentiating tumour from non-tumour causes in the initial evaluation of newly diagnosed brain lesions [39] (**Figure 6**). FET PET can also distinguish active tumour from radiation necrosis following treatment [40, 41].

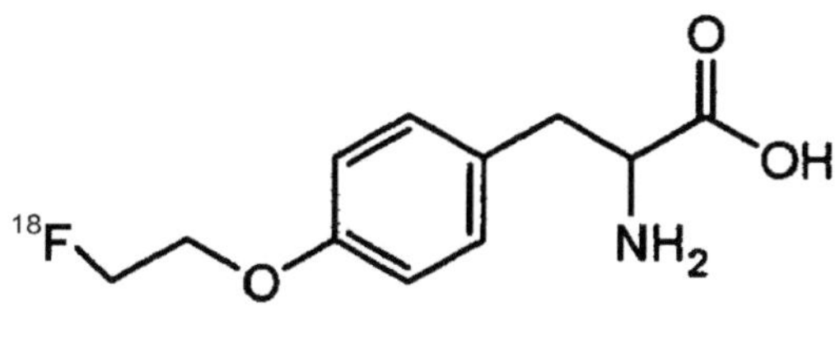

Figure 5. Chemical structure of F-18 fluoroethyltyrosine.

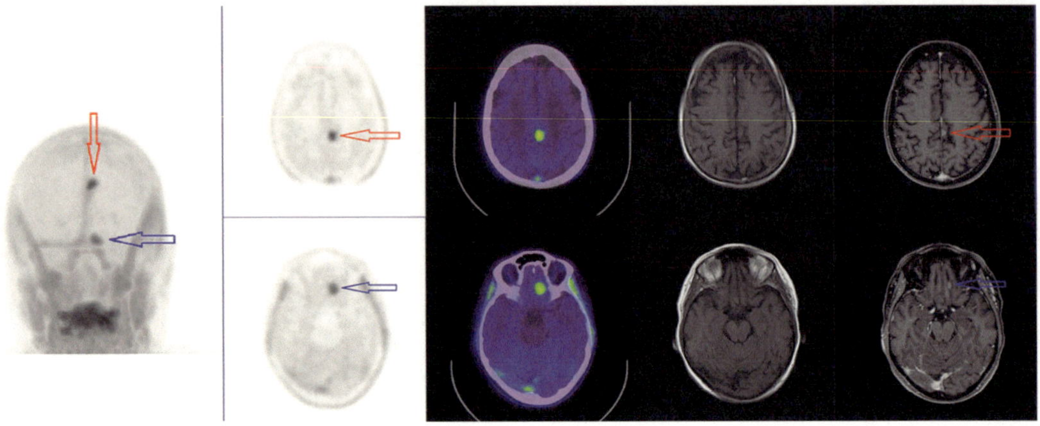

Figure 6. FET PET/CT (*left-sided panels*) and pre/post intravenous gadolinium MRI (*right-sided panels*) in a patient with two small cerebral melanoma metastases (*red and blue arrows*).

4.3. Fluorodihydroxyphenylalanine

FDOPA was originally developed for imaging the DOPA-decarboxylase pathway in Parkinson's disease and other neurodegenerative diseases. It is a fluorinated form of L-DOPA (**Figure 7**) which is used to increased dopamine concentrations in the treatment of Parkinson's disease. FDOPA has since been shown to be a marker of amino acid transport in brain tumours and metastases.

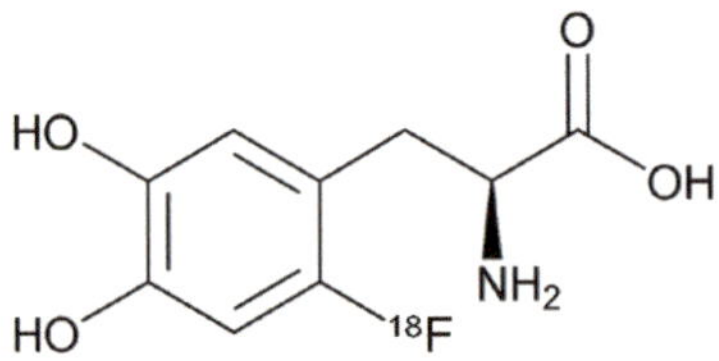

Figure 7. Chemical structure of F-18 fluorodihydroxyphenylalanine.

FDOPA uptake has been shown to correlate with tumour proliferation and grade [42], and more accurate than FDG for evaluating low-grade tumours and distinguishing tumour recurrence from radiation necrosis [43].

It also accumulates in neuroendocrine tumours (NETs) such as phaeochromocytomas and paragangliomas.

5. Fluorothymidine

Thymidine (T) is the pyrimidine deoxynucleoside in DNA that pairs with deoxyadenosine (A). F-18 fluorothymidine (FLT) is a thymidine analogue (**Figure 8**) and a substrate for thymi-

http://dx.doi.org/10.5772/62823

dine kinase 1 (responsible for synchronising cells in G1/early S phase), but unlike thymidine, FLT is a poor substrate for mitochondrial thymidine kinase 2 and its uptake is therefore specific to the cell cycle and a marker of cellular proliferation.

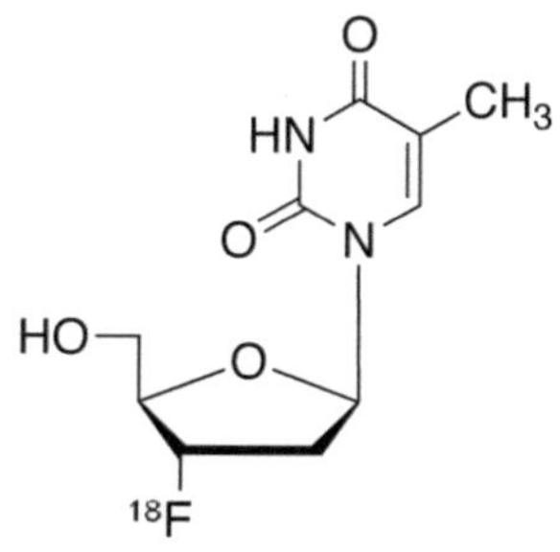

Figure 8. Chemical structure of F-18 fluorothymidine.

FLT uptake in normal brain cells is limited by the blood–brain barrier, thus FLT PET provides higher tumour-to-background contrast than FDG PET. FLT is more sensitive than FDG PET for the detection of recurrent high-grade glioma and also correlates better with tumour progression and survival [44].

However, its use as a quantitative marker of the activity of DNA synthesis in gliomas remains a subject of debate, particularly whether FLT can discriminate moderately proliferative tumours driven by thymidine salvage pathway utilisation from highly proliferative tumours primarily driven by de novo synthesis of thymidine. Quantitative FLT PET with kinetic modelling may also be useful for distinguishing glioma recurrence from radiation necrosis [45].

6. Choline

Choline is a water-soluble B-complex vitamin (**Figure 9**), normally found in blood, which is phosphorylated and subsequently integrated into lecithin, a component of cell membrane phospholipids. Malignant tumour cells demonstrate increased proliferation which results in increased cell membrane turnover and a greater demand for cell membrane components such as choline.

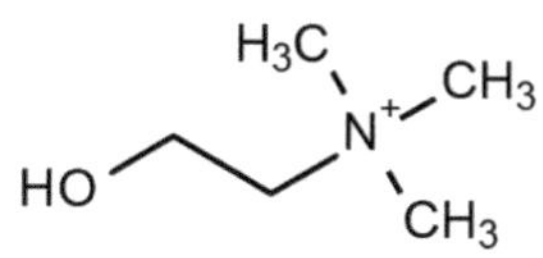

Figure 9. Chemical structure of choline.

Like the amino acid radiotracers, PET imaging with choline offers excellent delineation of tumour from brain with a 10:1 contrast ratio achievable within 5 min of radiotracer injection

[46]. Higher choline uptake generally corresponds with more malignant tumours, and choline PET also appears promising for radiotherapy planning because of more precise delineation of biological target volume [47]. It also has higher accuracy than FDG PET and MRI for the differentiating radiation necrosis and tumour recurrence [47].

Choline can be radiolabelled with C-11 or F-18, permitting its use in centres without an on-site cyclotron.

It has also been investigated extensively for imaging in prostate cancer, with some studies also suggesting a potential role in oesophageal and lung cancer [46, 48–50].

7. Hypoxia radiotracers

Hypoxia is an important factor in the malignant progression of tumour and its resistance to therapy. The majority of hypoxia PET radiotracers belong to a group of compounds known as nitroimidazoles that freely cross the blood–brain barrier, enter cells by diffusion and are subsequently reduced by nitroreductases at a rate inversely proportional to oxygen tension. Thus, in an oxygen-rich environment, they are able to diffuse back out of the cell again, whereas under hypoxic conditions, they are reduced and become irreversibly trapped in the cell. Another favourable property of the nitroimidazoles is their rapid equilibration within the brain parenchyma independently of perfusion.

7.1. Fluoromisonidazole

F-18 fluoromisonidazole (FMISO) was the first of the nitroimidazole radiotracers (**Figure 10**) to be developed for imaging with PET and has been widely used in preclinical and clinical studies.

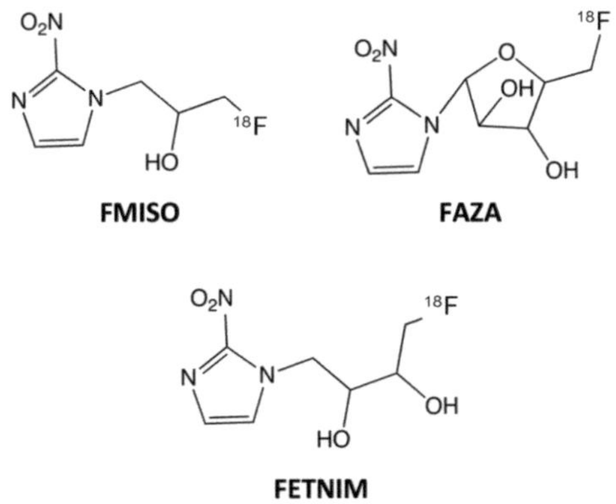

Figure 10. Nitroimidazoles are the most commonly used hypoxia PET radiotracers. FMISO: fluoromisonidazole; FAZA: fluoroazomycin; FETNIM: fluoroerythronitroimidazole.

Hypoxia can be quantified by analysing FMISO PET images using a simple tissue-to-blood ratio of radiotracer activity, with a ratio of 1.2 or greater useful for discriminating and quantifying hypoxic tissue. Hypoxic tumour volume and maximal tumour-to-blood ratio calculated in this way has been shown to predict worse prognosis independent of other factors [51]. FMISO can also differentiate lower from higher grade gliomas better than FDG [52].

More recently, an image-derived region to assess blood activity on FMISO PET has been shown to be an accurate surrogate for serial blood sampling in the quantification of hypoxia [53] and this may obviate the need for routine venous sampling in patients undergoing FMISO PET in the future.

7.2. Fluoroazomycin

F-18 fluoroazomycin (FAZA) is a second-generation nitroimidazole derivative (Figure 10) with more favourable pharmacokinetics than FMISO. FAZA demonstrates faster clearance of unbound radiotracer from non-hypoxic areas (thereby resulting in shorter waiting time for imaging) and improved biodistribution (does not cross the intact blood–brain barrier due to its increased hydrophilicity). Consequently, there is improved hypoxia-to-normoxia contrast, and FAZA shows considerable promise and is expected to overcome the disadvantages of FMISO for imaging hypoxia in brain tumours.

8. Meningiomas

Meningiomas are predominantly benign tumours in adults arising from the meningothelium of the arachnoid mater. Consequently, they occur at the brain surface—over the cerebral convexity, parafalcine region or along the skull base. Rarely, they can occur in intraventricular or intraosseous locations. Meningiomas account for 20–25% of all intracranial neoplasms, with women affected more commonly than men. They are commonly associated with loss of heterozygosity of the long arm of chromosome 22.

On CT and MRI, meningiomas typically appear as rounded or ovoid avidly enhancing masses with dural tails at the tumour margins, variable compressive effect on adjacent brain parenchyma (mainly depending on tumour size) and occasional hyperostosis of the adjacent skull.

Molecular imaging of meningiomas can be accurately performed using somatostatin analogue radiotracers [54] (**Figure 11**).

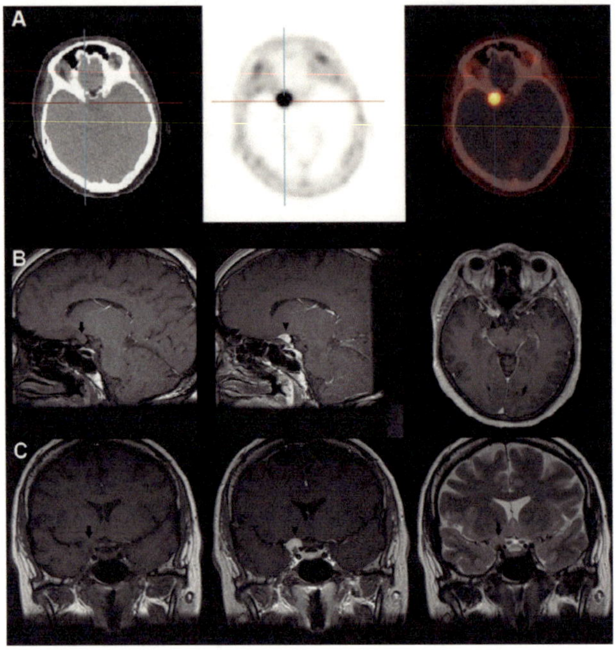

Figure 11. *Row A*: Fusion PET/CT shows a Ga-68 DOTATATE-avid focus directly adjacent to the right anterior clinoid process of the sphenoid bone. *Rows B and C*: Multiplanar MRI sequences show characteristic features of an intracranial meningioma on non-enhanced (*arrows*) and gadolinium-enhanced (*arrowheads*) imaging.

8.1. Somatostatin analogue radiotracers

Currently, the primary indication for using gallium-68 (Ga-68)-labelled somatostatin analogue radiotracers is for PET imaging of carcinoid and other NETs which usually express a high density of somatostatin receptors to which these peptides bind with high affinity [55]. Some non-NETs are also known to express somatostatin receptors, including meningiomas [56–58] which express all of the five somatostatin receptor (SSTR) subtypes but predominantly SSTR1 and SSTR2.

Traditional scintigraphic imaging of meningiomas utilised indium-111-labelled octreotide and single-photon emission computed tomography (SPECT). However, PET imaging with Ga-68-labelled somatostatin analogue radiotracers such as 1,4,7,10-tetraazacyclododecane-1,4,7,10-tetraacetic acid (DOTA)-Tyr^{3}-octreotate (TATE), DOTA-1-Nal^{3}-octreotide (NOC) and DOTA-Phe^{1}-Tyr^{3}-octreotide (TOC) offers superior count statistics and spatial resolution compared with SPECT. It also provides much higher target-to-background ratio of radiotracer uptake and more detailed tumour characterisation and has largely replaced octreotide SPECT imaging. This detailed spatial characterisation of meningiomas, when coupled with anatomical imaging by CT and MRI (in particular), allows for more accurate radiotherapy planning in patients with large, non-resectable tumours.

The demonstration of DOTATATE avidity in an intracranial lesion with only some features of meningioma on CT or MRI could permit differentiation of a meningioma from other tumours such as metastasis or craniopharyngioma, which can have a significant impact on clinical management.

There are also emerging data that DOTATATE uptake on PET improves diagnostic accuracy by delineating meningioma from tumour-free tissue [58] that can potentially enhance on CT and MRI especially in the setting of previous therapy.

FET PET in the late phase may be useful for the non-invasive grading of meningiomas [59].

9. Lymphoma

Almost all patients with primary CNS lymphoma have brain parenchymal lesions which have a predilection for the periventricular and superficial regions. Contrast-enhanced MRI remains the technique of choice when CNS lymphoma is suspected, although it is usually not possible to conclusively differentiate CNS lymphoma from other malignant brain lesions on MRI.

FDG remains the most widely explored radiotracer for PET imaging in CNS lymphoma, though its utility is limited compared with FDG PET in extracranial lymphoma, due to the poor tumour-to-background contrast in the brain. FDG uptake is typically intense in lymphoma—metabolic imaging with PET may help to differentiate lymphoma in the brain from low-grade gliomas and meningiomas [60–62] and may also be suitable for early evaluation of post-treatment response [60]. Infectious pathologies in the brain of immunocompromised subjects can be discerned from lymphoma by their usually hypometabolic nature on FDG PET [63], and high uptake ratio on thallium-201 (Tl-201) imaging [64]. Steroid treatment can cause false-negative results by reducing FDG uptake in CNS lymphoma [62].

MET PET typically shows intense uptake in CNS lymphomas which often involves a larger area than the corresponding enhancing abnormality on CT and MRI and may more accurately delineate the actual tumour margins [65]. It may also be more accurate for the detection of residual or recurrent lymphoma after treatment [65].

10. Other non-glial neoplasms

There is currently a limited role of PET in other non-glial brain neoplasms including neuronal tumours, pineal and pituitary tumours, germ cell tumours and embryonal tumours (PNET, neuroblastoma), although anecdotal evidence, case reports and series exist for some of these tumours.

PET imaging with MET, for example, detected all but one CNS germinoma in a case series of 10 patients [66], and choline uptake correlated with residual intracranial non-seminomatous germ cell tumour in a series of four patients [67].

Pituitary adenomas can appear as hypermetabolic lesions on FDG PET [68, 69], with higher uptake seen in macroadenomas than in microadenomas [69]. Increased DOTATATE uptake has been reported in intracranial metastases of pituitary carcinoma and may be useful in the decision to treat with peptide receptor radionuclide therapy [70, 71]. MET successfully detected all cases of craniopharyngioma in 10 patients [72].

11. PET/MRI

PET/MRI is a relatively novel hybrid diagnostic imaging device that can simultaneously acquire PET and MR images of the brain and other body regions. PET images show the distribution of an intravenously injected radiotracer, whilst MRI depicts the local responses of atomic nuclei to high-frequency radio waves when placed in a strong magnetic field. PET/MRI represents an advance on hybrid PET/CT imaging systems that are currently used in routine clinical practice for the assessment of patients with cancer and other diseases.

The integration of PET with MRI rather than CT has several advantages:

a. ***Reduced radiation exposure for patients.*** The use of MRI to correct PET images for the attenuation of emitted radiation by overlying tissue avoids the ionising radiation of CT. Because the acquisition time for MRI often exceeds that for PET, there are also opportunities to reduce the amount of radiotracer administered, by increasing PET acquisition time.

b. ***More accurate anatomical localisation of areas of radiotracer uptake.*** The simultaneous acquisition of MR and PET images reduces the likelihood of patient movement causing misregistration of the two image sets.

c. ***Compensation for some limitations of PET.*** The ability of PET to identify tumour sites is constrained by background physiological tracer uptake in some organs. For the most commonly used clinical PET radiotracer, FDG, these organs include the brain (as well as the liver and bone marrow) which are frequent sites of tumour recurrence after initial treatment. PET interpretation is also complicated by processes other than tumour infiltration that can cause radiotracer uptake, the most notably inflammation which can be particularly problematic when assessing cancer status after treatment, especially surgery or radiotherapy.

Many of these advantages are particularly relevant to brain tumour imaging, and indeed, the first exploration of feasibility of hybrid PET/MRI in clinical oncology was in brain tumours [73].

PET/MRI could theoretically harness the advantages of PET imaging with various radiotracers to accurately distinguish tumours from surrounding normal brain tissues—and the ability of advanced MRI techniques such as fMRI and diffusion tensor imaging to map the spatial relationship between tumours and adjacent functional brain tissues and white matter tracts—at the same time.

To date, studies in PET/MRI have shown that it can diagnose, grade and evaluate treatment response in glioma patients [74, 75]. Other studies have also shown that PET/MRI can identify areas of greater cellular proliferation and vascularity in brain tumours using a combination of advanced MRI techniques and PET radiotracers for treatment targeting [76–78]. FMISO PET/MRI can quantify hypoxia in recurrent glioma for risk stratification prior to commencement of angiogenesis inhibitor therapy (such as bevacizumab) and assess response to treatment [79, 80].

PET/MRI may gradually replace PET/CT in paediatric oncology due to the radiation dose saving achieved with performing MRI in place of CT, and more specifically in the field of neurooncology, the superior characterisation of brain tumours afforded by MRI over CT. In this arena, PET/MRI with choline and FDOPA have shown promise in the imaging of paediatric astrocytomas [81, 82].

The major disadvantages of PET/MRI currently relate to its high cost and consequent lack of access in many centres, need for optimisation of workflow and image acquisition parameters, and a greater body of evidence to evaluate its perceived superiority over existing techniques in neurooncology such as PET/CT, MRI or indeed PET/CT and MRI with software fusion of PET and MRI data. This would presumably require the results of large randomised controlled trials that should be a focus of future research efforts.

12. Conclusion

Whilst MRI remains the gold standard for imaging of brain tumours, future applications integrating PET—with its enlarging gamut of radiotracers—and MRI are likely forthcoming. This chapter briefly summarised the current status of the most commonly used radiotracers for the molecular imaging of brain tumours (**Table 2**). It will hopefully also serve as a useful guide that the reader can refer back to and build upon with future reading.

Radiotracer	Mechanism	Advantages	Disadvantages
FDG	Glucose analogue, active transport into cell mediated by GLUT transport proteins; phosphorylated by hexokinase and trapped intracellularly	Most widely used and explored radiotracer in PET	Poor tumour-to-background contrast due to intense physiological uptake in normal brain
MET	Essential amino acid transported into malignant glioma cells by LAT1 transporter and incorporated into proteins	Generally regarded as reference in glioma diagnosis, grading, prognosis, imaged-guided biopsy and	Short half-life (20 min) due to C-11 radiolabelling limits use to centres with cyclotron on-site or very nearby

Radiotracer	Mechanism	Advantages	Disadvantages
		radiotherapy planning, and detection of tumour recurrence in PET	
FET	Artificial amino acid transported into upregulated glioma cells but not incorporated into proteins	Overall accuracy for diagnosis of glioma comparable to MET; can distinguish active tumour from radiation necrosis; late phase FET PET may be useful for grading meningiomas	Use in grading of gliomas requires dynamic analysis of activity over time since not incorporated into proteins
FDOPA	Fluorinated form of L-DOPA, the precursor of dopamine that is transported physiologically into brain and abnormally (increased) into glioma	Uptake correlates with tumour proliferation and grade; more accurate than FDG for evaluating low-grade tumours and distinguishing tumour recurrence from radiation necrosis	Limited data outside of use for initial diagnosis of glioma
FLT	Thymidine analogue and substrate for cellular thymidine kinase 1 but poor substrate for mitochondrial thymidine kinase 2	More sensitive than FDG for detection of recurrent high-grade glioma; correlates better with tumour progression and survival	May accumulate in benign brain lesions with disrupted blood–brain barrier
Choline	Water-soluble B-complex vitamin phosphorylated and subsequently integrated into lecithin, a component of cell membrane phospholipids	Can be radiolabelled with C-11 and F-18; higher uptake generally corresponds with higher grade; more accurate than FDG for distinguishing tumour recurrence from radiation necrosis	May accumulate in benign inflammatory lesions
FMISO	First-generation nitroimidazole; enters cells by diffusion and subsequently reduced at a rate inversely proportional to oxygen tension	Permits quantification of hypoxia which has been shown to predict worse prognosis; can differentiate low from high grade gliomas	Requires venous blood sampling for quantification of hypoxia
FAZA	Second-generation nitroimidazole	Better hypoxia-to-normoxia contrast than FMISO	Requires venous blood sampling for quantification of hypoxia
Somatostatin analogues	Bind with high affinity to somatostatin receptors expressed richly by neuroendocrine tumours and some non-neuroendocrine tumours including meningiomas	Excellent tumour-to-background contrast for neuroendocrine tumours; appears promising for tumour delineation in radiotherapy planning	Limited data for use in radiotherapy planning

Table 2. Summary of radiotracers most commonly used in PET imaging of brain tumours.

http://dx.doi.org/10.5772/62823

Acknowledgements

W.P.L is supported by a Princess Alexandra Hospital Research Foundation grant.

Author details

W. Phillip Law*

Address all correspondence to: phil.law.au@gmail.com

Medical Imaging Department, Princess Alexandra Hospital, School of Medicine, University of Queensland, Brisbane, QLD, Australia

References

[1] Kumar V, Abbas AK, Aster JC. Robbins & cotran pathologic basis of disease. 9th ed. Philadelphia: Saunders; 2015.

[2] Louis DN, Ohgaki H, Wiestler OD, Cavenee WK (eds). WHO classification of tumours of the central nervous system. Lyon: IARC; 2007

[3] Cavaliere R, Schiff D. Cerebral metastases: a therapeutic update. Nat Clin Pract Neurol. 2006;2:426–436.

[4] Kato T, Shinoda J, Nakayama N, et al. Metabolic assessment of gliomas using 11C-methionine, [18F] fluorodeoxyglucose, and 11C-choline positron-emission tomography. AJNR Am J Neuroradiol. 2008;29:1176–1182.

[5] Pauleit D, Stoffels G, Bachofner A, et al. Comparison of (18)F-FET and (18)F-FDG PET in brain tumors. Nucl Med Biol. 2009;36:779–787.

[6] Spence AM, Muzi M, Mankoff DA, et al. ^{18}F-FDG PET of gliomas at delayed intervals: improved distinction between tumor and normal gray matter. J Nucl Med. 2004;45:1653–1659.

[7] Di Chiro G, Oldfield E, Bairamian D, et al. In vivo glucose utilization of tumors of the brain stem and spinal cord. In: Greitz T, Ingvar DH, Widen L, eds. The Metabolism of the Human Brain Studied with Positron Emission Tomography. New York: Raven Press;1985:351–361.

[8] Di Chiro G. Positron emission tomography using [18F] fluorodeoxyglucose in brain tumors: a powerful diagnostic and prognostic tool. Investig Radiol. 1987;22:360–371.

[9] Di Chiro G, DeLaPaz RL, Brooks RA, et al. Glucose utilization of cerebral gliomas measured by [18F] fluorodeoxyglucose and positron emission tomography. Neurology. 1982;32:1323–1329.

[10] Padma MV, Said S, Jacobs M, et al. Prediction of pathology and survival by FDG PET in gliomas. J Neurooncol. 2003;64:227–237.

[11] De Witte O, Levivier M, Violon P, et al. Prognostic value of positron emission tomography with [^{18}F]fluoro-2-D-glucose in the low-grade glioma. J Neurosurg. 1996;39:470–477.

[12] Goldman S, Levivier M, Pirotte B, et al. Regional glucose metabolism and histopathology of gliomas: a study based on positron emission tomography-guided stereotactic biopsy. Cancer. 1996;78:1098–1106.

[13] Hanson MW, Glantz MJ, Hoffman JM, et al. FDG PET in the selection of brain lesions for biopsy. J Comput Assist Tomogr. 1991;15:796–801.

[14] Herholz K, Pietryzk U, Voges J, et al. Correlation of glucose consumption and tumor cell density in astrocytomas: a stereotactic PET study. J Neurosurg. 1993;79:853–858.

[15] Pirotte B, Goldman S, David P, et al. Stereotactic brain biopsy guided by positron emission tomography (PET) with [F-18]fluorodeoxyglucose and [C-11]methionine. Acta Neurochir Suppl. 1997;68:133–138.

[16] Spence AM, Mankoff DA, Muzi M. Positron emission tomography imaging of brain tumors. Neuroimaging Clin N Am. 2003;13:717–739.

[17] Wen PY, Macdonald DR, Reardon DA, et al. Updated response assessment criteria for high-grade gliomas: response assessment in neuro-oncology working group. J Clin Oncol. 2010;28:1963–1972.

[18] Macdonald DR, Cascino TL, Schold SC Jr, Cairncross JG. Response criteria for phase II studies of supratentorial malignant glioma. J Clin Oncol. 1990;8:1277–1280.

[19] van den Bent MJ, Wefel JS, Schiff D, et al. Response assessment in neuro-oncology (a report of the RANO group): assessment of outcome in trials of diffuse low-grade gliomas. Lancet Oncol. 2011;12:583–593.

[20] Kim DK, Kim IJ, Hwang S, et al. System L-amino acid transporters are differently expressed in rat astrocyte and C6 glioma cells. Neurosci Res. 2004;50:437–446.

[21] Isselbacher KJ. Sugar and amino acid transport by cells in culture—differences between normal and malignant cells. N Engl J Med. 1972;286:929–933.

[22] Jager PL, Vaalburg W, Pruim J, de Vries EG, Langen KJ, Piers DA. Radiolabeled amino acids: basic aspects and clinical applications in oncology. J Nucl Med. 2001;42:432–445.

[23] Ogawa T, Shishido F, Kanno I, et al. Cerebral glioma: evaluation with methionine PET. Radiology. 1993;186:45–53.

[24] Herholz K, Holzer T, Bauer B, et al. ^{11}C-methionine PET for differential diagnosis of low-grade gliomas. Neurology. 1998;50:1316–1322.

[25] Chung JK, Kim YK, Kim SK, et al. Usefulness of ^{11}C-methionine PET in the evaluation of brain lesions that are hypo- or isometabolic on ^{18}F-FDG PET. Eur J Nucl Med Mol Imaging. 2002;29:176–182.

[26] De Witte O, Goldberg I, Wikler D, et al. Positron emission tomography with injection of methionine as a prognostic factor in glioma. J Neurosurg. 2001;95:746–750.

[27] Braun V, Dempf S, Weller R, Reske SN, Schachenmayr W, Rihter HP. Cranial neuronavigation with direct integration of 11C methionine positron emission tomography (PET) data—results of a pilot study in 32 surgical cases. Acta Neurochir (Wien). 2002;144:777–782.

[28] Kracht LW, Miletic H, Busch S, et al. Delineation of brain tumor extent with [11C]L-methionine positron emission tomography: local comparison with stereotactic histopathology. Clin Cancer Res. 2004;10:7163–7170.

[29] Pirotte B, Goldman S, Massager N, et al. Combined use of 18F-fluorodeoxyglucose and 11C-methionine in 45 positron emission tomography-guided stereotactic brain biopsies. J Neurosurg. 2004;101:476–483.

[30] Matsuo M, Miwa K, Shinoda J, et al. Target definition by C11-methionine-PET for the radiotherapy of brain metastases. Int J Radiat Oncol Biol Phys. 2009;74:714–722.

[31] Grosu A, Weber WA. PET for radiation treatment planning of brain tumours. Radiother Oncol. 2010;96:325–327.

[32] Terakawa Y, Tsuyuguchi N, Iwai Y, et al. Diagnostic accuracy of 11C-methionine PET for differentiation of recurrent brain tumors from radiation necrosis after radiotherapy. J Nucl Med. 2008;49:694–699.

[33] Tsuyuguchi N, Takami T, Sunada I, et al. Methionine positron emission tomography for differentiation of recurrent brain tumor and radiation necrosis after stereotactic radiosurgery—in malignant glioma. Ann Nucl Med. 2004;18:291–296.

[34] Tsuyuguchi N, Sunada I, Iwai Y, et al. Methionine positron emission tomography of recurrent metastatic brain tumor and radiation necrosis after stereotactic radiosurgery: is a differential diagnosis possible? J Neurosurg. 2003;98:1056–1064.

[35] van Waarde A, Elsinga PH. Proliferation markers for the differential diagnosis of tumor and inflammation. Curr Pharm Des. 2008;14:3326–3339.

[36] Popperl G, Kreth FW, Mehrkens JH, et al. FET PET for the evaluation of untreated gliomas: correlation of FET uptake and uptake kinetics with tumour grading. Eur J Nucl Med Mol Imaging. 2007;34:1933–1942.

[37] Weber WA, Wester HJ, Grosu AL, et al. O-2(18F)Fluorethyl-L-tyrosine and L-(methyl-11C)-methionine uptake in brain tumors: initial results of a comparative study. Eur J Nucl Med. 2000;27:542–549.

[38] Kunz M, Thon N, Eigenbrod S, et al. Hot spots in dynamic 18FET-PET delineate malignant tumor parts within suspected WHO grade II gliomas. Neuro-Oncology. 2011;13:307–316.

[39] Dunet V, Rossier C, Buck A, Stupp R, Prior JO. Performance of ^{18}F-fluoro-ethyl-tyrosine (^{18}F-FET) PET for the differential diagnosis of primary brain tumor: a systematic review and metaanalysis. J Nucl Med. 2012;53:207–214.

[40] Galldiks N, Rapp M, Stoffels G, et al. Response assessment of bevacizumab in patients with recurrent malignant glioma using [18F] fluoroethyl-L-tyrosine PET in comparison to MRI. Eur J Nucl Med Mol Imaging. 2013;40:22–33.

[41] Popperl G, Gotz, C, Rachinger W, Gildehaus FJ, Tonn JC, Tatsch K. Value of O-(2-[18F]fluoroethyl)-L-tyrosine PET for the diagnosis of recurrent glioma. Eur J Nucl Med Mol Imaging. 2004;31:1464–1470.

[42] Fueger BJ, Czernin J, Cloughesy T, et al. Correlation of 6-18F-fluoro-L-dopa PET uptake with proliferation and tumor grade in newly diagnosed and recurrent gliomas. J Nucl Med. 2010;51:1532–1538.

[43] Chen W, Silverman DH, Delaloye S, et al. ^{18}F-FDOPA PET imaging of brain tumors: comparison study with ^{18}F-FDG PET and evaluation of diagnostic accuracy. J Nucl Med. 2006;47:904–911.

[44] Chen W, Cloughesy T, Kamdar N, et al. Imaging proliferation in brain tumors with ^{18}F-FLT PET: comparison with ^{18}F-FDG. J Nucl Med. 2005;46:945–952.

[45] Spence AM, Muzi M, Link JM, et al. NCI-sponsored trial for the evaluation of safety and preliminary efficacy of 3′-deoxy-3′-[^{18}F]fluorothymidine (FLT) as a marker of proliferation in patients with recurrent gliomas: preliminary efficacy studies. Mol Imaging Biol. 2009;11:343–355.

[46] DeGrado TR, Baldwin SW, Wang S, et al. Synthesis and evaluation of ^{18}F-labeled choline analogs as oncologic PET tracers. J Nucl Med. 2001;42:1805–1814.

[47] Giovannini E, Lazzeri P, Milano A, Gaeta MC, Ciarmiello A. Clinical applications of choline PET/CT in brain tumors. Curr Pharm Des. 2015;21:121–127.

[48] Vallabhajosula S. ^{18}F-labeled positron emission tomographic radiopharmaceuticals in oncology: an overview of radiochemistry and mechanisms of tumor localization. Semin Nucl Med. 2007;37:400–419.

[49] Hara T. 18F-fluorocholine: a new oncologic PET tracer. J Nucl Med. 2001;42:1815–1817.

[50] Reske SN. [11C]Choline uptake with PET/CT for the initial diagnosis of prostate cancer: relation to PSA levels, tumour stage and anti-androgenic therapy. Eur J Nucl Med Mol Imaging. 2008;35:1740–1741.

[51] Spence AM, Muzi M, Swanson KR, et al. Regional hypoxia in glioblastoma multiforme quantified with [^{18}F]fluoromisonidazole positron emission tomography before radiotherapy: correlation with time to progression and survival. Clin Cancer Res. 2008;14:2623–2630.

[52] Hirata K, Terasaka S, Shiga T, et al. ^{18}F-fluoromisonidazole positron emission tomography may differentiate glioblastoma multiforme from less malignant gliomas. Eur J Nucl Med Mol Imaging. 2012;39:760–770.

[53] Muzi M, Peterson LM, O'Sullivan JN, et al. ^{18}F-Fluoromisonidazole quantification of hypoxia in human cancer patients using image-derived blood surrogate tissue reference regions. J Nucl Med. 2015;56:1223–1228.

[54] Law WP, Fiumara F, Fong W, Macfarlane DJ. The 'double pituitary hot spot' sign of skull base meningioma on gallium-68-labelled somatostatin analogue PET. J Med Imaging Radiat Oncol. 2013;57:680–683.

[55] Khan MU, Khan S, El-Refaie S, et al. Clinical indications for Gallium-68 positron emission tomography imaging. Eur J Surg Oncol. 2009;35:561–567.

[56] Klutmann S, Bohuslavizki KH, Brenner W, et al. Somatostatin receptor scintigraphy in postsurgical follow-up examinations of meningioma. J Nucl Med. 1998;39:1913–1917.

[57] Arena S, Barbieri F, Thellung S, et al., Expression of somatostatin receptor mRNA in human meningiomas and their implication in in vitro antiproliferative activity. J Neurooncol. 2004;66:155–166.

[58] Rachinger W, Stoecklein VM, Terpolilli NA, et al. Increased 68Ga-DOTATATE uptake in PET imaging discriminates meningioma and tumor-free tissue. J Nucl Med. 2015;56:347–353.

[59] Cornelius JF, Stoffels G, Filb C, et al. Uptake and tracer kinetics of O-(2-(18)F-fluoroethyl)-L-tyrosine in meningiomas: preliminary results. Eur J Nucl Med Mol Imaging. 2015;42:459–467.

[60] Go JL, Lee SC, Kim PE. Imaging of primary central nervous system lymphoma. Neurosurg Focus. 2006;21:E4.

[61] Palmedo H, Urbach H, Bender H, et al. FDG-PET in immunocompromised patients with primary central nervous system lymphoma: correlation with MRI and clinical follow-up. Eur J Nucl Med Mol Imaging. 2006;33:164–168.

[62] Rosenfeld SS, Hoffman JM, Coleman RE, et al. Studies of primary central nervous system lymphoma with fluorine-18-fluorodeoxyglucose positron emission tomography. J Nucl Med. 1992;33:532–536.

[63] Kasamon YL, Ambinder RF. AIDS-related primary central nervous system lymphoma. Hematol Oncol Clin N Am. 2005;19:665–687.

[64] Ruiz A, Ganz WI, Post MJ, et al. Use of thallium-201 brain SPECT to differentiate cerebral lymphoma from toxoplasma encephalitis in AIDS patients. AJNR Am J Neuroradiol. 1994;15:1885–1894.

[65] Ogawa T, Kanno I, Hatazawa J, et al. Methionine PET for follow-up of radiation therapy of primary lymphoma of the brain. Radiographics. 1994;14:101–110.

[66] Okochi Y, Nihashi T, Fujii M, et al. Clinical use of (11)C-methionine and (18)F-FDG-PET for germinoma in central nervous system. Ann Nucl Med. 2014;28:94–102.

[67] Tsouana E, Stoneham S, Fersht N, et al. Evaluation of treatment response using integrated 18F-labeled choline positron emission tomography/magnetic resonance imaging in adolescents with intracranial non-germinomatous germ cell tumours. Pediatr Blood Cancer. 2015;62:1661–1663.

[68] Ryu SI, Tafti BA, Skirboll SL. Pituitary adenomas can appear as hypermetabolic lesions in (^{18}F) F-FDG PET imaging. J Neuroimaging. 2010;20:393–396.

[69] Jeong SY, Lee S-W, Lee HJ, et al. Incidental pituitary uptake on whole-body 18F-FDG PET/CT: a multicentre study. Eur J Nucl Med Mol Imaging. 2010;37:2334–2343.

[70] Xiao J, Zhu Z, Zhong D, Ma W, Wang R. Improvement in diagnosis of metastatic pituitary carcinoma by 68Ga DOTATATE PET/CT. Clin Nucl Med. 2015;40:e129–131.

[71] Maclean J, Aldridge M, Bomanji J, Short S, Fersht N. Peptide receptor radionuclide therapy for aggressive atypical pituitary adenoma/carcinoma: variable clinical response in preliminary evaluation. Pituitary. 2014;17:530–538.

[72] Laser BS, Merchant TE, Indelicato DJ, Hua CH, Shulkin BL, Synder SE. Evaluation of children with craniopharyngioma using carbon-11 methionine PET prior to proton therapy. Neuro-oncology. 2013;15:506–510.

[73] Boss A, Bisdas S, Kolb A, et al. Hybrid PET/MRI of intracranial masses: initial experiences and comparison to PET/CT. J Nucl Med. 2010;51:1198–1205.

[74] Yoon JH, Kim JH, Kang WJ, et al. Grading of cerebral glioma with multiparametric MR imaging and 18F-FDG-PET: concordance and accuracy. Eur Radiol. 2014;24:380–389.

[75] Dunet V, Maeder P, Nicod-Lalonde M, et al. Combination of MRI and dynamic FET PET for initial glioma grading. Nuclearmedizin. 2014;53:155–161.

[76] Weber MA, Henze M, Tuttenberg J, et al. Biopsy targeting gliomas: do functional imaging techniques identify similar target areas? Investig Radiol. 2010;45:755–768.

[77] Widhalm G, Krssak M, Minchev G, et al. Value of 1H-magnetic resonance spectroscopy chemical shift imaging for detection of anaplastic foci in diffusely infiltrating

gliomas with non-significant contrast-enhancement. J Neurol Neurosurg Psychiatry. 2011;82:512–520.

[78] Bisdas S, Ritz R, Bender B, et al. Metabolic mapping of gliomas using hybrid MR-PET imaging: feasibility of the method and spatial distribution of metabolic changes. Investig Radiol. 2013;48:295–301.

[79] Barajas RF Jr, Pampaloni MH, Clarke JL, et al. Assessing biological response to bevacizumab using 18F-fluoromisonidazole PET/MR imaging in a patient with recurrent anaplastic astrocytoma. Case Rep Radiol. 2015;73:1361.

[80] Kickingereder P, Radbruch A, Burth S, et al. MR perfusion-derived hemodynamic parametric response mapping of bevacizumab efficacy in recurrent glioblastoma. Radiology. 2015. doi:10.1148/radiol.2015151172

[81] Fraioli F, Shankar A, Hargrave D, et al. 18F-fluoroethylcholine (18F-Cho) PET/MRI functional parameters in pediatric astrocytic brain tumors. Clin Nucl Med. 2015;40:e40–e45.

[82] Morana G, Piccardo A, Milanaccio C, et al. Value of 18F-3,4-dihydroxyphenylalanine PET/MR image fusion in pediatric supratentorial infiltrative astrocytomas: a prospective pilot study. J Nucl Med. 2014;55:718–723.

Chapter 9

Intraoperative Neurophysiological Monitoring in Neuro-oncology

Lorena Vega-Zelaya, Rafael G. Sola and Jesús Pastor

Additional information is available at the end of the chapter

http://dx.doi.org/10.5772/63241

Abstract

Neurosurgery can be considered a radical method to treat some illnesses and can seriously damage the nervous system. To avoid deleterious effects, such injuries must be detected during their initial development by means of intraoperative neurophysiological techniques (including intraoperative neurophysiological monitoring (IONM) and functional mapping).

In this chapter, we review the most relevant and frequently performed IONM/mapping techniques. Some insight about the electrophysiological basis of stimulation and recording of the nervous system are provided. Intraoperative neurophysiological techniques can be divided into free running or evoked elicited. Among the first we discuss EMG, EEG and ECoG. Evoked potentials discussed include somato-sensory (SSEPs), auditory (BAEPs), visual (VEPs), motor (MEPs) and stimulated EMG. We are especially interested in the clear and concise exposition of the methodological peculiarities, the fields of application and the flaws associated with the different techniques discussed, with a focus on practical applications. Therefore, we show examples of real operations performed at our institution.

We conclude that IONM and mapping are some of the techniques with more relevance during recent decades for oncological neurosurgery. The widespread use and improvement of these techniques have allowed a safer removal of a radical tumour, reducing the risk of permanent postoperative deficits and better functional postsurgical outcomes during neuro-oncological surgery.

Keywords: anaesthetized craniotomy, awake craniotomy, intraoperative neurophysiology, motor evoked potentials, multimodal evoked potentials

1. Introduction

Neuro-oncology is a great challenge for neurosurgeons from two perspectives: first, in some types of tumours, gross total resection (GTR) is the best predictor of outcome in terms of life expectancy [1,2]; second, a main goal of every surgery is to avoid introducing new iatrogenic lesions. The relative weight of every one of these principles can be changed based on individual considerations of the type of tumour, the structures affected, the life expectancy and even the social considerations of each patient. These features are particularly relevant to patients suffering from high-grade gliomas, for whom survival is directly related to the degree of tumour removal. Therefore, to maintain an adequate quality of life, the primary goal of surgery is to achieve GTR without compromising neurological function.

Central nervous system tumours are relatively common in adults; they are the second most common form of cancer and the most common type of solid tumour in children. Although more than half of these tumours are benign, they can cause substantial morbidity. The most common tumours in adolescents and adults aged 15–34 years are gliomas and meningiomas [3]. Glioblastoma multiforme (GBM) is the most common type of glioma. Meningiomas derive from meningothelial cells and comprise approximately 20 percent of primary brain tumours. GBM are more commonly located in the supratentorial region, with the frontal lobe being the most common site [3].

Advances in surgical techniques, such as intraoperative neurophysiological monitoring (IONM), intraoperative magnetic resonance imaging (MRI), diffusion tensor imaging (DTI), stereotactic guidance and fluorescent-guided resection (FGR), have facilitated the delineation of tumour borders and can aid in optimizing safe surgical resection [4–6].

Neurosurgery can be considered a radical method to treat some illnesses and can seriously damage the nervous system (NS). These injuries may not be apparent by visual inspection by the surgeon in the operating room but subsequently evolve into a definite lesion [7]. To avoid deleterious effects, such injuries can be detected during their initial development by IONM. Therefore, IONM is a powerful set of techniques that provide increased functional knowledge during a surgical operation, resulting in the safer removal of a radical tumour [8,9].

The operating room is an aggressive environment to perform recordings due to the presence of several sources of noise. Therefore, it is very important to identify the source of electromagnetic noise and to determine how to manage it. Unfortunately, this subject is beyond the scope of this chapter, but we refer the reader to Pastor J, 2014, [10] for a detailed discussion of these topics.

In this chapter, we review the most relevant and frequently performed IONM techniques. We are especially interested in the clear and concise exposition of the methodological peculiarities, the fields of application and the flaws associated with the different techniques discussed, with a focus on practical applications. Therefore, we show examples of real operations performed at our institution.

2. Neurophysiological techniques

The possibility of using neurophysiological techniques to study the physiology of the NS is based on the way of function of the NS. Therefore, before introducing the techniques, we must understand, at least in a general manner, the function of this system for recording signals because all of the information that can be obtained and used clinically ultimately depends on both features.

2.1. Some insight regarding the function and recordings of the nervous system

The basic functional unit of the NS is the action potential (AP), which is the stereotypical change in the transmembrane voltage of a neuron [11–13]. In general, the AP originates in the neural soma or axon hillock and is transmitted by the axon to the synapse. All potentials originate from closed circuits of current [14], and the extracellular component can be recorded using the appropriate electrodes. In general, small metal electrodes are used to detect these currents.

Bioelectrical signals coming from the brain originate from synaptic currents in the cortex [13,14], or in deep nuclei of the thalamus or brainstem. These currents (clearly together with their intracellular components) form closed circuits that spread via volume conduction. The relationship between the current density (mA/cm^2) and the electric field ($\vec{E}$, in V/cm) is given by the generalized Ohm's law:

$$\vec{J} = \sigma\vec{E} \tag{1}$$

where σ is the tensor of conductivity (mS/cm). Considering that conductivity is the inverse of resistivity, ϱ (kΩ cm). In the electrostatic approach, the electric field can be expressed in terms of the electrostatic potential (∅, in V) by the following expression:

$$\vec{E} = -\nabla\varnothing \tag{2}$$

where ∇ is the symbol for the gradient operator.[1] Substituting this expression into the first equation, we obtain the following:

$$\vec{J} = -\sigma\nabla\varnothing \tag{3}$$

which provides the current in terms of the potential. We want to highlight the presence of symbol σ. In the real head, conductivity depends on position (inhomogeneity) and direction (anisotropy). Therefore, it is not possible avoid the vectorial approach in Eq. (3) that can be written in the three spatial dimensions (x, y, z) as follows:

[1] The gradient operator is the partial derivative for the space and is given by $\nabla = \frac{\partial}{\partial x}\vec{i} + \frac{\partial}{\partial y}\vec{j} + \frac{\partial}{\partial z}\vec{k}$

$$\begin{pmatrix} J_x \\ J_y \\ J_z \end{pmatrix} = -\begin{bmatrix} \sigma_{xx} & \sigma_{xy} & \sigma_{xz} \\ \sigma_{yx} & \sigma_{yy} & \sigma_{yz} \\ \sigma_{zx} & \sigma_{zy} & \sigma_{zz} \end{bmatrix} \begin{pmatrix} \frac{\partial \varnothing}{\partial x} \\ \frac{\partial \varnothing}{\partial y} \\ \frac{\partial \varnothing}{\partial z} \end{pmatrix} \quad (4)$$

This tensorial equation can be represented for every spatial dimension *x, y, z* as follows:

$$\vec{J}_i = -\sigma_{ix}\frac{\partial \varnothing}{\partial x}\vec{i} - \sigma_{iy}\frac{\partial \varnothing}{\partial y}\vec{j} - \sigma_{iz}\frac{\partial \varnothing}{\partial z}\vec{k}; i = x, y, z \quad (5)$$

Hence, for the same voltage source, the current obtained depends on the conductivity of the different structures. Consequently, structures with higher resistivity, such as the skull and the skin, will only allow a lower current [14]. Similarly, if we recall that higher frequency oscillations of the cortex imply smaller synchronized regions, we can understand why frequencies above the beta band (13–30 Hz) are extremely difficult to record from the scalp. The necessity to record very small currents is the main reason why a low impedance is needed at the patient–electrode interface.

In general, two types of recordings can be distinguished in neurophysiology [15]: near-field and far-field potentials. These concepts are completely different from the same words used in electromagnetic theory. The generators of near-field potentials are located in the cerebral cortex with limited spreading on the scalp. That is, we assume that the neurons responsible for the potential are in the immediate proximity of the region in which this potential is observed. However, far-field potentials originate from the deepest structures (white matter, basal ganglia or brainstem nuclei), and their distribution throughout the scalp is more extensive.

We can divide the neural response recorded by electrodes into three types according to the type of stimuli that induces the response in the neural tissue [13]: (i) electrically induced responses. We apply a controlled stimulation to activate different structures. Among these, we have all the types of evoked potentials or the response of a muscle after electrical stimulation of its innervating nerve (stimulated electromyography or sEMG); (ii) neural response by involuntary stimulation. Those responses appearing in the neural tissue after surgical aggression, e.g., mechanical compression or torsion, ischemia or heating induced by electrocoagulation, must be included in this group. A typical example of this is the neurotonic discharge of a muscle (free electromyography or fEMG) induced by stretching or overheating of a cranial nerve (CN); (iii) physiological response of the NS. These are spontaneously induced responses that are intrinsically generated by the neural activity, either as a physiological or pathological expression of the activity, and can include electrocorticography (ECoG) or electrocardiography (EKG).

http://dx.doi.org/10.5772/63241

Neurophysiological techniques can be classified according to the manner by which the signals can be obtained, by means of a previous stimulation (a) or without that stimulus (b and c).

2.2. Free-running techniques

The recordings obtained using these techniques can be acquired continuously and do not require a command from the neurophysiologist to be released.

2.2.1. Electromyography (EMG)

Free EMG (or fEMG) is the recording of the bioelectrical activity from muscles. Usually, fEMG is recorded by a pair of intramuscular stainless steel electrodes that are inserted into the muscle separated by a distance of 2 cm.

Although we may be interested in the state of the muscle, the most common use of the fEMG signal is to identify changes in the CN or peripheral nerves. In fact, we used nerve-induced electrical activity of the muscle as a measure of the state of that nerve. In this way, we could be aware of irritative activity originating in the nerve as a consequence of traction, torsion, compression, or heat injury, among others. In addition, the patient should not be curarized during most of the surgery. It is important to distinguish between mechanical activity induced by surgical activity, which is usually transient, and neurotonic discharges, which are continuous and persist after the surgeon leaves the surgical field.

Settings that are used to record fEMG depend on the muscle being recorded, the size of the electrodes and the objective. However, it is quite common to use a 10–3000 Hz bandwidth, with either the notch on or off (in this case, the high pass filter should be increased up to 50 Hz), a gain always greater than 30 μV/div (the most common is 50 μV/div), and a time base between 100 ms/div (for small periods) and 750 ms/div (for longer periods). In the last case, we are aware that the shape of the muscle activity can be distorted (depending on the screen resolution) and could be misinterpreted as an artefact.

2.2.2. Electroencephalography (EEG) and electrocorticography (ECoG)

The difference between EEG and ECoG resides in the location of the recording electrodes. However, this difference is sufficient great to warrant separate discussion of the methods. As a result of the analysis of volume conduction, among other dissimilarities that are not discussed herein, EEG and ECoG will be differentiated based on the magnitude of the current and the frequency composition.

2.2.2.1. EEG

Recording electrodes are placed onto the skin of the scalp. The most common types are subdermal stainless steel needles that are placed inside the skin or cork-screw electrodes, which are more easily fixed to the patient but are clearly also more aggressive. Subdermal electrodes allow low impedance (less than 5 kΩ is fine), which is important for acquiring a good recording. We can use the International System 10–20 [16] to position the electrodes, but it is more common to use a reduced version of this system.

EEG can be used to monitor the state of the cerebral cortex, and the main indications in IONM are blood flow alterations and epileptic activity. Bioelectrical activity directly depends on blood flow, and a reduction of this variable will be observed as a slowing of the brain activity denoted by the appearance of theta/delta activity [17]. Epileptic activity can appear after a perfusion alteration or as a consequence of an insult to the cortex (mechanical, chemical or electrical). Considering that high-voltage electrical stimulation is common during IONM, EEG should be used in all patients with an increased risk of epileptic seizure. Similarly, we must be aware that general anaesthetics can increase the likelihood of seizures [18]. Customarily, some degree of quantification should be useful.

The bandwidth filter should be at least 0.5–30 Hz, with the notch on. For this type of recording, higher frequencies are uncommon in the presence of anaesthesia. The gain must be set between 7 and 15 μV/div and the time base at approximately 15–30 mm/s.

2.2.2.2. ECoG

ECoG is used to record the bioelectrical activity directly from the cortical surface. Several types of tumours that are located in the cortex can induce epilepsy or irritative activity, which are defined by the presence of a spike or sharp waves and its combinations. Hence, it is very relevant to assess the presence of these activities. In this sense, ECoG can discriminate between different functional regions in the cortex, namely [9,19] (i) the spiking area, where the irritative activity can be observed; (ii) the lesional area, where abnormal slowing or loss of activity is observed; and (iii) the non-pathological area, which is defined by the absence of the above-mentioned activities. The identification of these regions helps the surgeon to select the cortical region through which to approach the tumour [6,20].

As we have stated previously, it is very important to monitor the presence of epileptic activity during electrical stimulation of the cerebral cortex.

The settings for ECoG should consist of a bandwidth filter of 0.5–100 Hz, with the notch on, a gain of 750–1500 μV/div and a time base of 15–30 mm/s. As stated previously, some type of mathematical analysis can be helpful for the assessment of ECoG [5,6].

2.3. Evoked potentials

The signals recorded using these techniques have the common feature that a previous stimulation must be elicited. Some of these, due to a very small amplitude, must be averaged. Before each technique is discussed in detail, we shall briefly explain why an average is needed [21,22]. Averaging is an extraordinarily powerful tool to separate the signal from its noisy environment.

A neurophysiological measurement (m) consists of the signal to be acquired (s) and the noise (n) [23]. Consider $m(t)=s(t)+n(t)$. In many cases, the noise amplitude is greater than the signal ($n > s$). Therefore, to reduce the noise and enhance the signal we perform several rounds of stimulation (say M), such that, for each kth stimulus, the expression of the measure will be as follows:

$$m_k(t) = s_k(t) + n_k(t); k = 1,2,\ldots M \tag{6}$$

We can see that the average of M leads to $m(t)$, $s(t)$ and $n(t)$, denoted by, $\bar{m}$, $\bar{s}$, $\bar{n}$, and can be written as follows:

$$\bar{m} = \frac{1}{M}\sum_{i=1}^{M} m_i(t) = \frac{1}{M}\sum_{i=1}^{M} s_i(t) + \frac{1}{M}\sum_{i=1}^{M} n_i(t) = \bar{s} + \bar{n} \tag{7}$$

This expression embodies the justification of the method. However, to be truly useful, it is necessary that two conditions are met: (i) there is no causal relationship between the signal and the noise and (ii) the noise varies randomly from one stimulus to the next. The mean for any variable that varies randomly is $\bar{n}=0$; therefore, the greater the stimulus number, then the greater will be the similarity between $\bar{m}$ and $\bar{s}$. Furthermore, it is easy to prove (see Van Drongelen), but omitted here, the signal estimated from the measurement, improves by a factor of $1/\sqrt{M}$.

2.3.1. Somato-sensory evoked potentials (SSEPs)

These are potentials that are generated at several points of the somato-sensory pathway.

Electrical stimulation is performed along the path of a peripheral nerve. In the upper limb, the median nerve or ulnar nerve (at wrist or elbow) is commonly used. In the lower limb, the posterior tibial nerve is commonly used. In general terms, nerve stimulation is achieved in the region closest to the cathode (i.e., negative electrode), where it produces a cationic output current [24] that depolarizes the membrane. To avoid anodic block, it is very important to place the anode distally and the cathode proximally.

Stimulation can be performed through the use of auto-adherence electrodes or subdermal needles [23].

It is customary to name the recorded waves (potentials) according to two criteria: polarity; the downward deflection of the wave is considered to be positive (P) and upward deflection negative (N) and latency; the time (measured in milliseconds) during which the potential appears with greater frequency.

Different points will be used throughout the path that reflect the activity of various nerve structures [15]. Recording is performed by placing and properly fixing subdermal electrodes (other types, such as cork-screws or discs, can clearly also be used) according to the 10–20 IS.

2.3.1.1. Upper limb SSEP

- Erb's point. The active electrode is located on the midclavicular line, 2 cm above the clavicle. The reference electrode can be placed several centimetres away. A wave called N9 is recorded. It represents the near-field generated by the afferent arrival of CNAP in the brachial plexus.

- Cervical. The active electrode is located on the second spinose apophysis (C2) or fifth (C5) cervical vertebra, with the reference electrode in the Fz. At this location, we can identify several potentials as follows: (a) N11. This potential is likely a presynaptic travelling wave arising near the root entry zone of C6 and C7 and action potentials ascending in the dorsal columns. It is also known as the dorsal column volley. (b) N13. This potential is generated by the synapse of neurons spanning from dorsal columns onto the nucleus cuneatus. (c) P/N14. This is a distant potential generated by the caudal part of the medial lemniscus at the location of the brainstem. Latency and morphology can vary between individuals (i.e., they can be positive or negative) and may have one or more phases.

- Scalp. The active electrode is placed 5 cm in the lateral direction and 2 cm caudally in relation to the vertex (C4′/C3′ for right/left). The reference electrode is located on Fz. Typically, several potentials are registered as follows: (a) N18. Reflecting the postsynaptic potential activity of the ventrocaudal nucleus of the thalamus. (b) N20. This is a near-field potential that is generated by postsynaptic potentials at the hand cortical region. (c) P25 may be an average of the independent posterior frontal and parietal generators. (d) The N35 peak is attributed to the sense of pain and temperature (conveyed by small myelinated fibres).

2.3.1.2. Lower limb SSEP

- Popliteal fossa. Labelled N8.

- Lumbar point. The reference electrode is located in the spinous process of L1 with the reference electrode on the iliac crest. It is called LP (lumbar point) or N22.

- Cervical. It is known as N30.

- Scalp. The active electrode is located in the midline, 2 cm caudal to the vertex (Cz′), with the reference electrode located at Fz. The waves are called P37 and originate from the cortical area of the foot. A potential can also be registered in the fronto-central region with a latency of 38 ms (N38). Because the orientation of the dipole inside the longitudinal fissure is variable, P38 is sometimes maximal over the ipsilateral scalp (paradoxical localization).

The most common parameters employed for stimulation are trains between 4.18 and 7.1 Hz, with a 200–300 μs pulse width and an amplitude that is double the threshold of the motor

http://dx.doi.org/10.5772/63241

response. In general, the amplitudes are approximately 15–30 mA, and 200–300 pulses/train is recommended. The recording will have a bandwidth of 10–1500 Hz, with the notch off, a gain of 0.1–2 μV/div and a base time of 5–10 ms/div for the upper and the lower limbs, respectively. It is very important to recall that impedances must be below 5 kΩ.

Warning criteria include increase the latency greater than 10% and/or a decrease in amplitude to less than 50% with respect to baseline.

2.3.1.3. Cortical SSEP

During surgery of the cortex, it is very common to use phase reversal of SSEP to identify the transition between motor and somato-sensory areas, which usually occurs at the central sulcus (CS).

Thalamo-cortical projections from the ventrocaudal nucleus synapse in layer IV of the primary somato-sensory area. However, the rostral part of area 3 is located in the anterior wall of the central sulcus, and thus the current sources generated by these afferents can be modelled by a dipole oriented parieto-frontally rather than in a normal position relative to the surface.

We always use cortical SSEP when we need to identify the primary somato-sensory region and/or the motor area (Brodmann area 4). It is very important to keep in mind that in the case of tumours, a significant distortion of the anatomy can be observed [25,26].

The somato-sensory region corresponding to the forearm can be easily identified by the greater amplitude of the complex N1/P1/N2 waves [25].

The recording will have a bandwidth of 10–1500 Hz, with the notch off, a gain of 10–30 μV/div and a base time of 5–10 ms/div for the upper and the lower limbs, respectively. A 20-electrode grid placed at the lateral region of the fronto-parietal transition can be very helpful. By contrast, for the lower limb SSEP, a 4-8-electrode strip is placed at the medial region. The reference electrode should be placed as far as possible, i.e., at the contralateral earlobe, whereas the ground electrode should be as close as possible, e.g., at the ipsilateral earlobe [13,20].

2.3.2. Auditory evoked potentials (AEPs)

Brainstem AEPs (BAEP) are generated by different relay nuclei along the auditory pathway. They are far-field potentials that originate from very deep structures.

2.3.2.1. Brainstem auditory evoked potentials (BAEPs)

BAEPs are the set of waveforms that are recorded at the scalp after auditory stimulation of the middle ear. They are formed by the following potentials [26]: (a) wave I. Originates at the distal action potential of cranial nerve (CN) VIII, typically has a latency of 1.5 ms; (b) wave II. This potential is generated at the entry of CN VIII into the brainstem; (c) wave III. Synapse at the ipsilateral superior olivary nucleus. Latency of 3.5 ms; (d) wave IV is produced by activation of the nucleus or axons of the lateral lemniscus; (e) wave V appears to result from activation of the inferior colliculus; (f) waves VI and VII are presumed to be generated by the medial geniculate body and the thalamo-cortical pathways, respectively.

BAEPs are indicated when tumours affect the auditory system (mainly schwannomas of CN VIII) and tumours affecting the brainstem.

A high intensity (greater than 80 dB) is usually used during IONM. The frequency is 21.14 Hz, and a bandwidth of 10/30–1500 Hz is optimal (a broader bandwidth can allow too much noise), with the notch on. A minimum of 1000 stimuli/train are needed to obtain reproducible and stable waveforms.

2.3.2.2. Cortical auditory evoked potentials (cAEPs)

These potentials were initially thought to be generated in the primary auditory cortex (PAC), located deeply in the white matter of the lateral fissure of the transverse gyrus of Heschl. However, other different areas, including the second auditory cortex (SAC) and the insula are capable of eliciting cAEPs. There is considerable inter-subject and inter-hemispheric variability [27], and the whole structure remains to be elucidated.

cAEPs are characterized by a series of waves, which can be systematized as follows: (a) short latency waves: N13/P17/N30. These waves are typically recorded from the PAC. This complex is absent in the SAC and (b) intermediate latency waves: peak between 60 and 100 ms. These waves, which are always present in the SAC, can also be present in the PAC.

A stimulation frequency of 2.18 would be adequate. The bandwidth filter is 0.5–1500 Hz, with the notch filter off, and a minimum intensity of 70 dB (sensation level) is applied to the contralateral ear.

2.3.3. Visual evoked potentials (VEPs)

These waves exhibit the characteristics of near-field potentials generated from the primary visual cortex. In the surgery room, the most widely (and probably the only) technique used for stimulation is the application of flashes of light. A normal VEP in response to a pattern-reversal checkerboard is a positive midoccipital peak that occurs at a mean latency of 100 ms with three separate phases: an initial negative deflection (Nl or N75), a prominent positive deflection (P1 or P100) and a later negative deflection (N2 or N145).

Although we think that VEP has undeniable utility, there have been some questions about its efficacy. However, more recent results have demonstrated stable recordings and a strong correlation with the postoperative visual function [28,29]. Therefore, intraoperative VEP monitoring will be mandatory for surgeries harbouring a risk of visual impairment [30].

Stimulation is performed by flashing light-emitting diodes at 2.18 Hz, with 10 μs pulse width, and a bandwidth of 10–1000 Hz. We considered an increase in latency of 10% or a reduction in amplitude greater than 50% amplitude compared with baseline as alarm criteria [6].

In some cases, VEP can be directly recorded from the cortical surface. In these cases, potentials are much more stable, require fewer stimuli (in fact, a very small number of stimuli can induce the response) and are 2–3 orders of magnitude higher than the scalp recording [31].

2.3.4. *Motor evoked potentials (MEPs)*

Motor evoked potentials are the recordings that are obtained from muscles in response to stimulation of the motor system at different levels (cortex, inner capsule, corticospinal/corticobulbar tracts or spinal cord) [22]. Considering the amplitude of the response, these types of evoked potentials do not need to be averaged.

2.3.4.1. *Transcranial electrical stimulation (TES)*

This technique consists of the stimulation of the motor pathway by an electrical current delivered through electrodes placed outside the cranium, usually in the scalp [32]. The introduction of TES revolutionized the field of IONM [33].

It is commonly believed that TES excites the white matter of the inner capsule (IC) rather than cortical neurons. In fact, an increase in the magnitude of the current provides stimulation at the level of the brainstem [34]. This possibility must be recognized and kept in mind by the neurophysiologist, especially in the case of surgery at the supratentorial level.

Electrodes can be subdermal needles or cork-screws and are placed at different sites, depending on the region to be stimulated. The most common sites are as follows [35].

- C3/C4, positioned 6 cm from the vertex and in the same plane. These are adequate to elicit responses from the contralateral body, especially from the upper member.
- C1/C2, positioned in the same plane but separated 3 cm from the vertex. This configuration is suitable to elicit response from the lower limbs. However, it has the inconvenience of eliciting too much movement in the patient.
- Fz–Cz′: this configuration is adequate to elicit responses from the lower limbs simultaneously. Unfortunately, the response is more variable than the above configurations.
- M1/M2: the electrodes are located 9 cm from the vertex and usually 1 cm in the rostral direction. This configuration is suitable to elicit responses from facial and cranial nerves starting from the brainstem.
- C3/C4–Cz: in this montage, a hemispheric stimulation is elicited with an anode located 6 cm lateral from the vertex and a cathode at Cz. We have modified this configuration with a cathode located 2 cm from the vertex in the contralateral hemisphere [36]. This modification allowed a response not only from the face and contralateral upper limb but also from the lower member.

The parameters used to elicit MEP through TES are variable, but we use trains of 4–6 pulses, with a 50–75 μs pulse width, an inter-stimulus interval (ISI) of 2 ms (i.e., 500 Hz) and a voltage ranging from 120 to 450 V. It is extremely unusual to use a higher voltage. The recording should be performed with at least 50 μV/div, although it is quite common to use up to 500 μV/div for some muscles.

In some tumours located in the brainstem, cervical or upper thoracic cord, it can be useful to use a D wave recording rather than MEP. This wave reflects the travel wave of CNAP from the lateral cortico-spinal tract and must be recorded through electrodes placed in the immediacy of the spinal cord [32]. This technique is very useful because it can be performed under total neuromuscular relaxation and elicited by only one pulse. However, it cannot be used for vascular pathology of the spinal cord and must be cautiously considered when tumours are located near the anterior horns.

There is a false dispute, in our opinion, regarding the superiority of constant-current over constant-voltage stimulation. Of course, there are benefits and flaws of both techniques, but safe and reliable monitoring can be performed using voltage stimulation. Moreover, using a current of 61 mA with a pulse width of 500 μs [35], the total charge applied is 30.5 μC. However, a current of 340 mA over 50 μs [36] supplies a charge of 17 μC, which is approximately half of the total charge supplied with longer pulses.

2.3.4.2. Direct cortical stimulation (DCS)

For this technique, electrodes are applied directly to the cortical/subcortical surface. Direct cortical stimulation (DCS) to identify the primary motor cortex (PMC) is accomplished using paired electrodes. Stimulation is performed using 4–6 pulse trains at 500 Hz (the reason we denote this paradigm high frequency; this technique is also known as multipulse, which is misleading), with biphasic pulses of 150–200 μs in the duration/phase. Motor evoked potentials are assessed using pairs of subdermal needles spaced approximately 2 cm apart that are inserted into the contralateral muscles, but surface electrodes attached to the skin can also be used. Depending on the location of the tumour, it is customary to use the following muscles: the orbicularis oculi, orbicularis oris, deltoid, brachial biceps, extensor digitorum carpal flexor, abductor pollicis brevis, abductor digiti minimi, quadriceps, tibialis anterior and abductor hallucis.

Stimulation is initiated at 4 mA and increased continuously in increments of 1–2 mA until a stable compound muscle action potential (CMAP) is recorded, at a minimum amplitude of 30 μV or until an upper limit of 30 mA is achieved without eliciting a CMAP [5,6].

An alternative strategy entails the use of Ojemann's stimulation or low-frequency stimulation, which consists of a 50–60 Hz train that is 3–5 seconds in length and has a pulse width as high as 0.5 ms [37,38].

Although a systematic comparison between both strategies remains to be performed, it is important to be aware that neither electrical thresholds nor muscle response or electrical safety are equivalent.

In this sense, it is important at this point to consider some electrophysiological variables concerning patient safety. The effect of any type of electrical stimulation over the neural tissue is mediated by the total amount of charge applied to the system and the duration of application [39]. The electric current (*i*, in mA) is defined as follows:

http://dx.doi.org/10.5772/63241

$$i(t) = \frac{dq}{dt} \tag{8}$$

where q is the charge (in μC) and t is time (in ms). Thus, the total charge applied during time t_{pw} (time of pulse width) can be calculated from Eq. (8) as $q(t)=\int_0^{t_{pw}} i(t)dt$. For square pulses (which are the most common), the integral equals the amplitude × duration, e.g.:

$$q(t) = i \times t_{pw} \tag{9}$$

However, this expression only provides information about the charge/pulse. Therefore, to elucidate the total charge administered to the tissue (q_{total}), we must multiply by the number of pulses (N) as follows:

$$q_{total} = i \times t_{pw} \times N \tag{10}$$

Another relevant feature concerning safety is the maximum charge density (ρ_{max}), which is defined as q_{max}/A (μC/cm²/phase), where A is the area (usually in cm²). This parameter directly depends on the size and shape of the stimulation electrode.

A comparison of these magnitudes is provided in **Table 1** for three different stimulation paradigms.

Technique	**i_{max} (mA)**	**Pulse width (μs)**	**Number of pulses**	**Surface (cm²)**	**q_{max}/pulse (μC)**	**q_{total}/train (μC)**	**ρ_{max} (μC/cm²)**
HF	25	300	6	0.0133*	7.5	45	563.9
Awake craniotomy	10	1000	1	0.0079**	10.0	10	1265.8
Ojemann	10	500	240	0.0079	5.0	120	632.9

HF, high frequency.
*The surface is calculated from a 1.3 mm diameter disk electrode.
**The surface is calculated from a 1 mm diameter spherical electrode, assuming that only 1/4th of the surface is in contact with the cortex.

Table 1. Comparison of magnitudes.

Although there are no well-defined limits for the above-mentioned magnitudes, from the table we can observe that Ojemann's technique is the paradigm with the highest q_{total}/train, and the stimulation for awake craniotomy has the highest ρ_{max}.

2.3.5. Stimulated electromyography (sEMG)

For this technique, EMG is induced by an electrical shock that is delivered consciously, in contrast to the application described for fEMG. The pulses are usually delivered through bipolar (either concentric or parallel) or monopolar probes. In the latter case, it is important to use a cathodal current to stimulate the nerve and place the anode at a non-stimulated tissue.

The parameters must include pulses of a short length to avoid diffusion of the current. Normally, 50–100 μs should be adequate. The current must be maintained as low as possible to avoid injury to the neural tissue and diffusion. The latter effect must be considered in particular when a functional block is apparent because a high current or a long pulse (or both) can stimulate a region of the nerve distal in the damaged or blocked area and result in misleading information.

It is common to use sEMG in the next situation: (i) to explore a region to identify the proximity of nerves that are not easily visible (e.g., when the CN runs inside a schwannoma); (ii) to determine the identity of a nerve; (iii) to evaluate the functionality of the nerve. We usually measure the threshold to elicit a muscular response at two different points (proximal and distal to the region at risk or more damaged by the surgery) and calculate the ratio of $i_{distal}/i_{proximal}$. The closer this ratio is to 1, the better the function of the nerve.

The settings used to record sEMG depend on the muscle being recorded, but it is quite common to use a 50–3000 Hz bandwidth, with the notch off, a gain consistently greater than 30 μV/div (typically 50 μV/div), and a time base between 1.5 and 4.5 ms/div.

2.4. Cortical and subcortical surgery in awake patients

In recent years, there has been a renewed interest in surgery in awake patients [38,40,41]. This procedure uses the asleep–awake–sleep anaesthetic technique, which consists of induction with propofol + sevoflurane and topical blocking with svedocain + lidocaine around the skin incision. During exploration, the patient must be awaken slowly by removing the sedation. In recent years, a new anaesthetic, dexmedetomidine, has been introduced for this type of surgery and is considered the most effective [18].

Cortical stimulation is usually performed through a bipolar probe with ball-tips that are separated by 0.5 cm. It is common to use 60 Hz trains over 1–4 s. The pulse width is usually 1 ms, with a current intensity of 2.5–10 mA [42,43].

A low rate of intraoperative seizures has been reported (approximately 3–3.4%) [44], and some authors have concluded that control by ECoG is not mandatory [42]. However, this conclusion has been debated and remains to be validated.

In addition to this prevention, some authors have focussed on possible secondary effects derived from this technique. A normal human response to such an exceptional situation as awake craniotomy can, for instance, result in the delayed appearance of unintentional distressing recollections of the event or some type of post-traumatic stress disorder (as yet undescribed), despite the satisfaction of the patient concerning the procedure [45].

The limitations of awake surgery must be considered seriously. During such surgeries, the patient is awake with the head fixed and covered with cloth; and the patient may be kept awake for up to 2 h. Hence, patients must have both adequate cognitive function and the emotional maturity necessary to withstand such an environment. In fact, the Japan Society for Awake Surgery Guidelines limits the target patient population to those ranging from 15 to 65 years of age. Although with some limitations, awake craniotomy can be used in the paediatric population [50]. Nevertheless, use in mentally handicapped patients remains problematic or impossible.

However, no differences in the immediate postoperative motor status, extent of resection, or threshold intensity were found between IONM in anaesthetized patients and stimulation during awake craniotomy [46], although a detailed evaluation has not been performed for the different techniques or surgeries.

For selected patients, an awake craniotomy presents an option to reduce the risk of surgery-related neurological deficits, especially for language mapping. However, the benefits and risks of this type of procedure should be carefully considered, and the decision should serve the interests of the patient.

3. Different features of intraoperative neurophysiology

From a conceptual perspective, intraoperative clinical neurophysiology can be divided into two features: mapping and monitoring [47,48]. The characteristics of these features will be briefly described because neither their requirements nor the expectations associated with each are equivalent. The main differences between the features are the duration of study, the objectives and the modifications introduced to the surgery. However, in clinical practice, both features very often largely overlap or are used at different epochs of the same surgery.

3.1. Functional mapping

Functional mapping generally consists of the topographic assessment (although sometimes it is merely qualitative) of various structures to determine the functions that lead to or sit on the structures [9].

From the perspective of duration, it is usually short so that mapping ceases as soon as the function is positively identified. The objectives, as mentioned previously, are purely descriptive.

The changes during surgery are usually minor, especially because the surgery has a limited duration.

A typical example of mapping is the identification of eloquent areas in cortical surgery. In this case, the issue is to identify the eloquent regions. Thus, the surgeon knows the function of each region so he/she can decide where to position the incision or how far it can be moved prior to the detection of eloquent structures.

3.2. Intraoperative monitoring

Monitoring consists of the surveillance of the functional state(s)/structure(s) that is(are) being monitored for all or most of the surgical action, given the risk of iatrogenic injury [9].

Therefore, the duration of monitoring is considerably greater than in the case of mapping, and it usually lasts as long as the surgery itself. This condition naturally requires more dramatic changes than those used for mapping, beyond the modification of anaesthesia.

The objectives in this case are not just the functional identification but also the preservation of functional integrity, which can be compromised by many medical/surgical procedures, ranging from problems related to tissue perfusion (for example, by actively inducing hypotension or bleeding) to inadvertent surgical injuries such as the placement of spatulas.

In general, neurophysiological monitoring is widely employed in oncological or vascular neurosurgery.

4. Topographical approach to IONM

4.1. Cortical surgery

4.1.1. Anatomical and surgical considerations

IONM of cortical tumours is indicated when the lesion is in or near an eloquent area (areas responsible for carrying out basic neurological functions) such as the sensorimotor cortex or the language cortex. IONM enables clinicians to access the function of the motor and sensory systems of the patient during surgery to preserve neurological function, and it increases the success of radical tumour resection [6].

Functional mapping is initially performed to identify functional areas and their relationship with the tumour. This procedure might help the surgeon to determine the site at which to initiate resection of the tumour. Mapping is then followed by monitoring of the structures requiring continuous vigilance.

4.1.2. Particularities of IONM

As mentioned previously, ECoG is used to define functional areas. Moreover, electrical stimulation can elicit epileptiform discharges before, after and during mapping and IONM, considering that seizures in brain tumour patients are a common phenomenon accounting for 20–40 percent of cases [49].

Following the identification of functional areas via ECoG (**Figure 1B**), the location of the CS is determined by cSSEP phase reversal (**Figure 1C**). Accurate identification of the CS is extremely important because it permits identification of the PMC (**Figure 1C**) [5,6]. There is evidence that cSSEP phase reversal increases both the efficiency and the safety of PMC identification

[50]. Thereafter, DCS for the identification of PMC is performed. Of course, the motor map reference is always the Penfield homunculus [51]. However, when performing motor mapping, we must not forget that it does not conform strictly to reality [52]. It is a scheme upon which there are local movements in different directions [53].

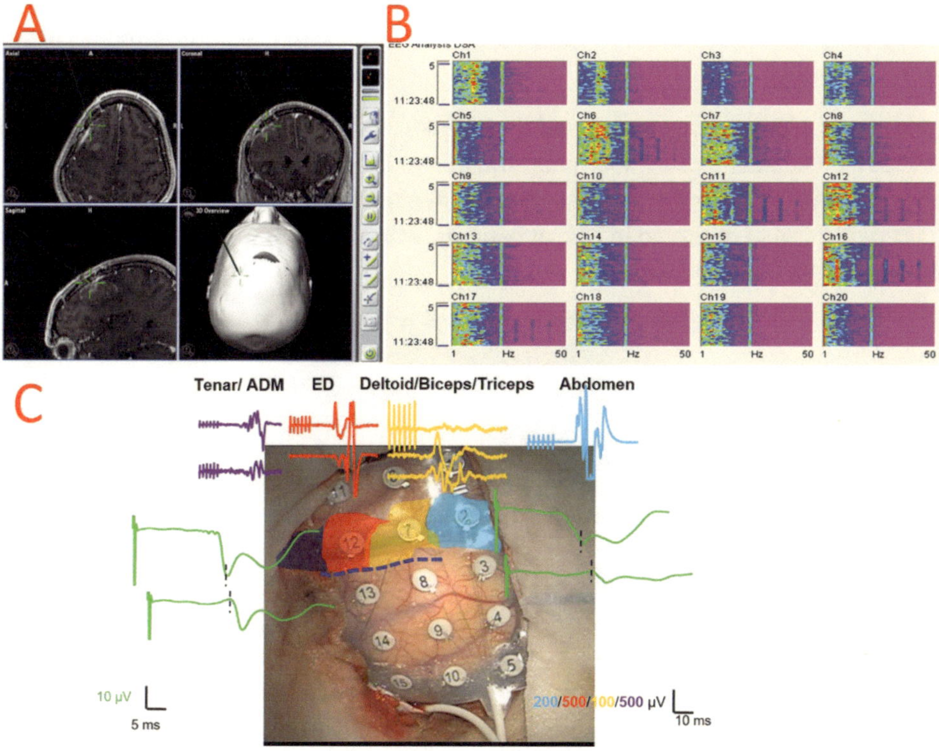

Figure 1. Cortical surgery in a patient with a left frontal glioma. (A) Neuronavigator showing coronal, frontal and sagittal views of left cortical tumour. (B) DSA of electrocorticography. For each electrode, there is a colour-coded plot showing the power spectral density for every frequency in the abscissa axis along the time shown in the ordinate axis. For electrodes 3–5, the power of all frequencies is lower than that for the rest of the grid. (C) Placement of the grid over the cortex with sensory and motor mapping. The coloured areas show the motor regions of the abdomen, arm, forearm and hand, and they correspond to the MEPs with the same colour. The dashed line in blue shows the area of the central sulcus, with the phase reversal illustrated in SSEPs in green.

4.1.3. Cortical language mapping

Locating the functional cortical regions related to language is the goal of intraoperative language mapping stimulation, which is performed during awake surgery. DCS is the technique of choice, as has been widely discussed in the previous section. Concerning this area of the cortex, we have provided additional information about the procedure employed for this type of surgery. The cortex is mapped every 5–10 mm, and positive stimulation sites responsible for language impairment are marked; the same technique is utilized during resection of the tumour via subcortical stimulation. A series of language tasks is conducted by a trained neuropsychologist throughout the duration of the tumour resection.

Although the risk of intraoperative seizures related to DCS is low, it is a real possibility. Additionally, considering that the patients are awake, this complication seems to be a particularly undesirable effect, not only from the perspective of patient discomfort but also because it would interfere with mapping by post-ictal hyperpolarisation. Using ECoG in this type of surgery could prevent, by monitoring and identifying discharges, the occurrence of seizures (**Figure 2**).

The identification of language areas and their fibres is not as successful as the localization of the cortical white matter in the PMC. Sanai and Berger [54] successfully identified the language areas in 145 (58%) of 250 patients with gliomas. Regarding neurological outcome, temporary language deficits were observed in 22% of patients, whereas permanent language deficits were observed in only 1.6% of patients.

A

B

C

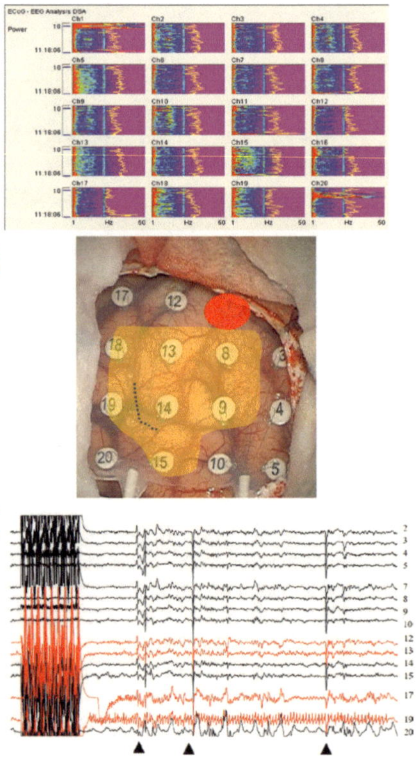

Figure 2. Mapping language in a patient with a cavernoma in Wernicke's area. (A) DSA showing a relative loss of cortical fast rhythms in electrodes 12 and 17. (B) Image showing the cortical mapping results. Red: Wernicke's area to 13 mA. Orange: region with negative results above 12 mA. The dotted line indicates the cortical incision for approaching. (C) Recording showing long-term after-discharges following stimulation by electrodes 18/1 –9 mA. The widespread artefact (arrowhead) corresponds to the moment at which cool serum was administered. The channels affected by after-discharges are shown in red.

http://dx.doi.org/10.5772/63241

4.1.4. Continuous IONM techniques

Following the determination of the relationship between the tumour and the PMC, continuous monitoring is performed via DCS using pairs of grid electrodes and employing high-frequency stimulation (**Figure 2B**).

It is accepted that the primary criterion for monitoring MEP in the setting of supratentorial surgery is an amplitude reduction of >50%. Temporary motor deficits have been linked to reversible declines in MEP amplitude of >50%, whereas irreversible declines and losses in MEP are predictors of permanent motor deficits [5]. Pastor et al. [5] described a study involving 34 patients who underwent surgical resection of glioma that was guided using 5-aminolevulinic acid (5-ALA) with no false-negative results. Nevertheless, postoperative neurological deficits without alterations in MEP are possible. This scenario, may be explained by secondary events such as postoperative oedema, haemorrhage and tumour resection from the supplementary motor area (SMA) [55].

An interesting issue for discussion is whether patients who harbour tumours in a region of the eloquent cortex other than the language area must be operated under general anaesthesia. As we have highlighted, there has recently been a renewed use of awake craniotomies [40,41]. In our experience, no new neurological deficits are observed in anaesthetized patients [5,20]. Accordingly, surgery near motor and somato-sensory cortical areas can be performed safely with the concomitant use of intensive neurophysiological mapping and monitoring [5]. Moreover, this combined approach is much more comfortable for both the patient and the surgical team.

When sensory function monitoring is also required, cSSEP are directly recorded from the grid. Monitoring the electrode entails the selection of higher amplitude responses for N1/P1/N2 potentials.

4.2. Semi-oval centre surgery

4.2.1. Anatomical and surgical considerations

The white matter in each hemisphere located between the cerebral cortex and deep nuclei together has a semi-oval shape. It consists of an association, a commissural and projecting cortical fibres. It contains, among others, the corticospinal, thalamo-cortical (containing somato-sensory and visual projections) or corticobulbar tracts.

In these patients, surgical removal of the tumour is performed far away from the motor cortex but near the subcortical structures such as the basal ganglia and the IC.

4.2.2. Particularities of IONM

As stated, DCS in these cases is usually precluded, and TES is the technique of choice. Because there is a risk of stimulation beneath the lesion, hemispheric TES must be performed. The somato-sensory pathway should also be monitored through the SSEP and, in a number of cases, even the VEP.

An interesting point is that warning criteria for the motor response may occur segmentally in isolated muscles. As previously described, these segmented changes are the most commonly observed changes [5] (**Figure 3**).

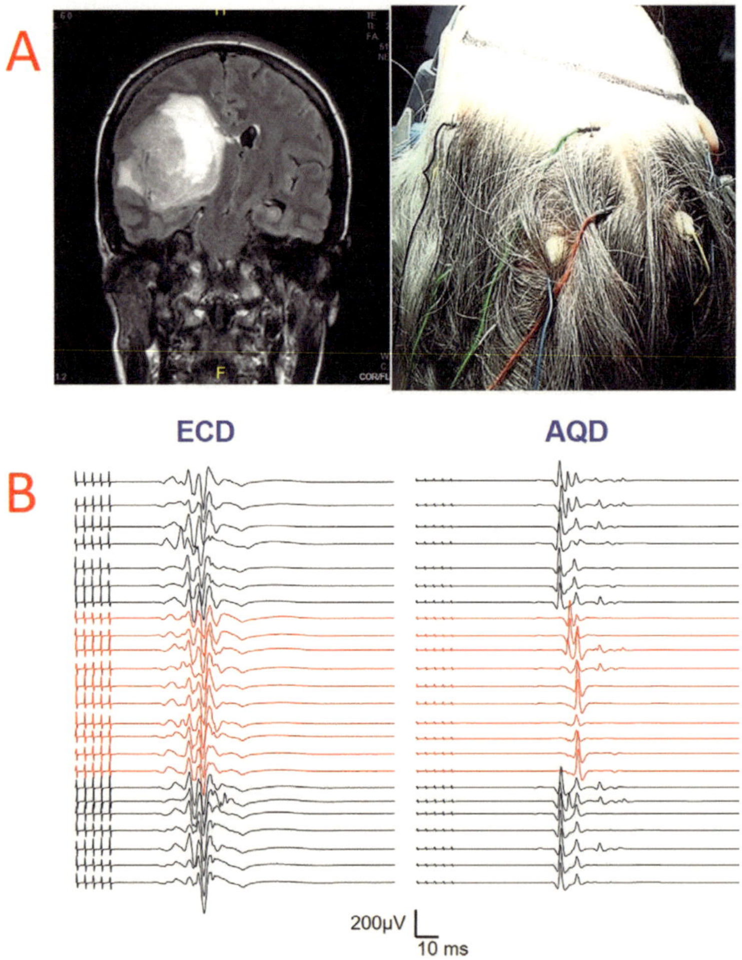

Figure 3. Monitoring of a patient with a tumour in the right semi-oval centre. (A) Frontal MRI before surgery, and an image indicating the placement of the electrodes for TES (B) MEPs monitoring of the upper limb at the moment a reversible segmental alteration occurred in the MEPs of the hand is shown in red.

Subcortical electrical stimulation is an important technique for the identification of the corticospinal tract [35]. The most accepted technique to date, in terms of effectiveness with respect to subcortical activation with a lower motor threshold (MT), is monopolar cathodal stimulation [39].

In general, a linear relationship is considered to be present among the five monopolar 0.2–0.5 ms pulses and the 3–4 ms ISI, as well as a threshold of 1 mA of stimulation, which is equivalent to approximately 1 mm of distance from the CST [56]. Some studies have attempted to determine the lowest intensity of stimulation allowed before resection should be terminated to prevent injury to the CST. This safety margin has not been standardized and has been defined as 6 mA in some studies, whereas other studies have suggested that both significant signal changes in MEP and permanent motor deficits do not occur below a threshold of 1–3 mA [57]. Regardless, it seems reasonable to follow these motor threshold safety margins provided that no alterations in MEP are observed during continuous motor monitoring; otherwise, the resection must be stopped immediately.

VEP are needed when the tumour is located in the occipito-parietal region due to the risk of injury to the thalamo-cortical projections to the visual cortex. In fact, we noted that up to 50% of patients monitored by VEP during semi-oval centre surgery displayed warning criteria [5].

4.3. Cranial base and anterior fossa surgery

4.3.1. Anatomical and surgical considerations

In general terms, the skull base consists of five bones: ethmoid, sphenoid, occipital, paired frontal and paired temporal bones. The anterior limit of the anterior fossa is the posterior wall of the frontal sinus. The anterior clinoid processes and the planum sphenoidale, which forms the roof of the sphenoid sinus, mark the posterior limit. The frontal bone forms the lateral boundaries.

The posterior aspect includes the optic canal, the superior orbital fissure (SOF), and the inferior orbital fissure (IOF). The SOF conveys the oculomotor (CN III), trochlear (CN IV), abducens (CN VI), ophthalmic nerves and V1, as well as the ophthalmic veins. An understanding of the relationship of the tumour to vital structures is essential to preserve these structures and to minimize morbidity associated with treatment.

The greater wing of the sphenoid forms the anterior limit of the middle skull base. The posterior limit is the clivus. The SOF, foramen rotundum, foramen ovale, and foramen spinosum lie in an anteroposterior and medio-lateral plane [58].

A significant structure that can be found lateral to the sphenoid sinus is the cavernous sinus. Along it lateral wall runs the internal carotid artery (ICA), CNs III, IV, V, and VI and the maxillary nerve (CN V2).The facial nerve (CN VII) and vestibule cochlear nerve (CN VIII) originate from the caudal pons. They course through the subarachnoid space and enter the porus acusticus and IAC.

With a suitable understanding of skull base anatomy and surgical access, diverse IONM techniques has been steadily improving the outcome of surgery, both in terms of disease-free survival and morbidity associated with treatment.

4.3.2. Particularities of IONM

According to the anatomy of the anterior and middle fosses, the main structures to monitor are the CNs. Therefore, the standard technique is recording fEMG to identify different discharge patterns related to either irritative or injury activity. Several criteria have been advanced to identify patterns that predict transitory or permanent nerve injury, but these criteria lack uniformity, and the correlation with the postoperative outcome is often unsatisfactory [59]. sEMG is a functional technique that is also essential during these types of surgeries.

Various techniques have been used for the placement and recording of the superior rectus muscle for CN III and the lateral rectus muscle for CN VI. These include the manual placement of bipolar needles, or single-shafted bipolar needles using an orbital ultrasound [60] or image guidance [61].

Corticobulbar tract (CBT) MEP monitoring is a neurophysiological technique that has improved greatly over time and is increasingly used in brainstem tumour surgery. Although the correlation between the intraoperative corticobulbar response and the postoperative outcome may not be completely accurate due to the possibility of false-positive and false-negative responses [62], experience seems to indicate that the complete disappearance of a corticobulbar MEP usually correlates with a severe, mostly irreversible, postoperative deficit. Conversely, when the corticobulbar MEP remains unchanged at the end of surgery, a transient deficit may not be prevented, but the great majority of these patients have recovered their preoperative status at the time of follow-up [59].

The vestibulocochlear nerve (CN VIII) and, to a greater extent, the auditory pathways as they pass through the brainstem are especially at risk during cerebellopontine angle (CPA), posterior/middle fossa or brainstem surgery. CN VIII can be damaged by several mechanisms, from vascular compromise to mechanical injury by stretch, compression, dissection and heat injury. Additionally, the cochlea itself can be significantly damaged during temporal bone drilling, by noise, mechanical destruction, or infarction, and due to rupture, occlusion or vasospasm of the internal auditory artery. CN VIII monitoring can be successfully achieved by live recording of the function of one of its parts, the cochlear or auditory nerve (AN), using the BAEPs [63].

The necessity to protect the optic tract is not uncommon in this setting, and thus intraoperative monitoring of the VEP is mandatory. Although such monitoring techniques were previously not well-established, high rates of feasibility have recently been reported in a number of publications, and stable VEPs have been associated with good postoperative visual function [30].

From a neurophysiological perspective the ICA emits at the supraclinoid segment, an important collateral branch: the posterior communicating. This artery is of paramount importance because in addition to providing branches to the optic chiasm and oculomotor

http://dx.doi.org/10.5772/63241

nerve, it is also responsible for irrigating the thalamus. Therefore, in this type of surgery, the MEP and SSEP must be monitored.

4.4. Posterior fossa surgery

4.4.1. Anatomical and surgical considerations

The posterior cranial fossa is the deepest and most capacious fossa of the skull base. It contains the cerebellum, pons and medulla oblongata. Recent advances in diagnostic and surgical techniques have increased the accessibility of this region to surgery, providing new and neurologically safer treatments for these patients [64].

Tumours of the skull base show a tendency to be large in size, they are critical brain lesions because they extend inside and around the brainstem, placing not only the CNs and/or their motor nuclei at risk of injury but also the motor and somato-sensory pathways.

The particular approach is determined not simply by the location of the lesion but largely by the path that allows access to the lesion while minimally disturbing critical structures. The surgeon must select a cranial approach that provides line-of-sight access to the lesion while avoiding excessive manipulation; however, this achievement is not simple due to the high density of critical structures in the brainstem, and even a mild manoeuvre can result in the injury to the delicate nuclei, tracts, or nerves.

4.4.2. Particularities of IONM

There is a critically high potential risk of damage to neural structures during the resection of these tumours, and therefore IONM is an indispensable tool for posterior fossa surgery. The decision to monitor certain structures depends on both the anatomical location of the tumour and the surgical approach selected by the surgeon.

In general, IONM consists of three procedures (**Figure 4**): (i) brainstem mapping (BSM), (ii) CBT-MEP monitoring and (iii) monitoring of ascending and descending long pathways and transverse auditory radiations. BSM is a neurophysiological technique that is used to locate cranial nerves and their motor nuclei on the floor of the fourth ventricle [65] through sEMG. During resection of brainstem tumours involving incision of the fourth ventricle, the facial colliculus (intramedullary roots of the CN VII around the abducens nucleus) and motor nuclei of the lower CNs nucleus are especially prone to injury because the tumour often grossly distorts the brainstem anatomy, and the normal landmarks on the floor of the fourth ventricle are missing. If the neurosurgeon cannot identify these landmarks, he will not be able to make a safe incision. Hence, the mapping assists surgeons in locating these important structures.

The recording technique used for targeted muscles is the same as discussed previously, and the standard set of muscles used to record muscle activity are as follows: the orbicularis oris, orbicularis oculi, and mentalis for the VII cranial motor nucleus (CMN), the posterior pharyngeal wall for CMN IX, the cricothyroid or vocalis muscle for X and the intrinsic tongue muscles for CMN XII. Electrical stimulation of the floor of the fourth ventricle is delivered through a monopolar hand-held probe using the same parameters described above for the stimulated EMG technique. It is important to stress that during this procedure, the threshold intensity is essential for proper localization of the CMN.

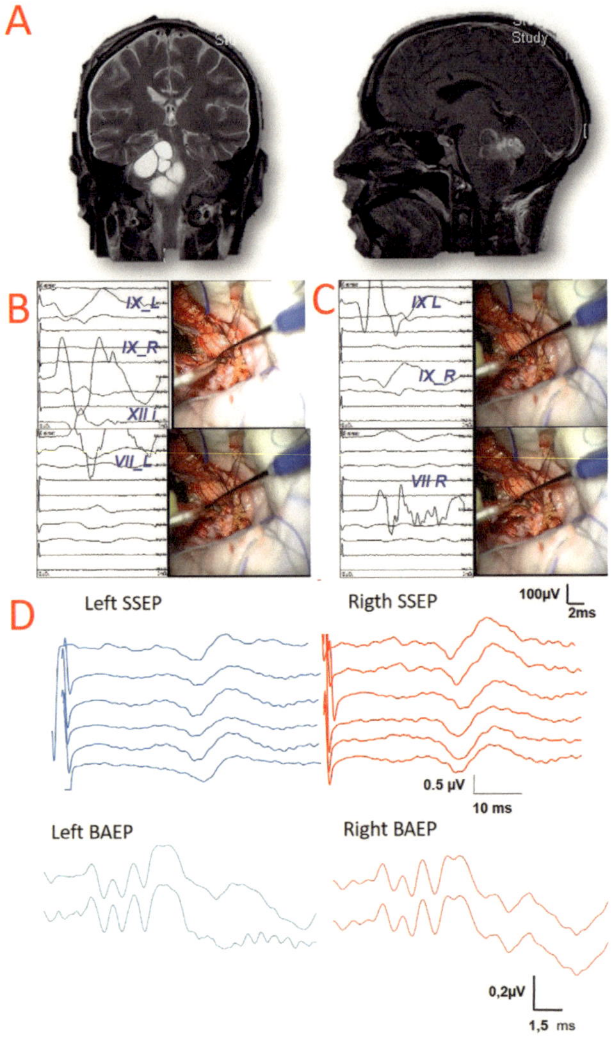

Figure 4. Brain stem mapping in a patient with a tumour locate on the floor of the fourth ventricle. (A) Frontal and sagittal MRI before surgery. (B) Stimulated EMG during identification of the right CN IX (above) and the left CN VII (below). (C) Identification of the left CN IX (above) and the right CN VII (below). (D) Brain stem monitoring comprising SSEPs (top) and BAEPs (bottom).

This technique is very valuable because although there has been a recent advancement of neuroimaging techniques, BSM remains the only way to reveal the surgical anatomy in the operative field [65,66]. We must not forget that it is a functional localization technique and can be performed only intermittently. Moreover, discrepancies between the final intraoperative recordings and postoperative function may occur. This situation can be explained by an injury to the afferent fibres during resection, in which the lower motoneuron is still intact or a nuclear injury results from a stimulation-elicited response activating the intramedullary root. Both instances can produce false-negative results [59,65]. A similar situation may occur during monitoring of the IX and X cranial nerve, difficulties in coughing or swallowing can occur postoperatively despite positive and normal CMAP recordings at the end of surgery. This phenomenon may be explained by BSM responses reflecting only the functional preservation of the efferent arc of these reflexes, but no information has been provided regarding the integrity of the sensory afferents.

For lesions that compress the brainstem ventrally or laterally, BSM provides a minimal contribution. In these cases, CBT-MEP monitoring is the neurophysiological technique indicated to monitor the entire CMN motor pathway from the cerebral cortex to the targeted muscle [59]. Likewise, when motor CN monitoring is considered, as mentioned previously, recording of fEMG with the identification of different discharge patterns will allow the identification of injury activity.

Electrical stimulation must be performed with extreme care due to the presence of vital structures within a very small space. Therefore, the frequency should be approximately 2.45 Hz, and the pulse width should be maintained as low as possible to provide specific stimulation and avoid current spreading. However, a compromise between current intensity and pulse width is essential, and therefore 100 μs and a current lower than 2 mA should be desirable.

Regarding the remaining critical neural structures, the ascending sensory pathways are monitored by BAEPs as well as SSEP, which together can be used to monitor approximately 20% of the brainstem [59]. Information concerning the descending motor pathways is provided by the use of MEP.

4.5. Spinal cord surgery

4.5.1. Anatomical and surgical considerations

Intramedullary spinal cord tumours (ISCTs) comprise 15% of intradural spinal tumours in adults [67]. Tumours of glial origin represent approximately 68% of ISCTs, most of which are ependymomas or astrocytomas [68].

Microsurgery plays a central role in the treatment of these tumours, and the main goal is the complete surgical removal. This aim is limited because preservation of spinal cord function with minimum neurological morbidity it is also desired, representing another challenge of these surgeries.

Microsurgical resection and the surgical strategy may vary, depending on the histological type of each tumour. However overall, there are well-defined steps during the surgical approach to ISCTs: opening of the posterior median sulcus, exposure and initial tumour debulking with separation between the sidewall of the tumour and spinal cord tissue and complete removal of the tumour, which requires the dissection and coagulation of the vascular afferences from the anterior spinal artery.

4.5.2. Particularities of IONM

During the resection of ISCT, lesions in neural structures can inadvertently occur, potentially creating severe neurological deficits. IONM of the spinal cord plays an important role in facilitating the resection of these tumours [69].

As previously described, an effective strategy could be to adapt IONM to the steps of the surgery to protect the somato-sensory and motor pathways [70]. Therefore, monitoring with SSEP and MEP is indicated.

Additionally, for spinal cord surgery, D wave recording is widely used and recommended. In well-documented studies of more than 100 ISCT surgeries, a preserved D wave up to 50% of the original amplitude, with a complete loss of muscle MEPs, has been shown to result in only transient paraplegia [71].

Although it also has disadvantages, we generally consider that under those circumstances in which the mechanism of injury to the spinal cord is purely ischemic, D wave monitoring does not add a significantly value to muscle MEP monitoring. Grey matter is more sensitive than white matter to cord ischemia, and both clinical and experimental data suggest that both peripheral and myogenic MEP disappear earlier than the D wave when spinal cord vascularisation is acutely compromised [72]. Regarding this issue, it seems logical to postulate that the nerve structures most likely to be affected during an ischemic alteration in ISCT surgery are the anterior horns (AH).

It is important to note that previous observations of EMG may improve the reliability of IONM during spinal cord surgery [73, 74]. Skinner and Transfeldt [75] have reported experience with EMG for monitoring ISCT in 14 patients. They described segmental and suprasegmental elicitation of neurotonic discharges that could anticipate the loss of MEP and predict a postoperative motor deficit. Moreover, some studies have associated spinal cord mechanical and thermal injury with EMG activity and motor conduction block (MEP loss) in animals [75, 76].

In our experience, we can define three different phases of the surgical approach to ISCTs that must be followed by the neurophysiological techniques used (**Figure 5**).(i) Phase A: during posterior median sulcus opening, it is important to protect the dorsal columns by monitoring the somato-sensory evoked potentials (SSEPs). (ii) Phase B: working at the cleavage plane, monitoring of motor evoked potentials (MEPs) is mandatory, mainly to protect the corticospinal tract in the lateral cords during the separation between the sidewall of the tumour and the spinal cord tissue. (iii) Phase C: the final phase of complete tumour removal during which, as previously mentioned, the anterior vascular supply is threatened and consequently there is a certain risk of injuring the AH. Thus, fEMG is critical during this phase.

http://dx.doi.org/10.5772/63241

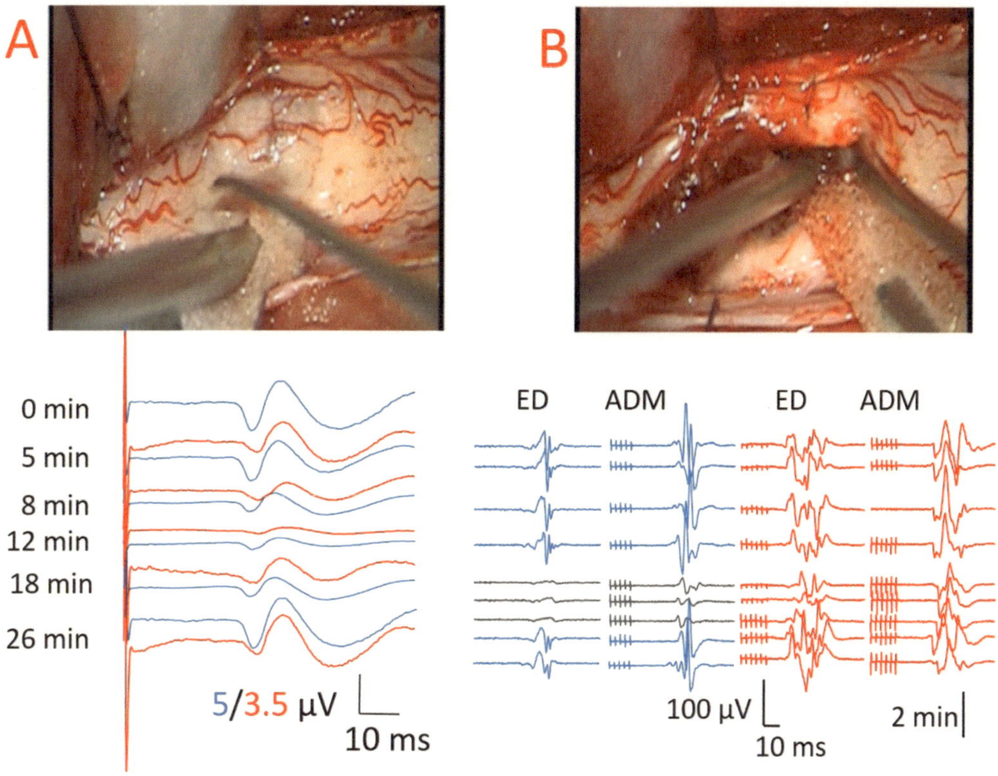

Figure 5. Two different times during monitoring of ISCT surgery. (A) (Top) Microphotograph during incision of the dorsal median raphe. (Bottom) SSEPs for the left (blue) and right (red) sides. Times are shown on the left. Zero min indicates opening of the dura. Between 8 and 18 min, both SSEPs, displayed a decrease in amplitude and an increase in latency (right SSEPs at 8 min). (B) (Top) Microphotograph during tumour removal from the lateral walls. (Bottom) MEPs for the left (blue) and right (red) sides. Grey lines indicate significant changes in MEPs. Times are shown on the left.

5. Conclusion

IONM is a cheap and effective method for reducing the risk of permanent postoperative deficits in many different operations in which NS is undergoing manipulation. It provides real-time monitoring of function to an extent that makes it superior to imaging methods that provide information about structures but not about the physiological state of the patient.

Intraoperative neurophysiology must be conducted by teams of experts that include a clinical neurophysiologist with a thorough understanding of neuroscience and the pathophysiology of the disorders that are to be treated.

Therefore, we can conclude without exaggerating that IONM and mapping are some of the techniques with more relevance during recent decades for oncological neurosurgery. The widespread use and improvement of these techniques have allowed better functional post-surgical outcomes, increasing life expectancy together with better functionality.

However, different topics have been debated that must be clarified. Among these are parameters for stimulation, indications regarding awake versus anaesthetized craniotomy, different types of DCS, and a better definition of the warning criteria or the prognostic utility of some surgeries. Future investigations will clarify most of these features and will undoubtedly contribute to improve outcomes in neuro-oncology.

Acknowledgements

This work was supported by a grant from the Plan Nacional de Investigación Científica, Desarrollo e Innovación Tecnológica (I+D+I), Instituto de Salud Carlos III, Subdirección General de Evaluación y Fomento de la Investigación PI12/02839 and partially supported by F.E.D.E.R.

Author details

Lorena Vega-Zelaya[1,3], Rafael G. Sola[2] and Jesús Pastor[1,3*]

*Address all correspondence to: jesus.pastor@salud.madrid.org

1 Clinical Neurophysiology, Hospital Universitario de la Princesa, Madrid, Spain

2 Neurosurgery, Hospital Universitario de la Princesa, Madrid, Spain

3 Biomedical Research Institute, Hospital Universitario de la Princesa, Madrid, Spain

References

[1] Stummer W, Reulen HJ, Novotny A, Stepp H, Tonn JC. Fluorescence-guided resections of malignant gliomas–an overview. Acta Neurochir Suppl. 2003; 88: 9–12.

[2] Stummer W, Pichlmeier U, Meinel T, Wiestler OD, Zanella F, Reulen HJ. Fluorescence-guided surgery with 5-aminolevulinic acid for resection of malignant glioma: a randomized controlled multicenter phase III trial. Lancet Oncol. 2006; 7: 392–401.

[3] Thakkar JP, Dolecek TA, Horbinski C, Ostrom QT, Lightner DD, Barnholtz-Sloan JS, et al. Epidemiologic and molecular prognostic review of glioblastoma. Cancer Epidemiol Biomarkers Prev. 2014 Oct; 23(10): 1985–1996. doi: 10.1158/1055-9965.

[4] Perry J, Okamoto M, Guiou M, Shirai K, Errett A, Chakravarti A. Novel therapies in glioblastoma. Neurol Res Int. 2012; 428565. http://dx.doi.org/10.1155/2012/428565.

[5] Pastor J, Vega-Zelaya L, Pulido P, Garnés-Camarena O, Abreu A, Sola RG. Role of intraoperative neurophysiological monitoring during fluorescence-guided resection surgery. Acta Neurochir (Wien). 2013; 155(12): 2201–2213.

[6] Vega-Zelaya L, Pastor J. Intraoperative neurophysiological monitoring techniques for the resection of malignant brain tumors located in eloquent cortical areas. Austin J Neurosurg. 2015; 2(4): 1038.

[7] Møller AR. Introduction. Intraoperative Neurophysiological Monitoring. 2nd edition. Humana Press, Totowa, 2006; pp: 1–8.

[8] Krieg SM, Shiban E, Droese D, Gempt J, Buchmann N, Pape H, et al. Predictive value and safety of intraoperative neurophysiological monitoring with motor evoked potentials in glioma surgery. Neurosurgery. 2012; 70(5): 1060–1071.

[9] Pastor J. Conceptos de Neurofisiología en Neurocirugía Funcional, in Navarrete EG y Sola RG (ed): Neurocirugía Funcional y Estereotáxica. Barcelona: Viguera Editores, 2011, pp. 17–27.

[10] Pastor J. Quirófano: Neurofisiología intraoperatoria. En: Cirugía raquimedular. Eds. C Botella, RG Sola, A Isla. Viguera Editores, Barcelona, 2014; pp. 157–170 ISBN 978-84-92931-26-2

[11] Koester J, Siegelbaum SA. Propagated signalling: the action potential. In: Principles of Neural Sciences, 5th edition, Eds: Kandel ER, Schwartz JH, Jessell TM, Siegelbaum SA, Hudspeth AJ. Elsevier, New York, 2013; pp. 148–176.

[12] Pastor J. Biophysical foundations of neural activity. Rev Neurol. 2000; 30(8): 741–755.

[13] Pastor J: Neurofisiología Intraoperatoria, in Navarrete EG y Sola RG (ed): Neurocirugía Funcional y Estereotáxica. Barcelona: Viguera Editores, 2011, pp. 589–604

[14] Nunez P, Srinivasan R. The physics-EEG interface. In: Electric Fields of the Brain, 2nd Edition. Oxford University Press, New York, 2006; pp. 3–55.

[15] Stevens JC. Somatosensory evoked potentials. In: Clinical Neurophysiology, 2nd ed., Ed: Daube JR. Oxford University Press; 2002. pp. 181–203.

[16] Nuwer MR, Comi C, Emerson R, Fuglsang-Frederiksen A, Guérit J-M, Hinrichs H, et al. IFCN standards for digital recording of clinical EEG. Electroencephalogr Clin Neurophysiol. 1998; 106: 259–261.

[17] Finnigan S, Wong A, Read S. Defining abnormal slow EEG activity in acute ischaemic stroke: delta/alpha ratio as an optimal QEEG index. Clin Neurophysiol. 2016; 127(2): 1452–1459. doi: 10.1016/j.clinph.2015.07.014. Epub 2015 Jul 22.

[18] Smith DJ, Howie MB. General anesthesia: intravenous and inhalational agents. In: Modern Pharmacology with Clinical Applications, 6th ed. Eds: Craig Ch R, Stitzel RE. Lippincott, Williams, Wilkins; Philadelphia; 2003; pp. 291–309.

[19] Vega-Zelaya L, Torres CV, Garnes-Camarena O, Ortega GJ, García-Navarrete E, Navas M, et al. Electrocorticographic evidence and surgical implications of different physiopathologic subtypes of temporal epilepsy. Clin Neurophysiol. 2014; 125: 2349–2357.

[20] Pastor J, Pulido P, Sola RG. Neurophysiological assisted transsulcal approach to a high grade glioma without affect neither motor nor somatosensory function. Rev Neurol. 2013; 56(7): 370–374.

[21] Van Drongelen W. Noise. In: Signal Processing for Neuroscientists. Amsterdam, Elsevier, 2004; pp. 34–53.

[22] Pastor J. Diagnóstico funcional: Neurofisiología. En: Cirugía raquimedular. Eds. C Botella, RG Sola, A Isla. Viguera Editores, Barcelona; pp. 99–114. ISBN 978-84-92931-26-2, 2014.

[23] Pastor J. Quirófano: Neurofisiología intraoperatoria. En: Cirugía raquimedular. Eds. C Botella, RG Sola, A Isla. Viguera Editores, Barcelona; pp. 157–170. ISBN 978-84-92931-26-2, 2014

[24] Pastor J, Reina MA. Fisiología del nervio periférico normal y patológico. In Wikinski JA, Reina MA, Bollini C, De Andrés JA, Salas X, Salgueiro C, et al, eds. Complicaciones neurológicas asociadas con la anestesia regional periférica y central. Buenos Aires: Ed. Panamericana; 2011. p. 87–103.

[25] Mauguière F. Somatosensory evoked potentials: normal responses, abnormal waveforms and clinical applications in neurological diseases. In: EEG, basic principles, clinical applications and related fields, Eds. Niedermeyer E, Lopes da Silva A.. Baltimore: Lippincott, Williams & Wilkins; 1993. pp. 1014–1058.

[26] Sala F, Lanteri P. Brain surgery in motor areas: the invaluable assistance of intraoperative neurophysiological monitoring. J Neurosurg Sci. 2003; 47: 79–88.

[27] Liégeois-Chauvel C, Trécuchon-Dafonseca A, Régis J, Marquis P, Chauvel P. Auditory evoked potentials in the definition of eloquent cortical areas. In: Presurgical Assessment of the Epilepsies with Clinical Neurophysiology and Functional Imaging. Eds: Rosenow F, Lüders HO. Elsevier, Amsterdam, 2004; 305–316.

[28] Wiedemayer H, Fauser B, Armbruster W, Gasser T, Stolke D. Visual evoked potentials for intraoperative neurophysiologic monitoring using total intravenous anesthesia. J Neurosurg Anesthesiol. 2003; 15: 19–24.

[29] Ota T, Kawai K, Kamada K, Kin T, Saito N. Intraoperative monitoring of cortically recorded visual response for posterior visual pathway. J Neurosurg. 2010; 112: 285–294.

[30] Kodama K, Goto T, Sato A, Sakai K, Tanaka Y, Hongo K. Standard and limitation of intraoperative monitoring of the visual evoked potential. Acta Neurochirurgica. 2010; 152: 643–648. doi:10.1007/s00701010-0600-2.

[31] Torres Díaz C, Pastor J, Rocio E, Sola RG. Continuous monitoring of cortical visual evoked potentials by means of subdural electrodes in surgery on the posterior optic pathway. A case report and review of the literature. Rev Neurol. 2012; 55(6): 343–348.

[32] Deletis, V. Intraoperative Neurophysiology and methodologies used to monitor the functional integrity of the motor system. In: Neurophysiology in Neurosurgery. Eds: Deletis V, Shils JL. Academic Press, London, 2002; pp: 25–54.

[33] Taniguchi M, Cedzich C, Schramm J. Modification of cortical stimulation for motor evoked potentials under general anesthesia: technical description. Neurosurgery. 1993; 32: 219–226.

[34] Rothwell J, Burke D, Hicks R, Stephen J, Woodforth I, Crawford M. Transcranial electrical stimulation of the motor cortex in man: further evidence for the site of activation. J Physiol. 1994; 481: 243–250.

[35] Szelényi A, Kothbauer KF, Deletis V. Transcranial electric stimulation for intraoperative motor evoked potential monitoring: stimulation parameters and electrode montages. Clin Neurophysiol. 2007; 118: 1586–1595.

[36] Pastor J, Perla-Perla P, Pulido-Rivas P, Sola RG. Hemispheric transcranial electrical stimulation: clinical results. Rev Neurol. 2010; 51: 65–71.

[37] Chang EF, Clark A, Smith JS, Polley MY, Chang SM, Barbaro NM, et al. Functional mapping-guided resection of low-grade gliomas in eloquent areas of the brain: improvement of long-term survival. Clinical article. J Neurosurg. 2011; 114(3): 566–573.

[38] De Witt Hamer PC, Robles SG, Zwinderman AH, Duffau H, Berger MS. Impact of intraoperative stimulation brain mapping on glioma surgery outcome: a meta-analysis. J Clin Oncol. 2012; 30: 2559–2565.

[39] Merrill DR, Bikson M, Jefferys JGR. Electrical stimulation of excitable tissue: design of efficacious and safe protocols. J Neurosci Methods. 2005; 141: 171–198.

[40] Peruzzi P, Puente E, Bergese S, Chiocca EA. Intraoperative MRI (ioMRI) in the setting of awake craniotomies for supratentorial glioma resection. Acta Neurochir. 2011; Suppl 109: 43–48.

[41] Duffau H, Capelle L, Sichez J, Faillot T, Abdennour L, Law Koune JD, et al. Intraoperative direct electrical stimulations of the central nervous system: the Salpetrier experience with 60 patients. Acta Neurochir (Wien). 1999; 141: 1157–1167.

[42] Boetto J, Bertram L, Moulinié G, Herbet G, Moritz-Gasser S, Duffau H. low rate of intraoperative seizures during awake craniotomy in a prospective cohort with 374

supratentorial brain lesions: electrocorticography is not mandatory. World Neurosurg. 2015 Dec; 84(6): 1838–1844. doi: 10.1016/j.wneu.2015.07.075.

[43] Li T, Bai H, Wang G, Wang W, Lin J, Gao H, et al. Glioma localization and excision using direct electrical stimulation for language mapping during awake surgery. Exp Ther Med. 2015 May; 9(5): 1962–1966.

[44] Hervey-Jumper SL, Li J, Lau D, Molinaro AM, Perry DW, Meng L, et al. Awake craniotomy to maximize glioma resection: methods and technical nuances over a 27-year period. J Neurosurg. 2015; 123(2): 325–339. doi: 10.3171/2014.10.JNS141520.

[45] Milian Ml, Tatagiba M, Feigl GC. Patient response to awake craniotomy— a summary overview. Acta Neurochir (Wien). 2014; 156(6): 1063–1070. doi: 10.1007/s00701-014-2038-4.

[46] Delion M, Terminassian A, Lehousse T, Aubin G, Malka J, N'Guyen S, et al. specificities of awake craniotomy and brain mapping in children for resection of supratentorial tumors in the language area. World Neurosurg. 2015; 84(6): 1645–1652. doi: 10.1016/j.wneu.2015.06.073.

[47] Bello L, Fava E, Cascaceli G, Bertani G, Carrabba G, Papagno C, et al. Intraoperative mapping for tumor resection. Neuroimag Clin N Am. 2009; 19: 597–614.

[48] Bertani G, Fava E, Casaceli G, Carrabba G, Casarotti A, Papagno C, et al. Intraoperative mapping and monitoring of brain functions for the resection of low-grade gliomas: technical considerations. Neurosurg Focus. 2009; 27(4): E4.

[49] Lwu S, Hamilton MG, Forsyth PA, Cairncross JG, Parney IF. Use of peri-operative anti-epileptic drugs in patients with newly diagnosed high grade malignant glioma: a single center experience. J Neurooncol. 2010 Feb; 96(3): 403–408.

[50] Simon MV, Sheth SA, Eckhardt CA, Kilbride RD, Braver D, Williams Z, et al. Phase reversal technique decreases cortical stimulation time during motor mapping. J Clin Neurosci. 2014; 21: 1011–1017.

[51] Porter R, Lemon R. Corticospinal function and voluntary movement. Oxford: Oxford University Press; 1993.

[52] Cuadrado ML, Arias JA, Palomar MA, Linares R. The pyramidal tract: new pathways. Rev Neurol. 2001; 32(12): 1151–1158.

[53] Schott GD. Penfield's homunculus: a note on cerebral cartography. J Neurol Neurosurg Psychiatry. 1993; 56: 329–333.

[54] Sanai N, Berger MS. Intraoperative stimulation techniques for functional pathway preservation and glioma resection. Neurosurg Focus. 2010; 28: E1.

[55] Krieg SM, Schäffner M, Shiban E, Droese D, Obermüller T, Gempt J, et al. Reliability of intraoperative neurophysiological monitoring using motor evoked potentials during

resection of metastases in motor-eloquent brain regions. J Neurosurg. 2013; 118: 1269–1278.

[56] Kamada K, Todo T, Ota T, Ino K, Masutani Y, Aoki S, et al. The motor-evoked potential threshold evaluated by tractography and electrical stimulation. J Neurosurg. 2009; 111(4): 785–795.

[57] Seidel K, Beck J, Stieglitz L, Schucht P, Raabe A. The warning-sign hierarchy between quantitative subcortical motor mapping and continuous motor evoked potential monitoring during resection of supratentorial brain tumors. J Neurosurg. 2013; 118(2): 287–296.

[58] Lang DA. Surgery of the cranial base. In: Surgery of Cranial Base Tumors, Eds.: Sekhar LN, Janecka IP. New York, Raven Press, 1993; pp. 93–121.

[59] Sala F, Manganotti P, Tramontano V, Bricolo A, Gerosa M. Monitoring of motor pathways during brain stem surgery: what we have achieved and what we still miss? Neurophysiol Clin. 2007; 37(6): 399–406.

[60] Schlake HP, Goldbrunner R, Siebert M, Behr R, Roosen K. Intra-Operative electromyographic monitoring of extra-ocular motor nerves (Nn. III, VI) in skull base surgery. Acta Neurochir (Wien). 2001; 143(3): 251–261.

[61] Alberti O, Sure U, Riegel T, Bertalanffy H. Image-guided placement of eye muscle electrodes for intraoperative cranial nerve monitoring. Neurosurgery. 2001; 49(3): 660–663; discussion 663–664.

[62] Dong CC, Macdonald DB, Akagami R, Westerberg B, Alkhani A, Kanaan I, et al. Intraoperative facial motor evoked potential monitoring with transcranial electrical stimulation during skull base surgery. Clin Neurophysiol. 2005; 116(3): 588–596.

[63] Simon MV. Neurophysiologic intraoperative monitoring of the vestibulocochlear nerve. J Clin Neurophysiol. 2011; 28(6): 566–581

[64] Bricolo A, Turazzi S. Surgery for gliomas and other mass lesions of the brainstem. Adv Tech Stand Neruosurg. 1995; 22: 261–341.

[65] Morota N, Deletis V, Epstein FJ, Kofler M, Abbott R, Lee M, et al. Brain stem mapping: neurophysiological localization of motor nuclei on the floor of the fourth ventricle. Neurosurgery. 1995; 37: 922–930.

[66] Sola RG, Pulido P, Pastor J, Ochoa M, Castedo J. Surgical treatment of symptomatic cavernous malformations of the brainstem. Acta Neurochir (Wien). 2007; 149(5): 463–470

[67] Wong AP, Dahdaleh NS, Fessler RG, Melkonian SC, Lin Y, Smith ZA, et al. Risk factors and long-term survival in adult patients with primary malignant spinal cord astrocytomas. J Neurooncol. 2003; 115(3): 493–503.

[68] Chamberlain MC, Tredway TL. Adult primary intradural spinal cord tumors: a review. Curr Neurol Neurosci Rep. 2011; 11(3): 320–328.

[69] Deletis V, Sala F. Intraoperative neurophysiological monitoring of the spinal cord during spinal cord and spine surgery: a review focus on the corticospinal tracts. Clin Neurophysiol. 2008; 119(2): 248–264.

[70] Sala F, Bricolo A, Faccioli F, Lanteri P, Gerosa M. Surgery for intramedullary spinal cord tumors: the role of intraoperative (neurophysiological) monitoring. Eur Spine J. 2007; 16 Suppl 2: S130–9.

[71] Kothbauer K, Deletis V, Epstein FJ. Intraoperative spinal cord monitoring for intramedullary surgery: an essential adjunct. Pediatr Neurosurg. 1997: 247–254.

[72] de Haan P, Kalkman CJ, Ubags LH, Jacobs MJ, Drummond JC. A comparison of the sensitivity of epidural and myogenic transcranial motor-evoked responses in the detection of acute spinal cord ischemia in the rabbit. Anesth Analg. 1996; 83: 1022–1027.

[73] Hyun SJ, Rhim SC. Combined motor and somatosensory evoked potential monitoring for intramedullary spinal cord tumor surgery: correlation of clinical and neurophysiological data in 17 consecutive procedures. Br J Neurosurg. 2009; 23(4): 393–400.

[74] Skinner SA, Nagib M, Bergman TA, Maxwell RE, Msangi G. The initial use of free-running electromyography to detect early motor tract injury during resection of intramedullary spinal cord lesions. Neurosurgery. 2005; 56 (2 Suppl): 299–314.

[75] Skinner SA, Transfeldt EE. Electromyography in the detection of mechanically induced spinal motor tract injury: observations in diverse porcine models. J Neurosurg Spine. 2009; 11(3): 369–374.

[76] Skinner SA, Hsu B, Transfeldt EE, Mehbod AA, Rippe DM, Wu C, et al. Spinal cord injury from electrocautery: observations in a porcine model using electromyography and motor evoked potentials. J Clin Monit Comput. 2013; 27(2): 195–201.

Chapter 10

Neurocognitive Effects of Primary Brain Tumors

Mohammad Abu-Hegazy and
Hend Ahmed El-Hadaad

Additional information is available at the end of the chapter

http://dx.doi.org/10.5772/62924

Abstract

Cognitive impairment, a common finding with the brain tumors, may result from the tumor itself or the treatment used: surgery, chemotherapy, or radiotherapy. Surgery for brain tumors improves the cognitive function due to reduction of compression as in case of removal of noninvasive tumors. Stability of cognitive function also was observed after tumor resection, such as tumors of third ventricle. Postoperative cognitive worsening was observed. Postoperative worsening of executive functions may correlate to volume of the operated area. Cognitive deficits may follow radiotherapy by several months to many years. These deficits may be due to vascular injury, local radionecrosis, and cerebral atrophy. This usually involves multiple domains, including memory, attention, executive function, and intelligence. The irradiated volume of brain tissue has great impact on cognition. Intensity-modulated radiotherapy (IMRT) and proton beam therapy result in greater sparing of healthy brain tissue and allow for a more-targeted delivery of radiation and smaller penetration of tissue beyond the tumor consequently reduce the risk of cognitive deficit after radiotherapy. Chemotherapy treatment in brain tumor seems to have a role in cognitive dysfunction deficits. The toxicity of chemotherapy increased when was given during or after radiotherapy. Chemotherapeutic agents, such as BCNU, CDDP, cytosine arabinoside, and intrathecal or intravenous methotrexate, have toxic effect to the CNS. Glioblastoma patients undergoing radiotherapy with concomitant and adjuvant temozolomide treatment do not develop cognitive deterioration. Patients with brain tumors face the challenge of cognitive impairment due to the tumor itself or treatments. Cognitive deficits in processing speed, memory, attention, and executive functions interfere with patients' daily life activities. Cognitive rehabilitation program has proven to be effective in patients with primary brain tumors. Cognitive impairments have a large impact on self-care, social and professional functioning, and consequently on quality of life. Preventing these late effects is a challenge for the medical team, psychologists, and rehabilitation specialists. Prevention depends in part on being able to predict those at greatest risk. Advances in neurosurgery, chemotherapy, and radiotherapy techniques are helping to a great extent, but may not be totally successful at preventing these late effects.

Keywords: Cognition, cognitive deficits, brain tumor, cognitive rehabilitation, brain tumor treatment

1. Introduction

1.1. Background

The term intellect designates the totality of the mental or cognitive operations that comprise human thought, and the higher cortical functions that make up the human mind. Memory is a specific cognitive function: the storage and retrieval of information. Other "higher" functions, such as language, calculations, spatial topography and reasoning, music, and creativity, all represent the functions of specific brain systems [1].

Cognitive functioning of brain tumor patients is an increasingly important outcome measure, because cognitive impairments can have a large impact on self-care, social and professional functioning, and consequently on quality of life (QOL) [2]. Patients with brain tumors often experience cognitive dysfunction associated with the disease itself and its treatment, as well, including surgery, radiotherapy (RT), and chemotherapy. Cognitive dysfunction has been recognized as the most frequent complication among long-term survivors. Despite the many advances made in the treatment modalities and surgical techniques, primary malignant brain cancer is a devastating illness, characterized by poor survival rates and significant morbidity as the disease progresses [3]. For many patients, cognitive changes are part of the disease process, but the pattern of impairment can vary markedly in different patients.

Resection of brain tumors may result in improvement of cognitive functions. Teixidor et al. [4] reported long-term improvement of verbal memory, after a transient immediate postoperative worsening, following frontal premotor and anterior temporal area resection, usually after a transient immediate postoperative worsening. Cognitive improvement has also been observed after surgical resection of high-grade gliomas [5], and in some studies stable, cognitive performance was observed after brain tumor resection, for instance, patients with tumors of the third ventricle [6].

Specific cognitive domain deficits after brain tumor removal were observed in some studies. A study conducted by Goldstein et al. [7] reported minimal deterioration in attention after right parenchymal frontal or precentral tumors resection. Another study [8] concluded that right rather than left prefrontal cortex resection was associated with, stroop performance test, selective attentional decline.

Radiation-induced cognitive impairment in some series is reported to occur in up to 50–90% of adult patients with brain tumor who survive >6 months after fractionated partial or whole-brain irradiation [9]. Moreover, because patients with brain tumor are surviving longer because of improved radiation therapy techniques and systemic therapies [10], the patient population experiencing these significant late effects is growing rapidly. Radiation-induced cognitive impairment is marked by decreased verbal memory, spatial memory, attention, and novel problem-solving ability [11]. Modern radiation therapy techniques have resulted in decreased acute and early delayed brain injury as well as late demyelination and white matter necrosis with less cognitive functional deficits, including progressive memory impairments, attention, and executive function that finally led to less impact on QOL of most survivors [12].

Neurocognitive sequelae of chemotherapy are less well documented than radiation effects [13]. Chemotherapy-related neurotoxicity to the central nervous system may be increased by intra-arterial administration, especially in combination with osmotic blood–brain barrier disruption, meant to increase the local concentration of chemotherapy in the brain [14]. Neurotoxicity may also be increased by chemotherapy given after, or even during, RT [15]. Primary central nervous system lymphoma is chemoresponsive, such as anaplastic oligodendroglioma (AO) and oligoastrocytoma (OA) tumors, chemotherapeutic agents are often ineffective due to limited ability to cross the BBB. Use of radiation therapy is often associated with significant neurotoxicity [16].

Advances in neurosurgery, chemotherapy, and RT are helping to a great extent in preventing cognitive deficit. Prevention depends in part on being able to predict the risky factors [17].

1.2. Objectives

The chapter examines:

– Cognition and its evaluation

– Brain tumors and cognition

– Brain tumor surgery and cognition

– Effect of adjuvant therapies (radio/chemotherapy) on cognition

– Prevention or reduction of cognitive deficits during the treatment of brain tumors

– Follow-up care and cognitive rehabilitation

2. Cognition and its evaluation

2.1. Cognition

Higher brain function may be subclassified into: (a) distributed functions, which do not localize to a particular brain region but instead require the concerted action of multiple parts on both sides of the brain, for example, attention and concentration, memory, higher-order executive function, social conduct, and personality; (b) localized functions, which are dependent on the normal structure and function of a particular part of one cerebral hemisphere, for example, language and praxis in dominant hemisphere the nondominant hemisphere hemisphere is largely, though not exclusively, responsible for visuospatial skills [18]. Cognitive impairment without crossing the threshold for dementia has been termed "mild cognitive impairment" (MCI) [19]. The MCI syndrome, as an expression of an incipient neurodegenerative disorder that may lead to dementia, is extremely heterogeneous and may coexist with systemic, neurologic, or psychiatric disorders that can cause cognitive deficits [20]. The criteria for MCI encompassed all possible cognitive manifestations of the syndrome and four subgroups have been proposed: deficits only in memory functions; memory deficits plus deficits in another cognitive domain; deficits in a single nonmemory domain; and deficits in more than one nonmemory domain [21].

2.2. Evaluation of cognitive functions

2.2.1. The Montreal cognitive assessment (MoCA)

MOCA was used as test of cognition, measure cognitive function, its cognitive domains: visuospatial/ executive function; naming; memory; language; abstraction; and attention. MoCA is scored out of 30 points. A normal score is 26 or above [22].

2.2.2. Mini Mental State Examination (MMSE)

MMSE is used for global cognitive functioning measurement [23].

2.2.3. Other cognitive domain-specific areas neuropsychological tests: focus on domain-specific areas of cognition:

(1) Hayling Sentence Completion Test, Word Span and Corsi's Test to test working memory [24], verbal and visual memory—Recognition Memory Tests, Words, and Topography [25]. (2) Rey Auditory Verbal Learning Test—RAVLT and logical memory to assess episodic memory, immediate and delayed recall [26], abstract reasoning: nonverbal—Raven's advanced progressive matrices [27, 28], verbal—Proverb Interpretation Test [29]. (3) Attention—Digit Span sub-test from the Wechsler Adult Intelligence Scale-III [30], Elevator Counting with Distraction from the Test of Everyday Attention [31], Trail Making test, part A and part B to test simple speed processing and complex attention, respectively, [32]. (4) Visual perception—Incomplete Letters Test from the Visual Object and Space Perception Battery [33], Rey–Osterrieth Complex Figure recall, to test visuospatial long-term memory, Rey–Osterrieth Complex Figure, copy to test visuoconstructional abilities [34]. (5) Phonemic and semantic fluency [35], language—Graded Naming Test [36], Word Comprehension—Synonyms Test [37]. (6) Executive functions—phonemic word fluency [38]. (7) Frontal Assessment Battery—FAB to assess frontal functionality [39].

For neuropsychological measures, age-, gender-, and education-corrected scores and equivalent scores should be calculated from the raw scores according to normative standards.

3. Brain tumors and cognition

Cognitive impairment, a common finding with the brain tumors, may result from the tumor itself or the treatment used surgery, chemotherapy, or RT.

3.1. Cognitive impairment due to tumor

More than 90% of patients with brain tumors showed impairments in the cognition at least in one area. The reported impairments of executive function were observed in 78%, while impairments of memory and attention were presented in more than 60% of patients [40].

Zucchella et al. [41] reported cognitive impairment in 54.4% of brain tumor patients, (53.75%) presented with multidomain impairment, while (46.25%) of the patients revealed cognitive deficits 16.25% of them limited to language, 13.75% to memory, 8.75% to attention, 6.25% to logical-executive functions, and 1.25% to visuospatial abilities.

Talacchi et al. [5] reported cognitive impairment in glioma patients 79% of patients have cognitive deficit in at least one test, (24, 3, 31, and 21% in one, two, three, four, or more tests, respectively, and this was correlated with edema, tumor grade, and size. Verbal memory, visuospatial memory, and word fluency were the most frequently affected functions.

3.2. Pathophysiology

Cognitive impairment associated with brain tumors can be induced by direct or indirect compression of normal brain tissue by reactive edema [42].

Tumor tissue can also invade directly into functional brain regions or indirectly disconnect the structures which can further contribute to cognitive deficits [43].

The mechanisms via which brain tumors affect brain function varied, highly malignant tumors grow quickly so they tend to infiltrate and displace the normal brain tissue, while the lower grade tumors tend to grow and infiltrate slowly disrupting brain function causing cognition deficit.

Tumors of ventricular system causes increase in intracranial pressure and hence affect the cognitive function; also large ventricular tumors affect the cognition directly through its compression effect. Functioning brain tumors which secrete hormones may have role in cognitive deficit through endocrine disturbance [44].

The main pathophysiology causes of cognitive dysfunction are not well known, different hypotheses were placed; progression of brain tumors seems to be the predominant one [45], also late treatment effects, for example, surgery, RT, chemotherapy, uses of antiepileptic drugs or corticosteroids), the psychological distress also may contribute in cognitive dysfunction [46].

The cognitive function disturbance in brain tumors may be due to combination of these factors.

4. Brain tumor surgery and cognition

In brain tumors, the first treatment modality is surgery. The aim was to balance the neurological outcomes (minimize the neurological deficits) and oncological outcome [2].

- Does brain surgery improve cognitive deficit?

Surgery for brain tumors improves the cognitive function due to the reduction of compression as after removal of noninvasive tumors, such as meningiomas, improvement of attentional function occur [42]. Patients with high-grade glioma have worse cognitive dysfunction than patients with low-grade glioma (LGG) [47]. The worse cognitive deficits in patients with high-grade gliomas have been attributed to higher incidence of intracranial hypertension, the rapid growth, and the infiltrative nature.

Sweet et al. [48] reported that the localization is associated with cognitive effects. Tumors of the pineal region associated with memory impairment, visuospatial function, attention, visuomotor function, problem-solving, and affective disorders.

Medial temporal lobe epilepsy caused by tumor is associated with cognitive deficit (long-term memory dysfunction, difficulties in learning, attention, naming, visuospatial abilities, executive functions, and intelligence) [49].

Less extensive surgery of the mesiotemporal structures correlates with better memory outcome than in the extensive temporal lobe surgery [50].

Verbal memory decline was observed in dominant temporal lobe resection [51], while visuospatial memory decline associated with nondominant temporal lobe resection [52].

Cognitive improvement has been observed after tumor resection, and improvement of verbal memory has been observed after LGG resections in frontal premotor and anterior temporal areas [4], usually after a transient postoperative worsening. This improvement was related to tumor lateralization [53].

Some studies reported postoperative cognitive worsening in (38%) of patients versus 24% rate of improved patients. Worsening associated with executive functions while improvement was observed with memory function. This worsening may correlate to volume of the operated area (tumor size) rather than the location. The postoperative improvement of memory function, the most frequent preoperative cognitive deficit, occurs due to release of the mass effect [54].

Teixidor et al. [4] reported immediate postoperative worsening for working memory in 96% of cases, and Giovagnoli et al. [55] reported that postoperative scores for cognitive tests were not significantly lower than the preoperative.

Talacchi et al. [5] found unexpected low incidence of additional deficits (38%) immediate postoperative and a considerable rate of early improvement (24%), and this correlated with tumor size and histology. This study reported also that postoperative worsening seems to be due to a generic mechanical effect and to manipulation/removal of tumor periphery rather than to discrete focal injury.

Yoshii et al. [53] reported that the cognitive functions in patients with LGG and meningiomas (MGs) in the right brain were normal preoperative and postoperative whereas it decreased preoperative and did not return to the normal scores postoperative in left brain MGs. Temporal and spatial orientation, similarities, first recall, writing, mental reversal decreased after operation.

The explanation of mild cognitive effects in MGs preoperatively is the ability of normal brain tissue to compensate as the slow growth of tumor provides enough time for this compensation, but after surgical decompression decline in brain function occurs due to remodeling of normal brain tissue [56]. Another explanation is that extracerebral tumor causes compression on brain tissues but local anatomical and functional integrity maintained before surgery.

Stability of cognitive function also was observed after tumor resection, like tumors of third ventricle; the preoperative cognitive impairment in executive function, memory, and fine manual speed did not improve or worsen postoperatively [57].

Postoperative cognitive defects in specific domains were observed, for example, some patients with frontal or precentral tumors showed postoperative minor deterioration in attention [58].

Right prefrontal cortex resection in one study [8] was associated with selective attention impairment (Stroop test performance).

5. Effect of brain RT on cognition

Cognitive deficits following RT are irreversible and progressive complication that may follow RT by several months to many years. These deficits may be due to vascular injury, local radionecrosis, and cerebral atrophy, the severity ranges from mild or moderate to progressive mental slowing, occurring in at least 12% of patients who were treated with radiation therapy [59].

5.1. Hypothesis of radiation-induced cognitive impairment

There are many hypotheses that explain how the cognitive deficits following radiation therapy occur, direct damage and subsequent death of parenchymal cells (oligodendrocytes, neurons, astrocytes, and microglia) or indirect through reactive oxygen species (ROS) production.

Dynamic interactions between the multiple cell types (astrocytes, endothelial cells, microglia, neurons, and oligodendrocytes) within the brain may be the cause of radiation-induced cognitive impairment [60]. Another hypothesis is that the RT can inhibit hippocampal neurogenesis causing the cognitive impairment.

Irradiation of the hippocampus results in loss of neuronal stem cells (NSCs) which are responsible on self-renewal and generating neurons, astrocytes, and oligodendrocytes [61]. The radiation injury to NSCs is dose-dependent [62] and results in decrease in proliferation of NSCs and decrease in its differentiation into neurons [63]. Radiation therapy for brain tumors may lead to a significant reduction in the number of neurogenic cells [64].

Direct damage of parenchymal brain cells due to RT and subsequent death of these leads to cognitive impairment; damage to oligodendrocytes, responsible for myelination, has been thought to play a role [65]. Neuronal irradiation of rodent causes altered expression of the gene activity-regulated cytoskeleton-associated protein, N-methyl-D-aspartate (NMDA) receptors, glutaminergic transmission, and also hippocampal long-term potentiation [66].

Disruption of the blood–brain barrier (BBB) as a result of brain RT has been associated with impaired cognition. This disruption and alteration of the BBB is likely due to imbalance between matrix metalloproteinase-2 and the metalloproteinase-2 tissue inhibitor levels [67], activation of microglial cells plays an important role in phagocytosis of dead cells, sustained activation is thought to contribute to a chronic inflammatory state in the brain [68]. Subsequent inflammation following RT and cell death usually associated with up regulation of cytokines, which are thought to be expressed by microglia, and pro-inflammatory transcription factors in the brain which contribute to endothelial cell dysfunction [69]. Glial and endothelial cells appear to have independent and overlapping roles in the pathogenesis.

Ionizing radiation produces its effect by direct DNA damage or indirect through generating ROS, leading to DNA damage to and activation of early response transcription factors and signal transduction pathways [70]. Activation of these pathways leads to the following: changes in cytokine milieu; the activation/influx of inflammatory cells, particularly microglia; marked increase in expression of the pro-inflammatory genes tumor necrosis factor (TNF)-α, interleukin (IL)-1β, IL-6, and Cox-2, and the chemokines, Monocyte Chemoattractant Protein-1 (MCP-1), intercellular adhesion molecule (ICAM)-1 and the development of post-irradiation complications [71].

Radiation injury to astrocytes makes them to undergo proliferation, exhibit hypertrophic nuclei/cell bodies, and show increased expression of glial fibrillary acidic protein .These reactive astrocytes secrete a host of pro-inflammatory mediators such as cyclooxygenase (Cox)-2 and the ICAM-1, which may lead to infiltration of leukocytes into the brain via BBB breakdown [72].

RT affects large- and medium-sized blood vessels of the brain. Vascular hypothesis predicts that blood-vessel dilatation, wall thickening with hyalinization, endothelial cell loss and a decrease in vessel density, all these finally lead to white-matter necrosis [73].

The severity of cognitive deficit following radiation therapy appears to be proportional to the dose of radiation therapy received by the hippocampus region [74].

5.2. Predisposing factors

Older ages more than 60 years and in some studies more than 40 years old have increased risk to develop leukoencephalopathy specifically in patients with genetic predisposition to leukoencephalopathy [75] with subsequent cognitive deficit. Also patient with white matter disease such as multiple sclerosis have increased risk, also vascular diseases such as hypertention carry risk [76].

Beside the previous patient-related factors, also there are factors related to treatment include the dose of RT received, dose per fraction and volume of irradiated brain, 5% of patients treated with more than 5000 cGy develop radiation necrosis [77], high radiation dose increases the risk of leukoencephalopathy, daily doses >200 cGy have a significantly increased risk of cognitive damage [75]. The large irradiated volume of brain tissues carries increased risk of cognitive impairment, and whole brain radiation has threefold to fourfold increased risk of encephalopathy [76].

Additional treatments to RT such as chemotherapy have increased risk on cognition than RT alone, systemic and intrathecal treatments have been implicated. Methotrexate chemotherapy when received intravenously or intrathecally after cranial irradiation has an effect on cognition in children and also on adults [78].

5.3. Neuropsychological assessments

Folstein MMSE is brief test that assess delirium or significant dementia. It does not adequately measure all the cognitive areas affected by radiation, and it is not a sensitive tool for detecting cognitive impairment in patients receiving RT [79].

Among the patients who have impaired cognitive function by neuropsychological testing, only 50% were considered abnormal on the MMSE [80].

The National Cancer Institute (NCI) Radiation Oncology Branch adapted the Meyers et al. [45] test battery by adding few measures to assess processing speed, working memory, and attention, which are functions that can be affected by RT [81].

Measurement of quality of life and daily activities of living is an important issue beside the neuropsychological testes, such as the Barthel index to assess the daily living skills and the Functional Assessment of Cancer Therapy-Brain (FACT-Br), to address the quality of life issues concerning brain tumor patients undergoing treatment The Barthel Index assesses daily living skills [82], and the FACT-Br was developed specifically to address the quality of life issues concerning brain tumor patients undergoing treatment [83].

5.4. Cognitive impairment following RT

RT is the leading cause of cognitive deficits involving multiple domains, including memory, attention, executive function, and intelligence.

Patients who received RT performed worse in measures of executive function and information processing speed. Worse cognitive functioning also observed with white-matter hyperintensities and global cortical atrophy [84].

Several studies assed cognitive defects to specific tumor-type and tumor location. Aarsen et al. [85] reported cognitive deficit, with sustained speech and speed of speech in children treated with RT for pilocytic astrocytoma, 60% of patients had difficulty with academics 3 years after treatment.

Cognitive impairment observed in children with medulloblastoma who had treated with RT. These deficits were prominent attention deficits correlated with impaired math and reading performance [86].

Hoppe-Hirsch et al. [87] conducted a study comparing intellectual outcomes of children diagnosed with ependymomas or medulloblastomas, treated with whole-brain radiotherapy (WBRT), and found that only 10% of medulloblastoma patients had an IQ above 90 after 10 years compared to 60% of ependymoma patients, and this result attributed to cerebral hemisphere radiation.

Posteroir fossa irradiation with 35 Gy was associated with lower cognitive scores than that irradiated with a dose 25 Gy, and IQ and verbal comprehension seems to be dose-dependent in posterior fossa tumors [88].

Large-sample controlled clinical trial conducted by Klein et al. [75] assed mid-term and long-term neuropsychological function following the RT in LGG. In the study, 195 patients with LGG compared with 195 healthy controls and 100 patients with hematological malignancies with mean follow-up period of 6 years. The results revealed that patients with LGG had lower scores in all cognitive domains than the controls and hematological patients, and the main cause of cognitive deficits was the tumor, but cognitive deficits of memory domain was observed only in patients who received RT with dose per fraction more than 2 Gy.

Another study was conducted on those patients after 12-year follow-up and found that the attentional deficits deteriorated in patients who received RT. The progressive decline was found even in patients received <2 Gy dose per fraction [89].

Decline in nonverbal memory was observed in patients with LGGs years post-RT, despite the long-term improvements which observed in verbal memory, attention, and executive function [84]. Postoperative RT in LGG was found to have a significant risk of long-term leukoencephalopathy and cognitive impairment [90].

The irradiated volume of brain tissue has great impact on cognition. A study conducted by Jalali et al. [91] reported that patients who treated with stereotactic conformal RT presented with unchanged overall mean full-scale IQ, while one third of patients showed a >10% decline in full-scale IQ as compared to baseline.

Chang et al. [92] found that cognitive deficits after the treatment with sterotactic radiosurgery (SRS) had lower incidence than that in patients treated with whole-brain radiotherapy (WBRT). The cognitive deficit in learning and memory function was (24%) in patients treated with SRS and (52%) in patients treated with WBRT and SRS.

Intensity-modulated radiotherapy (IMRT) is a type RT technique in which more sparing of normal brain tissue can be achieved and precise contouring to the tumor tissue.

Hippocampal sparing with IMRT reduced doses delivered to hippocampus by 87% (0.49 Gy) and 81% (0.73 Gy) [93].

Proton beam therapy results in greater sparing of healthy brain tissue and allows for a more-targeted delivery of radiation and smaller penetration of tissue beyond the tumor [94]. The mean dose of radiation to the hippocampus could be reduced much more, and it could be half that of IMRT and consequently reduce the risk of cognitive deficit after RT [95].

6. Effect of chemotherapy on cognition

Chemotherapy treatment in brain tumor seems to have a role in cognitive deficits. There is association between chemotherapy used in the treatment of brain tumor and an increased risk for cognitive dysfunction especially, if it is administered with RT.

6.1. Pathogenesis of cognitive impairment

The mechanisms by which chemotherapy-induced cognitive impairment are unclear [96].

Chemotherapy may reduce the number of neural stem/progenitor cells, which have role in memory and learning ability [97], and neural precursor cells are chemo-sensitivity, neural stem, and line age-restricted progenitor cells that form, among other cell types, the myelinating oligodendrocytes in the frontal white matter [98].

Primary pathological lesions including demyelination, inflammation, and microvascular injury [99]. Also mature oligodendrocytes are chemo-sensitive at lower dosage than those required to kill tumor cells [100].

Multiple chemotherapeutic agents affect hippocampal neurogenesis causing decrease in cell proliferation within the germinal region of the hippocampus and development of cognitive deficit [101].

Genetic role in chemotherapy-induced cognitive decline may be impilicated, and there is increased risk of cognitive impairment after RT with the apolipoprotein E4 alleles [102].

6.2. Cognitive impairment of chemotherapeutic agents

Chemotherapy added to slow the tumor progression especially in children to postpone radiation therapy or to reduce the dose of radiation therapy to decrease the neurocognitive sequelae of increasing doses of RT. Neurotoxic side-effects of chemotherapy alone can be difficult, because most patients of brain tumor have been treated with RT and chemotherapy [103].

The evidence that chemotherapy alone causes neurocognitive effects is not consistent. Studies have concluded that chemotherapy effects are negligible and not clinically significant compared to craniospinal irradiation (CSI) [104].

Neurotoxicity of chemotherapy arises during, or shortly after, chemoterapy. RT causes disturbance in BBB, so the toxicity of chemotherapy increased when was given during or after RT. In these cases, the chemotherapeutic drugs reach higher concentrations in brain tissue because of leakage of the blood–brain barrier due to RT. Intrathecal chemotherapy has higher CNS toxicity compared to systemic chemotherapy [105].

Chemotherapeutic agents, such as BCNU, CDDP, cytosine arabinoside, and intrathecal or intravenous methotrexate, have toxic effect to the CNS. Chemotherapy-related cognitive impairment in primary CNS lymphoma was observed in one or more domains: (attention, executive function, memory, psychomotor speed, and language). Other studies have shown that cognitive stability or cognitive improvement during chemotherapy provided that the tumor was responsive to chemotherapy treatment [106, 107]. Uses of high-dose IV methotrexate or interathecal methotrexate with radiation therapy result in dementia particularly when the radiation is given prior to the methotrexate. Leukoencephalopathy more commonly occurs. MRI shows bilateral periventricular white matter changes. The radiation therapy disrupts the BBB and results in increased permeability of the white matter to the methotrexate [108].

Copeland et al. [109] concluded that chemotherapy had only a slight effect on neurocognitive status and was confined to perceptual motor skills with observed age effect on performance IQ.

Chemotherapeutic agents, such as BCNU, cisplatin, and cytarabine, have proved to be more toxic to neural precursor cells than cancer cells [110]. Carmustine, methotrexate, and cytarabine have been found to induce central neurotoxicity to neural stem cell populations located in the subventricular zone and dentate gyrus [99].

Prabhu et al. [111] conducted a study on LGG patients and concluded that the addition of chemotherapy procarbazine, lomustine, and vincristine (PCV) to RT for LGGs did not result in significant MMSE score decline when compared to RT alone.

Regarding the HRQOL, there is a short-lasting negative impact of PCV chemotherapy on HRQOL during and shortly after treatment, but no long-term effects on HRQOL have been established [112].

Patients with previously untreated anaplastic astrocytoma, OA, or oligodendroglioma were evaluated for the long-term efficacy and safety of accelerated fractionated RT combined with intravenous carboplatin. In a phase II study conducted by Levin et al. [113], they found that after RT, patients received procarbazine, lomustine (CCNU), and vincristine (PCV) for 1 year or until tumor progression, 10% of those patients developed serious clinical neurologic deterioration and/or dementia requiring full-time caregiver attention.

Hilverda et al. [114] reported that glioblastoma patients undergoing RT with concomitant and adjuvant temozolomide treatment did not develop cognitive deterioration.

In LGG patients, temozolomide is not only successful in terms of extending the survival duration but also has been proven to maintain or even improve HRQOL while patients are on treatment [115].

Patients with recurrent high-grade glioma (HGG), successfully treated with temozolomide, achieved significant improvement in the HRQOL domains, whereas patients with disease progression had significant deterioration in most HRQOL domains [116].

7. Prevention or reduction of cognitive deficits during treatment of brain tumors

Reduction in treatment-related brain tissue toxicity has occurred with advances in neurosurgical techniques, advances in radiation therapy techniques, and use of neuroprotective agents.

7.1. Pharmacological prevention of neurocognitive impairment

Neuroprotective agents may be used to protect healthy tissue against neuronal cell death or degeneration caused by the treatment of brain tumor.

Lithium can be used to protect progenitor cells in the hippocampus through inhibition of radiation-induced apoptosis and induction of the DNA repair, and the tumor cells not included in this protection process. A study conducted by Yang et al. [117] found that neurocognitive performance in mice was improved after receiving lithium concomitant with RT, anthor neuroprotective drug; fenofibrate which prevents activation of microglia. Administration of fenofibrate during whole-brain RT prevents effects on hippocampal neurogenesis in mice, as it enhances survival of newborn neurons in the dentate gyrus [118].

7.2. New treatment techniques

The use of image-guided surgery such as the intraoperative magnetic resonance imaging resulted in improvement in tumor resection and reduction of residual [119]. The use of endoscopic biopsy is a minimally invasive method can be performed safely in conjunction with diversion of cerebrospinal fluid in cases of obstructive hydrocephalus and decrease neurocognitive decline [120].

New radiation techniques such as IMRT are able to minimize the radiation to healthy brain structures. With using IMRT, hippocampus can be localized and hence the dentate gyrus can be spared, resulting in prevention or decrease neurocognitive decline to some extent [121]. Lin et al. [122] reported significantly lower rates of memory loss posttreatment and with no treatment-related decline in quality of life with IMRT RT.

Insignificant neurocognitive decline was found in a study conducted by Wahba et al. [123] after use of reduced CSI followed by adjuvant chemotherapy in patients with average-risk medulloblastoma.

With proton beam RT, there is less radiation to surrounding normal brain tissues and decrease the area at risk for radiation injury, therefore, sparing of neurocognitive functioning [124].

7.3. Stem cell implantation

Mesenchymal stem cell implantation may reduce the cognitive impairment by two mechanisms: First, reversal of inflammatory process, as implanted mesenchymal stem cells can migrate to the site of damaged brain tissue and then release growth factors, [125]. Second, human mesenchymal stem cells can differentiate into neurons in the hippemocampal area and prevent radiation-induced late cognitive impairment [126].

8. Rehabilitation

Patients with brain tumors face the challenge of cognitive impairment due to the tumor itself or treatments. Cognitive deficits in processing speed, memory, attention, and executive functions interfere with patients' relationships, occupational activities and daily life activities.

8.1. Pharmacologic treatment of neurocognitive impairment

Methylphenidate (MPH) is a CNS stimulant that increases synaptic concentration of dopamine and noradrenaline in the brain [127]. De-Long et al. [128] conducted a pilot study on children with ALL or brain tumor, they found that approximately 75% of those patients had response to treatment with MPH regarding neuropsychological dysfunction.

Meyers et al. [129] reported significant improvements in processing speed, memory, mental flexibility, and even mood, in adult patients with brain tumors and receiving MPH. Conklin et al. showed encouraging results in the use of psychostimulant medication. On 122 survivors of childhood brain tumors or ALL who were enrolled in a double-blinded, cross-over trial comparing the acute efficacy and adverse effects of MPH and placebo.

Donepezil is acetylcholinesterase inhibitor and has efficacy in the treatment of cognitive functions impairment; uses of donepezil in adult patients with brain tumors treated with RT demonstrate improvements in cognition impairment such as attention, concentration, and verbal memory [130].

However, stimulant medication is short-acting and is not expected to result in long-term improvement in academic achievement and neurocognitive functioning once it is discontinued; on the other hand, newer pscyhostimulant medications have been widely used in children with attention-deficit hyperactivity disorder (ADHD) and have proven to have fewer side effects and a longer half-life than MPH, for these reasons further studies are needed [131].

8.2. Cognition rehabilitation program

Cognitive rehabilitation program has proven to be effective in in-patients with primary brain tumors. The program consists of psychoeducation, teaching of strategies to compensate for problems in attention, memory, and executive functioning in daily life.

Cognitive remediation program (CRP) highly structured and individualized regimen, included traditional massed practice rehabilitation, instruction in metacognitive strategies, and cognitive-behavioral psychotherapy focused primarily on improving resistance to distraction. Butler and Copeland tested the effectiveness of CRP. Thirty-one subjects who had been treated from CNS tumors included in the study, and they were suffering from cognitive impairment such as attention deficits documented by continuous performance test (CPT). Cognitive behavioral psychotherapy was used. Significant improvement in focused attention and attention/concentration was observed in those who underwent the CRP, but no significant benefit was measured with regard to arithmetic computation. The authors concluded that the intervention produced improved neurocognitive functioning on measures of attention, but that it was too early to expect a downstream effect on the desired end result of improved academic achievement [132].

A study conducted by Butler et al. all patients was offered the CRP treatment, improvement neurocognitive variables were observed but this was not statistically significant. The study results demonstrated highly significant improvement in academic achievement for those who completed the CRP, and significant gains in their child's or adolescent's attention/concentration in activities of daily living [133].

The majority of the participants of cognitive rehabilitation program found the program to be useful. However, older participants found the program more burdensome than younger participants [134].

Richard et al. [135] conduct a study to compare two cognitive rehabilitation program, goal management training (GMT) which is a neuroscience-based integration of mindfulness and strategy training and the Brain Health Workshop (BHW) which offers supportive psychoeducation about living with a brain tumor. They found that significant improvement in executive functions and greater attainment of pre-training functional goals in the GMT group while The BHW group showed in significant improvement in mood and behavioral regulation.

Author details

Mohammad Abu-Hegazy[1,3*] and Hend Ahmed El-Hadaad[2]

*Address all correspondence to: mhegazy@mans.edu.eg

1 Neurology Department, Mansoura University, Mansoura, Egypt

2 Clinical Oncology and Nuclear Medicine Department, Mansoura University, Mansoura, Egypt

3 Faculty of Medicine, Mansoura University, Mansoura, Egypt

References

[1] Kirshner HS. Approaches to Intellectual and Memory Impairments. In: Bradley WG, Daroff RB, Fenichel GM, Jankovic J, editors. Neurology in Clinical Practice: Principles of Diagnosis and Management. 4th Ed. Chichester: Elsevier Inc; 2004. pp. 65–74

[2] Klein M, Duffau H, Hamer PD. Cognition and resective surgery for diffuse infiltrative glioma: an overview. J Neurooncol. 2012;108:309–318

[3] Wrensch M, Minn Y, Chew T, Bondy M, et al. Epidemiology of primary brain tumors: current concepts and review of the literature. Neuro-oncology. 2002;4:278–299

[4] Teixidor P, Gatignol P, Leroy M, et al. Assessment of verbal working memory before and after surgery for low-grade glioma. J Neurooncol. 2007;81:305–313

[5] Talacchi A, Santini B, Savazzi S, et al. Cognitive effects of tumour and surgical treatment in glioma patients. J Neurooncol. 2011;103:541–549

[6] Friedman MA, Meyers CA, Sawaya R. Neuropsychological effects of third ventricle tumor surgery. Neurosurgery. 2003;52:791–798

[7] Goldstein B, Armstrong CL, John C, et al. Attention in adult intracranial tumors patients. J Clin Exp Neuropsychol. 2003;25:66–78

[8] Vendrell P, Junque C, Pujol J, et al. The role of prefrontal regions in the Stroop task. Neuropsychologia. 1995;33:341–352

[9] Meyers CA, Brown PD. Role and relevance of neurocognitive assessment in clinical trials of patients with CNS tumors. J Clin Oncol. 2006;24:1305–1309

[10] Cochran DC, Chan MD, Aklilu M, et al. The effect of targeted agents on outcomes in patients with brain metastases from renal cell carcinoma treated with Gamma Knife surgery. J Neurosurg. 2012;116:978–983

[11] Roman DD, Sperduto PW. Neuropsychological effects of cranial radiation: current knowledge and future directions. Int J Radiat Oncol Biol Phys. 1995;31:983–998

[12] Greene-Schloesser D, Robbins ME. Radiation-induced cognitive impairment from bench to bedside. Neuro-oncology. 2012;14:iv37–iv44. doi:10.1093/neuonc/nos196

[13] Anderson FS, Kunin-Batson AS, Perkins JL, et al. White versus gray matter function as seen on neuropsychological testing following bone marrow transplant for acute leukemia in childhood. Neuropsychiatr Dis Treat. 2008;4:283–288

[14] Shapiro WR, Green SB, Burger PC, et al. A randomized comparison of intra-arterial versus intravenous BCNU, with or without intravenous 5-fluorouracil, for newly diagnosed patients with malignant glioma. J Neurosurg. 1992;76:772–781

[15] DeAngelis LM, Yahalom J, Thaler HT, et al. Combined modality therapy for primary CNS lymphoma. J Clin Oncol. 1992;10:635–643

[16] Angelov L, Doolittle ND, Kraemer DF, et al. Blood–brain barrier disruption and intra-arterial methotrexate-based therapy for newly diagnosed primary CNS lymphoma: a multi-institutional experience with 149 patients. J Clin Oncol. 2009;27:3503–3509

[17] Askins MA, Moore BD 3rd. Preventing neurocognitive late effects in childhood cancer survivors. J Child Neurol. 2008;23:1160–1171

[18] Ginsberg L. Lecture Notes: Neurology, Lionel Ginsberg, 9th Ed. Chichester: John Wiley & Sons, Ltd., India, New delhi; Printed in Singapor; 2010. pp. 11–16.

[19] Lopez OL, Jagust WJ, DeKosky ST, et al. Prevalence and classification of mild cognitive impairment in the Cardiovascular Health Study Cognitive Study: part 1. Arch Neurol. 2003;60(10):1385–1389

[20] Ganguli M, Dodge HH, Shen C, DeKosky ST. Mild cognitive impairment, amnestic type: an epidemiologic study. Neurology. 2004;63(1):115–121

[21] Winblad B, Palmer K, Kivipelto M, et al. Mild cognitive impairment beyond controversies, towards a consensus: report of the International Working Group on Mild Cognitive Impairment. J Intern Med. 2004;256(3):240–246

[22] Nasreddine ZS, Phillips NA, Bédirian V, Charbonneau S, Whitehead V, Collin I, et al. The Montreal cognitive assessment, MoCA: a brief screening tool for mild cognitive impairment. J Am Geriatr Soc. 2005;53:695–9

[23] Folstein MF, Folstein SE, Mc Hugh PR. "Mini-mental state". A practical method for grading the cognitive state of patients for the clinician. J Psychiatry Res. 1975;12:189–198

[24] Orsini A, Grossi D, Capitani E, Laiacona M, Papagno C, Vallar G. Verbal and spatial immediate memory span: normative data from 1355 adults and 1112 children. Ital J Neurol Sci. 1987;8(6):539–548

[25] Warrington EK. The Camden Memory Tests. Hove: Psychology Press; 1996

[26] Carlesimo GA, Buccione I, Fadda L, Graceffa A, Mauri M, Lo Russo S, Bevilacqua G, Caltagirone C. Standardization of two memory tests for clinical use: short story and figure rey. Nuova Rivista Neurol. 2002;12:1–13

[27] Raven J. Advanced Progressive Matrices Set 1. Oxford: Oxford Psychologists Press; 23, 1976

[28] Caffarra P, Vezzadini G, Zonato F, Copelli S, Venneri A. A normative study of a shorter version of Raven's progressive matrices. Neurol Sci. 2003;24(5):336–339

[29] Murphy P, Shallice T, Robinson G, Mac Pherson SE, Turner M, Woollett K, etal. Impairments in proverb interpretation following focal frontal lobe lesions. Neuropsychologia. 2013;51(11):2075–86. doi:10.1016/j.neuropsychologia.2013. 06.029

[30] Wechsler D. Adult Intelligence Scale—Third Edition. San Antonio, TX: The Psychological Corporation; 1997

[31] Robertson IH, Ward T, Ridgeway V, Nimmo-Smith I. The structure of normal human attention: the test of every day attention. J Int Neuropsychol Soc. 1996;2(6):525–534

[32] Giovagnoli AR, Del Pesce M, Mascheroni S, Simoncelli M, Laiacona M, Capitani E. Trail making test: normative values from 287 normal adults controls. Ital J Neurol Sci. 1996;17:305–309

[33] Warrington EK, James M. The Visual Object and Space Perception Battery. Bury St Edmunds: Thames Valley Test Company; 1991

[34] Caffarra P, Vezzadini G, Dieci F, Zonato F, Venneri A. Rey–Osterrieth complex figure: normative values in an Italian population sample. Neurol Sci. 2002;22:443–447

[35] Novelli G, Papagno C, Capitani E, Laiacona M, Cappa SF, Vallar G. Tre test clinici di ricerca e produzione lessicale. Taratura su soggetti normali. Arch Psicol Neurol Psichiatr. 1986;47:477–506

[36] McKenna P, Warrington EK. Testing for nominal dysphasia. J Neurol Neurosurg Psychiatry. 1980;43:781–788. doi:10.1136/jnnp.43.9.781

[37] Warrington EK, McKenna P, Orpwood L. Single word comprehension: a concrete and abstract words synonym test. Neuropsychol Rehabil. 1998;8(2):143–154. doi: 10.1080/713755564

[38] Benton AL. Differential behavioral effects in frontal lobe disease. Neuropsychologia. 1968;6(1):53–60. doi:10.1016/0028-3932(68)90038-9

[39] Apollonio I, Leone M, Isella V, Piamarta F, Consoli T, Villa ML, Forapani E, Russo A, Nichelli P. The Frontal Assessment Battery (FAB): normative values in an Italian population sample. Neurol Sci. 2005;26:108–116

[40] Tucha O, Smely C, Preier M, Lange KW. Cognitive deficits before treatment among patients with brain tumors. Neurosurgery. 2000;47:324–334

[41] Zucchella C, Bartolo M, Di Lorenzo C, Villani V, Pace A. Cognitive impairment in primary brain tumors outpatients: a prospective cross-sectional survey. J Neurooncol. 2013;112(3):455–460. doi:10.1007/s11060-013-1076-8. Epub 2013 Feb 16

[42] Tucha O, Smely C, Preier M, Becker G, Paul GM, Lange KW. Preoperative and postoperative cognitive functioning in patients with frontal meningiomas. J Neurosurg. 2003;98(1):21–31

[43] Bosma I, Vos MJ, Heimans JJ, Taphoorn MJB, Aaronson NK, Postma TJ, van der Ploeg HM, Muller M, Vandertop WP, Slotman BJ, Klein M. The course of neurocognitive functioning in high-grade glioma patients. Neuro-oncology. 2007;9(1):53–62

[44] Kayl AE, Meyers CA. Does brain tumor histology influence cognitive function? Neuro-oncology. 2003;5(4):255–60

[45] Meyers CA, Smith JA, Bezjak A, Mehta MP, Liebmann J, Illidge T, Kunkler I, Caudrelier JM, Eisenberg PD, Meerwaldt J, Siemers R, Carrie C, Gaspar LE, Curran W, Phan SC, Miller RA, Renschler MF. Neurocognitive function and progression in patients with brain metastases treated with whole-brain radiation and motexafin gadolinium: results of a randomized phase III trial. J Clin Oncol. 2004;22:157–165

[46] Taphoorn MJ, Klein M. Cognitive deficits in adult patients with brain tumours. Lancet Neurol. 2004;3(3):159–168

[47] Busch E. Psychical symptoms in neurosurgical disease. Acta Psychiatr Neurol. 1940;15:257–290

[48] Sweet JJ, Nies KJ, Lorber R, Vick NA. Relative absence of neuropsychological deficit in patients with low-grade astrocytomas. J Clin Psychol Med Settings. 1994;1:83–104

[49] Allegri RF, Drake M, Thomson A. Neuropsychological findings in patients with middle temporal lobe epilepsy. Rev Neurol. 1999;29:1160–1163

[50] Helmstaedter C, Richter S, Roske S, Oltmanns F, Schramm J, Lehmann TN. Differential effects of temporal pole resection with amygdalohippocampectomy versus selective amygdalohippocampectomy on material-specific memory in patients with mesial temporal lobe epilepsy. Epilepsia. 2008;49(1):88–97

[51] Joo EY, Han HJ, Lee EK, Choi S, Jin JH, Kim JH, Tae WS, Seo DW, Hong SC, Lee M, Hong SB. Resection extent versus postoperative outcomes of seizure and memory in mesial temporal lobe epilepsy. Seizure. 2005;14(8):541–551

[52] Dulay MF, Levin HS, York MK, Mizrahi EM, Verma A, Gold smith I, Grossman RG, Yoshor D. Predictors of individual visual memory decline after unilateral anterior temporal lobe resection. Neurology. 2009;72(21):1837–1842

[53] Yoshii Y, Tominaga D, Sugimoto K, Tsuchida Y, Hyodo A, Yonaha H, et al. Cognitive function of patients with brain tumor in pre- and postoperative stage. Surg Neurol. 2008;69:51–61

[54] Broglio PS, Puetz TW. The effect of sport concussion on neurocognitive function, self-report symptoms and postural control. Sports Med. 2008;38(1):53–67

[55] Giovagnoli AR, Boiardi A. Cognitive impairment and quality of life in long-term survivors of malignant brain tumors. Ital J Neurol Sci. 1994;15:481–488

[56] Shen C, Bao WM, Yang BJ, Xie R, Cao XY, Luan SH, Mao Y. Cognitive deficits in patients with brain tumor. Chin Med J (Engl). 2012;125(14):2610–2617

[57] Petrucci RJ, Buchheit WA, Woodruff GC, et al. Transcallosal parafornicial approach for third ventricle tumors: neuropsychological consequences. Neurosurgery. 1987;20:457–464

[58] Braun V, Albrecht A, Kretschmer T, et al. Brain tumour surgery in the vicinity of short-term memory representation–results of neuronavigation using fMRI images. Acta Neurochir (Wien). 2006;148:733–739

[59] Crossen JR, Garwood D, Glatstein E, Neuwelt EA. Neurobehavioral sequelae of cranial irradiation in adults: a review of radiation-induced encephalopathy. J Clin Oncol. 1994;12:627–642

[60] Tofilon PJ, Fike JR. The radioresponse of the central nervous system: a dynamic process. Radiat Res. 2000;153:357–370

[61] Gage FH, Kempermann G, Palmer TD, Peterson DA, Ray J. Multipotent progenitor cells in the adult dentate gyrus. J Neurobiol. 1998;36:249–266

[62] Bellinzona M, Gobbel GT, Shinohara C, Fike JR. Apoptosis is induced in the subependyma of young adult rats by ionizing irradiation. Neurosci Lett. 1996;208:163–166

[63] Mizumatsu S, Monje ML, Morhardt DR, Rola R, Palmer TD, Fike JR. Extreme sensitivity of adult neurogenesis to low doses of X-irradiation. Cancer Res. 2003;63:4021–4027

[64] Monje ML, Vogel H, Masek M, Ligon KL, Fisher PG, Palmer TD. Impaired human hippocampal neurogenesis after treatment for central nervous system malignancies. Ann Neurol. 2007;62:515–520

[65] Shi L, Linville MC, Iversen E, Molina DP, Yester J, Wheeler KT, Robbins ME, Brunso-Bechtold JK. Maintenance of white matter integrity in a rat model of radiation-induced cognitive impairment. J Neurol Sci. 2009;285(1–2):178–84

[66] Greene-Schloesser D, Robbins ME, Peiffer AM, Shaw EG, Wheeler KT, Chan MD. Radiation-induced brain injury: a review. Front Oncol. 2012;2:73

[67] Lee WH, Warrington JP, Sonntag WE, Lee YW. Irradiation altersMMP-2/TIMP-2system and collagen type iv degradation in brain. Int J Radiat Oncol Biol Phys. 2012;82:1559–1566

[68] Gebicke-Haerter PJ. Microglia in neurodegeneration: molecular aspects. Microsc Res Tech. 2001;54:47–58

[69] Gaber MW, Sabek OM, Fukatsu K, Wilcox HG, Kiani MF, Merchant TE. Differences in ICAM-1 and TNF-alpha expression between large single fraction and fractionated irradiation in mouse brain. Int J Radiat Biol. 2003;79(5):359–366

[70] Dent P, Yacoub A, Fisher PB, Hagan MP, Grant S. MAPK pathways in radiation responses. Oncogene. 2003;22:5885–5896

[71] Lee WH, Sonntag WE, Mitschelen M, Yan H, Lee YW. Irradiation induces regionally specific alterations in pro-inflammatory environments in rat brain. Int J Radiat Biol. 2010;86:132–144

[72] Zhou H, Liu Z, Liu J, Wang J, Zhou D, Zhao Z, Xiao S, Tao E, Suo WZ. Fractionated radiation-induced acute encephalopathy in a young rat model: cognitive dysfunction and histologic findings. AJNR Am J Neuroradiol. 2011;32:1795–1800

[73] Monje ML, Palmer T. Radiation injury and neurogenesis. Curr Opin Neurol. 2003;16:129–134

[74] Shors TJ, Miesegaes G, Beylin A, Zhao M, Rydel T, Gould E. Neurogenesis in the adult is involved in the formation of trace memories. Nature. 2001;410:372–376

[75] Klein M, Heimans JJ, Aaronson NK, et al. Effect of radiotherapy and other treatment-related factors on mid-term to long-term cognitive sequelae in low-grade gliomas: a comparative study. Lancet. 2002;360:1361–1368

[76] Swennen MH, Bromberg JE, Witkamp TD, et al. Delayed radiation toxicity after focal or whole brain radiotherapy for low-grade glioma. J Neurooncol. 2004;66:333–339

[77] Schultheiss TE, Kun LE, Ang KK, Stephens LC. Radiation response of the central nervous system. Int J Radiat Oncol Biol Phys. 1995;31:1093–1112

[78] Taphoorn, Martin JB, Bromberg, Jacoline EC. Neurological effect of therapeutic irradiation. Continuum. 2005;11:93–115

[79] Meyers CA, Wefel JS. The use of the mini-mental state examination to assess cognitive functioning in cancer trials: no ifs, ands, buts, or sensitivity. J Clin Oncol. 2003;21:3557–3558

[80] Meyers CA, Hess KR, Yung WK, Levin VA. Cognitive function as a predictor of survival in patients with recurrent malignant glioma. J Clin Oncol. 2000;18:646–650

[81] Wefel JS, Kayl AE, Meyers CA. Neuropsychological dysfunction associated with cancer and cancer therapies: a conceptual review of an emerging target. Br J Cancer. 2004;90:1691–1696

[82] Mahoney FI, Barthel DW. Functional evaluation: the Barthel index. Md State Med J. 1965;14:61–65

[83] Weitzner MA, Meyers CA, Gelke CK, Byrne KS, Cella DF, Levin VA. The Functional Assessment of Cancer Therapy (FACT) scale. Development of a brain subscale and revalidation of the general version (FACT-G) in patients with primary brain tumors. Cancer. 1995;75:1151–1161

[84] Armstrong CL, Hunter JV, Ledakis GE, Cohen B, Tallent EM, Goldstein BH, et al. Late cognitive and radiographic changes related to radiotherapy: initial prospective findings. Neurology. 2002;59:40–48

[85] Aarsen FK, Paquier PF, Arts WF, Van Veelen ML, Michiels E, Lequin M, Catsman-Berrevoets CE. Cognitive deficits and predictors 3 years after diagnosis of a pilocytic astrocytoma in childhood. J Clin Oncol. 2009;27(21):3526–3532

[86] Reeves CB, Palmer SL, Reddick WE, Merchant TE, Buchanan GM, Gajjar A, Mulhern RK. Attention and memory functioning among pediatric patients with medulloblastoma. J Pediatr Psychol. 2006;31(3):272–280

[87] Hoppe-Hirsch E, Brunet L, Laroussinie F, Cinalli G, Pierre-Kahn A, Rénier D, Sainte-Rose C, Hirsch JF. Intellectual outcome in children with malignant tumors of the posterior fossa: influence of the field of irradiation and quality of surgery. Childs Nerv Syst. 1995;11(6):340–345

[88] Shortman RI, Lowis SP, Penn A, McCarter RJ, Hunt LP, Brown CC, Stevens MC, Curran AL, Sharples PM. Cognitive function in children with brain tumors in the first year after

diagnosis compared to healthy matched controls. Pediatr Blood Cancer. 2014;61(3):464–72

[89] Douw L, Klein M, Fagel SS, van den Heuvel J, Taphoorn MJ, Aaronson NK, et al. Cognitive and radiological effects of radiotherapy in patients with low-grade glioma: long-term follow-up. Lancet Neurol. 2009;8:810–818

[90] Surma-aho O, Niemela M, Vilkki J, Kouri M, Brander A, Salonen O, et al. Adverse long-term effects of brain radiotherapy in adult low-grade glioma patients. Neurology. 2001;56:1285–1290

[91] Jalali R, Mallick I, Dutta D, Goswami S, Gupta T, Munshi A, et al. Factors influencing neurocognitive outcomes in young patients with benign and low-grade brain tumors treated with stereotactic conformal radiotherapy. Int J Radiat Oncol Biol Phys. 2010;77:974–979

[92] Chang EL, Wefel JS, Hess KR, Allen PK, Lang FF, Kornguth DG, Arbuckle RB, Swint JM, Shiu AS, Maor MH, Meyers CA. Neurocognition in patients with brain metastases treated with radiosurgery or radiosurgery plus whole-brain irradiation: a randomised controlled trial. Lancet Oncol. 2009;10(11):1037–1044

[93] Gondi V, Tolakanahalli R, Mehta MP, Tewatia D, Rowley H, Kuo JS, Khuntia D, Tomé WA. Hippocampal-sparing whole-brain radiotherapy: a "how-to" technique using helical tomotherapy and linear accelerator-based intensity-modulated radiotherapy. Int J Radiat Oncol Biol Phys. 2010;78(4):1244–1252

[94] Weber DC, Ares C, Lomax AJ, et al. Radiation therapy planning with photons and protons for early and advanced breast cancer: an overview. Radiat Oncol. 2006;1:22–57

[95] Blomstrand M, Brodin NP, Munck Af Rosenschöld P, Vogelius IR, Sánchez Merino G, Kiil-Berthlesen A, Blomgren K, Lannering B, Bentzen SM, Björk-Eriksson T. Estimated clinical benefit of protecting neurogenesis in the developing brain during radiation therapy for pediatric medulloblastoma. Neuro-oncology. 2012;14(7):882–889

[96] Mitchell T, Turton P. 'Chemobrain': concentration and memory effects in people receiving chemotherapy—a descriptive phenomenological study. Eur J Cancer Care. 2011;20:539–548

[97] Gong X, Schwartz PH, Linskey ME, Bota DA. Neural stem/progenitors and glioma stem-like cells have differential sensitivity to chemotherapy. Neurology. 2011;76:1126–1134

[98] Dietrich J, Han R, Yang Y, Mayer-Proschel M, Noble M. CNS progenitor cells and oligodendrocytes are targets of chemotherapeutic agents in vitro and in vivo. J Biol. 2006;5(7):22

[99] Saykin AJ, Ahles TA, McDonald BC. Mechanisms of chemotherapy-induced cognitive disorders: neuropsychological, pathophysiological, and neuroimaging perspectives. Semin Clin Neuropsychiatry. 2003;8:201–216

[100] Han R, Yang YM, Dietrich J, Luebke A, Mayer-Proschel M, Noble M. Systemic 5-fluorouracil treatment causes a syndrome of delayed myelin destruction in the central nervous system. J Biol. 2008;7(4):12

[101] Seigers R, Schagen SB, Beerling W, et al. Long-lasting suppression of hippocampal cell proliferation and impaired cognitive performance by methotrexate in the rat. Behav Brain Res. 2008;186(2):168–175

[102] Ahles TA, Saykin AJ, Noll WW, et al. The relationship of APOE genotype to neuropsychological performance in long-term cancer survivors treated with standard dose chemotherapy. Psychooncology. 2003;12:612–619

[103] Keime-Guibert F, Napolitano M, Delattre JY. Neurological complications of radiotherapy and chemotherapy. J Neurol. 1998;245:695–708

[104] der Weid N, Mosimann I, Hirt A, et al. Intellectual outcome in children and adolescents with acute lymphoblastic leukaemia treated with chemotherapy alone: age- and sex-related differences. Eur J Cancer. 2003;39:359–365

[105] Wen PY. Central nervous system complications of cancer therapy. In: Schiff D, Wen PY, editors. Cancer neurology in clinical practice. Chichester: Totowa: Humana Press; 2003. pp. 215–231

[106] Herrlinger U, Kuker W, Uhl M, Blaicher HP, Karnath HO, Kanz L, et al. NOA-03 trial of high-dose methotrexate in primary central nervous system lymphoma: final report. Ann Neurol. 2005;57:843–847

[107] Fliessbach K, Helmstaedter C, Urbach H, Althaus A, Pels H, Linnebank M, et al. Neuropsychological outcome after chemotherapy for primary CNS lymphoma: a prospective study. Neurology. 2005;64:1184–1188

[108] Nolan CP, DeAngelis LM. Neurologic complications of chemotherapy and radiation therapy. Continuum. 2015;2:429–451

[109] Copeland DR, Moore BD, Francis DJ, et al. Neuropsychologic effects of chemotherapy on children with cancer: a longitudinal study. J Clin Oncol. 1996;14:2826–2835

[110] Dietrich J, Han R, Yang Y, Mayer-Proschel M, Noble M. CNS progenitor cells and oligodendrocytes are targets of chemotherapeutic agents in vitro and in vivo. J Biol. 2006;5(7):22

[111] Prabhu RS, Won M, Shaw EG, Hu C, Brachman DG, Buckner JC, Mehta MP. Effect of the addition of chemotherapy to radiotherapy on cognitive function in patients with low-grade glioma: secondary analysis of RTOG 98–02. J Clin Oncol. 2014;32:535–541. doi:10.1200/JCO.2013.53.1830)

[112] Taphoorn MJ1, Sizoo EM, Bottomley A. Review on quality of life issues in patients with primary brain tumors. Oncologist. 2010;15(6):618–626. doi:10.1634/theoncologist.2009–0291. Epub 2010 May 27

[113] Levin VA, Yung WK, Bruner J, et al. Phase II study of accelerated fractionation radiation therapy with carboplatin followed by PCV chemotherapy for the treatment of anaplastic gliomas. Int J Radiat Oncol Biol Phys. 2002;53:58–66

[114] Hilverda K, Bosma I, Heimans JJ, Postma TJ, Peter Vandertop W, Slotman BJ, et al. Cognitive functioning in glioblastoma patients during radiotherapy and temozolomide treatment: initial findings. J Neurooncol. 2010;97:89–94

[115] Liu R, Solheim K, Polley MY, et al. Quality of life in low-grade glioma patients receiving temozolomide. Neuro-oncology. 2009;11:59–68

[116] Osoba D, Brada M, YungWK, et al. Health-related quality of life in patients with anaplastic astrocytoma during treatment with temozolomide. Eur J Cancer. 2000;36:1788–1795

[117] Yang ES, Wang H, Jiang G, et al. Lithium-mediated protection of hippocampal cells involves enhance-ment of DNA-PK-dependent repair in mice. J Clin Investig. 2009;119:1124–1135

[118] Ramanan S, Kooshki M, Zhao W et al. The PPARa agonist fenofibrate preserves hippocampal neurogenesis and inhibits microglial activation after whole-brain irradiation. Int J Radiat Oncol Biol Phys. 2009;75:870–877

[119] Kuhnt D, Ganslandt O, Schlaffer SM, et al. Quantification of glioma removal by intraoperative high-field magnetic resonance imaging: an update. Neurosurgery. 2011;69:852–862

[120] Ahn ES, Goumnerova L. Endoscopic biopsy of brain tumors in children: diagnostic success and utility in guiding treatment strategies. J Neurosurg Pediatr. 2010;5:255–262

[121] St Clair WH, Adams JA, Bues M, et. Al. Advantage of protons compared to conventional X-ray or IMRT in the treatment of a pediatric patient with medulloblastoma. . Int J Radiat Oncol Biol Phys. 2004;58:727–734

[122] Lin SY, Yang CC, Wu YM, Tseng CK, Wei KC, Chu YC, Hsieh HY, Wu TH, Pai PC, Hsu PW, Chuang CC. Evaluating the impact of hippocampal sparing during whole brain radiotherapy on neurocognitive functions: a preliminary report of a prospective phase II study. Biomed J. 2015;38(5):439–449. doi:10.4103/2319-4170.157440

[123] Wahba HA, Abu-Hegazy M, Wasel Y, Ismail EI, Zidan AS. Adjuvant chemotherapy after reduced craniospinal irradiation dose in children with average-risk medulloblastoma: a 5-year follow-up study. JBUON. 2013;18(2):425–429

[124] Merchant TE, Hua CH, Shukla H, et al. Proton versus photon radiotherapy for common pediatric brain tumors: comparison of models of dose characteristics and their relationship to cognitive function. Pediatr Blood Cancer. 2008;51:110–117

[125] Kim YJ, Park HJ, Lee G, et al. Neuroprotective effects of human mesenchymal stem cells on dopami-nergic neurons through anti-inflammatory action. Glia. 2009;57:13–23

[126] Acharya MM, Christie LA, Lan ML, et al. Human neural stem cell transplantation ameliorates radiation-induced cognitive dysfunction. Cancer Res. 2011;71:4834–4845

[127] Berridge CW, Shumsky JS, Andrzejewski ME, et al. Differential sensitivity to psychostimulants across prefrontal cognitive tasks: differential involvement of noradrenergic a1- and a2-receptors. Biol Psychiatry. 2012;71:467–473

[128] DeLong R, Friedman H, Friedman N, Gustafson K, Oakes J, Methylphenidate in neuropsychological sequelae of radiotherapy and chemotherapy of childhood brain tumors and leukemia. J Child Neurol. 1992;7(4):462–463

[129] Meyers CA, Weitzner MA, Valentine AD, Levin VA. Methylphenidate therapy improves cognition, mood, and function of brain tumor patients. J Clin Oncol. 1998;16(7):2522–2527

[130] Shaw EG, Rosdhal R, D'Agostino RB Jr, et al. Phase II study of donepezil in irradiated brain tumor patients: effect on cognitive function, mood, and quality of life. J Clin Oncol. 2006;24:1415–1420

[131] Nazemi KI, Butler RW. Neuropsychological rehabilitation for survivors of childhood and adolescent brain tumors: a view of the past and a vision for a promising future: an interdisciplinary approach. J Pediatr Rehabil Med. 2011;4:37–46

[132] Butler RW, Copeland DR, Fairclough DL, et al. A multicenter, randomized clinical trial of a cognitive remediation program for childhood survivors of a pediatric malignancy. J Consult Clin Psychol. 2008;76(3):367–378

[133] Butler RW, Copeland RR. Interventions for cancer late effects and survivorship, In: Brown R. editor. Comprehensive Handbook of Childhood Cancer and Sickle Cell Disease. Chichester: New York, NY: Oxford University Press, Inc.; 2006. p. 297

[134] Gehring K, Aaronson N, Taphoorn M, Sitskoorn M. A description of a cognitive rehabilitation programme evaluated in brain tumour patients with mild to moderate cognitive deficits. Clin Rehabil. 2011;25(8):675–692. doi:10.1177/0269215510395791

[135] Richard NM, Bernstein LJ, Mason WP, Laperriere N, Chung C, Millar BA, Maurice C, 25 Edelstein K. Cognitive rehabilitation for brain tumor survivors: a pilot study. 2016 Cancer Survivorship Symposium.http://meetinglibrary.asco.org/content/119165?media=vm&poster=1

Section 3

Management

Chapter 11

Current Trends in High-Grade Gliomas

Maleeha Ahmad, MD, FRCS SN,
Scott G. Turner, MD and Steven A. Toms, MD, FACS

Additional information is available at the end of the chapter

http://dx.doi.org/10.5772/63297

Abstract

This is an overview of the current trends in the management of high-grade gliomas based on the current evidence available at the time of compiling this chapter in the first quarter of 2016, by a dedicated, high-volume Neurosurgical Oncology team of clinical and surgical Neuro-Oncologists based in central Pennsylvania.

Keywords: High-grade glioma, glioblastoma, malignant brain tumor, brain tumor, intrinsic glioma

1. Introduction

The year 2016 continues to be both an enlightening and an exciting year for advances in the investigation and management of high-grade gliomas. The hallmark of glioblastomas is their molecular and genetic heterogeneity, the ability to infiltrate diffusely and undergo rapid neoangiogenesis, while actively challenging our current combinatorial therapeutic approach. At the time of writing, over 230 clinical trials were open in the USA, with ongoing recruitment or due to start. This overview of current trends will involve the details of the molecular markers now in use for both the diagnosis and prognostication of high-grade gliomas, updates on neuroimaging guidelines for both de novo and secondary high-grade gliomas, and the discussion of potential adjuvant therapies to the current standard of care.

2. Twenty-first century epidemiological trends

The most recent 2015 Statistical Report of the Central Brain Tumor Registry [1] documents the epidemiology of glioblastomas from 2008 to 2012. Glioblastomas remain the most common malignant histology (46.1%) of all primary malignant brain tumors, with an age-proportional incidence peaking at the ninth decade of life (age range 75-84 years). Of interest, glioblastomas have been shown to be 1.6 times more common in males, twice as common in Caucasians, and only 5.1% of patients survive five years after diagnosis.

3. The genetic risk of glioma

The lifetime risk of gliomas is 4-5 per 1000 of the general population. Thus, inheriting of one of the low penetrance glioma risk variants may increase the risk by 20-40% to approximately 6 per 1000 [2]. The risk loci of glioma variants have been identified as ten inherited variants near eight genes, 2 with stratification leading to an increase in the risk of developing gliomas.

The common inherited variants are named for the nearby genes of TERC, TERT, EGFR, CDKN2B, PHLDB1, CCDC26, TP53 and RTEL1, and are not directly involved in protein coding [3]. Of interest, these variants increase the odds ratio of gliomagenesis on a scale of 1.2–1.4. TERT, TERC, and RTEL1 are involved in telomere maintenance, and it has been hypothesized that a longer telomere length may possibly contribute to risk of gliomas [4, 5]. Additionally, of note, is the predictive and prognostic value of gliomas with TERT gene promoter mutations in association with isocitrate dehydrogenase (IDH) mutations and loss of heterozygosity of 1p/19q [4]. The less common risk loci are noted to correlate with higher odds ratios, and these are located near TP53 (2.4-fold increase in relative risk) and CCDC26 (6.3-fold increase in relative risk) especially in the presence of an IDH mutation or an oligodendroglial component. Moreover, the UCSF Adult Glioma Study noted that population screening for the risk loci near the CCDC26 yielded significantly more false positives than true positives, and hence the yield for undertaking this screening test of risk loci was extremely low [2].

At this point, with our current knowledge arsenal, the authors advise the following three acquired molecular glioblastoma markers to be identified and then further correlate to survival and outcome: IDH mutation, 1p/19q, and TERT promoter mutation. These molecular glioblastoma markers are then further subdivided into five glioma subgroups to further elicit the pathways of gliomas in pathways: TERT mutated only (most common in approximately half of the cases), IDH mutated only, TERT and IDH mutation (least common), triple negative and triple positive [6, 7]. Of note, the IDH mutation status was analyzed in the BELOB trial, which showed a lower median overall survival for patients with wild-type IDH (8 months) compared with median survival of 20 months for patients with an IDH mutational status [8]. We also note here, in our clinical role as Neurosurgical Oncologists, of the recent landmark paper associating a definite survival benefit after maximal surgical resection, including both enhancing and nonenhancing tumor, resulting in an improved prognosis observed in the IDH1 mutant subgroup [9]. Thus, individualized surgical strategies for high-grade gliomas must be considered on the molecular IDH marker status of the tumor [10].

The recent development of a targeted next-generation sequencing panel (GlioSeq) provides simultaneous, highly accurate and comprehensive genetic profiling of a wide array of central nervous system (CNS) tumors on an increasingly smaller volumes of biopsies in a single workflow format [11]. This next-generation assay allows simultaneous detection of the major mutations (>1360 hot spots in 30 CNS tumor-related genes) in addition to 14 gene fusions and 24 gene copy number changes in a rapid and cost-effective manner. We look forward to the incorporation of the versatile GlioSeq as a high throughput technological advance to rapidly identify a variety of genetic alterations and small deletions, thereby assisting in diagnosis and prognostic stratification of brain tumors.

Finally, the Neuro-Oncology community looks forward to the Glioma International Case-Control Consortium undertaking the important task of identification of new risk loci by the genotyping of 4000 glioma and 4000 nonglioma patients in the Epi4K project (epgb.org/epi4k).

4. Neuro-radiological updates for high-grade gliomas

The updated aims of the working group of the Response Assessment in Neuro-Oncology (RANO) continue to provide guidelines for a uniform criteria for the assessment of determining the progression and treatment response of high-grade gliomas [12]. RANO guidelines will be discussed in detail here, as it is imperative to emphasize the clinical need for consistency and standardization of imaging, for a reliable assessment of tumor burden and progression.

The RANO guidelines refer to the reliability of imaging data and reproducibility of the acquired results to be undertaken no later than 72 hours postsurgical resection and is determined by the standardization of gadolinium dose, slice thickness ≥5 mm or no more than twice the thickness of a measurable lesion. We now describe RANO guidelines nomenclature as per the updated guidelines [12, 13]:

- **Measurable lesions** are bidimensionally contrast-enhancing, with clearly defined margins in two perpendicular diameters, each measuring at least 10 mm in diameter.
- **Nonmeasurable lesions** refer to those with maximal diameters of <10 mm, masses with poorly defined margins (cysts, necrotic lesions, and leptomeningeal tumors) and nonenhancing lesions only seen on FLAIR/T2. Hence, for nonmeasurable lesions, continued radiological surveillance may indicate only the attainment of clinical plateau of stable disease, versus the response rate of measurable lesions as a response or failure to therapy in radiological follow-up.

Furthermore, there are four RANO categories to treatment response:

- Complete response

  This refers to the lack of all enhancing lesions for a minimum of four weeks and the appearance of new lesions, this should be married to the patients' clinical picture of stability or response, whilst weaning or off steroids.

- Partial response

This refers to no progression of nonmeasurable lesions and no new lesions. Specifically, this is defined as ≥50% decrease in sum of all products of diameters (SPD) of all target lesions with stable clinical symptomatology and a stable steroid dose.

- Progressive disease

  This differs from partial response with having ≥25% increase in the sum of target lesions, with significant increase in nonenhancing lesions, with clinical deterioration with no decrease in steroid dose and/or a new radiological lesion.

- Stable disease

  This is the radiological diagnosis of exclusion of neither complete nor partial response, with lack of progression seen.

As per the RANO guidelines, criteria for progressive disease is met when the majority of new enhancement is noted beyond the 80% isodose line of radiotherapy or on histopathological confirmation. This is an important point for us to bear in mind, as a third of glioblastoma patients may be reported on as undergoing pseudoprogression, thus this term needs to be utilized in accordance with the RANO guidelines. Also of importance, is the pseudoresponse seen post-antiangiogenic therapy (anti-vascular endothelial growth) which decrease the permeability of the blood-brain barrier thereby decreasing the gadolinium enhancement [14]. *Radiological surveillance with T2/FLAIR is sensitive in identifying vasogenic edema and used in combination with DWI is a increases the likelihood of identifying tumor burden* [15]. *An improvement in T2/FLAIR is associated with improved survival and decreased mortality, DWI remains an independent predictor of progression free survival at 6 months* [12, 15].

RANO guidelines state that all radiological responses must persist for four weeks prior to be considered 'true' progression or response: this is the crux of the RANO guidelines.

5. Immunotherapy

Glioblastomas undertake a host of immunosuppressive mechanisms, resulting in challenges for the immunotherapeutic interventions [16]. In this subsection, we discuss the immunotherapy and the use and rationale of trials and their application.

Optimal antitumor therapy needs to have an antigen as an immunological target along with the activation of the immune system for facilitating trafficking and infiltration of the now activated immune system targeting the tumor.

Let us start by overviewing the multiple key immunosuppressive mechanisms existing within the highly plastic glioblastoma microenvironment. Regulatory T cells (Tregs) are produced within the thymus (nTregs) or are induced (iTregs). Of the two, nTregs are noted in higher concentration within the glioblastoma tumor clusters [16]. Immunosuppressive mechanisms have been directly correlated to, by identifying the cytokines within the tumor cysts fluid secreted by the Tregs: transforming growth factor beta [TGF-β] and interleukin 10 [IL-10]. Inhibitors of TGF-β receptor kinase are currently in preclinical testing. Up to a tenth of the mass of glioblastomas consist of the tumor-associated macrophages (M2 linage) and microglia. The aggressiveness of glioma-stem cells is enhanced by the secretion of TGF-β by the tumor-associated macrophages. The glioblastoma stem cells increase the number of circulating Tregs and also activate the signal transducer and activator of transcription 3 (STAT 3), which is found to be ubiquitously expressed in glioblastoma cells [16].

High-grade glioma progression has also been shown to be enhanced in the presence of glioma-secreted colony stimulating factor 1 (CSF-1) to cause polarization of tumors toward the glioma-supportive (M2) phenotype [17]. Of note, the vascular endothelial growth factor (VEGF) has multiple functions of tumorigenesis and simultaneously of inhibition of dendritic cell function. We discuss the role of anti-VEGR receptor agents in further detail below in subsection 6.

Immune checkpoint programmed death PD-1 binds the ligand for PD-1 (PD-L1) to suppress CD4+ and CD8+ cells. PD-L1 is upregulated in gliomas, specifically the mesenchymal subtype of glioblastomas and has been associated with inhibition and apoptosis of T cells. Anti-PD1 blockade has been undertaken in the murine glioblastoma models successfully with an increase in survival, in combination with radiotherapy [18].

Cytotoxic T-Lymphocyte-associated protein 4 (CTLA-4) is an inhibitory surface receptor found on constitutionally active Tregs, and hence, is the other immune checkpoint inhibitor of great clinical interest [19, 20]. The FDA has recently approved ipilimumab, a monoclonal antibody directed against CTLA-4, after Phase III trials for melanoma patients showed an objective increase in survival. In the murine model, anti-CTLA-4 and IL-12 administration demonstrated a reduction in Tregs and increased immune effector response, which is now under investigation for glioblastoma therapies [21, 22].

An investigational immunotherapeutic agent that has been in the limelight for the past couple of years is RINTEGA® (Rindopepmut CDX-110). RINTEGA® is administered intradermally and consists of the EGFRv*III*-specific peptide sequence conjugated to keyhole limpet hemocyanin, thereby stimulating pronounced EGFRvIII-specific humoral and cellular responses resulting in the production of anti-EGFRv*III* antibodies infiltrating and attacking the tumor. EGFR*vIII* is a tumor-specific oncogene and a mutated form of the epidermal growth factor receptor (EGFR), which is noted in one-third of all GBM cases with aggressive tumor proliferation and correspondingly poor median survival compared with other glioblastoma cases [23–25]. EGFR*vIII* is not expressed in normal tissue, hence making it a unique immunotherapeutic target.

Hence, at this point, we will dedicate a few lines to the discontinuation of the ACT IV study in March 2016 based on the recommendation of the Data Safety and Monitoring Board and an update has appeared on the Celldex Therapeutics website. ACT IV was a Phase III study conducted in newly diagnosed EGFRvIII-positive glioblastoma patients with RINTEGA® and granulocyte-macrophage colony stimulating factor added to standard of care temozolamide with the control arm regimen undergoing standard of care temozolamide plus intradermal keyhole limpet hemocyanin. The control arm significantly outperformed expectations (hazard ratio = 0.99; median OS: RINTEGA 20.4 months vs. control 21.1 months) and hence the study showed an inability to meet the primary outcome survival endpoint.

The ReACT study is the randomized, Phase II trial of RINTEGA® in combination with bevacizumab (Avastin®) in patients with recurrent EGFRvIII-positive glioblastoma. In November 2015, Celldex Therapeutics reported long-term survival data in group 1 (bevacizumab-naive patients randomized to receive either RINTEGA or a control injection of KLH in a blinded fashion; all patients also received bevacizumab) at the Society for Neuro-Oncology Annual Meeting. At two years, the survival rate was 25% for patients in the RINTEGA arm versus 0% for patients in the control arm, with continuing advantage shown across multiple endpoints [26].

6. Anti-angiogenic treatments

The pathological angiogenesis of glioblastomas is a hallmark of the disease process, with multiple mechanisms hypothesized, including the transdifferentiation of tumor cells into endothelial cells, vascular mimicry, and vessel co-opting [27]. Tumor angiogenesis has been shown to be associated with the recruitment of hematopoietic and circulating precursor cells [28].

The VEGF (vascular endothelial growth factor) pathway is highly expressed in glioma angiogenesis with overexpression of VEGF-A. There have been a multitude of factors identified to propagate and inhibit the VEGF pathway, including hypoxia inducible angiogenic factors, and endogenous factors like placenta growth factor. The anti-VEGF/VEGR compounds inhibit the proliferation of endothelial cells and neoangeogenesis, with a corresponding decrease in the permeability of the blood–brain barrier. Within 48 hours of anti-VEGF-A therapy with bevacizumab (Avastin®), there is decreased contrast enhancement, which may be misleading and hence to be read as a pseudoresponse. In contrast the T2/FLAIR progression is seen on serial radiological imaging, which has been postulated to be a nonangiogenic invasive growth pattern and the likelihood of T2 progress predicting subsequent T1 and in turn tumor progression [14, 29]. Hence, our above discussion on RANO criteria will be called upon here to be borne in mind while analysing the imaging characteristics of patients on antiangiogenic therapy.

Bevacizumab (Avastin®) is the antibody to VEGF-A which has been utilized in Phase I, II and III trials to investigate its role in both newly diagnosed and recurrent glioblastoma. Of note, the AVAglio (Avastin® in Glioblastoma) study was undertaken in a for newly diagnosed glioblastoma patients in a randomized manner (bevacizumab versus placebo) with double-blinding. Postsurgical resection, the patients were commenced on the Stupp protocol (concurrent radiotherapy 2 Gy 5 days a week and temozolomide 75 mg/kg) in combination with intravenous bevacizumab 10 mg/kg (or placebo) every fortnight. After a 28-day treatment break, the patients were commenced on a maintenance dose of temozolomide (150–200 mg/kg) and fortnightly intravenous bevacizumab (10 mg/kg) or placebo for 6 weeks. This was followed by bevacizumab (10 mg/kg) every three weeks as monotherapy. The patients were assessed clinically at predetermined, regular time points. The results of the AVAglio study echoed those of the Phase III Radiation Therapy Oncology Group (RTOG-0825) with both studies showing a trend toward increase in progression free survival but no significant difference in overall survival [30, 31]. It is important to note, as with other previous studies, the adverse effects of the bevacizumab group were noted to be higher than in the placebo group and noted to include hypertension, proteinuria, and (arterial) thromboembolism. The question arises regarding the failure of progression-free survival to overall survival, and it is postulated there are possible escape mechanisms in the anti-VEGF pathway and treatment which results in an aggressive, recurrent tumor [29]. The crossover seen in the AVAglio trial may have had considerable impact on the true survival data, and in comparison the BELOB [single-agent bevacizumab or lomustine versus a combination of bevacizumab plus lomustine in patients with recurrent glioblastoma] Phase II trial had virtual exclusion of patient cross-over to the bevacizumab arm, and also surprisingly there were fewer of the above-described adverse effects of bevacizumab [8]. Additionally, while the predictive value of MGMT promoter methylation and treatment with temozolomide is well known [32], the prognostic significance in association with anti-angiogenic or other chemotherapeutic agents is less well understood. Thus, in increasingly more of the recent trials, the MGMT status is included and required to allow the study of temozolomide-free arms [29]. It has also been noted in preliminary clinical trial data that angiopoietin-1/-2 may potentially destabilize vessel and when used in association with VEGF-A, angiogenic synergy is exhibited and further clinical trials being undertaken with this hypothesis in mind [27].

Moreover, genetic expression data of glioblastoma subgroups has been recently retrospectively explored using the AVAglio trial data. To recap, the Cancer Genome Atlas subdivides the heterogeneous entity of glioblastoma into the following subtypes: proneural, classical, and mesenchymal (with the previously known neural subtype possibly being an artefact) [33]. In this most recent study, the addition of bevacizumab is shown to be associated with increased overall survival in the proneural subtype GBM, with naïve, nonmutated IDH [34]. This report came as a welcome surprise to the Neuro-Oncology community, as patients with the proneural subtype lacking IDH mutations have historically a poorer survival compared with proneural subtype with IDH mutations.

We also note that on preclinical GBM models, it has been shown that bevacizumab induces hypoxia in treated tumors, which is accompanied by increased glycolytic activity and tumor invasiveness [35]. This is an area for further research to exploit in view of anaerobic glycolytic dependency of glioblastomas and is discussed below in subsection 8 in further detail.

7. Glioma virus therapies

Glioma virus therapies are broadly divided into two categories. Replication-deficient viral vectors to be used as delivery vehicles for therapeutic, antitumor genes. Second, are the replication-competent oncolytic viruses that target, infect, and replicate within the host glioma cell with the intent of destroying the tumor host cells with progeny particle release [36, 37]. The two viruses studied most widely are the adenovirus and herpes simplex (HSV-1) virus. There are double-stranded DNA viruses, whereby extensive modification may be carried out in order for the virus vectors to carry the therapeutic genes under investigation [36]. While there are multiple Phase I and II clinical trials underway (clinicaltrials.gov), an impetus remains on the parallel to streamline the efficacy of these viruses to ensure the potency of the viral vectors without overtly impairing the host immune system response (may want to note that the mechanism of some of these virus such as the Duke polio virus may be by immune system induction). Convection enhanced delivery using continuous, positive pressure bulk flow of the therapeutic virus to the glioma may be undertaken to improve delivery [38, 39]. Specificity may be enhanced for viral entry into the glioma on modification of attachment-mediating surface proteins and chimeric capsids [25]. Of most interest, are the viral genes being engineered to be enhanced using hypoxia-responsive promoters in areas of low-hypoxia, a known glioma phenotype [37, 39].

Of note is the Toca511 trial, with an estimated completion date of November 2017. This is a multicenter, randomized, Open label Phase II/III study of Toca 511 and Toca FC versus standard of care. This comprises investigator's choice of single-agent chemotherapy (lomustine or temozolomide) or bevacizumab administered to patients with recurrent high-grade gliomas. Toca 511 (vocimagene amiretrorepvec) is an investigational injectable retroviral replicating vector (RRV) encoding a yeast-derived prodrug activator enzyme, cytosine deaminase (CD). Toca 511 selectively infects and spreads through the high-grade glioma cells, thereby delivering the CD gene and the tumor cells can then produce the CD enzyme.

Toca FC is an orally administered, extended-release version of prodrug 5-fluorocytosine (5-FC) which is absorbed and carried through the bloodstream. This crosses the blood–brain barrier and is then converted by the CD enzyme into the active 5-FU, at high concentrations within the glioma cells infected by Toca 511. 5-FU in turn causes tumor cell apoptosis and activation of the immune system by the release of tumor-associated antigens and viral proteins from the dying cells. We look forward to the results of this retroviral replicating vector against high-grade gliomas and the possible extrapolation to other solid cancers.

8. Tumor treating fields

In 2015, Optune™ became the first FDA-approved therapy for newly diagnosed glioblastomas in over a decade to demonstrate statistically significant extension of progression free and overall survival. Optune™ is the brand name for the NovoTTF™ 100A system manufactured by the commercial stage oncology company Novocure™.

Optune™ is a portable, noninvasive device delivering low-intensity, intermediate frequency, alternating bidirectional electric fields referred to as Tumor Treating Fields (TTF). The electric fields are delivered locoregionally via transducer arrays through the shaved scalp. The mechanism of action is the antimitotic action of the tumor treating fields interfering with cell division and organelle assembly within the rapidly replicating tumor cells. While microphotography has shown examples of prolonged mitoses and proliferation arrest, the specificity of the tumor treating fields for tumor cells only in the absence of an exact mechanism has raised skepticism within the Neuro-Oncology and Oncology clinician community [40].

What is undeniable, however, is the two-year survival rate among patients treated with Optune™ in combination with temozolomide was 48% higher than in patients compared with patients treated with temozolomide alone [41]. In 2014, the multinational, randomized Phase III EF-14 trial was halted after successful demonstration of superior progression-free and overall survivals in patients receiving Optune™ in combination with temozolomide, compared with temozolomide alone. Patients treated with Optune™, in combination with temozolomide, demonstrated a statistically significant increase in progression-free survival compared with temozolomide alone (median progression-free survival of 7.2 months compared with 4.0 months, hazard ratio = 0.62, p = 0.001. There was also a statistically significant increase in overall survival compared with temozolomide alone (median overall survival of 20.5 months compared with 15.6 months, hazard ratio = 0.66, p = 0.004) [40–42]. It is noted that patients in the control arm received a median of four cycles of temozolamide, whereas patients in the Optune™ arm received six cycles of temozolamide, which is an additional confounding factor (patients lived longer therefore they got more temo).

The bottom line here is the availability of Optune™ as a viable option for all patients with newly diagnosed glioblastoma after successful chemoradiation and stable disease at potential initiation of treatment with tumor treating fields [42]. We look forward to the incorporation of Optune™ in future trials as a standard arm and with permutations of other combinatorial therapies.

9. Glycolysis in glioblastomas

Glioblastomas appear to thrive and proliferate in a hypoxic environment, thus relying upon anaerobic glycolysis [43]. Thus research efforts over the past decade have been toward maximizing of glycolytic inhibition within the hypoxic glioma environment [44–47].

In their 2015 paper, Sanzey et al. undertook genome-wide transcriptomic analysis of patient-derived glioblastoma and stem cells to demonstrate a strong upregulation of glycolysis-related genes in response to severe hypoxia. Glioblastoma xenografts were used to identify seven glycolytic genes, with knockdown that led to a dramatic murine survival benefit, with phosphofructokinase-1 [PFK1] and pyruvate dehydrogenase kinase-1 [PDK1] as the most promising therapeutic targets to address the metabolic escape mechanisms of glioblastomas [44]. At this point, it is instructive to correlate the high glycolytic states of tumor cells to the increase in the radioresistance of glioblastomas [48]. A pyruvate dehydrogenase kinase inhibitor [Dichloroacetate] is used to treat lactic acidosis and is noted to modify tumor metabolism by activating mitochondrial activity and thus, force glycolytic tumor cells into oxidative phosphorylation. Dichloroacetate alone demonstrated modest antitumor effects in both in vitro and in vivo models of glioblastoma and reversed the radiotherapy-induced glycolytic shift, thereby improving the survival of orthotopic glioblastoma-bearing mice [46]. We look forward to clinical trials modulating the metabolic state of glioblastoma cells and thus, modify their sensitization to radiotherapy.

10. Conclusion

The past several decades have seen an explosion of information on the molecular biology of gliomas and immune environment of cancer. There have been a proliferation of trials involving novel signal transduction inhibitors, neoangiogenic, and immune modulatory targets. Novel methods of delivery of therapeutic molecules and genes have been developed, including a novel device to deliver nonionizing energy to inhibit mitosis. Imaging criteria have been developed to better assess response to therapy and aid the clinician and researcher in evaluating the tumor response to these diverse therapeutic modalities. New genetic testing has been developed in order to predict prognosis and will soon be incorporated into clinical trials as Neurooncology moves toward the goal of more personalized cancer therapy.

Author details

Maleeha Ahmad, MD, FRCS SN*, Scott G. Turner, MD and Steven A. Toms, MD, FACS

*Address all correspondence to: mahmad@geisinger.edu

Department of Neurosurgery, Geisinger Medical Center, Danville, Pennsylvania, USA

References

[1] Ostrom QT, Gittleman H, Fulop J, Liu M, Blanda R, Kromer C, et al. CBTRUS statistical report: primary brain and central nervous system tumors diagnosed in the United States in 2008-2012. Neuro-Oncology Supplement. 2015 2015;17(4):24.

[2] Rice T, Lachance DH, Molinaro AM, Eckel-Passow JE, Walsh KM, Barnholtz-Sloan J, et al. Understanding inherited genetic risk of adult glioma—a review. Neuro-Oncology Practice. 2016;3(1):10.

[3] Labussiere M, Boisselier B, Mokhtari K, Di Stefano A, Rahimian A, Rossetto M, et al. Combined analysis of TERT, EGFR, and IDH status defines distinct prognostic glioblastoma classes. Neurology. 2014;83(13):1200–6.

[4] Killela PJ, Reitman ZJ, Jiao Y, Bettegowda C, Agrawal N, Diaz LAJ, et al. TERT promoter mutations occur frequently in gliomas and a subset of tumors derived from cells with low rates of self-renewal. Proc Natl Acad Sci U S A. 2013;110(15):6021–6.

[5] Labussiere M, Di Stefano AL, Gleize V, Boisselier B, Giry M, Mangesius S, et al. TERT promoter mutations in gliomas, genetic associations and clinico-pathological correlations. Br J Cancer. 2014;111(10):2024–32.

[6] Eckel-Passow JE, Lachance DH, Molinaro AM, Walsh KM, Decker PA, Sicotte H, et al. Glioma Groups Based on 1p/19q, IDH, and TERT Promoter Mutations in Tumors. N Engl J Med. 2015;372(26):2499–508.

[7] Tabouret E, Chinot O, Sanson M, Loundou A, Hoang-Xuan K, Delattre J, et al. Predictive biomarkers investigated in glioblastoma. Expert Rev Mol Diagn. 2014;14(7):883–93.

[8] Taal W, Oosterkamp HM, Walenkamp AME, Dubbink HJ, Beerepoot LV, Hanse MCJ, et al. Single-agent bevacizumab or lomustine versus a combination of bevacizumab plus lomustine in patients with recurrent glioblastoma (BELOB trial): a randomised controlled phase 2 trial. Lancet Oncol. 2014;15(9):943–53.

[9] Beiko J, Suki D, Hess KR, Fox BD, Cheung V, Cabral M, et al. IDH1 mutant malignant astrocytomas are more amenable to surgical resection and have a survival benefit associated with maximal surgical resection. Neuro-oncol. 2014;16(1):81–91.

[10] Agnihotri S, Aldape KD, Zadeh G. Isocitrate dehydrogenase status and molecular subclasses of glioma and glioblastoma. Neurosurgical Focus. 2014;37(6):E13.

[11] Nikiforova MN, Wald AI, Melan MA, Roy S, Zhong S, Hamilton RL, et al. Targeted next-generation sequencing panel [GlioSeq] provides comprehensive genetic profiling of central nervous system tumors. Neuro-oncolgy. 2016;18(3):379.

[12] Yang D. Standardized MRI assessment of high-grade glioma response: a review of the essential elements and pitfalls of the RANO criteria. Neuro-Oncol Pract. 2016;3(1):59.

[13] Chang SM, Wen PW, Vogelbaum MA, Macdonald DA, van den Bent MJ. Response Assessment in Neuro-Oncology (RANO): more than imaging criteria for malignant glioma. Neuro-Oncol Pract. 2015;2(4):205.

[14] Gerstner ER, Frosch MP, Batchelor TT. Diffusion magnetic resonance imaging detects pathologically confirmed, nonenhancing tumor progression in a patient with reurrent glioblastoma receiving bevacizumab. J Clin Oncol. 2010;28(6):e91.

[15] Furuta T, Nakada M, Ueda F, Watanabe T, Arakawa Y, Higashi R, et al. Prognostic paradox: brain damage around the glioblastoma resection cavity. J Neurooncol. 2014;118(1):187–92.

[16] Nduom EK, Weller M, Heinberger A.B. Immunosuppressive mechanisms in glioblastoma. Neuro-oncology. 2015;17(7):vii9.

[17] Pyonteck SM, Akkari L, Schuhmacher AJ, Bowman RL, Sevenich L, Quail DF, et al. CSF-1R inhibition alters macrophage polarization and blocks glioma progression. Nat Med. 2013;19(10):1264–72.

[18] Zeng J, See AP, Phallen J, Jackson CM, Belcaid Z, Ruzevick J, et al. Anti-PD-1 blockade and stereotactic radiation produce long-term survival in mice with intracranial gliomas. Int J Radiat Oncol Biol Phys. 2013;86(2):343–9.

[19] Wainwright DA, Chang AL, Dey M, Balyasnikova IV, Kim CK, Tobias A, et al. Durable therapeutic efficacy utilizing combinatorial blockade against IDO, CTLA-4, and PD-L1 in mice with brain tumors. Clini Cancer Res. 2014;20(20):5290–301.

[20] Curry WT, Lim M. Immunomodulation:checkpoint blockade etc. Neuro-Oncol Supplement. 2015;17(7):vii26.

[21] Vom Berg J, Vrohlings M, Haller S, Haimovici A, Kulig P, Sledzinska A, et al. Intratumoral IL-12 combined with CTLA-4 blockade elicits T cell-mediated glioma rejection. J Exp Med. 2013;210(13):2803–11.

[22] Cloughesy TF, Cavenee WK, Mischel PS. Glioblastoma: from molecular pathology to targeted treatment. Annu Rev Pathol. 2014;9:1–25.

[23] Inda M, Bonavia R, Mukasa A, Narita Y, Sah DWY, Vandenberg S, et al. Tumor heterogeneity is an active process maintained by a mutant EGFR-induced cytokine circuit in glioblastoma. Genes Dev. 2010;24(16):1731–45.

[24] Emlet DR, Gupta P, Holagdo-Madruga M. Targeting a glioblastoma cancer stem-call population defined by EGF receptor variant III. Cancer Res. 2013;74:1238.

[25] Sampson JH, Mitchell DA. Vaccination strategies for neuro-oncology. Neuro-Oncol Supplement. 2015;7(7):vii15.

[26] Reardon DA, Desjardins A, Schuster J. ReACT: Long-term survival from a randomized phase II study of rindopepimut (CDX-110) plus bevacizumab in relapsed glioblastoma. Annual Conference for the Society of Neuro-Oncology;San Antonio, TX, USA November 2015.

[27] Carmeliet P, Jain RK. Molecular mechanisms and clinical applications of angiogenesis. Nature. 2011;473(7347):298–307.

[28] Lyden D, Hattori K, Dias S, Costa C, Blaikie P, Butros L, et al. Impaired recruitment of bone-marrow-derived endothelial and hematopoietic precursor cells blocks tumor angiogenesis and growth. Nat Med. 2001;7(11):1194–201.

[29] Wick W, Platten M, Wick A, Hertenstein A, Radbruch A, Bendszus M, et al. Current status and future directions of anti-angiogenic therapy for gliomas. Neuro-Oncology. 2016;18(3):315.

[30] Chinot OL, Wick W, Mason W, Henriksson R, Saran F, Nishikawa R, et al. Bevacizumab plus radiotherapy-temozolomide for newly diagnosed glioblastoma. N Engl J Med. 2014;370(8):709–22.

[31] Gilbert MR, Dignam JJ, Armstrong TS, Wefel JS, Blumenthal DT, Vogelbaum MA, et al. A randomized trial of bevacizumab for newly diagnosed glioblastoma. N Engl J Med. 2014;370(8):699–708.

[32] Berghoff AS, Hainfellner JA, Marosi C, Preusser M. Assessing MGMT methylation status and its current impact on treatment in glioblastoma. CNS Oncoly. 2015;4(1):47–52.

[33] Verhaak RGW, Hoadley KA, Purdom E, Wang V, Qi Y, Wilkerson MD, et al. Integrated genomic analysis identifies clinically relevant subtypes of glioblastoma characterized by abnormalities in PDGFRA, IDH1, EGFR, and NF1. Cancer Cell. 2010;17(1):98–110.

[34] Sandmann T, Bourgon R, Garcia J. Patients with proneural glioblastoma may derive overall benefit from the addition of bevacizumab to first line radiotherapy and temozolamide: Retrospective analysis of the AVAglio trial. J Clin Oncol. 2015;33(25): 2735.

[35] Keunen O, Johansson M, Oudin A, Sanzey M, Rahim SAA, Fack F, et al. Anti-VEGF treatment reduces blood supply and increases tumor cell invasion in glioblastoma. Proc Natl Acad Sci U S A. 2011;108(9):3749–54.

[36] Kane JR, Miska J, Young JS, Kanojia D, Kim JW, Lesniak MS. Sui generis: gene therapy and delivery systems for the treatment of glioblastoma. Neuro-oncology. 2015;17(Suppl 2):24–36.

[37] Kaufmann JK, Chiocca EA. Glioma virus therapies between bench and bedside. Neuro-oncology. 2014;16(3):334–51.

[38] Vogelbaum MA, Aghi MK. Convection-enhanced delivery for the treatment of glioblastoma. Neuro-oncology. 2015;17(Suppl 2):3–8.

[39] Oberoi RK, Parrish KE, Sio TT, Mittapalli RK, Elmquist WF, Sarkaria JN. Strategies to improve delivery of anticancer drugs across the blood–brain barrier to treat glioblastoma. Neuro-oncology. 2015;18(1):27.

[40] Sampson JH. Alternating Electric Fields for the Treatment of Glioblastoma. JAMA. 2015;314(23):2511–3.

[41] Stupp R, Taillibert S, Kanner AA, Kesari S, Steinberg DM, Toms SA, et al. Maintenance therapy with tumor-treating fields plus temozolomide vs temozolomide alone for glioblastoma: A randomized clinical trial. JAMA. 2015;314(23):2535–43.

[42] Wick W. TTFields: where does all the skepticism come from? Neuro-oncology. 2016;18(3):303.

[43] Nagy A, Eder K, Selak MA, Kalman B. Mitochondrial energy metabolism and apoptosis regulation in glioblastoma. Brain Res. 2015;1595:127–42.

[44] Sanzey M, Abdul Rahim SA, Oudin A, Dirkse A, Kaoma T, Vallar L, et al. Comprehensive analysis of glycolytic enzymes as therapeutic targets in the treatment of glioblastoma. PLoS ONE [Electronic Resource]. 2015;10(5):e0123544.

[45] Mathews EH, Liebenberg L. Is knowledge of brain metabolism the key to treating highly glycolytic cancers and metastases?. Neuro-oncology. 2013;15(6):649.

[46] Shen H, Hau E, Joshi S, Dilda PJ, McDonald KL. Sensitization of glioblastoma cells to irradiation by modulating the glucose metabolism. Mol Cancer Ther. 2015;14(8):1794.

[47] Agnihotri S, Zadeh G. Metabolic reprogramming in glioblastoma: the influence of cancer metabolism on epigenetics and unanswered questions.Neuro Oncol. 2016;18(2): 160–72.

[48] Debus J, Abdollahi A. For the next trick: new discoveries in radiobiology applied to glioblastoma. American Society of Clinical Oncology Educational Book. 2014 ASCO Educational Book Errata asco.org/edbook © 2014 American Society of Clinical Oncology, Alexandria, VA 95–9.

Chapter 12

Laser Ablation in Neuro-oncology

Mayur Sharma, Danilo Silva,
Suresh Balasubramanian, Gene H. Barnett and
Alireza M. Mohammadi

Additional information is available at the end of the chapter

http://dx.doi.org/10.5772/62771

Abstract

Laser interstitial thermal therapy (LITT) has emerged as a potential tool in the armamentarium of neurosurgeons managing patients with deep-seated and difficult-to-access brain tumors. Advances in stereotactic neurosurgery coupled with neuroimaging tools have led to the resurgence of interest in laser therapy for a variety of neurosurgical indications. Stereotactic placement of laser probe using minimally invasive techniques and the ability to monitor the tissue ablation in real time using MR thermometry are two distinct advantages of LITT. Patients with recurrent gliobastoma multiforme (GBM) or newly diagnosed gliomas with significant medical comorbidities, radiation necrosis, radiosurgery-resistant brain metastasis and cancer-related pain pose significant challenges in the field of neuro-oncology. LITT offers an opportunity to obtain stereotactic biopsy and cytoreduction in a minimally invasive nature. In this chapter, we have described the current applications of LITT in neuro-oncology, including malignant gliomas, brain metastatic disease, radiation necrosis and other indications such as cancer-related pain and epilepsy. We have also described the principles, technical nuances and LITT systems currently available in the clinical practice. With growing interest and acceptance of LITT in neuro-oncology, we are likely to obtain high-quality evidence supporting the utility of this modality in patients with a variety of neuro-oncological conditions in the near future.

Keywords: laser therapy, thermal therapy, gliomas, radiation necrosis, brain metastasis, epilepsy, cancer pain

1. Introduction

Laser interstitial thermal therapy (LITT) has established itself as a new treatment modality in neurosurgery due to its minimally invasiveness nature, safety and efficacy. Nowadays, LITT has become a reality in the world of neuro-oncology [1–4], epilepsy surgery [5–7], and is also emerging as an attractive option in the fields of spine surgery [8–10] and chronic pain syndromes[10–12]. In neuro-oncology, LITT has emerged as an option for malignant gliomas, refractory brain metastatic disease and radiation necrosis. LITT is best suited, but not limited, for patients with tumors located in deep-seated, difficult-to-access areas that could develop significant postoperative neurological deficits and poor performance status with traditional microsurgical resection. It is a FDA-approved treatment option for intracranial lesions including recurrent glioblastomas [4]. Concerning brain metastatic disease, although stereotactic radiosurgery (SRS) has become the standard of care for most patients, the failure rate associated with SRS is up to 23% [13–15]. Additionally, the potential risk of developing radiation necrosis following SRS can vary from 1.4 to 24% [16–18], and this complication can be refractory to standard therapeutic options like steroids and Bevacizumab. LITT has been effective in managing both radiosurgery-resistant brain metastasis [2, 3, 19–22] and radiation necrosis [3, 21–24].

The surgical applications of lasers are represented by three distinct functionalities of this technology: photocoagulation, photovaporization and photosensitization [25]. LITT is referred to the first one, photocoagulation, which implies tissue damage by thermal energy provided by a source of constant and continuous laser delivery to a planned target volume. It was first introduced in 1983 by Bown and colleagues [26], who used a neodymium-doped yttrium aluminum garnet (Nd:YAG) laser and achieved focal tissue coagulation in an experimental brain tumor model without tissue vaporization. Research using experimental animal models demonstrated the brain tissue changes in response to hyperthermia and confirmed that coagulation necrosis could result from the application of thermal energy to brain tissue [27–30]. However, the inability to monitor and control the laser-induced thermal effects limited the widespread application of this technology. Recent advances in magnetic resonance (MR) thermography [31] allowed real-time image feedback of laser thermal energy delivery, making it possible to predict the thermal damage of a planned target in the brain.

In the present chapter, the authors describe the current applications of LITT in neuro-oncology, including malignant gliomas, brain metastatic disease and radiation necrosis together with the basic principles and technical nuances related to the surgical procedure and the current LITT systems available in clinical practice. We also touched upon other applications of LITT such as cancer-related refractory pain and epilepsy. Future directions are also discussed in this chapter.

2. Laser interstitial thermal therapy: principles and rationale

Treating cancers with heat energy dates back to 1960s when Rosomoff et al. [32] first reported the application of ruby pulsed laser beam in two patients with GBM and in experimental animals. They reported that in normal brains of experimental animals, laser application was associated with total cellular destruction with vacuolization secondary to vaporization and hemorrhage. The sensitivity to laser can be increased by Cardio-green and Evans blue injections. Whereas on brain tumors in patients with GBM, laser therapy induced cellular necrosis without hemorrhage and inflammation. Laser bursts were given at 2 min interval at estimated 3 cm depth from the cortical surface, followed by progressive 1 cm depth till approximately 9 cm depth from the surface was reached. Differential susceptibility of normal and tumor to laser application was noted in this study. However, given that the precise application and delivery of laser energy were not feasible at that time, this therapy has fallen out of favor and did not get acceptance in routine clinical practice. In 1985, Winter et al. [33] used microwave hyperthermia for treating brain tumors. Later, brain tumors were treated with focused ultrasound by Britt and coworkers [34]. Following these reports, another study [35] investigated the use of interstitial hyperthermia and iridium brachytherapy in malignant gliomas.

Without the availability of technology to safely monitor the extent of hyperthermia, these techniques remained largely experimental and were unable to be integrated in mainstream clinical practice. When the technological advancements overcome these limitations, thermal ablation using LITT was considered as a more viable, practical and cost-effective approach in treating brain tumors in selected patients. Using LITT, otherwise surgically inaccessible tumors were made amenable to surgical ablation with good outcomes [36, 37]. Though earlier generation probes like Nd-YAG lasers had limitations such as charring of adjacent tissue, thus limiting energy penetration and uncertainties in the extent of tissue ablation [37, 38], new-generation probes have protective mechanisms to prevent charring and also use real-time MR imaging (MR thermometry) to monitor the extent of ablation for minimizing thermal damage to normal surrounding brain parenchyma.

3. Histopathological and biological effects of LITT

Delivering thermal injury with LITT causes some major biological changes in the tissues [39]. Laser photons in the near-infrared range, when directed to the target tissue, get absorbed and converted to heat energy. Aided by abundant blood flow, conduction, convection and refraction all play a significant role in distributing the heat energy around the target tissue [39]. The inherent biology of the surrounding structures and the physical properties of the laser determine the uniformity in the distribution of the heat applied. Ablation of the entire target lesion is the primary aim of using LITT [40].

Cellular homeostasis is usually not disturbed with mild elevation in temperature to approximately 40°C. However, when the temperature is increased in the range of 42 to 45°C (hyperthermia), there is a substantial increase in susceptibility to cellular damage [40, 41]. When the temperature is increased from 46 to 60°C, marked cytotoxicity and cell death ensue with considerably decreased time needed to kill the cells [42, 43]. Above 60°C, there is substantial damage to the mitochondrial enzymes, cytosol and the nucleic acid proteins that culminate to coagulation necrosis [44]. Super boiling temperatures like 105°C results in charring, tissue boiling, vaporization, and carbonization which if not released immediately might culminate in increased intracranial pressure. Apart from the true values of the temperature used, the time of exposure to such temperatures is also important. For example, 43°C for 2 min causes reversible damage to the tissue, while the same temperature for 10 min causes permanent tissue damage and for 60 min causes coagulative necrosis [22, 45]. Based upon the Arrhenius equation, only shorter intervals are needed when using high temperatures to get the same results [46].

The target lesion usually undergoes central coagulation necrosis following LITT therapy, surrounded by a zone of edema next to the undamaged tissue [36]. By the end of 1st week, granulation tissue gradually replaces the zone of necrosis. The targeted lesion then develops into a cystic lesion with remnant necrotic debris surrounded by reactive gliosis with mesenchymal deposits [47, 48].

Three distinct zones can be identified on MRI following LITT. The first central zone represents the zone of coagulation necrosis and if the temperature inadvertently exceeds 100°C, then there is a chance of charring and vaporization followed by a pseudo cavity formation. Just outside the core area lays a non-viable part with increased interstitial fluid called the intermediate zone. The outermost marginal zone is viable consisting of edematous viable surrounding brain parenchyma following thermal exposure and sharply delineates itself from the inner two zones. The ultra-structure of the inner two zones of thermal injury show disrupted organelles and evidence of apoptosis, whereas the outer zone shows only axonal swelling, neuronal shrinkage and hypertrophied endothelial cells with no evidence of vessel thrombosis [4, 49–51]. Following LITT therapy, the target lesions might exhibit an increase in size due to necrosis and perilesional edema, but eventually will shrink and form a rim of granulation tissue.

4. Technical aspects and commercially available components of LITT

4.1. MR thermometry

After numerous attempts of measuring the thermal energy delivery to the target tissue during LITT, including the use of skin thermometers, subcutaneous and interstitial probes, infrared detectors and thermographic cameras [28, 29, 52–56], it was the addition of MR thermometer that played the most significant role in allowing real-time monitoring and quantification of thermal energy delivery leading to thermal ablation [27]. MR thermography based on the temperature-dependent water proton resonance frequency (PRF) is capable of providing visual imaging together with a quantification model of thermal deposition with accurate temporal and spatial resolution. The theory behind PRF is based on the fact that as temperature increases during LITT, the number of free H_2O molecules also increases due to breakage of hydrogen bonds between H_2O molecules. The hydrogen nuclei (proton) are mobilized more efficiently within the gradient field when in the free H_2O molecule state, producing real-time imaging that can be interpreted and visualized using the proper computer software in the treatment workstation [57, 58].

4.2. Lasers and probes used for LITT

The two most common types of lasers used for LITT are the continuous-wave neodymium-doped yttrium aluminum garnet (Nd:YAG), with a wavelength of 1064 nm, and diode lasers with wavelengths between 800–980 nm, which operate at a wide range of powers [1, 59, 60]. Nd:YAG lasers are capable to achieve deeper tissue penetration compared to diode lasers, especially in soft tissues with high blood perfusion at wavelengths between 1000–1100 nm [59, 61]. Diode lasers have the advantage of producing lesions faster, but typically with less penetration [2].

LITT probes have three main components: an optical fiber with a 600 μm diameter, a heat-resistant terminal tip made of sapphire or quartz, measuring around 10 mm [59] and a cooling system, which is required to avoid overheating, tissue carbonization and optical fiber damage [61]. The current cooling mechanisms use either a cooled gas system (CO_2) or a constant stream of fluid (water or saline) delivered to the tip of the probe through a sheath associated to the optic fiber [60, 62]. The thermal energy delivery at the probe tip has been classically described as a symmetrical ellipsoid shape centered along the axis of the probe. Recent advances in probe design, most specifically by the NeuroBlate® System (Monteris Medical Corporation, Plymouth, MN, USA), also led to the development of side firing laser probes, which allows the surgeon to control the laser ablation of complex shaped tumors in a real-time fashion.

4.3. Commercially available LITT systems used in neurosurgery

Currently, there are two commercially available FDA-cleared LITT systems for neurosurgery in the United States: the NeuroBlate® System (Monteris Medical Corporation, Plymouth, MN, USA) and the Visualase Thermal Therapy System (Medtronic Inc., Minneapolis, MN, USA).

The Visualase Thermal Therapy System uses a 15 W 980 nm diode laser generator that supplies energy to a disposable 1.65-mm diameter outer cooling catheter, which contains a 1cm-long fiber optic with a light diffusing, tip [2, 63]. The cooling mechanism is provided by circulating sterile saline [2] and limits the duration of laser application to several minutes. Thermal energy is delivered in an ellipsoid-cylindrical fashion. The system is a MRI-guided laser ablation system, which is connected to a computer workstation capable of displaying real-time thermography data at the target location. Thermal information produces color-coded "thermal" and "damage" images [3, 27]. Limit temperatures can be designated as safety points on the pre-treatment MRI such that if during treatment an increase in temperature beyond the designated limit is detected at those points, the laser is automatically deactivated.

The NeuroBlate® system consists of a solid-state Dornier diode laser operating at the Nd:YAG wavelength (1064 nm) with a laser output of 30 W. The probes are available at diameters of 3.2 and 2.2 mm. The cooling mechanism is provided by a CO_2 gas-cooled system [22, 45]. One unique feature of this system is that both side-firing and diffuse-tip probes are available. The NeuroBlate® directional side-firing laser probe is aimed for contoured ablation of complex shaped targets while the diffusing-tip laser probe is designed to provide fast volumetric ablation in a concentric fashion. The probes are inserted using frameless stereotactic guidance. The Monteris® Mini-Bolt provides rigid skull fixation and allows a direct interface to the NeuroBlate laser probe. The system is a MRI-guided laser ablation system, which is connected to a computer workstation capable of displaying real-time thermography data at the target location. The NeuroBlate software displays the extent of thermal energy delivered as thermal-damage-threshold (TDT) lines. The yellow line surrounds the target volume that has received the thermal energy equivalent of 43°C for at least 2 min; the blue line surrounds the target volume that has been exposed to 43°C for at least 10 min; finally, the white line corresponds to tissue exposed to 43°C for 60 min. Tissues located outside the yellow TDT line are expected to have no permanent damage, while tissue volume inside the blue line undergoes severe thermal damage and tissue volume within the white line experiences coagulation necrosis [22, 45] (**Figure 1**).

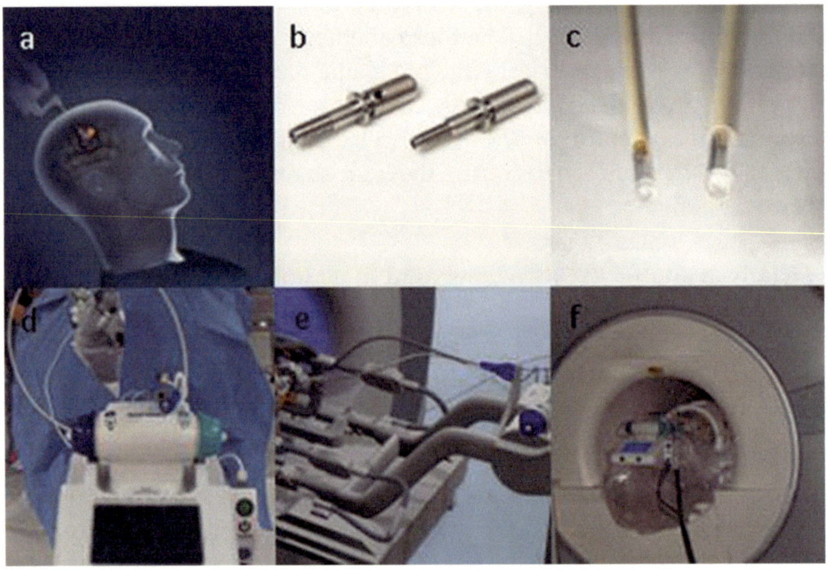

Figure 1. (a–d) show the individual components of NeuroBlate® System including the bolts (b), laser probes (c) and robotic motor drive (d). Figures 1e–f depict the integration of robotic motor drive with the MRI scanner. *(Images used by permission from Monteris Medical Corporation, Plymouth, MN, USA. The use of any Monteris Medical photo or image does not imply Monteris' review or endorsement of any article or publication).*

Disclosures: Drs. Gene Barnett and Alireza Mohammadi are consultants of Monteris Medical Company (NeuroBlate System). Figure 1 is provided by Monteris Medical Company and is the only contribution of this company in this chapter.

5. Animal models and preclinical studies

Various canine [32, 64, 65] and murine [48, 66–68] animal models of brain tumors have been used to investigate the efficacy of laser thermal therapy on tumors and surrounding brain tissue, as well as to evaluate the thermal dose models. First, animal experiments evaluating the impact of laser energy on normal murine brains can be dated back to 1960s. Fine et al. [68] used ruby pulsed laser delivering 100 J of energy to the forehead of mice, which resulted in a mortality rate of 75% within a day of exposure. Later, Earle et al. [67] showed that 20–40 J of energy delivered using ruby laser was not lethal and resulted in sub-arachnoid and intracerebral hemorrhage with minimal neurological effects. Later, Rosomoff et al. [32] reported similar findings using 8 J ruby laser in a rat and dog experiment models. They also reported that the sensitivity to laser could be increased by Cardio-green and Evans blue injections. Kangasniemi et al. [64] reported the feasibility and utility of MR-guided laser (980 nm diode) ablation of tumors (transmissible venereal tumors) in seven canines. Utility of LITT was studied in Lewis mice implanted with glioma cells [48] and neoplastic lesion was monitored using MRI. In addition, proliferation of implanted tumor cells, gliosis and apoptosis was monitored using immunohistological techniques. LITT caused necrosis of neoplastic cells; however, apoptosis of residual tumor cells at the margin (more vascularized compared to pre-treatment) was noted following LITT [48]. Canine models have also been used to establish various thermal dose models, so as to reliably predict post-LITT tissue damage as well as to monitor tissue ablation in real time [65]. Localized interstitial thermal therapy using magnetic nanoparticles (dextran- or aminosilane-coated iron-oxide nanoparticles) have been described in a rat model of GBM [69]. Interestingly, rats treated with aminosilane-coated nanoparticles showed improvement in survival (4.5 times prolongation), whereas those treated with dextran-coated particles did not show any difference in survival compared to controls. These animal experiments paved a way to the development of LITT and future therapeutic options for gliomas.

6. Use of LITT in gliomas

High-grade glioma or glioblastoma multiforme (GBM, WHO grade IV), in particular, is a significant clinical challenge in the field of neuro-oncology with a high rate of morbidity and mortality. GBM constitutes approximately 45% of all malignant primary glial neoplasms [70]. Gross total surgical resection with concurrent chemo-radiotherapy is the mainstay treatment modality for this aggressive tumor [71]. However, even with the best available treatment options, 5-year overall survival (OS), progression-free survival (PFS) and median survival have been reported to be 9.9%, 6.9 months and 14.6 months, respectively [59, 71, 72]. The median survival decreases to 12.1 months with post-resection radiotherapy alone instead of concurrent chemo-radiotherapy and to 6.2 months in patients with progressive disease following standard treatment regimen [71, 72]. There is controversial data regarding optimal management (surgical vs. medical) in patients with recurrent GBM. Extent of resection greater than 80% has been shown to have improved overall survival in carefully selected patients with recurrent GBM [73–75]. Young patients with good performance status have been shown to have improved overall survival following surgical resection for recurrent GBM [76, 77]; however, after adjusting for age, no significant benefit was achieved following repeat surgery [77]. In addition, redo craniotomy for progressive GBM is associated with increased risk of per-operative complications including neurological deficits (18–22%) [78, 79]. Also, there is a cumulative risk of these complications following each craniotomy with maximum risk between first and second procedures [80]. There is insufficient evidence supporting the role of radiosurgery, stereotactic fractionated radiation therapy or interstitial brachytherapy in patients with recurrent GBM [81, 82]. Of note, radiosurgery has also been shown to be associated with increased toxicity in patients with recurrent disease [81]. Survival benefit of 9.3 months have been reported in patients (good performance status) receiving interstitial brachytherapy for recurrent GBM [82]. Given a high incidence of this primary brain tumor with lack of effective therapies and dismal outcome, significant research is directed toward developing effective medical and surgical treatment modalities to improve overall and progression free survival. Laser interstitial thermal therapy (LITT) is one of the advancements in the surgical management of these tumors. LITT is a minimally invasive procedure, which involves stereotactic-guided placement of laser probe and utilizes thermal energy to cause protein coagulation and cell death [83, 84]. Advances in neuroimaging coupled with stereotactic techniques have led to the resurgence of interest in the utility of laser thermacoagulation in patients with brain tumors. In addition, integration of MR thermography to LITT made it possible to deliver thermal energy under real-time monitoring, thus avoiding injury to surrounding normal brain tissue [85]. Given these advantages of LITT, this technique has been utilized for a variety of neurosurgical indications such as deep-seated gliomas [1, 4, 86, 87], epilepsy [20, 88], brain metastasis with radiation necrosis [19, 23, 24, 49] and cingulotomy for intractable pain [12, 89].

First report of utilization of Nd-YAG laser thermal therapy in five patients with deep-seated brain tumors was published in 1990 [90]. Later, several studies with a smaller ($n < 8$) sample size reported the utility of this modality in patients with grade II/III gliomas [36, 87, 91–93]. In 2001, Leonardi et al. [94] reported the utility of stereotactic-guided laser-induced interstitial thermotherapy (SLITT) in 24 patients with residual/recurrent brain tumors [94]. Twenty-four patients with primary glial tumors (17 high grade and 7 low grade gliomas) underwent 30 Nd-YAG laser (1064 nm) procedures under local anesthesia using 0.2T MRI guidance [94]. Interestingly, the tumor ablation was monitored using 3D turbo-FLASH T-1W MRI while laser was applied in steps. Two different lesion architectures at 1108, 1393 J and tissue necrosis at 2979 J were observed on MR imaging during laser ablation. No correlation between the tissue response to thermal treatment and the grade of the tumor was observed in this study [94]. Of note, tumor response rate and clinical outcomes were not reported in this study [94]. Complications such as neurological deficits ($n = 4$), seizures ($n = 2$) and superficial wound infection ($n = 1$) were reported following LITT in this study. A year later, same investigators reported an overall survival of 34, 30 and 9 months in patients with low-grade astrocytoma, anaplastic gliomas and GBM, respectively, following LITT in 24 patients with brain tumors. Similarly, mean time to progression (PFS) for low-grade astrocytoma, anaplastic gliomas and GBM was reported to be 16, 10 and 4 months, respectively, in this study [86]. In 2005, Schwarzmaier et al. [95] reported MR-guided (0.5T) partial ablation using LITT in two patients with recurrent GBM. One of these patients had multifocal GBM, which was found during follow up of primary tumor and underwent LITT for the second focus, whereas second patient had GBM recurrence after standard treatment. Survival of 16 and 20 months following GBM recurrence was reported in this study, thus implicating the role of LITT in achieving improved tumor control and overall survival [95]. A year later, same investigators reported the results of MRgLITT in 16 patients with recurrent GBM with a mean follow up of 9.1 ± 6.3 months [1]. The mean tumor volume treated was 21.6±18.6 cm^3, six patients had two procedures and three patients had three LITT procedures. Of these 16 patients, 15 had surgery, 16 had radiotherapy and 6 had chemotherapy prior to LITT and all patients received chemotherapy following LITT. Authors have reported median survival of 5.2 and 11.2 months after recurrence in first the 10 and later 6 patients, respectively, with an overall median survival of 9.4 months after recurrence and 6.9 months after LITT. Authors have attributed this difference in median survival between the first (n = 10) and the later cohort (n = 6) of patients to the "learning curve" in terms of delay between the tumor recurrence and LITT (2 months vs. 0.3 months in first and later group) [1]. Neurological complications including transient weakness in right upper limb in one patient and non-neurological complications such as neutropenia (n = 3), thrombocytopenia (n = 1) and deranged liver function tests (n = 1) following LITT was reported in this study [1]. Of note, the length of hospital stay was 12.0±4.2 days with no ICU stay and 12 out of 16 patients were dead at the end of the study (7 deaths were due to tumor progression and 5 deaths were due to pulmonary embolism, septic mycosis, gastrointestinal bleeding, sigmoid perforation with peritonitis). Carpentier et al. [96] reported utility of MRgLITT (1.5 T) as a salvage therapy in four patients with recurrent GBM following standard treatment regimen. Five recurrent tumors in four patients (two temporal, one corpus callosum, one centrum semiovale and one temporal) with mean diameter of 16.4 mm under total ablation using Visualase system in this study. All patients except one underwent complete resection prior to salvage LITT. Recurrence was noted following a mean progression-free survival of 37 days and mean overall survival of 10.5 months following LITT, which is longer than the overall survival in patients with recurrent GBM (approximately 4–6 months) [71, 72]. Of note, local recurrence was noted in two patients (45, 30 and 19 days) and another two patients (30 and 60 days) had distant recurrences following LITT. The procedure was well tolerated in all patients with transient adverse effects such as single episode of seizure (n = 1), supplementary motor syndrome (n = 1) and CSF leak (n = 1) [96]. In 2013, the first human phase I study investigating the safety and efficacy of escalating dose of thermal energy using LITT in patients with recurrent GBM was published [4]. This was a multicenter study and enrolled 11 patients at two centers (Cleveland Clinic and UH-case Western Medical Center) from September 2008 to October 2009. Inclusion criterion sued in this study was: adult patients with recurrent GBM following standard treatment regimen, KPS≥ 60, tumor size 15–40 mm cross-sectional dimension, supratentorial location of the tumor, stable medical comorbidities and no concurrent adjunct therapies. Of note, the primary end point of the study was the safety and feasibility of the NeuroBlate® system whereas the overall survival, progression-free survival, improvement in KP score and change in tumor volumes were the secondary end points [4]. Three thermal dose threshold lines [TDT, yellow (43°C for 2 min), blue (43°C for 10 min) and white lines (43°C for 60 min)] were chosen for the study based on previous animal studies. Ten patients underwent LITT procedure and were followed up for a minimum of 6 months or until death, which ever was earlier. All patients died secondary to disease progression following LITT therapy with a median follow up of 8 months. Three patients were initially enrolled for yellow thermal dose threshold line (43°C for 2 min) to the tumor margin. These three patients were followed for 14 days and assessed for any toxicity (defined as decrease of 20 or more points on KPS score). If an independent committee in two out of three patients noted toxicity, the thermal dose was either modified or the trial was halted. If there were no consequences during the follow up of 14 days, another three patients were enrolled for blue and white thermal dose threshold lines subsequently using the same protocol [4]. Mean total and treated tumor volume in all treated patients were 6.8 ± 5 cm^3 and 5± 3.2 cm^3 (78% of total tumor volume), respectively, in this study [4]. The procedure took approximately 2–8 mins/slice and was well tolerated in all the patients with a median hospital stay of 3 days. One entry site infection at 147 days following LITT was reported with no other significant procedure-related complications. Adverse events such as dysphasia with upper limb weakness (n = 1), homonymous hemianopia with contralateral weakness (n = 1), intracerebral hemorrhage due to rupture of pseudo aneurysm (n = 1, 6 weeks after LITT and was managed by endovascular coil placement), white matter injury with hemiparesis (n = 1), deep vein thrombosis (n = 3), pulmonary embolism (n = 1) and grade 3 neutropenia (n = 1) were reported following LITT in this study. Post-LITT edema was noted at 48 h MRI and was managed with steroids. Interestingly, one patient with gliosarcoma developed tumor seeding along the biopsy tract involving the skull and epicranial tissue 9 months after the LITT procedure [4]. The median progression-free survival at 6 months and median overall survival were reported to be ≥ 30 % (compared to 15% reported in the literature) and 316 days, respectively, following LITT in this study. Two deaths were reported during the follow up and the authors concluded LITT to be safe and effective (especially with blue and white TDT ablated zones) in carefully selected patients with recurrent deep-seated GBMs. DTI tractography and angiography might improve the safety profile of LITT, by delineating the critical neural and vascular structures along the tract of laser probe [4]. Mohammadi et al. [97] investigated the efficacy of LITT in 34 patients with high-grade gliomas HGG (GBM, n = 24 and anaplastic astrocytoma/oligodendroglioma, n = 10) in difficult-to-access (DTA) areas in a multicenter retrospective study. Of these 34 patients, 16 patients (16 procedures) underwent LITT as an upfront therapy and 18 patients (19 procedures) underwent LITT for recurrent disease. Median time from initial diagnosis of HGG was 29 months for LITT therapy in patients with recurrent disease with a median follow up of 7.2 months following LITT. Following LITT, all patients had standard adjunct treatment and were monitored with serial follow-up MRIs every 3 months. Progression-free survival was the primary end point, whereas overall survival and complications were considered as secondary end points in this study. Frontal lobe was the most common location (n = 15), followed by thalamus (n = 7), parietal and temporal (n = 5 each) and corpus callosum in a single patient. The median tumor volume that was treated using LITT was 10.13 cm^3 and 3 cm was the maximum tumor diameter in this study [97]. And, 98% of tumor volume was covered with yellow TDT lines and 91% with blue TDT lines, with median hospital stay of 3 days. Progression-free survival during the median follow up of 7.2 months was 5.1 months and 71% of treated patients had progressive disease. Majority (52%) of tumor progression following LITT was noted at the periphery of tumor, followed by at the center of the ablated zone (22%), outside the treatment field (22%) and in the contralateral hemisphere (4%). One year estimated survival was 68± 9 % and 12 patients (35%) expired due to disease progression during the follow up. Based on the volume of tumor covered by yellow and blue TDT lines, patients were stratified as favorable (<0.05 cm^3 tumor volume missed by yellow TDT lines and <1.5 cm^3 of tumor volume between yellow and blue TDT lines) and unfavorable groups (≥0.05 cm^3 tumor volume missed by yellow TDT lines and ≥1.5 cm^3 of tumor volume between yellow and blue TDT lines) [97]. The median PFS in favorable group was 9.7 months, whereas it was 4.6 months in unfavorable group. Interestingly, when controlled for tumor volume of >10 cc, the effect of TDT line coverage on PFS did not reach significance in this study. In terms of adverse events, 13 adverse events (37%) were noted in this study. Transient ($n = 5$) and permanent ($n = 2$) worsening of preoperative neurological deficits, superficial infection ($n = 1$), deep vein thrombosis ($n = 1$), ventriculitis ($n = 1$), seizure ($n = 1$), hyponatremia ($n = 1$), hydrocephalus ($n = 1$), intracerebral hematoma ($n = 3$) and mortality due to intracerebral hematoma ($n = 1$) were the complications following LITT noted in this study [97]. This study showed LITT to be an efficacious therapy in patients with primary or recurrent high-grade gliomas in difficult to access areas. However, major limitations of this study were its retrospective nature and small sample size. A recent single center retrospective study reported the utility of LITT in patients with a variety of intracranial pathologies including gliomas ($n = 34$) [98]. Total operative time and ablation time were 2.9±0.6 hrs and 9.3±6.5 mins, respectively. Median ICU and hospital stay was 1.0 day each and average hospital stay was 3.6±5.4 days following LITT in this study. There was an overall increase in size of lesion immediately following LITT, followed by a gradual reduction in size 24 h after the procedure which was similar to that at first follow up [98]. Postoperative complications such as neurological worsening ($n = 7$), hemorrhage ($n = 2$), edema ($n = 4$), infection ($n = 1$), inaccurate catheter placement ($n = 2$) and deaths ($n = 2$) were reported [98]. Mortality occurred in two patients with glioblastoma multiforme (midbrain/pons in one patient) who developed malignant cerebral edema following LITT. One patient underwent hemicraniectomy with no successful outcome and died in the same admission. The 30-day readmission rate was 5.6% in this study. Of note, outcome measures such as overall survival, progression-free survival or recurrence were not reported in this study [98].

Although there is no Class 1 evidence supporting the efficacy of LITT in patients with high-grade gliomas, there is also paucity of high-quality data supporting the role of craniotomy and surgical resection in such patients [99]. Given the minimally invasive nature of LITT coupled with advances in neuroimaging stereotactic techniques and thermography, LITT can be a useful treatment modality in patients with poor performance status or medical comorbidities and high-grade glioma. The advantages of LITT have led to the exploration of this technique for a variety of intracranial tumors. LITT has been investigated in various prospective case-controlled studies and there is a likelihood to have Class 2 evidence data in the next couple of years.

7. Use of LITT in brain metastasis and radiation necrosis

Brain metastasis is a common and challenging clinical scenario affecting up to 40% of patients with systemic malignancies [100–102]. Lung carcinoma (16–19%) is the leading systemic cause of brain metastasis followed by renal (6–9%), melanoma (7–7.4%), breast (5%) and colorectal cancers (1.2–1.8%) [103, 104]. Prognosis in patients with brain metastasis is often dismal, due to limited therapeutic options. Majority of chemotherapeutic agents and targeted immunotherapies do not cross the blood brain barrier, hence limited applicability of these agents in management of patients with brain metastasis. Stereotactic radiosurgery (SRS) has emerged as a primary therapeutic modality in patients with single or multiple brain metastases with an improvement in overall survival and quality of life [13, 14, 105, 106]. However, there is a subset of patients (up to 23%) who fail SRS with progression of metastatic disease and subsequent mortality [13, 15]. Brain metastasis from radio-resistant systemic tumors such as renal cell carcinoma, sarcoma, melanoma and triple negative breast carcinoma carries a worse prognosis, despite better control rates with SRS as compared to conventional radiotherapy [107]. Stereotactic radiosurgery is also associated with adverse radiation effects (AREs) with a 1-year cumulative incidence of 13–14%, which increases with size and volume of the tumor [108–111]. Of these adverse radiation effects, radiation necrosis (RN) is the most challenging in terms of diagnosis and management with a reported incidence ranging between 1.4% and 25% [16–18, 112]. Imaging modalities such as MR perfusion, MR spectroscopy, 6-[(18)F]-fluoro-L-3,4-dihydroxyphenylalanine (F-DOPA)/FDG PET, l-methyl-(11)C-methionine ((11)C-MET) and SPECT scan have been shown to be useful in differentiating radiation necrosis from recurrent metastasis or tumor [113–116]. The sensitivity, specificity, accuracy of perfusion MRI and F-DOPA PET have been reported to be 86.7, 68.2, 75.6 and 90, 92.3, 91.3%, respectively [114]. SPECT scan has been shown to have the highest specificity of 97.8% (sensitivity 87.6%) for differentiating tumor progression and radiation necrosis and may be preferred over other imaging modalities [116]. Medical therapeutic options for RN include corticosteroids, Bevacizumab, hyperbaric oxygen therapy, anticoagulation (heparin or warfarin) or vitamin E [117–125]. Surgical resection of RN can be considered in symptomatic patients with mass effect in accessible areas [125]. Therefore, there is always a scope for newer treatment strategies in the management of patients with brain metastasis to improve the clinical outcomes. LITT is a minimally invasive technique that offers an alternative therapeutic option in patients with either SRS-failed or radio-resistant brain metastasis. LITT also offers an opportunity to have a histological diagnosis before laser ablation in cases of suspicion between recurrence of metastasis and radiation-related changes. The minimally invasive nature of this technology permits its utility in patients with multiple medical comorbidities with poor Karnofsky performance status (KPS) and tumors in difficult-to-access locations.

First use of laser therapy for brain metastasis was reported in 1986, with successful-laser assisted ablation of a midbrain metastasis from primary lung adenocarcinoma [126]. In 1990, Sugiyama et al. [90] reported the utility of laser in patients with deep-seated tumors including metastasis. Later, Schulze et al. [36] studied the histological effects of laser thermotherapy in seven patients with brain metastasis and eight patients with glial tumors. In this study, authors reported that laser therapy created a unique pattern of architectural changes at the histological level with central zone of necrosis surrounded by edematous tissue. This surrounding edematous tissue tends to undergo cystic changes following regenerative and resorptive changes [36]. In addition to thermal coagulation, laser-induced tumor damage is caused by disruption of cellular membranes and organelles. Authors advocated this technique in older patients with significant medical comorbidities and brain tumors. First pilot clinical trial investigating the safety and feasibility of LITT in patients with resistant focal metastatic brain tumors was reported in 2008 [2]. Four patients with six metastatic brain tumors (temporal lobe, $n = 2$; parietal lobe, $n = 2$; frontal lobe, $n = 1$; and occipital lobe, $n = 1$) were enrolled in this trial. Follow-up MRI scans were performed at 7, 15, 30 and 90 days after the procedure to monitor the zone of thermal necrosis. LITT was well tolerated and all patients were discharged within 14 h after the procedure in this study [2]. There was an acute increase in the tumor volume immediately after the procedure followed by a gradual reduction in the volume during the follow-up imaging. No adverse events, complications or tumor recurrence within the ablated zones were noted during the follow up [2]. Results of this trial were published in 2011, which showed no tumor recurrence in ablated zones in all 7 patients (15 metastatic tumors) at a follow up of 30 months [19]. Mean age of patients enrolled in this study was 54 years, with breast or pulmonary adenocarcinoma and average number of metastasis per patient was 3.3. Total coverage of the tumor under TDT lines was achieved in nine patients and partial coverage in six patients. Single applicator for laser delivery was used in majority of patients ($n = 13$) and two applicators in another two due to complex tumor shape. Majority of tumors were less than 2 cm in size ($n = 10$) and another five were 2–3 cm in size. Mean duration of the procedure and hospital stay was 135 mins and 26 h, respectively, and all patients were discharged within 24 h of procedure [19]. Complications such as blood suffusion, probe misplacement, transient aphasia and cerebellar syndrome were reported following LITT therapy. Of note, there was a mean increase of 26% (range 0–124%) in tumor volume at a mean interval of 4.7 days (range 0–15 days) after the procedure, which returned to baseline volume within 20 days (range 0–75 days). Following LITT, contrast-enhancing rim of the metastasis disappeared in a mean interval of 12.2 months. Mean overall survival and progression-free survival following LITT were 17.4±3.5 months and 3.8±1.0 months, respectively [19].

Another study reported progression-free and overall median survival of 5.8 months each following LITT in five patients with metastasis (non-small cell lung carcinoma, $n = 2$; colon adenocarcinoma, $n = 1$, melanoma, $n = 1$, fallopian tube carcinoma, $n = 1$) [20]. Frontal lobe was involved in two patients, fronto-parietal in one, insula in one and parietal in one patient. Four patients had one trajectory and another two patients had double trajectories for laser therapy. Of note, mean hospital and ICU stay following LITT were 4.4 days and 1 day, respectively, in patients with metastasis [20]. This duration of hospital stay following LITT was significantly higher as compared to previous study by Carpentier et al. [19, 20]. Complications such as transient aphasia (insula) and hemiparesis (frontal) were noted following LITT, which improved gradually with steroids. Patient with melanoma metastasis showed stable tumor size with edema and decrease in size of lesion at 1 and 3 months, respectively, following LITT on follow-up MRI [20]. Two patients had systemic progression; other two had CNS progression and none of the patients required additional treatment in this study.

Torres-Reveron et al. [3] reported the utility of LITT in six patients with progressive brain metastatic tumors (non-small cell lung cancer, $n = 2$; melanoma, $n = 2$; small cell lung cancer, $n = 1$; ovarian cancer, $n = 1$) following SRS. Tumor recurrence was diagnosed using PET and SPECT imaging in two patients, each using these imaging modalities; however interestingly, stereotactic biopsy prior to ablation therapy was negative in all the patients [3]. There was an increase in length (63%) and width (64%) of the tumor on post-operative MRI at 2 weeks after LITT compared to preoperative size similar to previous studies [19, 20, 24]. However, in concordance with previous studies, tumor size returned to baseline within 4.5 to 6 months following the procedure in all the patients [3]. Interestingly, initial increase in size of lesion was not associated with increase in concurrent FLAIR signal changes on post-operative MRI at 2 weeks after the procedure. These radiological changes were also associated with improvement in clinical symptoms and thus the ability to wean off the patient from steroids. Satisfactory tumor control was achieved in four out of six patients; one patient had progression of systemic disease and died within 1 month of procedure. Another patient had progressive increase in tumor size 3 months after the procedure following initial response, and surgical resection of the tumor showed tumor progression. No significant complications were reported in this study. Similarly, another study investigated the efficacy of LITT in recurrent lesions following stereotactic radiosurgery for brain metastasis [21]. Of note, biopsy and histological diagnosis was not routinely performed in this study and authors advocated LITT irrespective of clinical diagnosis (tumor recurrence vs. radiation necrosis). Seventeen LITT procedures were performed in 16 patients and 14 patients (15 procedures) were available for follow up in this study. Non-small cell lung carcinoma (n = 12) was the most common systemic malignancy metastasizing to the brain, followed by breast and colon adenocarcinoma. Average time interval between SRS and LITT was 64.3 weeks [21]. Greater than 25% increase in tumor volume as compared to the immediate post-operative scan (after 24 h) was defined as local treatment failure or recurrence. Mean tumor size that was treated using LITT was 3.66 cm^3 and 3.3 lesions were treated per treatment [21]. Mean procedure time, mean duration of ablation and in-patient hospital stay were 136.0, 7.43 and 1.2 days, respectively, in this study. Interestingly, postoperative MRI (within 24 h) revealed an average increase of 278% in tumor volume size following LITT in 12/14 patients and the other two patients showed 74 and 91% decrease in preoperative tumor volume. Subsequently, greater than 10% reduction in tumor volume was observed in seven patients at a median interval of 24 weeks, achieving a local control rate of 75.8% (13 of 15 lesions). Two patients experienced recurrence at 4 and 18 weeks following LITT within the treated zone and underwent surgical resection of the recurrent tumor. The median progression-free survival and overall survival at 39 weeks follow up were 37 weeks and 57%, respectively. Mortality was related to extra cranial disease in five patients and intracranial disease distant from the treated site in one patient. Two complications including non-operative hemorrhage (n = 1) and new onset hemiparesis (n = 1) was noted following LITT; former patient expired secondary to extra cranial progression and the other patient improved with steroids [21].

A recent study reported delayed failure in two patients who underwent LITT following tumor progression and refractory cerebral edema after SRS [23, 49]. LITT was performed 7 months (breast adenocarcinoma) and 14 weeks (lung adenocarcinoma) after stereotactic radiosurgery. Patient with lung adenocarcinoma metastasis to the external capsule had significant perilesional edema following radiosurgery and also experienced severe side effects secondary to steroid therapy (refractory hyperglycemia, weight gain and bilateral proximal muscle weakness), therefore LITT was considered 14 weeks after SRS [23]. This patient had significant clinical improvement and steroid was weaned off in 2 weeks following ablation therapy.

However, first patient with parietal metastasis and second patient with external capsule metastasis demonstrated tumor recurrence at 6 and 11 months, respectively, which was histologically confirmed following surgical resection [49]. A recent review based on pooled 25 patients with brain metastasis who were treated with LITT reported a median overall survival (OS) of 12.6 months (range 9.0–19.8 months) and progression-free survival (PFS) to vary between 3.8–8.5 months [127]. Severe complication rate was reported to be 8% and included events such as perioperative hemorrhage (non-surgical) and blood suffusion. Intracranial progression of disease (excluding local progression, 8%) and extra cranial progression as the etiology of mortality was reported in 36 and 55% of patients respectively following LITT for brain metastasis. Median survival time (9.0–19.8 months) and severe complication rate of 8% following LITT are similar to 1.4–16.1 months and 6–19%, respectively, following surgical management of brain metastasis [128]. Given these comparable outcomes, LITT is an effective therapeutic option for patients with resistant brain metastasis in difficult-to-access areas. There is a paucity of literature on the utility of LITT in patients with radiation necrosis (RN). It is often difficult to distinguish patients with radiation necrosis and those with tumor recurrence following stereotactic radiosurgery. Therefore, the majority of reported cases could represent a mixture of these clinical conditions, even following stereotactic biopsy. In an anecdotal report, LITT was used for diagnosed RN following stereotactic biopsy (may represent a mixed lesion), as patient was refractory and not able to tolerate standard medical management (steroids and bevacizumab) for suspected RN [24]. Patient developed several steroid-related complications along with several medical comorbidities. In light of these facts and the presence of a lesion in a difficult-to-access area (left centrum semiovale), LITT was considered in this patient with RN following SRS for brain metastasis (non-small cell lung carcinoma). As demonstrated in earlier reports, there was a significant improvement in clinical symptoms following LITT and patient was weaned off the steroid in 2 weeks after the procedure. However, there was a mild increase in size of lesion with no significant FLAIR signal changes at 7 weeks postoperative MRI, which was consistent with the literature.

Patel et al. [98] reported the utility of LITT in patients with a variety of intracranial pathologies including patients with recurrent metastasis or radiation necrosis (n = 37) [98]. Total operative time and ablation time were 2.8±0.6 h and 8.7±8.1 mins, respectively. Postoperative complications such as neurological worsening (n = 7), hemorrhage (n = 1), edema (n = 1), infection (n = 1) and thermal injury to pituitary leading to secondary complications (n = 1) were reported [98]. Overall survival and progression-free survival or recurrence was not reported in this study [98].

LITT has shown initial promising results in patients with recurrent brain metastasis and RN (to some extent) following SRS. However, long-term prospective randomized controlled studies are warranted and required to validate the efficacy of LITT for these clinical indications.

8. Use of LITT in other intracranial tumors

Jethwa et al. [63] reported the application of Visualase laser system in 20 patients (33 procedures) with a variety of intracranial tumors over a period of 1 year. GBM was the most common pathology treated (*n* = 6), followed by metastasis (*n* = 4), ependymoma (*n* = 3), meningioma (*n* = 2), hemangioblastoma (*n* = 2), anaplastic astrocytoma (*n* = 1), chordoma (*n* = 1) and supratentotrial primitive neuroectodermal tumor (*n* = 1) in this study. LITT was considered primarily in patients with failed prior treatment (10 out of 20), in surgically inaccessible areas (*n* = 3), patient preference (*n* = 3) or in those in who conventional surgery was considered high risk (*n* = 4) [63]. Majority of patients were treated with single laser application; however, two patients with GBM, one each with metastasis, meningioma, ependymoma underwent two applications and one patient with GBM required three laser applications to cover the tumor volume. One patient each with ependymoma and GBM underwent staged LITT procedure 2 months apart and one with supratentotrial primitive neuroectodermal tumor underwent repeat procedure due to tumor recurrence. The average tumor volume and average tumor diameter treated was 7.0± 9.0 cm^3 and 2.4± 0.85 cm. The average ablation time was 13.9± 10.7 min and median hospital stay of 24 h (average stay of 2.27 days) in this study [63]. It was noted in the study that LITT was well tolerated in the majority of patients with four procedure-related complications. Inaccurate placement of laser probe (patient with cerebellum hemangioblastoma), placement-related hemorrhage (near right sylvian fissure meningioma), pituitary thermal injury (pediatric patient with third ventricle recurrent ependymoma) and significant periprocedural edema (patient with GBM) were reported following 33 LITT procedures in 20 patients. All these complications except pituitary thermal injury required open surgical procedure. Tumor control rates and follow-up imaging were not reported in this study. Another group reported the use of LITT in six patients with intracranial tumors (metastasis, *n* = 4; pituitary prolactinoma, *n* = 1; medullary ependymoma) and one patient with conus ependymoma [129]. Complete ablation was achieved in six out of seven patients and no procedure-related adverse effects were noted in these patients [129]. No long-term outcomes and follow-up results were reported following LITT for these tumors. Recently, Patel et al. [98] reported the utility of LITT using Visualase system in patients with a variety of intracranial tumors such as meningioma (*n* = 2), ependymoma (*n* = 3), hemangioblastoma (*n* = 2), primitive neuroectodermal tumor (*n* = 3), cavernoma (*n* = 2), chordoma (*n* = 1), teratoma (*n* = 1), CNS lymphoma (*n* = 1) and pineal tumor (*n* = 1) [98]. Total operative time and ablation time were 2.8±0.6 hrs and 8.7±8.1 mins, respectively, in all patients with intracranial tumors including glial tumors (GBM, ganglioglioma, pilocytic astrocytoma). Postoperative complications such as neurological worsening (*n* = 7), hemorrhage (*n* = 2), edema (*n* = 4), infection (*n* = 1), inaccurate catheter placement (*n* = 2) and two deaths following LITT were reported [98]. A major limitation of this study was that outcomes including tumor control rates and recurrence were not reported in this study [98]. The procedure was not completed in two patients, one with recurrent meningioma due to hemorrhage during probe insertion which required emergent evacuation and the second patient with hemangioblastoma had inaccurate placement of laser probe which led to abortion of the procedure.

9. Use of LITT in cancer-related pain

Cancer-related pain is a significant clinical problem affecting up to 60–90% of patients with cancer in terminal stages [130]. The first line of management in such patients is pharmacological including opioids; however, 10–20% of such patients are refractory to medical line of management and thus requires intervention for pain management [131–133]. Various neuromodulation and ablative procedures such as intrathecal morphine, myelotomy, cordotomy, DREZotomy, sympathetic blocks, paravertebral blocks and cingulotomy have been described for pharmacological-resistant, cancer-related and various refractory pain syndromes [131–137]. Ablative cingulotomy using radiofrequency [136] and neuromodulation using DBS [138] has been described in patients with various refractory pain syndromes. With the advances in neuroimaging and stereotactic techniques and introduction of LITT, this technique has been explored in patients with pharmacoresistant cancer-related pain [12, 98]. Patel et al. [12] describe the feasibility of MRgLITT in three patients (four procedures) with cancer-related pain. Ablation coordinates used in patients who underwent first-time ablation includes $x = 7.9$ mm (6.9–8.6mm range); $y = 20.5$ mm (20–22 mm range); $Z = 6.9$ mm (2.9–7.0 mm) above the lateral ventricles. Second ablation 1–2 cm above the first ablation was performed in patients with first-time ablation procedures. One patient who underwent ablation for recurrence had three ablations. Median ablation time and volume ablated were 257 seconds and 1.5 cm^3, respectively. Median pain severity score (PSS) decreased from 7.7 in preoperative period to 1.6 following the LITT procedure. Similarly, pain interference score (PIS) decreased from 9.9 to 2.0 following the procedure [12]. Median pain reduction was maintained for 5 weeks (2–16 weeks) following LITT and all patients had significant reduction in medication requirements during the period. No significant adverse effects related to the procedure were noted in this study. The advantage of LITT is that the ablation can be monitored in real-time using MR thermography, which was not feasible in earlier ablative techniques.

Another recent study reported the utility of LITT in five patients with chronic pain syndrome [98]. Total operative time and ablation time were 2.9±0.3 h and 4.3±0.6 mins, respectively. No postoperative complications were noted following LITT in patients with chronic pain [98]. Outcomes in terms of pain control was not reported in this study [98].

10. Use of LITT in epilepsy

Pharmacoresistant or drug-resistant epilepsy (DRE) is a significant clinical challenge with prevalence of approximately 28 to 40% in patients with epilepsy [139, 140]. In addition, approximately 10% of pediatric patients with epilepsy meet the criterion of DRE within 18 months of diagnosis [140]. Epilepsy surgery has been shown to have beneficial long-term effects in terms of seizure control (seizure free outcome rate of 67 and 26% at 5 and 15 years follow-up, respectively) and psychosocial outcomes in patients with DRE [141–143]. Based on a recent meta-analysis, the incidence of neurological deficits, permanent neurological deficits, wound infection/meningitis following temporal lobectomy with/without amygdalohippocampectomy and extratemporal lobar/multilobar resections have been reported to be 5.2, 0.8, 1.1 and 19.5, 3.2, 1.9%, respectively [144]. The complication rates have been shown to increase from 10% during first resective surgery in pediatric patients with complex refractory epilepsy to 50% during second respective surgery [145]. Given this success of epilepsy surgery in controlling seizures with associated morbidity in patients with DRE, there is always a need to improvise on surgical techniques so as to reduce the morbidity while improving the outcomes. Introduction of MRI-guided LITT in neurosurgery over the past decades have paved a way to exploration of this technique in patients with DRE. MRgLITT is a minimally invasive stereotactic technique that can be used to ablate the epileptogenic zone and associate fibers so as to simulate the resection and disconnection procedures, respectively. FDA approved Auto LITT in 2009, following a successful Phase 1 multicenter trial investigating the safety of this system in patients with recurrent GBM. In 2012, Curry et al. [146] first reported the use of MRI-guided (1.5T) LITT (Visualase thermal system) in five patents with DRE. In this study, they ablated six epileptic zones (cingulate tuber $n = 1$, mesial temporal sclerosis $n = 1$, hypothalamic hamartoma $n = 2$ and frontal cortical dysplasia $n = 2$) in five patients with DRE and all patients were reported to be seizure-free at 2–13 months of follow up [146]. No complications were reported in this study. Another study reported the use of this modality in a 3-year-old with a diagnosis of precocious puberty and pharmacoresistant gelastic seizures and MRI showed type III hypothalamic hamartoma (both pedunculated and sessile component) [88]. Patient underwent MRgLITT using Visualase system without perioperative complications. There was significant improvement in behavior and seizures at 2 weeks after the procedure. At 6 months follow up, patient remained seizure-free with improvement in behavior and self-indulging learning patterns such as playing and entertainment [88]. A year later, Wellmer et al. [147] reported the successful use of 3T MR-guided stereotactic radiofrequency thermal coagulation in two patients with DRE due to type IIB frontal focal cortical dysplasia. These focal cortical dysplasias were identified as epileptogenic zones prior to LITT and one of these lesions was in close proximity to the cortico-spinal tract as elicited by the motor-evoked potentials using in-depth electrodes. Both patients were seizure-free at 12 and 5 months with no persistent postoperative complications (one patient had transient mouth paresis) following thermal coagulation [147]. Authors emphasized the importance of precise placement of radiofrequency probe and destruction of epileptogenic zone, taking into account the surrounding eloquent area. Gonzalez-Martinez et al. [148] reported robot (ROSA, Medtech Surgical, Inc.) assisted placement of laser probe (Visualase Inc.) under intraoperative MRI guidance to ablate a periventricular heterotopic lesion in a 19-year-old female with DRE of 10-years duration. Authors reported that combination of robot, LITT and intraoperative MRI is a safe, accurate, efficacious and time-efficient minimally invasive technique that can be used for placement and ablation of epileptogenic zone in patients with DRE [148]. Esquenazi and colleagues [149] reported the utility and feasibility of stereotactic MRgLITT (3T) in two patients with DRE and periventricular nodular heterotopia. One patient underwent temporal lobectomy in addition to LITT and was seizure-free during the follow up and another patient had significant seizure control leading to adjustment in medications following the procedure [149]. Former patient with two procedures had transient visual deficit and no complications in another patient were reported during the follow up. Stereotactic placement of multiple trajectories to achieve conformity of complex tumor shapes at deeper locations was also described in this report. Recently, Lewis and colleagues [150] described the feasibility and efficacy of MRgLITT in 17 pediatric patients with DRE using Visualase system. In this retrospective study, 17 patients with DRE underwent 19 MRgLITT procedures with a mean follow up of 16.1 months. Focal cortical dysplasia (n = 12) was the most common pathology followed by tuberous sclerosis complex (n = 5), hypothalamic hamartoma (n = 1), mesial temporal sclerosis (n = 1), Rasmussen encephalitis (n = 1) and tumor (n = 1) [150]. One LITT procedure was aborted and one was partially completed leading to completion of LITT in 17 procedures. Nine patients had prior surgeries including two patients had three, one had two and the rest had one procedure each prior to LITT. Engel class I, class II, class III and class IV outcome were achieved in 41, 6, 18 and 35%, respectively, following LITT with an average postprocedure hospital stay of 1.56 days. 38% of patients with Engel class I/II outcomes and 56% of patients with Engel class III/IV outcomes had at least one resective surgery prior to LITT [150]. Inaccurate fiber placement, device malfunction, inaccurate fiber placement with IVH (aseptic meningitis and ventriculostomy) and post-ablation edema/drug-induced gastritis were noted in one patient each leading to eight individual complications in four patients [150]. Patients with lesions <2 cm in size, well-circumscribed solitary lesions and concordant EEG and presurgical data were considered optimal candidates for LITT ablation in this study [150]. Recently, Patel et al. [98] reported the utility of LITT in 10 patients with pharmacoresistant epilepsy [98]. Total operative time and ablation time were 2.6±0.4 h and 7.6±2.3 mins, respectively. No procedure-related complications were noted in this study. However outcome in terms of seizures control was not reported in this study [98]. Based on these studies, LITT has shown promising results in patients with DRE, especially those who require repeat resection surgery with favorable outcome while minimizing morbidity. However, long-term prospective randomized controlled studies are warranted to validate the efficacy of LITT in patients with DRE and to establish appropriate selection and inclusion criterion to achieve favorable outcomes.

11. Future trends

FDA approved AutoLITT in 2009, following a multicenter trial investigating the efficacy of this modality in patients with recurrent GBM. Laser ablation has currently been investigated as a potential treatment modality in patients with failed stereotactic radiosurgery for brain metastasis (NCT01651078, Laser Ablation after Stereotactic Radiosurgery, LAASR study). Following these results, LITT is likely to be explored in other areas of neuro-oncology.

12. Our experience

At Cleveland clinic we have an experience of about 150 patients, who underwent LITT for a variety of indications since 2011. At our center, we use NeuroBlate® System (Monteris Medical

Corporation, Plymouth, MN, USA) with a side firing probes (Figure 1). Regarding intra-axial tumors, we have used LITT in 30 patients with de novo GBM, 24 patients with recurrent GBM (following standard treatment), 22 patients with recurrent anaplastic tumors, upfront in 10 patients with anaplastic tumors, 24 patients with low-grade gliomas (7 upfront and 17 recurrent). We have also used this modality in 17 patients with radiation necrosis and 15 patients with metastasis. We are also participating in a multi-institutional study investigating the role of this modality in patients with failed SRS (LAASR study). We have also utilized this therapy in patients with recurrent meningioma ($n = 4$) and schwanomma ($n = 1$, upfront) as well as epilepsy surgery (more than five cases).

13. Conclusion

LITT is a stereotactic minimally invasive technique that involves ablation of pathological tissue using laser energy. This technique has shown promising results in a variety of neuro-oncological conditions such as recurrent GBM, upfront deep-seated GBM, recurrent metastasis following SRS, radiation necrosis and cancer-related pain. LITT was approved by FDA in 2009 for unlimited intracranial usage. Minimally invasive nature of the therapy coupled with real-time monitoring of thermal ablation are distinct advantages of LITT over traditional surgical approaches, especially for deep-seated tumors in patients with significant co-morbidities. Currently, there is Level III /Level IV evidence in the literature supporting the role of LITT in patients with recurrent GBM/high-grade gliomas, metastasis and radiation necrosis. There is a paucity of data regarding other indications of LITT. However, trials are underway and are likely to provide significant level of evidence supporting the efficacy of LITT in a variety of the above-mentioned indications in coming years.

Author details

Mayur Sharma, Danilo Silva, Suresh Balasubramanian, Gene H. Barnett and Alireza M. Mohammadi*

*Address all correspondence to: MOHAMMA3@ccf.org

The Rose Ella Burkhardt Brain Tumor Neuro-Oncology Center, Neurological Institute, Cleveland Clinic, Cleveland, Ohio

References

[1] Schwarzmaier HJ, Eickmeyer F, von Tempelhoff W, Fiedler VU, Niehoff H, Ulrich SD, Yang Q, Ulrich F. MR-guided laser-induced interstitial thermotherapy of recurrent

glioblastoma multiforme: preliminary results in 16 patients. European journal of radiology 2006;59(2):208–15.

[2] Carpentier A, McNichols RJ, Stafford RJ, Itzcovitz J, Guichard JP, Reizine D, Delaloge S, Vicaut E, Payen D, Gowda A, George B. Real-time magnetic resonance-guided laser thermal therapy for focal metastatic brain tumors. Neurosurgery 2008;63(1 Suppl 1):ONS21-8; discussion ONS8-9.

[3] Torres-Reveron J, Tomasiewicz HC, Shetty A, Amankulor NM, Chiang VL. Stereotactic laser induced thermotherapy (LITT): a novel treatment for brain lesions regrowing after radiosurgery. Journal of neuro-oncology 2013;113(3):495–503.

[4] Sloan AE, Ahluwalia MS, Valerio-Pascua J, Manjila S, Torchia MG, Jones SE, Sunshine JL, Phillips M, Griswold MA, Clampitt M, Brewer C, Jochum J, McGraw MV, Diorio D, Ditz G, Barnett GH. Results of the neuroblate system first-in-humans phase i clinical trial for recurrent glioblastoma: clinical article. Journal of neurosurgery 2013;118(6):1202–19.

[5] Kang JY, Wu C, Tracy J, Lorenzo M, Evans J, Nei M, Skidmore C, Mintzer S, Sharan AD, Sperling MR. Laser interstitial thermal therapy for medically intractable mesial temporal lobe epilepsy. Epilepsia 2016;57(2):325–34.

[6] Buckley R, Estronza-Ojeda S, Ojemann JG. Laser ablation in pediatric epilepsy. Neurosurgery clinics of North America 2016;27(1):69–78.

[7] Gross RE, Willie JT, Drane DL. The role of stereotactic laser amygdalohippocampotomy in mesial temporal lobe epilepsy. Neurosurgery clinics of North America 2016;27(1): 37–50.

[8] Tatsui CE, Stafford RJ, Li J, Sellin JN, Amini B, Rao G, Suki D, Ghia AJ, Brown P, Lee SH, Cowles CE, Weinberg JS, Rhines LD. Utilization of laser interstitial thermotherapy guided by real-time thermal MRI as an alternative to separation surgery in the management of spinal metastasis. Journal of neurosurgery. Spine 2015;23(4):400–11.

[9] Brouwer PA, Brand R, van den Akker-van Marle ME, Jacobs WC, Schenk B, van den Berg-Huijsmans AA, Koes BW, van Buchem MA, Arts MP, Peul WC. Percutaneous laser disc decompression versus conventional microdiscectomy in sciatica: a randomized controlled trial. The spine journal: official journal of the North American Spine Society 2015;15(5):857–65.

[10] Lee GW, Jang SJ, Kim JD. The efficacy of epiduroscopic neural decompression with Ho:YAG laser ablation in lumbar spinal stenosis. European journal of orthopaedic surgery & traumatology: orthopedie traumatologie 2014;24(Suppl 1):S231–7.

[11] Ammar TA. Monochromatic infrared photo energy versus low level laser therapy in chronic low back pain. Journal of lasers in medical sciences 2015;6(4):157–61.

[12] Patel NV, Agarwal N, Mammis A, Danish SF. Frameless stereotactic magnetic resonance imaging-guided laser interstitial thermal therapy to perform bilateral

anterior cingulotomy for intractable pain: feasibility, technical aspects, and initial experience in 3 patients. Neurosurgery 2015;11(Suppl 2):17–25; discussion.

[13] Flickinger JC, Kondziolka D, Lunsford LD, Coffey RJ, Goodman ML, Shaw EG, Hudgins WR, Weiner R, Harsh GRt, Sneed PK, et al. A multi-institutional experience with stereotactic radiosurgery for solitary brain metastasis. International journal of radiation oncology, biology, physics 1994;28(4):797–802.

[14] Kondziolka D, Patel A, Lunsford LD, Kassam A, Flickinger JC. Stereotactic radiosurgery plus whole brain radiotherapy versus radiotherapy alone for patients with multiple brain metastases. International journal of radiation oncology, biology, physics 1999;45(2):427–34.

[15] Petrovich Z, Yu C, Giannotta SL, O'Day S, Apuzzo ML. Survival and pattern of failure in brain metastasis treated with stereotactic gamma knife radiosurgery. Journal of neurosurgery 2002;97(5 Suppl):499–506.

[16] Minniti G, Clarke E, Lanzetta G, Osti MF, Trasimeni G, Bozzao A, Romano A, Enrici RM. Stereotactic radiosurgery for brain metastases: analysis of outcome and risk of brain radionecrosis. Radiation oncology (London, England) 2011;6:48.

[17] Jagannathan J, Petit JH, Balsara K, Hudes R, Chin LS. Long-term survival after gamma knife radiosurgery for primary and metastatic brain tumors. American journal of clinical oncology 2004;27(5):441–4.

[18] Kano H, Shuto T, Iwai Y, Sheehan J, Yamamoto M, McBride HL, Sato M, Serizawa T, Yomo S, Moriki A, Kohda Y, Young B, Suzuki S, Kenai H, Duma C, Kikuchi Y, Mathieu D, Akabane A, Nagano O, Kondziolka D, Lunsford LD. Stereotactic radiosurgery for intracranial hemangioblastomas: a retrospective international outcome study. Journal of neurosurgery 2015;122(6):1469–78.

[19] Carpentier A, McNichols RJ, Stafford RJ, Guichard JP, Reizine D, Delaloge S, Vicaut E, Payen D, Gowda A, George B. Laser thermal therapy: real-time MRI-guided and computer-controlled procedures for metastatic brain tumors. Lasers in surgery and medicine 2011;43(10):943–50.

[20] Hawasli AH, Bagade S, Shimony JS, Miller-Thomas M, Leuthardt EC. Magnetic resonance imaging-guided focused laser interstitial thermal therapy for intracranial lesions: single-institution series. Neurosurgery 2013;73(6):1007–17.

[21] Rao MS, Hargreaves EL, Khan AJ, Haffty BG, Danish SF. Magnetic resonance-guided laser ablation improves local control for postradiosurgery recurrence and/or radiation necrosis. Neurosurgery 2014;74(6):658–67; discussion 67.

[22] Sharma M, Balasubramanian S, Silva D, Barnett GH, Mohammadi AM. Laser interstitial thermal therapy in the management of brain metastasis and radiation necrosis after radiosurgery: An overview. *Expert review of neurotherapeutics*. 2016;16(2):223–232.

[23] Fabiano AJ, Alberico RA. Laser-interstitial thermal therapy for refractory cerebral edema from post-radiosurgery metastasis. World neurosurgery 2014;81(3–4):652.e1–4.

[24] Rahmathulla G, Recinos PF, Valerio JE, Chao S, Barnett GH. Laser interstitial thermal therapy for focal cerebral radiation necrosis: a case report and literature review. Stereotactic and functional neurosurgery 2012;90(3):192–200.

[25] Ryan RW, Spetzler RF, Preul MC. Aura of technology and the cutting edge: a history of lasers in neurosurgery. Neurosurgical focus 2009;27(3):E6.

[26] Bown SG. Phototherapy in tumors. World journal of surgery 1983;7(6):700–9.

[27] Chen L, Wansapura JP, Heit G, Butts K. Study of laser ablation in the in vivo rabbit brain with MR thermometry. Journal of magnetic resonance imaging: JMRI 2002;16(2): 147–52.

[28] Cheng MK, McKean J, Boisvert D, Tulip J, Mielke BW. Effects of photoradiation therapy on normal rat brain. Neurosurgery 1984;15(6):804–10.

[29] Elias Z, Powers SK, Atstupenas E, Brown JT. Hyperthermia from interstitial laser irradiation in normal rat brain. Lasers in surgery and medicine 1987;7(4):370–5.

[30] Tracz RA, Wyman DR, Little PB, Towner RA, Stewart WA, Schatz SW, Wilson BC, Pennock PW, Janzen EG. Comparison of magnetic resonance images and the histopathological findings of lesions induced by interstitial laser photocoagulation in the brain. Lasers in surgery and medicine 1993;13(1):45–54.

[31] De Poorter J. Noninvasive MRI thermometry with the proton resonance frequency method: study of susceptibility effects. Magnetic resonance in medicine 1995;34(3):359–67.

[32] Rosomoff HL, Carroll F. Reaction of neoplasm and brain to laser. Archives of neurology 1966;14(2):143–8.

[33] Winter A, Laing J, Paglione R, Sterzer F. Microwave hyperthermia for brain tumors. Neurosurgery 1985;17(3):387–99.

[34] Britt RH, Pounds DW, Lyons BE. Feasibility of treating malignant brain tumors with focused ultrasound. Progress in experimental tumor research 1984;28:232–45.

[35] Roberts DW, Coughlin CT, Wong TZ, Fratkin JD, Douple EB, Strohbehn JW. Interstitial hyperthermia and iridium brachytherapy in treatment of malignant glioma. A phase I clinical trial. Journal of neurosurgery 1986;64(4):581–7.

[36] Schulze PC, Vitzthum HE, Goldammer A, Schneider JP, Schober R. Laser-induced thermotherapy of neoplastic lesions in the brain—underlying tissue alterations, MRI-monitoring and clinical applicability. Acta neurochirurgica 2004;146(8):803–12.

[37] Svaasand LO, Ellingsen R. Optical properties of human brain. Photochemistry and photobiology 1983;38(3):293–9.

[38] Takizawa T. The carbon dioxide laser surgical unit as an instrument for surgery of brain tumours—its advantages and disadvantages. Neurosurgical review 1984;7(2–3):135–44.

[39] Jaunich M, Raje S, Kim K, Mitra K, Guo Z. Bio-heat transfer analysis during short pulse laser irradiation of tissues. International Journal of Heat and Mass Transfer 2008;51(23–24):5511–21.

[40] Goldberg SN, Gazelle GS, Mueller PR. Thermal ablation therapy for focal malignancy: a unified approach to underlying principles, techniques, and diagnostic imaging guidance. AJR. American journal of roentgenology 2000;174(2):323–31.

[41] Seegenschmiedt MH, Brady LW, Sauer R. Interstitial thermoradiotherapy: review on technical and clinical aspects. American journal of clinical oncology 1990;13(4):352–63.

[42] Goldberg SN, Gazelle GS, Halpern EF, Rittman WJ, Mueller PR, Rosenthal DI. Radiofrequency tissue ablation: importance of local temperature along the electrode tip exposure in determining lesion shape and size. Academic radiology 1996;3(3):212–8.

[43] Larson TR, Bostwick DG, Corica A. Temperature-correlated histopathologic changes following microwave thermoablation of obstructive tissue in patients with benign prostatic hyperplasia. Urology 1996;47(4):463–9.

[44] Thomsen S. Pathologic analysis of photothermal and photomechanical effects of laser-tissue interactions. Photochemistry and photobiology 1991;53(6):825–35.

[45] Mohammadi AM, Schroeder JL. Laser interstitial thermal therapy in treatment of brain tumors—the NeuroBlate System. Expert review of medical devices 2014;11(2):109–19.

[46] Laidler KJ. The development of the Arrhenius equation. Journal of chemical education 1984;61(6):494.

[47] Schober R, Bettag M, Sabel M, Ulrich F, Hessel S. Fine structure of zonal changes in experimental Nd:YAG laser-induced interstitial hyperthermia. Lasers in surgery and medicine 1993;13(2):234–41.

[48] Schulze PC, Adams V, Busert C, Bettag M, Kahn T, Schober R. Effects of laser-induced thermotherapy (LITT) on proliferation and apoptosis of glioma cells in rat brain transplantation tumors. Lasers in surgery and medicine 2002;30(3):227–32.

[49] Fabiano AJ, Qiu J. Delayed failure of laser-induced interstitial thermotherapy for postradiosurgery brain metastases. World neurosurgery 2014;82(3–4):e559–63.

[50] Hawasli AH, Ray WZ, Murphy RK, Dacey RG, Jr., Leuthardt EC. Magnetic resonance imaging-guided focused laser interstitial thermal therapy for subinsular metastatic adenocarcinoma: technical case report. Neurosurgery 2012;70(2 Suppl Operative):332–7; discussion 8.

[51] Murovic JA, Chang SD. The pathophysiology of cerebral radiation necrosis and the role of laser interstitial thermal therapy. World neurosurgery 2015;83(1):23–6.

[52] Berns MW, Coffey J, Wile AG. Laser photoradiation therapy of cancer: possible role of hyperthermia. Lasers in surgery and medicine 1984;4(1):87–92.

[53] Dougherty TJ, Grindey GB, Fiel R, Weishaupt KR, Boyle DG. Photoradiation therapy. II. Cure of animal tumors with hematoporphyrin and light. Journal of the national cancer institute 1975;55(1):115–21.

[54] Henderson BW, Waldow SM, Mang TS, Potter WR, Malone PB, Dougherty TJ. Tumor destruction and kinetics of tumor cell death in two experimental mouse tumors following photodynamic therapy. Cancer research 1985;45(2):572–6.

[55] Gomer CJ, Rucker N, Razum NJ, Murphree AL. In vitro and in vivo light dose rate effects related to hematoporphyrin derivative photodynamic therapy. Cancer research 1985;45(5):1973–7.

[56] Marchesini R, Andreola S, Emanuelli H, Melloni E, Schiroli A, Spinelli P, Fava G. Temperature rise in biological tissue during Nd:YAG laser irradiation. Lasers in surgery and medicine 1985;5(2):75–82.

[57] Rieke V, Butts Pauly K. MR thermometry. Journal of magnetic resonance imaging. JMRI 2008;27(2):376–90.

[58] McNichols RJ, Gowda A, Kangasniemi M, Bankson JA, Price RE, Hazle JD. MR thermometry-based feedback control of laser interstitial thermal therapy at 980 nm. Lasers in surgery and medicine 2004;34(1):48–55.

[59] Norred SE, Johnson JA. Magnetic resonance-guided laser induced thermal therapy for glioblastoma multiforme: a review. BioMed research international 2014;2014:761312.

[60] Rahmathulla G, Recinos PF, Kamian K, Mohammadi AM, Ahluwalia MS, Barnett GH. MRI-guided laser interstitial thermal therapy in neuro-oncology: a review of its current clinical applications. Oncology 2014;87(2):67–82.

[61] Stafford RJ, Fuentes D, Elliott AA, Weinberg JS, Ahrar K. Laser-induced thermal therapy for tumor ablation. Critical reviews in biomedical engineering 2010;38(1):79–100.

[62] Anvari B, Tanenbaum BS, Hoffman W, Said S, Milner TE, Liaw LH, Nelson JS. Nd:YAG laser irradiation in conjunction with cryogen spray cooling induces deep and spatially selective photocoagulation in animal models. Physics in medicine and biology 1997;42(2):265–82.

[63] Jethwa PR, Barrese JC, Gowda A, Shetty A, Danish SF. Magnetic resonance thermometry-guided laser-induced thermal therapy for intracranial neoplasms: initial experience. Neurosurgery 2012;71(1 Suppl Operative):133–44; 44–5.

[64] Kangasniemi M, McNichols RJ, Bankson JA, Gowda A, Price RE, Hazle JD. Thermal therapy of canine cerebral tumors using a 980 nm diode laser with MR temperature-sensitive imaging feedback. Lasers in surgery and medicine 2004;35(1):41–50.

[65] Yung JP, Shetty A, Elliott A, Weinberg JS, McNichols RJ, Gowda A, Hazle JD, Stafford RJ. Quantitative comparison of thermal dose models in normal canine brain. Medical physics 2010;37(10):5313–21.

[66] Day ES, Thompson PA, Zhang L, Lewinski NA, Ahmed N, Drezek RA, Blaney SM, West JL. Nanoshell-mediated photothermal therapy improves survival in a murine glioma model. Journal of neuro-oncology 2011;104(1):55–63.

[67] Earle KM, Carpenter S, Roessmann U, Ross MA, Hayes JR, Zeitler E. Central nervous system effects of laser radiation. Federation proceedings 1965;24(Suppl 14):129.

[68] Fine S, Klein E, Nowak W, Scott RE, Laor Y, Simpson L, Crissey J, Donoghue J, Derr VE. Interaction of laser radiation with biologic systems. I. Studies on interaction with tissues. Federation proceedings 1965;24(Suppl 14):35–47.

[69] Jordan A, Scholz R, Maier-Hauff K, van Landeghem FK, Waldoefner N, Teichgraeber U, Pinkernelle J, Bruhn H, Neumann F, Thiesen B, von Deimling A, Felix R. The effect of thermotherapy using magnetic nanoparticles on rat malignant glioma. Journal of neuro-oncology 2006;78(1):7–14.

[70] Ostrom QT, Bauchet L, Davis FG, Deltour I, Fisher JL, Langer CE, Pekmezci M, Schwartzbaum JA, Turner MC, Walsh KM, Wrensch MR, Barnholtz-Sloan JS. The epidemiology of glioma in adults: a "state of the science" review. Neuro-oncology 2014;16(7):896–913.

[71] Stupp R, Hegi ME, Mason WP, van den Bent MJ, Taphoorn MJ, Janzer RC, Ludwin SK, Allgeier A, Fisher B, Belanger K, Hau P, Brandes AA, Gijtenbeek J, Marosi C, Vecht CJ, Mokhtari K, Wesseling P, Villa S, Eisenhauer E, Gorlia T, Weller M, Lacombe D, Cairncross JG, Mirimanoff RO. Effects of radiotherapy with concomitant and adjuvant temozolomide versus radiotherapy alone on survival in glioblastoma in a randomised phase III study: 5-year analysis of the EORTC-NCIC trial. The Lancet. Oncology 2009;10(5):459–66.

[72] Stupp R, Mason WP, van den Bent MJ, Weller M, Fisher B, Taphoorn MJ, Belanger K, Brandes AA, Marosi C, Bogdahn U, Curschmann J, Janzer RC, Ludwin SK, Gorlia T, Allgeier A, Lacombe D, Cairncross JG, Eisenhauer E, Mirimanoff RO. Radiotherapy plus concomitant and adjuvant temozolomide for glioblastoma. The New England journal of medicine 2005;352(10):987–96.

[73] Oppenlander ME, Wolf AB, Snyder LA, Bina R, Wilson JR, Coons SW, Ashby LS, Brachman D, Nakaji P, Porter RW, Smith KA, Spetzler RF, Sanai N. An extent of resection threshold for recurrent glioblastoma and its risk for neurological morbidity. Journal of neurosurgery 2014;120(4):846–53.

[74] Hervey-Jumper SL, Berger MS. Reoperation for recurrent high-grade glioma: a current perspective of the literature. Neurosurgery 2014;75(5):491–9; discussion 8–9.

[75] Chaichana KL, Zadnik P, Weingart JD, Olivi A, Gallia GL, Blakeley J, Lim M, Brem H, Quinones-Hinojosa A. Multiple resections for patients with glioblastoma: prolonging survival. Journal of neurosurgery 2013;118(4):812–20.

[76] Barbagallo GM, Jenkinson MD, Brodbelt AR. 'Recurrent' glioblastoma multiforme, when should we reoperate? British journal of neurosurgery 2008;22(3):452–5.

[77] Ortega A, Sarmiento JM, Ly D, Nuno M, Mukherjee D, Black KL, Patil CG. Multiple resections and survival of recurrent glioblastoma patients in the temozolomide era. Journal of clinical neuroscience: official journal of the Neurosurgical Society of Australasia 2016;24:105–11.

[78] Chang SM, Parney IF, McDermott M, Barker FG, 2nd, Schmidt MH, Huang W, Laws ER, Jr., Lillehei KO, Bernstein M, Brem H, Sloan AE, Berger M. Perioperative complications and neurological outcomes of first and second craniotomies among patients enrolled in the Glioma Outcome Project. Journal of neurosurgery 2003;98(6):1175–81.

[79] Moiyadi AV, Shetty PM. Surgery for recurrent malignant gliomas: feasibility and perioperative outcomes. Neurology India 2012;60(2):185–90.

[80] Hoover JM, Nwojo M, Puffer R, Mandrekar J, Meyer FB, Parney IF. Surgical outcomes in recurrent glioma: clinical article. Journal of neurosurgery 2013;118(6):1224–31.

[81] Tsao MN, Mehta MP, Whelan TJ, Morris DE, Hayman JA, Flickinger JC, Mills M, Rogers CL, Souhami L. The American Society for Therapeutic Radiology and Oncology (ASTRO) evidence-based review of the role of radiosurgery for malignant glioma. International journal of radiation oncology, biology, physics 2005;63(1):47–55.

[82] Chan TA, Weingart JD, Parisi M, Hughes MA, Olivi A, Borzillary S, Alahakone D, Detorie NA, Wharam MD, Kleinberg L. Treatment of recurrent glioblastoma multiforme with GliaSite brachytherapy. International journal of radiation oncology, biology, physics 2005;62(4):1133–9.

[83] Anzai Y, Lufkin R, DeSalles A, Hamilton DR, Farahani K, Black KL. Preliminary experience with MR-guided thermal ablation of brain tumors. AJNR. American journal of neuroradiology 1995;16(1):39–48; discussion 9–52.

[84] Sakai T, Fujishima I, Sugiyama K, Ryu H, Uemura K. Interstitial laserthermia in neurosurgery. Journal of clinical laser medicine & surgery 1992;10(1):37–40.

[85] McDannold N. Quantitative MRI-based temperature mapping based on the proton resonant frequency shift: review of validation studies. International journal of hyperthermia: the official journal of European Society for Hyperthermic Oncology, North American Hyperthermia Group 2005;21(6):533–46.

[86] Leonardi MA, Lumenta CB. Stereotactic guided laser-induced interstitial thermotherapy (SLITT) in gliomas with intraoperative morphologic monitoring in an open MR: clinical expierence. Minimally invasive neurosurgery: MIN 2002;45(4):201–7.

[87] Kahn T, Bettag M, Ulrich F, Schwarzmaier HJ, Schober R, Furst G, Modder U. MRI-guided laser-induced interstitial thermotherapy of cerebral neoplasms. Journal of computer assisted tomography 1994;18(4):519–32.

[88] Tovar-Spinoza Z, Carter D, Ferrone D, Eksioglu Y, Huckins S. The use of MRI-guided laser-induced thermal ablation for epilepsy. Child's nervous system: ChNS: official journal of the International Society for Pediatric Neurosurgery 2013;29(11):2089–94.

[89] Sundararajan SH, Belani P, Danish S, Keller I. Early MRI characteristics after MRI-guided laser-assisted cingulotomy for intractable pain control. AJNR. American journal of neuroradiology 2015;36(7):1283–7.

[90] Sugiyama K, Sakai T, Fujishima I, Ryu H, Uemura K, Yokoyama T. Stereotactic interstitial laser-hyperthermia using Nd-YAG laser. Stereotactic and functional neurosurgery 1990;54–55:501–5.

[91] Roux FX, Merienne L, Fallet-Bianco C, Beuvon F, Devaux B, Leriche B, Cioloca C. Stereotaxic laser interstitial thermotherapy. A new alternative in the therapeutic management of some brain tumors. Neuro-Chirurgie 1992;38(4):238–44.

[92] Ascher PW, Justich E, Schrottner O. A new surgical but less invasive treatment of central brain tumours Preliminary report. Acta neurochirurgica. Supplementum 1991;52:78–80.

[93] Bettag M, Ulrich F, Schober R, Furst G, Langen KJ, Sabel M, Kiwit JC. Stereotactic laser therapy in cerebral gliomas. Acta neurochirurgica. Supplementum 1991;52:81–3.

[94] Leonardi MA, Lumenta CB, Gumprecht HK, von Einsiedel GH, Wilhelm T. Stereotactic guided laser-induced interstitial thermotherapy (SLITT) in gliomas with intraoperative morphologic monitoring in an open MR-unit. Minimally invasive neurosurgery: MIN 2001;44(1):37–42.

[95] Schwarzmaier HJ, Eickmeyer F, von Tempelhoff W, Fiedler VU, Niehoff H, Ulrich SD, Ulrich F. MR-guided laser irradiation of recurrent glioblastomas. Journal of magnetic resonance imaging: JMRI 2005;22(6):799–803.

[96] Carpentier A, Chauvet D, Reina V, Beccaria K, Leclerq D, McNichols RJ, Gowda A, Cornu P, Delattre JY. MR-guided laser-induced thermal therapy (LITT) for recurrent glioblastomas. Lasers in surgery and medicine 2012;44(5):361–8.

[97] Mohammadi AM, Hawasli AH, Rodriguez A, Schroeder JL, Laxton AW, Elson P, Tatter SB, Barnett GH, Leuthardt EC. The role of laser interstitial thermal therapy in enhancing progression-free survival of difficult-to-access high-grade gliomas: a multicenter study. Cancer medicine 2014;3(4):971–9.

[98] Patel P, Patel NV, Danish SF. Intracranial MR-guided laser-induced thermal therapy: single-center experience with the Visualase thermal therapy system. Journal of neurosurgery 2016:1–8.

[99] Metcalfe SE, Grant R. Biopsy versus resection for malignant glioma. The Cochrane database of systematic reviews 2001(3):Cd002034.

[100] Mintz A, Perry J, Spithoff K, Chambers A, Laperriere N. Management of single brain metastasis: a practice guideline. Current oncology (Toronto, Ont.) 2007;14(4):131–43.

[101] Colaco R, Martin P, Chiang V. Evolution of multidisciplinary brain metastasis management: case study and literature review. The Yale journal of biology and medicine 2015;88(2):157–65.

[102] Nayak L, Lee EQ, Wen PY. Epidemiology of brain metastases. Current oncology reports 2012;14(1):48–54.

[103] Barnholtz-Sloan JS, Sloan AE, Davis FG, Vigneau FD, Lai P, Sawaya RE. Incidence proportions of brain metastases in patients diagnosed (1973 to 2001) in the Metropolitan Detroit Cancer Surveillance System. Journal of clinical oncology: official journal of the American Society of Clinical Oncology 2004;22(14):2865–72.

[104] Schouten LJ, Rutten J, Huveneers HA, Twijnstra A. Incidence of brain metastases in a cohort of patients with carcinoma of the breast, colon, kidney, and lung and melanoma. Cancer 2002;94(10):2698–705.

[105] Soon YY, Tham IW, Lim KH, Koh WY, Lu JJ. Surgery or radiosurgery plus whole brain radiotherapy versus surgery or radiosurgery alone for brain metastases. The Cochrane database of systematic reviews 2014;3:Cd009454.

[106] Greto D, Scoccianti S, Compagnucci A, Arilli C, Casati M, Francolini G, Cecchini S, Loi M, Desideri I, Bordi L, Bono P, Bonomo P, Meattini I, Detti B, Livi L. Gamma Knife radiosurgery in the management of single and multiple brain metastases. Clinical neurology and neurosurgery 2015;141:43–7.

[107] Powell JW, Chung CT, Shah HR, Canute GW, Hodge CJ, Bassano DA, Liu L, Mitchell L, Hahn SS. Gamma Knife surgery in the management of radioresistant brain metastases in high-risk patients with melanoma, renal cell carcinoma, and sarcoma. Journal of neurosurgery 2008;109(Suppl):122–8.

[108] Yamamoto M, Hara M, Ide M, Ono Y, Jimbo M, Saito I. Radiation-related adverse effects observed on neuro-imaging several years after radiosurgery for cerebral arteriovenous malformations. Surgical neurology 1998;49(4):385–97; discussion 97–8.

[109] Chin LS, Ma L, DiBiase S. Radiation necrosis following gamma knife surgery: a case-controlled comparison of treatment parameters and long-term clinical follow up. Journal of neurosurgery 2001;94(6):899–904.

[110] Ganz JC, Reda WA, Abdelkarim K. Adverse radiation effects after Gamma Knife Surgery in relation to dose and volume. Acta neurochirurgica 2009;151(1):9–19.

[111] Sneed PK, Mendez J, Vemer-van den Hoek JG, Seymour ZA, Ma L, Molinaro AM, Fogh SE, Nakamura JL, McDermott MW. Adverse radiation effect after stereotactic radiosurgery for brain metastases: incidence, time course, and risk factors. Journal of neurosurgery 2015;123(2):373–86.

[112] Kohutek ZA, Yamada Y, Chan TA, Brennan CW, Tabar V, Gutin PH, Yang TJ, Rosenblum MK, Ballangrud A, Young RJ, Zhang Z, Beal K. Long-term risk of radionecrosis and imaging changes after stereotactic radiosurgery for brain metastases. Journal of neuro-oncology 2015;125(1):149–56.

[113] Chuang MT, Liu YS, Tsai YS, Chen YC, Wang CK. Differentiating radiation-induced necrosis from recurrent brain tumor using MR perfusion and spectroscopy: a meta-analysis. PloS one 2016;11(1):e0141438.

[114] Cicone F, Minniti G, Romano A, Papa A, Scaringi C, Tavanti F, Bozzao A, Maurizi Enrici R, Scopinaro F. Accuracy of F-DOPA PET and perfusion-MRI for differentiating radionecrotic from progressive brain metastases after radiosurgery. European journal of nuclear medicine and molecular imaging 2015;42(1):103–11.

[115] Terakawa Y, Tsuyuguchi N, Iwai Y, Yamanaka K, Higashiyama S, Takami T, Ohata K. Diagnostic accuracy of 11C-methionine PET for differentiation of recurrent brain tumors from radiation necrosis after radiotherapy. Journal of nuclear medicine: official publication, Society of Nuclear Medicine 2008;49(5):694–9.

[116] Shah AH, Snelling B, Bregy A, Patel PR, Tememe D, Bhatia R, Sklar E, Komotar RJ. Discriminating radiation necrosis from tumor progression in gliomas: a systematic review what is the best imaging modality? Journal of neuro-oncology 2013;112(2):141–52.

[117] Shaw PJ, Bates D. Conservative treatment of delayed cerebral radiation necrosis. Journal of neurology, neurosurgery, and psychiatry 1984;47(12):1338–41.

[118] Kohshi K, Imada H, Nomoto S, Yamaguchi R, Abe H, Yamamoto H. Successful treatment of radiation-induced brain necrosis by hyperbaric oxygen therapy. Journal of the neurological sciences 2003;209(1–2):115–7.

[119] Levin VA, Bidaut L, Hou P, Kumar AJ, Wefel JS, Bekele BN, Grewal J, Prabhu S, Loghin M, Gilbert MR, Jackson EF. Randomized double-blind placebo-controlled trial of bevacizumab therapy for radiation necrosis of the central nervous system. International journal of radiation oncology, biology, physics 2011;79(5):1487–95.

[120] Wong ET, Huberman M, Lu XQ, Mahadevan A. Bevacizumab reverses cerebral radiation necrosis. Journal of clinical oncology: official journal of the American Society of Clinical Oncology 2008;26(34):5649–50.

[121] Gonzalez J, Kumar AJ, Conrad CA, Levin VA. Effect of bevacizumab on radiation necrosis of the brain. International journal of radiation oncology, biology, physics 2007;67(2):323–6.

[122] Liu AK, Macy ME, Foreman NK. Bevacizumab as therapy for radiation necrosis in four children with pontine gliomas. International journal of radiation oncology, biology, physics 2009;75(4):1148–54.

[123] Matuschek C, Bolke E, Nawatny J, Hoffmann TK, Peiper M, Orth K, Gerber PA, Rusnak E, Lammering G, Budach W. Bevacizumab as a treatment option for radiation-induced cerebral necrosis. Strahlentherapie und Onkologie: Organ der Deutschen Rontgengesellschaft ... [et al] 2011;187(2):135–9.

[124] Glantz MJ, Burger PC, Friedman AH, Radtke RA, Massey EW, Schold SC, Jr. Treatment of radiation-induced nervous system injury with heparin and warfarin. Neurology 1994;44(11):2020–7.

[125] Parvez K, Parvez A, Zadeh G. The diagnosis and treatment of pseudoprogression, radiation necrosis and brain tumor recurrence. International journal of molecular sciences 2014;15(7):11832–46.

[126] Tobler WD, Sawaya R, Tew JM, Jr. Successful laser-assisted excision of a metastatic midbrain tumor. Neurosurgery 1986;18(6):795–7.

[127] Banerjee C, Snelling B, Berger MH, Shah A, Ivan ME, Komotar RJ. The role of magnetic resonance-guided laser ablation in neurooncology. British journal of neurosurgery 2015;29(2):192–6.

[128] Paek SH, Audu PB, Sperling MR, Cho J, Andrews DW. Reevaluation of surgery for the treatment of brain metastases: review of 208 patients with single or multiple brain metastases treated at one institution with modern neurosurgical techniques. Neurosurgery 2005;56(5):1021–34; discussion 34.

[129] Vadivelu S, Schulder M. MRI-guided interstitial laser therapy of brain tumours. In: Jolesz FA, ed. Intraoperative imaging and image-guided therapy. New York, NY, 2014.

[130] Daut RL, Cleeland CS. The prevalence and severity of pain in cancer. Cancer 1982;50(9): 1913–8.

[131] Bentley JN, Viswanathan A, Rosenberg WS, Patil PG. Treatment of medically refractory cancer pain with a combination of intrathecal neuromodulation and neurosurgical ablation: case series and literature review. Pain medicine (Malden, Mass.) 2014;15(9): 1488–95.

[132] Naja Z, Al-Tannir M, Ziade F, Daher M. Management of cancer pain: different intervention techniques. Le Journal medical libanais. The Lebanese medical journal 2008;56(2):100–4.

[133] Harsh V, Viswanathan A. Surgical/radiological interventions for cancer pain. Current pain and headache reports 2013;17(5):331.

[134] Christo PJ, Mazloomdoost D. Interventional pain treatments for cancer pain. Annals of the New York Academy of Sciences 2008;1138:299–328.

[135] Sloan PA. Neuraxial pain relief for intractable cancer pain. Current pain and headache reports 2007;11(4):283–9.

[136] Viswanathan A, Harsh V, Pereira EA, Aziz TZ. Cingulotomy for medically refractory cancer pain. Neurosurgical focus 2013;35(3):E1.

[137] Sharma M, Shaw A, Deogaonkar M. Surgical options for complex craniofacial pain. Neurosurgery clinics of North America 2014;25(4):763–75.

[138] Rasche D, Rinaldi PC, Young RF, Tronnier VM. Deep brain stimulation for the treatment of various chronic pain syndromes. Neurosurgical focus 2006;21(6):E8.

[139] Jobst BC. Consensus over individualism: validation of the ILAE definition for drug resistant epilepsy. Epilepsy currents/American Epilepsy Society 2015;15(4):172–3.

[140] Berg AT, Shinnar S, Levy SR, Testa FM, Smith-Rapaport S, Beckerman B. Early development of intractable epilepsy in children: a prospective study. Neurology 2001;56(11):1445–52.

[141] Wasade VS, Elisevich K, Tahir R, Smith B, Schultz L, Schwalb J, Spanaki-Varelas M. Long-term seizure and psychosocial outcomes after resective surgery for intractable epilepsy. Epilepsy & behavior E&B 2015;43:122–7.

[142] Tellez-Zenteno JF, Dhar R, Wiebe S. Long-term seizure outcomes following epilepsy surgery: a systematic review and meta-analysis. Brain: a journal of neurology 2005;128(Pt 5):1188–98.

[143] Spencer S, Huh L. Outcomes of epilepsy surgery in adults and children. The Lancet. Neurology 2008;7(6):525–37.

[144] Tebo CC, Evins AI, Christos PJ, Kwon J, Schwartz TH. Evolution of cranial epilepsy surgery complication rates: a 32-year systematic review and meta-analysis. Journal of neurosurgery 2014;120(6):1415–27.

[145] Bower RS, Wirrell EC, Eckel LJ, Wong-Kisiel LC, Nickels KC, Wetjen NM. Repeat resective surgery in complex pediatric refractory epilepsy: lessons learned. Journal of neurosurgery. Pediatrics 2015;16(1):94–100.

[146] Curry DJ, Gowda A, McNichols RJ, Wilfong AA. MR-guided stereotactic laser ablation of epileptogenic foci in children. Epilepsy & behavior: E&B 2012;24(4):408–14.

[147] Wellmer J, Kopitzki K, Voges J. Lesion focused stereotactic thermo-coagulation of focal cortical dysplasia IIB: a new approach to epilepsy surgery? Seizure 2014;23(6):475–8.

[148] Gonzalez-Martinez J, Vadera S, Mullin J, Enatsu R, Alexopoulos AV, Patwardhan R, Bingaman W, Najm I. Robot-assisted stereotactic laser ablation in medically intracta-

ble epilepsy: operative technique. Neurosurgery 2014;10(Suppl 2):167–72; discussion 72–3.

[149] Esquenazi Y, Kalamangalam GP, Slater JD, Knowlton RC, Friedman E, Morris SA, Shetty A, Gowda A, Tandon N. Stereotactic laser ablation of epileptogenic periventricular nodular heterotopia. Epilepsy research 2014;108(3):547–54.

[150] Lewis EC, Weil AG, Duchowny M, Bhatia S, Ragheb J, Miller I. MR-guided laser interstitial thermal therapy for pediatric drug-resistant lesional epilepsy. Epilepsia 2015;56(10):1590–8.

Chapter 13

Interstitial Chemotherapy for Malignant Gliomas

Ke Sai, Shu-xin Sun and Zhong-ping Chen

Additional information is available at the end of the chapter

http://dx.doi.org/10.5772/62838

Abstract

Glioma is the most common primary tumor in the central nervous system (CNS). Even with aggressive treatments, gliomas remain as one of the most devastating tumors. Chemotherapy through oral administration of temozolomide (TMZ) is currently the standard regimen for malignant gliomas. However, the systemic toxicity and drug resistance are frequently observed in glioma patients. In order to improve the efficacy and minimize side effects, multiple strategies have been developed. Interstitial chemotherapy is a promising one. By directly delivering chemotherapeutic agents in tumor bed, interstitial chemotherapy bypasses the blood–brain barrier (BBB) and therefore achieves a higher concentration with less systemic exposure. In this chapter, we will have a thorough review on the development and the application of interstitial chemotherapy in gliomas, with the focus on the biomaterial-based and convection-enhanced delivery system. In addition, the future of interstitial chemotherapy is also be shortly discussed.

Keywords: malignant gliomas, local therapy, surgery, adjuvant chemotherapy, temozolomide, Gliadel waffer

1. Introduction

Malignant gliomas account for more than 50% of primary central nervous system (CNS) tumors and are among the most formidable cancers in human beings (1). Although aggressive debulking surgery followed by radiation and chemotherapy is the mainstay for malignant gliomas, the prognosis of malignant gliomas remains far from satisfactory. The 5-year overall survival (OS) is as low as 9.8% for patients with glioblastoma multiforme (GBM), a malignancy classified as grade IV by the world health organization (WHO) (2). The recurrence seems to be inevitable for malignant gliomas. Most patients with recurred GBM will die within 6 months even with salvage treatments.

The exact mechanisms underlying the intractability of malignant gliomas have not been fully understood, but the inherent resistance and the sheltering environment of brain have been proposed to protect the disease from conventional treatments. First of all, the infiltrative growth pattern of glioma cells makes the complete surgical resection almost impossible. Second, the existence of blood–brain barrier (BBB), which is tightly formed by capillary endothelial cells together with astrocytes, restricts the entry of most systemically administered chemotherapeutic agents into the tumor parenchyma (3). Third, the inherent and acquired insensitivity to radiation and chemotherapy through the disturbance of signaling pathway in glioma cells results in the resistance to current therapies (4). Because gliomas seldom metastasize outside the CNS and usually recur within 1–2 cm from the original tumor site, it is reasonable to expect the efficacy of directly delivering potent chemotherapeutic drugs into the tumor mass and its adjacent area. By this means, not only a higher drug concentration around the tumor but also a minimal systemic toxicity can be achieved.

2. Early experience

2.1. Topical application

Various methods have been attempted for locoregional therapy. The initial experience started with topical application. In 1963, Heppner and Diemath (5) treated brain tumor patients with local chemotherapy by placing gelatin sponges soaked with endoxan. Similarly, Ringkjob applied gelatin sponges filled with cytostatic agents including 5-fluorouracile (5-FU), methylene hydrazine, and thiophosphoramide to the resection cavity in patients with gliomas and brain metastases (6). Although the adverse effects were minimal in both studies, the clinical benefits were either hard to define or inappreciable. As a result, topical application of chemotherapeutics was gradually disregarded.

2.2. Direct injection

Direct injection is another early strategy to give local therapy. A subcutaneous reservoir (e.g., Ommaya reservoir) is implanted with its catheter into the resection cavity during surgery of brain tumors. Repeated injection of multiple chemotherapeutic agents can be done trough the reservoir postoperatively. Because direct injection is easy and repeatable, a number of studies have been done to explore the efficacy. In a Phase I/II trial, Boiardi et al. (7) implanted Ommaya reservoir in 12 patients with recurred malignant glioma. Two cycles of mitoxantrone were directly delivered into intratumoral cavity through Ommaya reservoir with or without systemic chemotherapy. The treatment was well tolerated in all patients. Either response or stable disease was found in 9 of 12 patients. A Japanese group investigated the histopathological changes after local chemotherapy via Ommaya reservoir (8). Massive coagulation necrosis surrounded by abundant reactive collagenous tissues, gliomesenchymal tissue, and infiltrating lymphocytes was found in the tumor bed, especially in areas around the catheter tip of Ommaya reservoir. This finding suggested the effectiveness of local chemotherapy. In

2008, Boiardi and colleagues (9) reported a non-randomized study with a large sample size. Two hundred and seventy-six patients with recurrent GBM were enrolled. Among them, 161 cases (Group A) were only treated systemically with oral temozolomide (TMZ), while 50 patients (Group B) were re-operated and received TMZ therapy postoperatively, and 50 cases (Group C) were treated with re-operation, postoperative TMZ, and locoregional therapy with mitoxantrone. The overall survival for Group C, B, and A was 27, 26, and 15.5 months, respectively ($p = 0.1$). The median survival after tumor recurrence was 16.8, 12, and 6.6 months for Group C, B, and A ($p = 0.001$), respectively. The authors therefore suggested that a second surgery combined with local chemotherapy would prolong the survival of patients with recurrent malignant gliomas.

In addition to chemotherapeutics, other agents have also been investigated for local therapy via direct injection. For example, Mamelak and colleagues (10) evaluated the safety and biodistribution of iodine-131 (^{131}I)-TM-601, a synthetic radioiodinated targeting peptide, for recurrent malignant gliomas in a Phase I trial. A total of 18 patients received a single dose of ^{131}I-TM-601 from one of the three dosing panels (0.25, 0.50, or 1.0 mg of TM-601). The agent was injected into the tumor cavity via a subcutaneous reservoir 2 weeks after surgery. The dosimetry analysis demonstrated a long-term retention of the agents around the injection site. The median half-life in the cavity margin was more than 50 h. No severe adverse effects were found during the delivery. Among 11 patients who completed the 180-day follow-up, two patients with recurrent GBM survived more than 30 months. The median survival was as long as 77.6 weeks in a subgroup of patients who received 0.5-mg dose of ^{131}I-TM-601. In another study, Prados and colleagues investigated the safety and efficacy of local gene therapy in recurrent GBM patients. Virus-producing cells (VPC) containing the herpes simplex virus thymidine-kinase (HSV-Tk) gene were injected into tumor cavity directly during debulking surgery and postoperatively via reservoir, followed by ganciclovir treatment (11). Among 30 patients enrolled in the study, 16 had severe adverse events such as infection, skin necrosis, and myelosuppression. The median survival of the series of 30 patients was 8.4 months. Six patients (20%) survived more than 1 year from the date of enrollment. The authors concluded that the direct delivery of gene therapy demonstrated some evidence of efficacy, while the improvement of procedures was needed to decrease the toxicity. Other studies also evaluated the feasibility to treat gliomas locally with immunotherapeutic agents such as autologous lymphocytes and immunomodulators (12, 13).

Although antecdotal reports of success achieved by direct injection of chemotherapeutics for glioma patients can be frequently found in literatures, no large-scale well-designed Phase III trial has been ever performed. In fact, local chemotherapy through direct injection has its own limitations. Firstly, repeated puncture and injection through the reservoir are associated with increased risk of intracranial infection and hemorrhage. Secondly, the injected drugs heterogeneously distribute in the tumor cavity through this approach. A sharp drug distribution gradient has been found, with an extremely high concentration around the tip of the catheter and a significant drop in the adjacent area. Therefore, the clinical exploration of local chemotherapy via direct injection dramatically declined.

3. Polymeric drug delivery

3.1. History

In order to overcome the drawbacks mentioned above and to achieve the local controlled release of chemotherapeutics, efforts have been made to develop delivery system with synthetic polymers. Early in 1970s, an ethylene vinylacetate copolymer (EVAc) was employed to generate a poriferous matrix and incorporate macromolecules such as chemotherapeutics (14). The impregnated agents are released from the matrix in a predictable and sustained style by diffusion. The rate of release depends on the physicochemical property of the agents, such as solubility, charge, and molecular weight. However, EVAc was restricted by the non-degradable nature and was therefore seldom used in neuro-oncology.

3.2. Carmustine implants

3.2.1. Background information

Various biodegradable polymers, such as the 1,3-bis(p-carboxyphenoxy) propane and sebacic acid (PCPP-SA), the fatty acid dimer sebacic acid (FAD-SA), and poly(lactide-co-glycolide) (PLGA) polymers, have been investigated in the last 3 decades. But until now, PCPP-SA is the most successful and widely used polymer for brain tumors. This compound has several advantages as matrix (15). Firstly, PCPP-SA is hydrophobic and can therefore protect the impregnated drug from inactivation by the surrounding aqueous environment. Secondly, the two-stage degradation of PCPP-SA matrix results in the gradual release of the content. At the first stage, the bonds between sebacic acid and sebacic acid or those between sebacic acid and CPP rapidly hydrolyzed, whereas the bonds between CPP and CPP take a longer time to degrade. This initial degradation is followed by a process of inward erosion which starts at the surface of the matrix and goes interiorly into the core. By modulating the ratio of sebacic acid and CPP in the matrix, the speed of degradation can be adjusted from hours to days as required. In addition, the breakdown of the PCPP-SA does not leave foreign body behind. Currently, the only US Food and Drug Administration (FDA) approved local chemotherapeutical agent for brain tumors, that is, Gliadel wafer, is composed by PCPP-SA as matrix and 1,3-bis(2-chloroethyl)-1-nitrosurea (carmustine or BCNU) as content.

BCNU is one of the most effective chemotherapeutics against malignant brain tumors at the time when the first local polymeric drug delivery system was being developed. BCNU is a classic alkylating and exerts its anti-tumor effect by forming inter-strand crosslink in DNA and subsequently inhibiting the replication and transcription of DNA in tumor cells (16). The highly lipid-soluble and nonpolar nature of BCNU makes it ideal for cancers in CNS because the agent has a good penetration of BBB. The concentration of BCNU in cerebral spinal fluid (CSF) is as high as 30% of that in plasma after intravenous injection. Clinical studies have demonstrated that systemic administration of BCNU is capable of prolonging the survival of patients with malignant gliomas (17). As a result, BCNU alone or combined with other agents has once been the most frequently used chemotherapy regimens for malignant gliomas. Although effective, intravenously administered BCNU is limited by its toxicities (18).

Gastrointestinal adverse effects such as nausea and vomiting can be observed shortly after infusion of BCNU and last for hours. Systemic BCNU therapy also causes myelosuppression. The peak of hematologic suppression may occur 1 month after BCNU administration, and it may take weeks for the recovery of bone marrow. In addition, pulmonary injury is another toxicity caused by BCNU treatment. Although rare, with the occurrence of approximately 5% of the patients, the BCNU-associated pneumonitis induces restrictive pulmonary disorders and subsequently progressive lung fibrosis, even after the withdrawal of the agent. Some patients terminate the chemotherapy due to the severe and irreversible toxicities. Based on its clinical efficacy against malignant brain tumors and the undesirable adverse effects, BCNU was impregnated into the PCPP-SA polymers. The BCNU wafers were explored for preclinical testing followed by clinical investigation.

3.2.2. *Preclinical evidence*

Preclinical exploration established the safety of the wafers in the CNS. Brem and colleagues (19) implanted the PCCP-SA polymers in the frontal lobe of rabbits and evaluated the biocompatibility. No neurological deficits or behavioral abnormalities suggestive of toxicity were observed. All the tested animals survived to the date of sacrifice. The histological analysis revealed that the inflammatory reaction from PCCP-SA was not significantly different from that in the controlled group implanted with Gelform, a widely used hemostatic material in neurosurgical operations. In primate models, the interstitial chemotherapy with BCNU polymers alone or combined with external beam radiation was found to be safe. The localized inflammatory response induced by BCNU wafers was well tolerated and manageable (20).

The *in vivo* experiments were also performed to evaluate the pharmacokinetics of BCNU wafers. In a rat model, the concentration of radiolabelled BCNU on the coronal sections of the brains was measured (21). BCNU delivered by polymers was at a concentration of 1 mM around the implanted site for the entire 30-day experiment. On day one, after implantation, BCNU penetrated the brain at a radius of 5 mm at a significant concentration, which was defined as 10% of the maximum concentration at the brain/polymer interface. Grossman and colleagues (22) investigated the intra-cerebral drug distribution in rabbits after the implantation of BCNU wafers. Radiolabeled BCNU was detected in 50% the area of the brain sections 3 days after BCNU-polymer implantation. On day seven, the concentration of BCNU was as high as 6 mM at the distance of 10 mm from the implantation site, which is far more than the active concentration of 14–16 μM against glioma cells *in vitro*. Because BCNU impregnated in polymers is released in a controlled manner, Fung and colleagues (23) calculated and compared the area under curve (AUC, concentration over time) of BCNU delivered by polymers to monkey brain and that administered by intravenous injection. In that study, polymeric BCNU delivery was estimated to achieve a 4-fold larger AUC in distant sites of brain and as high as 1200-fold more at the brain/polymer interface, in comparison with the conventional intravenous administration.

The efficacy of interstitial chemotherapy with BCNU was then tested in animal models. Tamargo and colleagues (24) demonstrated that local delivery of BCNU via polymers significantly prolonged the survival of rats intracranially implanted with 9 L gliosarcoma cells, compared with intraperitonal injection of the agent. The median survival of animals treated with BCNU polymers was 62 days, which was more than double that for rats treated with systemic administration. In another study with the rat orthotopic glioma model, BCNU-impregnated polymers were found to be superior to extend the lifespan of tumor-bearing rats, compared with the direct injection of BCNU into the tumor tissues (25).

3.2.3. Clinical trials

The preclinical evidence of the safety and the effectiveness of polymeric BCNU delivery rationalized the investigation of the clinical benefit of this therapy. Brem and colleagues reported a multicenter Phase I–II trial with BCNU polymers in recurrent glioma patients. In that study, twenty-one patients with recurrent malignant glioma were enrolled (26). Up to 8 BCNU polymer wafers with three escalating concentrations, that is, 1.93, 3.85, and 6.35%, were implanted in the tumor beds. The authors demonstrated that the local treatment with BCNU was well tolerated, and no systemic adverse effects related to the therapy were observed in all patients. The study also recorded the survival outcome. The average survival time was 65, 64, and 32 weeks for patients treated with the low, medium, and high concentration of BCNU, respectively. Based on the result of this study, the further efficacy evaluation employed polymeric wafers with the 3.85% dose of BCNU. However, it is worth noting that patients treated with the highest dose of BCNU in the study had the shortest survival, which was not due to the adverse effects. In fact, the small sample size and the difference in the grade of gliomas among three groups account for the paradox. The group treated with the highest dose composed a higher proportion of GBM than the other two groups. In another multicenter single-arm Phase I trial, Brem and colleagues (27) demonstrated that the placement of polymeric BCNU wafers followed by the external radiation was safe for newly diagnosed malignant gliomas.

The role of interstitial chemotherapy with BCNU in recurrent malignant glioma was explored in a multicenter, double-blinded, placebo-controlled trial of 222 patients from 27 centers (28). Biodegradable polymers with 3.85% BCNU or empty polymer wafers were randomly implanted in the tumor site after resection. One hundred and ten patients received BCNU polymers and 112 had placebo-wafers. The median survival of patients with BCNU wafers was 31 weeks, which is superior to 23 weeks for patients with empty polymers (HR = 0.67, $p = 0.006$, after accounting for the effects of prognostic factors). Among 212 patients, 145 (65.3%) had pathologically confirmed GBM. Significantly reduced mortality at 6 months was observed in GBM patients treated with BCNU wafers (44%, 32 of 72 cases) than those treated with placebo implants (64%, 47 of 73 patients, $p = 0.02$). As a result, FDA approved the use of 3.85% BCNU wafers (Gliadel®) for recurrent malignant gliomas. However, a recent meta-analysis from the Cochrane library doubted the benefit of BCNU wafers in the treatment of recurrent malignant gliomas (29). No statistical difference in survival was found between patients treated with Gliadel® and those with placebo (HR = 0.83, 95% CI 0.62–1.10, $p = 0.2$). The acquired chemoresistant by the point of the implantation of BCNU wafers and the treatment-associated changes, such as the radiation-induced gliosis, which may restrict the diffusion of BCNU around the resection cavity, was suggested to be responsible for the ineffectiveness.

Efforts have also been put to investigate the efficacy of BCNU wafers as the initial treatment for newly diagnosed malignant gliomas. Two phase III multicenter, double-blinded, placebo-controlled trials drew the similar conclusions. In 1997, Valtonen and colleagues (30) published the study that was prematurely terminated due to the unavailability of the wafers. Thirty-two patients (16 in each group) with newly diagnosed malignant gliomas were randomly assigned to the active treatment group with BCNU wafers or the placebo group at the time of the primary surgery. An improved survival was observed in active treatment group (58.1 weeks), compared with the placebo group (39.9 weeks) ($p = 0.012$). For the subset of patients with GBM, BCNU wafers also offered survival benefit compared with placebo (53.3 vs. 39.9 weeks, $p = 0.008$). To confirm this positive result, a Phase III clinical trial with a larger sample size of 240 patients with newly diagnosed malignant glioma was subsequently performed (31). Patients randomly received the placement of either BCNU or empty polymers in the tumor bed, followed by the postoperative external radiation therapy. Prognostic factors, such as age, sex, Karnofsky performance status (KPS), and tumor grading, were balanced. The BCNU-treatment group had a significantly longer median survival (13.9 months) than placebo group (11.6 months) ($p = 0.03$). The risk of death was reduced by 29% in the treatment group. More adverse events including symptomatic intracranial hypertension (9.1 vs. 1.7%) and CSF leaking (5 vs. 0.8%) were observed in patients treated with BCNU wafers. In 2003, FDA granted the approval of Gliadel® wafers to treat newly diagnosed malignant gliomas. Until now, Gliadel® wafers are commercially available in the United States, Canada, Europe, and Japan for the adjuvant treatment of newly diagnosed malignant gliomas.

A preclinical works have revealed that the anti-glioma effect positively related to the loading dose of BCNU in biodegradable polymers in primate models (32). The question of whether a higher concentration of BCNU for interstitial chemotherapy is safe and capable of prolonging the overall survival of glioma patients was raised. The New Approaches to Brain Tumor Therapy (NABTT) CNS Consortium therefore investigated the safety of polymer wafers with higher concentrations of BCNU in a dose escalation trial (33). Forty-four patients with malignant gliomas were treated with polymer wafers containing BCNU at escalating doses of 6.5, 10, 14.5, 20, and 28%, respectively. The authors demonstrated that BCNU-impregnated wafers with a higher concentration of up to 20%, which was more than five times the dose of commercially available Gliadel®, were safe. The median OS of the patients after the placement of BCNU wafers was 251 days. Although further large-scale trials were suggested to explore the efficacy of high-dose BCNU wafers, the group has not initiated any of the studies. Recently, we evaluated the safety of high-dose BCNU-loaded biodegradable wafers in Chinese patients with recurrent malignant glioma (34). The wafers we used are comprised of poly (lactide-co-glycolide) (PLGA) containing 10% BCNU. PLGA is also a FDA approved material for drug delivery, which has more tunable mechanical properties and can be stored at 2–10°C in comparison with PCCP used in Gliadel®. In addition, PLGA degrades directly into water and carbon dioxide and does not need clearance in liver or kidney. The dosage of 10% BCNU is 2.5 times that of Gliadel®. Our study demonstrated that 12 implants with 240 mg

BCNU was well tolerated in tested patients. No dose-limiting toxicity was found. The median survival of this cohort of patients was 322 days. The 6-months, 1-year, and 2-year survival rates were 66.7, 40, and 13.3%, respectively. A registered double-blinded randomized Phase III trial is on-going to investigate the efficacy of the high-dose BCNU-impregnated PLGA wafers for recurrent malignant gliomas.

In 2005, Stupp and colleagues (35) published the milestone Phase III trial on the efficacy of adjuvant chemotherapy with temozolomide (TMZ) for GBMs. TMZ is a second generation alkylating agent, which can be administered orally. The Stupp regimen, that is, the concurrent chemoradiation with TMZ followed by six cycles of adjuvant TMZ, offered a modest but statistically significant extension of the survival of patients with GBM. As a result, TMZ is currently the standard-of-care for GBMs. The preclinical data presented by Plowman and colleagues (36) revealed that sequential administration of BCNU and TMZ resulted in a dramatic synergism and significantly inhibited the growth of glioma xenograft in mice. At the time when TMZ emerges, the safety profile and treatment outcome of TMZ with additional Gliadel® wafers was unclear. Gururangan and colleagues (37) investigated the safety of TMZ combined with BCNU wafers in a dose-escalation trial. Ten patients with recurrent malignant glioma were treated with BCNU implants followed by oral administration of TMZ at daily dose of 100, 150, and 200 mg/m^2, respectively. The combined treatment was well tolerated. Only one patient treated with TMZ at the highest daily dose of 200 mg/m^2 suffered from grade III thrombocytopenia. Until now, no randomized Phase III trial has been conducted to explore the efficacy of combined therapies in comparison with either TMZ or Gliadel® alone. Several prospective and retrospective studies with small number of patients indicated that sequential treatment with Gliadel® and TMZ resulted in an incremental gain of 2–3 months in median survival (38). Although the level of clinical evidence is not high enough, the combined treatment with Gliadel® and TMZ is currently recommended as an active option for newly diagnosed and recurrent malignant gliomas by the National Comprehensive Cancer Network (NCCN) guidelines (39).

3.2.4. Prevention for complications

The implantation of BCNU wafers is generally safe, but clinical lessons have been learned from the employment of Gliadel® for the management of malignant gliomas. The common adverse effects include healing abnormalities, seizures, and intracranial hypertension (40). Several strategies have been suggested to decrease the risks associated with BCNU implants (41). After the resection of the tumor, BCNU wafers should line up the surface of the tumor bed. Stack of the implants should be avoided because the stacking may result in an irregular release of BCNU due to the altered degradation kinetics of polymers. A large communication between resection cavity and ventricle is the contraindication for wafer implantation. The unexpected translocation of BCNU wafers into ventricle may lead to the life-threatening hydrocephalus. In addition, a watertight closure of the dura is critical to avoid CSF leak and decreases the risk of healing abnormalities and infection. Perioperative anti-convulsants are necessary to prevent seizures. Since the implantation of BCNU wafers is associated with

http://dx.doi.org/10.5772/62838

increased risk of cerebral edema and intracranial hypertension, steroid is suggested to continue for at least 2 weeks after surgery.

3.2.5. Economic consideration

Although effective, BCNU wafers are expensive for the treatment of malignant gliomas. Much attention should be paid to the financial implication of the use of BCNU wafers. Rogers and colleagues (42) conducted a cost-utility analysis. The authors demonstrated that neurosurgery with Gliadel® implantation followed by radiation therapy costs 54,500 English pounds per additional quality-adjusted life-year (QALY) gained in comparison with surgery combined with radiotherapy alone. Probabilistic sensitivity model revealed a <10% probability that Gliadel® would be considered as cost-effective at a willingness-to-pay threshold of 30,000 English pounds per QALY. The authors concluded that Gliadel® is not cost-effective for healthcare resources but can be considered as an alternative adoption for the dreadful disease with a shortage of effective treatments.

3.2.6. Future prospects

Gliadel® represents the first success of the interstitial chemotherapy with biodegradable polymers. With the increased understanding of glioma biology and the advances in pharmaceutical technology, exploration of how to improve the efficacy of polymeric drug delivery is on the way. For example, O^6-alkylguanine-DNA alkyltransferase (AGT) is a well-known DNA repair protein, which protects tumor cells from damage through removing O^6-alkylguanine lesions introduced by alkylating agents such as BCNU and TMZ (43). Brain tumors, especially malignant gliomas, are rich in AGT. The level of AGT is negatively associated with the prognosis of patients with malignant glioma, who receive BCNU therapy (44). Therefore, the inhibition of AGT is a promising strategy to reverse the resistance of glioma cells to BCNU. Quinn and colleagues (45) reported the results of a Phase II trial to test the efficacy of the combination of O^6-benzylguanine (O^6-BG), an AGT inhibitor, with BCNU implantation. Fifty-two patients with recurrent malignant glioma were treated with infusion of O^6-BG and implantation of Gliadel® wafers. The median OS was 50.3 weeks, and the 1- and 2-year OS was 47 and 10% respectively, which suggested the potential clinical benefit. In addition, various chemotherapeutic agents other than BCNU have been exploited to deliver through polymeric system. Preclinical studies demonstrated that many drugs such as temozolomide, paclitaxel, taxotere, and camptothecin were efficacious against gliomas through polymeric delivery (46–49). Further clinical investigation of the safety and efficacy is therefore warranted.

4. Convection-enhanced delivery

4.1. Basic concepts

Convection-enhanced delivery (CED) is a catheter-based direct drug microperfusion technique, which was introduced by Bobo (50). CED continuously infuses soluble therapeutic agents into targeted site in CNS through fine catheters implanted either by surgery or stereotaxis. The hydrostatic pressure gradient (bulk flow) in CED is generated through a motor-driven pump connected to the catheters. CED has several advantages as compared with other drug delivery methods. First of all, CED bypasses BBB and targets tumor bed through the implantation of catheters. The local concentration achieved by CED can be orders of magnitude higher than that produced via intravenous injection, while the systemic toxicity is minimal. Secondly, the pressure-driven CED creates a homogeneous distribution of infused agents in a large region in brain while the diffusion-driven drug delivery such as polymeric wafers usually leads to a limited penetration from the diffusive interface. A dramatic drop-off (250- to 1000-fold decrease) in concentration was observed with the polymeric delivery in the tissue 1–2 mm away from the surface (51). Thirdly, a very large volume of infusion can be achieved via CED. It has been demonstrated that a volume of 200 ml infusion into brain did not cause irreversible neurological deficits in patients with brain tumors (52). Finally, various agents with different molecular weights such as conventional chemotherapeutical drugs, small molecular inhibitors, and immunotoxins can be readily infused through CED. Whereas sophisticated technologies are required to integrate those agents into polymeric system.

4.2. Determining variables for infusate distribution

Several critical factors will influence the distribution of infusate delivered by CED. These include (i) infusion rate and volume; (ii) catheter features; (iii) anatomical structure and interstitial fluid pressure; (iv) intrinsic characteristics of infusate.

The concentration differential is the key driving force for diffusion-driven drug delivery such as polymeric chemotherapy. By contrast, CED is a method to deliver agents mainly dependent on pressure gradient in the interstitial space. As a result, the distribution volume of infusate is mainly determined by infusion volume and rate. In an animal model, the distribution volume correlates with infusion volume in a linear manner. However, this dependence of infusate distribution on volume of infusion disappears due to the infusate reflux along the catheter/brain interface (backflow) when the infusion rate reaches a threshold (e.g., >0.5 μl/min). Therefore, the optimal infusion rate and volume facilitate a better distribution of infusate.

Backflow is one of the major barriers for the clinical usage of CED. The reflux of infusate not only reduces the concentration of delivered drugs in the target location but also increases the risk of adverse effects such as chemical meningitis due to the leakage of the agents into the subarachoid spaces. The properties of the implanted catheters such as shape and size, and the implantation method of the catheters are associated with the incidence of backflow in CED. At the early stage of CED, the open-ended straight catheters were used, but the backflow was frequently observed even at a relatively low infusion rate. A systemic analysis demonstrated that the diameter of catheters positively correlates with the backflow (53). Catheters with the diameter of <1 mm significantly minimize the backflow and achieve better drug distribution (54). It has been suggested that a smaller size of the catheter introduces less tissue displacement and trauma, consequently reducing the backflow. Fiandaca and colleagues modified the shape of the catheter by developing a step design. The step catheter consists of 0.2 mm needle with a glued-in, internal silica tube (0.102-mm inner diameter) that extends beyond the end of

http://dx.doi.org/10.5772/62838

the needle by 5–10 mm (55). The authors demonstrated that the step catheter was reflux-resistant even when the infusion rate increased to as high as 5 μl/min. Gill and colleagues (56) evaluated the performance of CED with a recessed-step catheter, which incorporates an indwelling catheter with adjustable winged stop within a guide tube. This novel design showed a superior control of backflow in comparison with the conventional step catheter. Other catheter designs such as hollow fiber catheter, multiple port catheter, and balloon-tipped catheter have also been developed to minimize reflux and improve drug distribution (57).

The tissue structure and pathology at the targeting site are critical factors that influence the topography and the drug distribution achieved in CED. Normal brain tissues have significant heterogeneity and anisotropy in architecture and permeability for fluid flow. Anatomically, grey matter is mainly composed of glial cells and neuron somas, and the effective diffusivity is generally isotropic in grey matter. Whereas, white matter comprises bundles of axons connecting various grey matter areas to each other in brain. The permeability varies in white matter, primarily depending on the density and directional alignment of axon fibers (58). The diffusion of infusate is anisotropic in white matter. In addition, morphological analysis and mathematical models revealed that extracellular space is more easily extended by infusion fluid in white matter than that in grey matter (59, 60). As a result, white matter is more susceptible to extracellular bulk flow and infusate can travel a longer distance because of the higher permeability along the white matter. In pathological tissues such as gliomas, the bulk flow can be less predictable due to the heterogeneous cytoarchitecture and the treatment-related changes. GBM is characterized with the thriving growth of tumor cells, pseudopalisading necrosis, and glomeruloid vascular proliferation in histology (61). Interstitial fluid pressure (IFP) has been found to increase in intracranial tumors in preclinical models and patients (62). The leaky vasculature coupled with the resistance to bulk flow in the tortuous interstitial space of the surrounding grey and white matter is suggested to be the underlying mechanism for the increased IFP in GBMs (63). More importantly, IFP varies in different areas of the tumor. IFP elevates in the tumor center and dramatically drops toward the tumor periphery or the surrounding normal brain tissue. The outward pressure gradient restrains infusate to enter the tumor core, and the leaky tumor vasculature facilitates the rapid efflux of infused drugs into systemic circulation. Treatment-induced changes may also complicate the drug delivery in CED. For example, postoperative inflammatory reaction decreases the diffusion of drug with a larger molecular weight in extracellular spaces (64). In addition, to treat a residue tumor surrounding the resection cavity, which directly communicates with the subarachnoid space or ventricle, makes it more difficult to deliver drugs via CED. The numbers and placement of catheters should be carefully planned according to the postoperative tumor characteristics.

Besides, the intrinsic features such as the physical and chemical properties of infusate are highly related to the efficiency of CED. Drugs with small molecular weight can be employed in CED, but their faster clearance from CNS limits their diffusion. Agents that easily cross the BBB are not good choices for CED because they can be readily eliminated from the CNS and transported into the systemic circulation. Similarly, drugs that are rapidly taken up or metabolized in the CNS may reduce the distribution of the infusates. Viscosity is also an important factor for bulk flow in CED. Intuitively, the less viscous the infusate is, the more smoothly it diffuses in the extracellular space. Subsequently, a larger diffusion volume is expected from the low-viscosity drugs. However, Mardor and colleagues (65) demonstrated in a rat model that agents with high viscosity tend to have an increased volume of diffusion because they are more resistant to backflow. Therefore, when a drug is chosen as a candidate for CED, its physico-chemical characteristics such as molecular weight, viscosity, clearance rate should be taken into account. In addition, novel strategies are explored to improve the efficacy of CED through delaying the degradation or clearance of agents in the target sites. To achieve this goal, drugs are conjugated or encapsuled with nanoparticles or liposomes (66, 67).

4.3. Agents for convection-enhanced delivery

A wide range of therapeutic agents, such as conventional chemotherapies, targeted toxins, viruses and oligonucleotides, have been investigated on CED for the safety and efficacy in the treatment for gliomas in clinical trials.

4.3.1. Conventional chemotherapeutics

Topotecan, a topoisomerase I inhibitor, is an ideal conventional chemotherapeutic agent for CED. Firstly, topotecan is more readily to accumulate in gliomas than in normal brain tissue. Secondly, it specifically kills glioma cells and is less toxic to normal brain. In addition, topoisomerase I is a natural-product agent with a high molecular weight. As a result, topotecan is difficult to bypass BBB when administered intravenously. Whereas topotecan is less easily removed into systemic circulation and can be retained in the targeted site for a prolonged time when it is infused via CED. Jeffery and colleagues conducted a Phase Ib trial to deliver topotecan to recurrent malignant gliomas (68). Sixteen patients were enrolled in that dose-escalation trial. The treatment was well tolerated with the stable maintenance of quality of life and neurocognitive functioning of patients. Tumors substantially regressed without significant systemic and neurocognitive adverse effects in selected patients with recurrent malignant gliomas refractory to conventional treatment. The total response of the single topotecan infusion was 69%. The results were encouraging for relapse patients in whom previous treatment had failed, but the efficacy of this treatment requires to be confirmed in Phase II and III trials.

Another conventional chemotherapeutic agent, paclitaxel, has also been delivered through CED to treat malignant gliomas. In a Phase I/II trial, a total of 20 cycles of intratumoral CED of paclitaxel was administered to 15 patients with histologically confirmed recurrent GBM (69). Among these 15 patients, complete response was observed in five cases and partial response in six cases, respectively. The response rate reached 73%. The poor response seemed to be associated with the backflow of paclitaxel into subarachnoid spaces, ventricles, and resection cavities. Although effective, the local delivery of paclitaxel caused significant incidence of complications including transient chemical meningitis in six patients, infection in three patients and transient neurological deficits in four patients. The treatment-related side effects have been suggested to be the results of infusate reflux. Strategies such as sealing the burr hole with bone wax and adapting the concentration of paclitaxel were used to prevent the extracranial leakage of the cytotoxic drug and minimize the treatment-induced side effects (70).

4.3.2. Targeted cytotoxins

Targeted cytotoxins represent a novel class of agents with high specificity for brain tumors. The potent protein toxins produced by bacteria are conjugated to carrier ligands, which specifically bind to the receptors on the surface of glioma cells. Less resistance to targeted cytotoxins was observed in glioma cells because the agents kill glioma cells through irreversible *de novo* protein synthesis, independent of any malignancy-associated genetic alterations. The relatively small molecular weight and the highly soluble proteinaceous nature of targeted cytotoxins make them attractive for CED.

TF-CRM107 is the first targeted cytotoxin investigated in clinical trials. The agent is composed of diphtheria toxin conjugated to transferrin-C and preferentially targets glioma cells due to the increased expression of transferrin receptor in tumor tissue. Preclinical works demonstrated that TF-CRM107 eliminated glioma cells at picomolar concentrations *in vitro* and significantly inhibited the growth of subcutaneous glioma xenografts in a mouse model (71, 72). Delivery of TF-CRM107 through CED was safe for patients with malignant brain tumors. In a dose-escalating trial, the treatment was well tolerated (52). No significant neurological and systemic adverse events were observed. In the subsequent Phase II trial, 44 patients with refractory and recurrent malignant gliomas were enrolled (73). TF-CRM107 (concentration of 0.67 μg/ml) was delivered continuously through CED at a rate escalating up to 0.2 ml/h per catheter (a total of 0.4 ml/h for 2 catheters) until a volume of 40 ml was infused. The outcome was encouraging, with a total response of 35% and a median survival of 37 weeks. Unfortunately, the multicenter Phase III trial failed to confirm the efficacy of TF-CRM107 delivered by CED. The study was stopped because an intermediate futility analysis revealed that the chance of positive outcome was <20%.

Cintredekin besudotox (CB, also known as also known as IL13-PE38QQR), a recombinant chimera protein consisted of IL-13 coupled with a truncated form of *Pseudomonas* exotoxin (PE38QQR), is one of the most well-studied targeted toxins. The toxicity and safety profile were carefully reviewed by Kunwar and colleagues (74). Fifty-one patients with recurrent malignant glioma including 46 GBMs, who were infused with CB via CED after resection, were evaluated. The treatment was well tolerated, and the adverse effects were mostly transient and manageable. The authors categorized the adverse effects according to the onset time related to the procedures including the placement of catheters and delivery of the agents. Three symptomatic periods were defined: The first one was between surgery and CED; the second was during CED and up to 7 days after infusion; and the third period was 2–10 weeks after treatment. Adverse events including intracranial hemorrhage and infection were more likely observed in the first period, which was related to the placement of catheters. Whereas the mass effect due to the volume of infusion was responsible for neurological deficits during the second period. Neurological deficits were also found in patients during the third symptomatic period. It has been suggested that the treatment-induced inflammation or the non-specific toxicity for normal brain cells resulted in the side effects. This study not only confirmed the safety of the delivery of CB via CED but also provided important information about the pathophysiological mechanism underlying the adverse events observed in the clinical trial with CED, which is helpful to minimize the complications in further studies. A multicenter Phase III trial (Phase III Randomized Evaluation of CED of IL13-PE38QQR Compared to Gliadel® Wafer with Survival End Point in GBM Patients at First Recurrence, PRECISE) investigated the efficacy of CB infused via CED (75). Two hundred ninety-six patients with recurrent GBM were randomized to receive CED of CB or Gliadel® wafers. Unfortunately, although there was statistically significant improvement in progression-free survival between patients treated with CB and those with Gliadel® wafers (17.7 vs. 11.4 weeks, $p = 0.0008$), no survival benefit was found, with the median survival of 11.3 months for CB and 10 months for Gliadel® wafers for the efficacy evaluable population ($p = 0.310$). But it is worth noting that 32% of catheter placements were not performed per protocol specifications and drug distribution was not evaluated with image monitoring. These two limitations may be possible explanation for the failure of the trial. Lately, Sampson and colleagues (76) retrospectively analyzed the catheter positioning and drug distribution in the PRECISE trial using BrainLAB iPlan Flow software that was not available during the trial. The study demonstrated that more than 50% of catheters did not meet all positioning criteria among 174 cases with sufficient data. In addition, the simulation analysis revealed that the average coverage volume was very low, with only 20.1% of the 2-cm penumbra surrounding the resection cavity covered on average. Therefore, lessons learned from PRECISE trial clearly indicate that the accurate catheter positioning and the real-time monitoring of drug distribution are critical for the success of interstitial drug delivery via CED.

4.3.3. Future prospects

Until now, many other agents such as monoclonal antibodies (e.g., ^{131}I-chTNT-1/B mAb), oligonucleotides (e.g., TGF-beta2 antisense oligonucleotides) and viruses (e.g. LSFV-IL12) have been investigated via CED in early-stage clinical studies (77–79) and demonstrated benefit in selected patients. Well-designed randomized trials are required to confirm the efficacy. In the future, so as to fulfill an effective treatment strategy, CED will require optimized infusates, improved catheters, standardization of catheter placement, mathematical models to predict drug distribution, as well as the real-time monitoring of infusate delivery.

5. Conclusion

Malignant glioma, especially GBM, is still a devastating cancer in CNS. Despite of intensive treatment with neurosurgical resection, radiotherapy, and adjuvant chemotherapy with TMZ, the median survival is less than 2 years. Development of novel strategies against malignant gliomas is of urgent necessity. The advent of interstitial chemotherapy has definitely increased treatment options for patients with malignant glioma. Local delivery of chemotherapeutic agents bypasses the physiological barrier of normal brain, achieving a significantly increased concentration in targeted sites and a minimized systemic toxicity. Gliadel® wafers represent the success of interstitial chemotherapy for malignant gliomas. On the other hand, CED is a promising approach for local drug delivery, but improvement in the techniques is required. In addition, novel methods such as micro-chips and gene delivery is under investigation (80). In a word, interstitial chemotherapy conveys the opportunity of more efficiently and effectively delivering anti-glioma agents to the infiltrative tumors than conventional routes of administration.

Author details

Ke Sai, Shu-xin Sun and Zhong-ping Chen*

*Address all correspondence to: chenzhp@sysucc.org.cn

Department of Neurosurgery/Neuro-oncology, Sun Yat-sen University Cancer Center, State Key Laboratory of Oncology in South China, Collaborative Innovation Center for Cancer Medicine, 651 Dongfeng Road East, Guangzhou, People's Republic of China

References

[1] Ostrom QT, Gittleman H, Fulop J, Liu M, Blanda R, Kromer C, et al. CBTRUS statistical report: primary brain and central nervous system tumors diagnosed in the United States in 2008–2012. Neuro-oncology. 2015;17(Suppl 4):iv1–62.

[2] Li YM, Suki D, Hess K, Sawaya R. The influence of maximum safe resection of glioblastoma on survival in 1229 patients: can we do better than gross-total resection? J Neurosurg. 2016; 124(4):977–88.

[3] Bhujbal SV, de Vos P, Niclou SP. Drug and cell encapsulation: alternative delivery options for the treatment of malignant brain tumors. Advanced Drug Delivery Reviews. 2014;67–68:142–53.

[4] Lathia JD, Mack SC, Mulkearns-Hubert EE, Valentim CL, Rich JN. Cancer stem cells in glioblastoma. Genes & Development. 2015;29(12):1203–17.

[5] Heppner F, Diemath HE. Local chemotherapy of brain tumors. Acta Neurochirurgica. 1963;11:287–93.

[6] Ringkjob R. Treatment of intracranial gliomas and metastatic carcinomas by local application of cytostatic agents. Acta Neurologica Scandinavica. 1968;44(3):318–22.

[7] Boiardi A, Salmaggi A, Pozzi A, Broggi G, Silvani A. Interstitial chemotherapy with mitoxantrone in recurrent malignant glioma: preliminary data. Journal of Neuro-oncology. 1996;27(2):157–62.

[8] Shimura T, Teramoto A, Nakazawa S, Aihara K. A clinicopathological study of malignant glioma done after local administration of chemotherapeutic agents. Clinical Neuropathology. 1996;15(2):119–24.

[9] Boiardi A, Silvani A, Eoli M, Lamperti E, Salmaggi A, Gaviani P, et al. Treatment of recurrent glioblastoma: can local delivery of mitoxantrone improve survival? Journal of Neuro-oncology. 2008;88(1):105–13.

[10] Mamelak AN, Rosenfeld S, Bucholz R, Raubitschek A, Nabors LB, Fiveash JB, et al. Phase I single-dose study of intracavitary-administered iodine-131-TM-601 in adults with recurrent high-grade glioma. Journal of Clinical Oncology. 2006;24(22):3644–50.

[11] Prados MD, McDermott M, Chang SM, Wilson CB, Fick J, Culver KW, et al. Treatment of progressive or recurrent glioblastoma multiforme in adults with herpes simplex virus thymidine kinase gene vector-producer cells followed by intravenous ganciclovir administration: a phase I/II multi-institutional trial. Journal of Neuro-oncology. 2003;65(3):269–78.

[12] Brown CE, Badie B, Barish ME, Weng L, Ostberg JR, Chang WC, et al. Bioactivity and safety of IL13Ralpha2-redirected chimeric antigen receptor CD8+ T cells in patients with recurrent glioblastoma. Clinical Cancer Research. 2015;21(18):4062–72.

[13] Oshiro S, Tsugu H, Komatsu F, Ohnishi H, Ueno Y, Sakamoto S, et al. Evaluation of intratumoral administration of tumor necrosis factor-alpha in patients with malignant glioma. Anticancer Research. 2006;26(6A):4027–32.

[14] Fu JC, Moyer DL, Hagemeier C. Effect of comonomer ratio on hydrocortisone diffusion from sustained-release composite capsules. Journal of Biomedical Materials Research. 1978;12(3):249–54.

[15] Gallia GL, Brem S, Brem H. Local treatment of malignant brain tumors using implantable chemotherapeutic polymers. Journal of the National Comprehensive Cancer Network: JNCCN. 2005;3(5):721–8.

[16] Noll DM, Mason TM, Miller PS. Formation and repair of interstrand cross-links in DNA. Chemical Reviews. 2006;106(2):277–301.

[17] DeAngelis LM, Burger PC, Green SB, Cairncross JG. Malignant glioma: who benefits from adjuvant chemotherapy? Annals of Neurology. 1998;44(4):691–5.

[18] Jungk C, Chatziaslanidou D, Ahmadi R, Capper D, Bermejo JL, Exner J, et al. Chemotherapy with BCNU in recurrent glioma: analysis of clinical outcome and side effects in chemotherapy-naive patients. BMC Cancer. 2015;16(1):81.

[19] Brem H, Kader A, Epstein JI, Tamargo RJ, Domb A, Langer R, et al. Biocompatibility of a biodegradable, controlled-release polymer in the rabbit brain. Selective Cancer Therapeutics. 1989;5(2):55–65.

[20] Brem H, Tamargo RJ, Olivi A, Pinn M, Weingart JD, Wharam M, et al. Biodegradable polymers for controlled delivery of chemotherapy with and without radiation therapy in the monkey brain. Journal of Neurosurgery. 1994;80(2):283–90.

[21] Fung LK, Shin M, Tyler B, Brem H, Saltzman WM. Chemotherapeutic drugs released from polymers: distribution of 1,3-bis(2-chloroethyl)-1-nitrosourea in the rat brain. Pharmaceutical Research. 1996;13(5):671–82.

[22] Grossman SA, Reinhard C, Colvin OM, Chasin M, Brundrett R, Tamargo RJ, et al. The intracerebral distribution of BCNU delivered by surgically implanted biodegradable polymers. Journal of Neurosurgery. 1992;76(4):640–7.

[23] Fung LK, Ewend MG, Sills A, Sipos EP, Thompson R, Watts M, et al. Pharmacokinetics of interstitial delivery of carmustine, 4-hydroperoxycyclophosphamide, and paclitaxel from a biodegradable polymer implant in the monkey brain. Cancer Research. 1998;58(4):672–84.

[24] Tamargo RJ, Myseros JS, Epstein JI, Yang MB, Chasin M, Brem H. Interstitial chemotherapy of the 9L gliosarcoma: controlled release polymers for drug delivery in the brain. Cancer Research. 1993;53(2):329–33.

[25] Buahin KG, Brem H. Interstitial chemotherapy of experimental brain tumors: comparison of intratumoral injection versus polymeric controlled release. Journal of Neurooncology. 1995;26(2):103–10.

[26] Brem H, Mahaley MS, Jr., Vick NA, Black KL, Schold SC, Jr., Burger PC, et al. Interstitial chemotherapy with drug polymer implants for the treatment of recurrent gliomas. Journal of Neurosurgery. 1991;74(3):441–6.

[27] Brem H, Ewend MG, Piantadosi S, Greenhoot J, Burger PC, Sisti M. The safety of interstitial chemotherapy with BCNU-loaded polymer followed by radiation therapy in the treatment of newly diagnosed malignant gliomas: phase I trial. Journal of Neurooncology. 1995;26(2):111–23.

[28] Brem H, Piantadosi S, Burger PC, Walker M, Selker R, Vick NA, et al. Placebo-controlled trial of safety and efficacy of intraoperative controlled delivery by biodegradable polymers of chemotherapy for recurrent gliomas. The Polymer-brain Tumor Treatment Group. Lancet. 1995;345(8956):1008–12.

[29] Hart MG, Grant R, Garside R, Rogers G, Somerville M, Stein K. Chemotherapy wafers for high grade glioma. The Cochrane Database of Systematic Reviews. 2011(3):CD007294.

[30] Valtonen S, Timonen U, Toivanen P, Kalimo H, Kivipelto L, Heiskanen O, et al. Interstitial chemotherapy with carmustine-loaded polymers for high-grade gliomas: a randomized double-blind study. Neurosurgery. 1997;41(1):44–8; discussion 8–9.

[31] Westphal M, Hilt DC, Bortey E, Delavault P, Olivares R, Warnke PC, et al. A phase 3 trial of local chemotherapy with biodegradable carmustine (BCNU) wafers (Gliadel wafers) in patients with primary malignant glioma. Neuro-oncology. 2003;5(2):79–88.

[32] Sipos EP, Tyler B, Piantadosi S, Burger PC, Brem H. Optimizing interstitial delivery of BCNU from controlled release polymers for the treatment of brain tumors. Cancer Chemotherapy and Pharmacology. 1997;39(5):383–9.

[33] Olivi A, Grossman SA, Tatter S, Barker F, Judy K, Olsen J, et al. Dose escalation of carmustine in surgically implanted polymers in patients with recurrent malignant glioma: a New Approaches to Brain Tumor Therapy CNS Consortium trial. Journal of Clinical Oncology. 2003;21(9):1845–9.

[34] Sai K, Zhong MG, Wang J, Chen YS, Mou YG, Ke C, et al. Safety evaluation of high-dose BCNU-loaded biodegradable implants in Chinese patients with recurrent malignant gliomas. Journal of the Neurological Sciences. 2014;343(1–2):60–5.

[35] Stupp R, Mason WP, van den Bent MJ, Weller M, Fisher B, Taphoorn MJ, et al. Radiotherapy plus concomitant and adjuvant temozolomide for glioblastoma. The New England Journal of Medicine. 2005;352(10):987–96.

[36] Plowman J, Waud WR, Koutsoukos AD, Rubinstein LV, Moore TD, Grever MR. Preclinical antitumor activity of temozolomide in mice: efficacy against human brain tumor xenografts and synergism with 1,3-bis(2-chloroethyl)-1-nitrosourea. Cancer Research. 1994;54(14):3793–9.

[37] Gururangan S, Cokgor L, Rich JN, Edwards S, Affronti ML, Quinn JA, et al. Phase I study of Gliadel wafers plus temozolomide in adults with recurrent supratentorial high-grade gliomas. Neuro-oncology. 2001;3(4):246–50.

[38] Dixit S, Hingorani M, Achawal S, Scott I. The sequential use of carmustine wafers (Gliadel(R)) and postoperative radiotherapy with concomitant temozolomide followed by adjuvant temozolomide: a clinical review. British Journal of Neurosurgery. 2011;25(4):459–69.

[39] Chowdhary SA, Ryken T, Newton HB. Survival outcomes and safety of carmustine wafers in the treatment of high-grade gliomas: a meta-analysis. Journal of Neuro-oncology. 2015;122(2):367–82.

[40] Sabel M, Giese A. Safety profile of carmustine wafers in malignant glioma: a review of controlled trials and a decade of clinical experience. Current Medical Research and Opinion. 2008;24(11):3239–57.

[41] Giese A, Bock HC, Kantelhardt SR, Rohde V. Risk management in the treatment of malignant gliomas with BCNU wafer implants. Central European Neurosurgery. 2010;71(4):199–206.

[42] Rogers G, Garside R, Mealing S, Pitt M, Anderson R, Dyer M, et al. Carmustine implants for the treatment of newly diagnosed high-grade gliomas: a cost-utility analysis. PharmacoEconomics. 2008;26(1):33–44.

[43] Drablos F, Feyzi E, Aas PA, Vaagbo CB, Kavli B, Bratlie MS, et al. Alkylation damage in DNA and RNA—repair mechanisms and medical significance. DNA Repair. 2004;3(11):1389–407.

[44] Belanich M, Pastor M, Randall T, Guerra D, Kibitel J, Alas L, et al. Retrospective study of the correlation between the DNA repair protein alkyltransferase and survival of brain tumor patients treated with carmustine. Cancer Research. 1996;56(4):783–8.

[45] Quinn JA, Jiang SX, Carter J, Reardon DA, Desjardins A, Vredenburgh JJ, et al. Phase II trial of Gliadel plus O6-benzylguanine in adults with recurrent glioblastoma multiforme. Clinical Cancer Research. 2009;15(3):1064–8.

[46] Brem S, Tyler B, Li K, Pradilla G, Legnani F, Caplan J, et al. Local delivery of temozolomide by biodegradable polymers is superior to oral administration in a rodent glioma model. Cancer Chemotherapy and Pharmacology. 2007;60(5):643–50.

[47] Vellimana AK, Recinos VR, Hwang L, Fowers KD, Li KW, Zhang Y, et al. Combination of paclitaxel thermal gel depot with temozolomide and radiotherapy significantly prolongs survival in an experimental rodent glioma model. Journal of Neuro-oncology. 2013;111(3):229–36.

[48] Sampath P, Rhines LD, DiMeco F, Tyler BM, Park MC, Brem H. Interstitial docetaxel (taxotere), carmustine and combined interstitial therapy: a novel treatment for experimental malignant glioma. Journal of Neuro-oncology. 2006;80(1):9–17.

[49] Weingart JD, Thompson RC, Tyler B, Colvin OM, Brem H. Local delivery of the topoisomerase I inhibitor camptothecin sodium prolongs survival in the rat intracranial 9L gliosarcoma model. International Journal of Cancer. 1995;62(5):605–9.

[50] Bobo RH, Laske DW, Akbasak A, Morrison PF, Dedrick RL, Oldfield EH. Convection-enhanced delivery of macromolecules in the brain. Proceedings of the National Academy of Sciences of the United States of America. 1994;91(6):2076–80.

[51] Strasser JF, Fung LK, Eller S, Grossman SA, Saltzman WM. Distribution of 1,3-bis(2-chloroethyl)-1-nitrosourea and tracers in the rabbit brain after interstitial delivery by biodegradable polymer implants. The Journal of Pharmacology and Experimental Therapeutics. 1995;275(3):1647–55.

[52] Laske DW, Youle RJ, Oldfield EH. Tumor regression with regional distribution of the targeted toxin TF-CRM107 in patients with malignant brain tumors. Nature Medicine. 1997;3(12):1362–8.

[53] Chen MY, Lonser RR, Morrison PF, Governale LS, Oldfield EH. Variables affecting convection-enhanced delivery to the striatum: a systematic examination of rate of

infusion, cannula size, infusate concentration, and tissue-cannula sealing time. Journal of Neurosurgery. 1999;90(2):315–20.

[54] White E, Bienemann A, Malone J, Megraw L, Bunnun C, Wyatt M, et al. An evaluation of the relationships between catheter design and tissue mechanics in achieving high-flow convection-enhanced delivery. Journal of Neuroscience Methods. 2011;199(1):87–97.

[55] Krauze MT, Saito R, Noble C, Tamas M, Bringas J, Park JW, et al. Reflux-free cannula for convection-enhanced high-speed delivery of therapeutic agents. Journal of Neurosurgery. 2005;103(5):923–9.

[56] Gill T, Barua NU, Woolley M, Bienemann AS, Johnson DE, Sullivan SO, et al. In vitro and in vivo testing of a novel recessed-step catheter for reflux-free convection-enhanced drug delivery to the brain. Journal of Neuroscience Methods. 2013;219(1):1–9.

[57] Debinski W, Tatter SB. Convection-enhanced delivery for the treatment of brain tumors. Expert Review of Neurotherapeutics. 2009;9(10):1519–27.

[58] Linninger AA, Somayaji MR, Mekarski M, Zhang L. Prediction of convection-enhanced drug delivery to the human brain. Journal of Theoretical Biology. 2008;250(1): 125–38.

[59] Whittle IR, Miller JD. A rodent model of infusion brain edema: methodology and pathophysiological effects of saline and protein infusions. Acta Neurochirurgica. 1990;105(3-4):158–68.

[60] Basser PJ. Interstitial pressure, volume, and flow during infusion into brain tissue. Microvascular Research. 1992;44(2):143–65.

[61] Brat DJ, Van Meir EG. Glomeruloid microvascular proliferation orchestrated by VPF/VEGF: a new world of angiogenesis research. The American Journal of Pathology. 2001;158(3):789–96.

[62] Boucher Y, Baxter LT, Jain RK. Interstitial pressure gradients in tissue-isolated and subcutaneous tumors: implications for therapy. Cancer Research. 1990;50(15):4478–84.

[63] Navalitloha Y, Schwartz ES, Groothuis EN, Allen CV, Levy RM, Groothuis DR. Therapeutic implications of tumor interstitial fluid pressure in subcutaneous RG-2 tumors. Neuro-oncology. 2006;8(3):227–33.

[64] Voges J, Reszka R, Gossmann A, Dittmar C, Richter R, Garlip G, et al. Imaging-guided convection-enhanced delivery and gene therapy of glioblastoma. Annals of Neurology. 2003;54(4):479–87.

[65] Mardor Y, Rahav O, Zauberman Y, Lidar Z, Ocherashvilli A, Daniels D, et al. Convection-enhanced drug delivery: increased efficacy and magnetic resonance image monitoring. Cancer Research. 2005;65(15):6858–63.

[66] Xi G, Robinson E, Mania-Farnell B, Vanin EF, Shim KW, Takao T, et al. Convection-enhanced delivery of nanodiamond drug delivery platforms for intracranial tumor treatment. Nanomedicine: Nanotechnology, Biology, and Medicine. 2014;10(2):381–91.

[67] Huo T, Barth RF, Yang W, Nakkula RJ, Koynova R, Tenchov B, et al. Preparation, biodistribution and neurotoxicity of liposomal cisplatin following convection enhanced delivery in normal and F98 glioma bearing rats. Plos One. 2012;7(11):e48752.

[68] Bruce JN, Fine RL, Canoll P, Yun J, Kennedy BC, Rosenfeld SS, et al. Regression of recurrent malignant gliomas with convection-enhanced delivery of topotecan. Neurosurgery. 2011;69(6):1272–9; discussion 9–80.

[69] Lidar Z, Mardor Y, Jonas T, Pfeffer R, Faibel M, Nass D, et al. Convection-enhanced delivery of paclitaxel for the treatment of recurrent malignant glioma: a phase I/II clinical study. Journal of Neurosurgery. 2004;100(3):472–9.

[70] Tanner PG, Holtmannspotter M, Tonn JC, Goldbrunner R. Effects of drug efflux on convection-enhanced paclitaxel delivery to malignant gliomas: technical note. Neurosurgery. 2007;61(4):E880–2; discussion E2.

[71] Martell LA, Agrawal A, Ross DA, Muraszko KM. Efficacy of transferrin receptor-targeted immunotoxins in brain tumor cell lines and pediatric brain tumors. Cancer Research. 1993;53(6):1348–53.

[72] Laske DW, Ilercil O, Akbasak A, Youle RJ, Oldfield EH. Efficacy of direct intratumoral therapy with targeted protein toxins for solid human gliomas in nude mice. Journal of Neurosurgery. 1994;80(3):520–6.

[73] Weaver M, Laske DW. Transferrin receptor ligand-targeted toxin conjugate (Tf-CRM107) for therapy of malignant gliomas. Journal of Neuro-oncology. 2003;65(1):3–13.

[74] Kunwar S, Chang SM, Prados MD, Berger MS, Sampson JH, Croteau D, et al. Safety of intraparenchymal convection-enhanced delivery of cintredekin besudotox in early-phase studies. Neurosurgical Focus. 2006;20(4):E15.

[75] Kunwar S, Chang S, Westphal M, Vogelbaum M, Sampson J, Barnett G, et al. Phase III randomized trial of CED of IL13-PE38QQR vs Gliadel wafers for recurrent glioblastoma. Neuro-oncology. 2010;12(8):871–81.

[76] Sampson JH, Archer G, Pedain C, Wembacher-Schroder E, Westphal M, Kunwar S, et al. Poor drug distribution as a possible explanation for the results of the PRECISE trial. Journal of Neurosurgery. 2010;113(2):301–9.

[77] Hdeib A, Sloan A. Targeted radioimmunotherapy: the role of (1)(3)(1)I-chTNT-1/B mAb (Cotara) for treatment of high-grade gliomas. Future Oncology. 2012;8(6):659–69.

[78] Hau P, Jachimczak P, Schlingensiepen R, Schulmeyer F, Jauch T, Steinbrecher A, et al. Inhibition of TGF-beta2 with AP 12009 in recurrent malignant gliomas: from preclinical to phase I/II studies. Oligonucleotides. 2007;17(2):201–12.

[79] Ren H, Boulikas T, Lundstrom K, Soling A, Warnke PC, Rainov NG. Immunogene therapy of recurrent glioblastoma multiforme with a liposomally encapsulated replication-incompetent Semliki forest virus vector carrying the human interleukin-12 gene--a phase I/II clinical protocol. Journal of Neuro-oncology. 2003;64(1-2):147–54.

[80] Chaichana KL, Pinheiro L, Brem H. Delivery of local therapeutics to the brain: working toward advancing treatment for malignant gliomas. Therapeutic Delivery. 2015;6(3): 353–69.

Chapter 14

Oligoastrocytoma: A Vanishing Tumor Entity

Marta Mellai, Laura Annovazzi,
Marta Mazzucco and Davide Schiffer

Additional information is available at the end of the chapter

http://dx.doi.org/10.5772/63240

Abstract

Oligoastrocytoma (OA) was a glioma recognized in the current World Health Organization (WHO) classification of the central nervous system (CNS) tumors as a mixed tumor with an astrocytic and an oligodendroglial component. Its definability was, however, poor so that its prevalence varies in the various collections. A series of contributions of the literature and the "International Society of Neuropathology (ISN) – Haarlem *Consensus*" recently denied its existence as a tumor entity on the basis of 1p/19q, isocitrate dehydrogenase (IDH) and α-thalassemia/mental retardation syndrome X-linked (ATRX) status. Most tumors previously diagnosed as OAs were, therefore, reclassified as either oligodendrogliomas or astrocytomas.

We revised 40 OAs from our glioma series initially diagnosed with stringent histologic criteria. After the revision based on the above mentioned molecular markers, most of them changed diagnosis falling into the categories of oligodendroglioma or astrocytoma. Only one fulfilled the stringent criteria of the current classification system, whereas two cases remained undefined.

Since ATRX is constitutively expressed in microglia/macrophages, their number in the histologic sections has a paramount importance in recognizing the oligodendroglial component. The double ATRX/GFAP, ATRX/IDH1^{R132H} and ATRX/Iba-1 immunostainings greatly conditions the recognition of the oligodendroglial and astrocytic tumor cells.

Keywords: oligoastrocytoma, 1p/19q co-deletion, IDH, ATRX, prognosis

1. Introduction

In the 2007 World Health Organization (WHO) classification of the central nervous system (CNS) tumors [1], oligoastrocytoma (OA) was considered as a mixed glioma with an astrocytic and an oligodendroglial component [2, 3]. It could be easily recognized if the two components were clearly separated, as it rarely happened. Usually, the two cell types were found intermingled and the differential diagnosis towards astrocytomas and oligodendrogliomas was difficult and, frequently, it remained undefined. Since its first recognition [4] and confirmation [5], its definability was poor and the tumor was even considered as an oligodendroglioma with reactive astrocytes [6]. The poor tumor definability explains why the prevalence of OAs in the various collections of the literature has been so variable and it accounted for the need to establish criteria useful for the recognition of the tumor. It was suggested to rely on the occurrence of at least 10% neoplastic oligodendrocytes in astrocytic gliomas [7] or 10% neoplastic astrocytes in oligodendroglial gliomas [8], provided that oligodendrocytes were neoplastic and not normal, and that astrocytes were tumor and not reactive. These criteria, however, were too vague in the clinical practice and the definition of the tumor remained a subjective matter. In particular, the recognition of normal from tumor oligodendrocytes, especially in slightly infiltrating or diffuse growth where the cell density is low, remained unsolved [9].

As a matter of fact, the diagnostic uncertainties of OA were also due to the lack of a reliable marker for tumor oligodendrocytes in tissue sections. The prevailing diffuse and infiltrating growth of both oligodendrogliomas and the oligodendroglial component of OAs led to find the coexistence in the same tumor area of tumor and normal oligodendrocytes to the point that it was even difficult to establish, in some cases, whether a tumor infiltration existed or not. On the other hand, the difficulty to recognize a mild oligodendroglial infiltration in oligodendrogliomas themselves was already known, even exploiting the occurrence of abnormal nuclei or crowding of tumor cells along capillaries or around neurons.

Another critical point was the difficulty to distinguish reactive from tumor astrocytes and to recognize the real nature of minigemistocytes [10], glial fibrillary oligodendrocytes (GFOC) [11–13], real gemistocytes, and perineural satellites.

The origin of the tumor was referred to a progenitor stage preceding the astrocytic and oligodendroglial differentiation and, therefore, tumor suppressor protein p53 (TP53) mutations were searched for in the astrocytic component and the 1p/19q co-deletion in the oligodendroglial one and a genetic analysis was suggested [14]. Anyway, the variability of OA prevalence in the various collections remained high. It was observed that the absence of 1p/19q co-deletion, typical of oligodendrogliomas, entailed the occurrence of TP53 mutations [15], but also that it could be present or absent in both tumor components and that all tumor cells seemed to share the same genetic aberrations [14].

2. Epidemiology and demographics

2.1. Incidence

OA was the third most common glioma. It accounted for 1% of all brain tumors and 5–10% of all glial neoplasms. The incidence of OA was approximately 0.03 *per* 100,000 individuals in the United States. Young and middle-aged adult population was affected. The median age of diagnosis was 42 years. Males were more commonly affected than females; the male to female ratio was approximately 1.43–1. OA usually affected individuals of the Caucasian race with a higher incidence rate in developed countries [1].

2.2. Etiology

Common risk factors in the development of OA included family history of brain tumors, ionizing radiation, and allergic diseases.

2.3. Location

OA preferentially developed in the cerebral hemispheres with a frequency that corresponded to the relative size of the cerebral lobes (frontal, temporal, parietal, and occipital) [1]. It commonly arose in the supratentorial regions. Occasional locations were insula, diencephalon, and spinal cord whereas cerebellar location was very uncommon.

2.4. Clinical features

The most common symptoms were seizure, headache, and personality changes.

2.5. Neuroradiological features

On magnetic resonance imaging (MRI), OA was described as characterized by a mass which is typically hypointense on T1-weighted images and hyperintense on T2-weighted images. No enhancement is observed on Gadolinium enhanced T1-weighted images (**Figure 1A**, **B**).

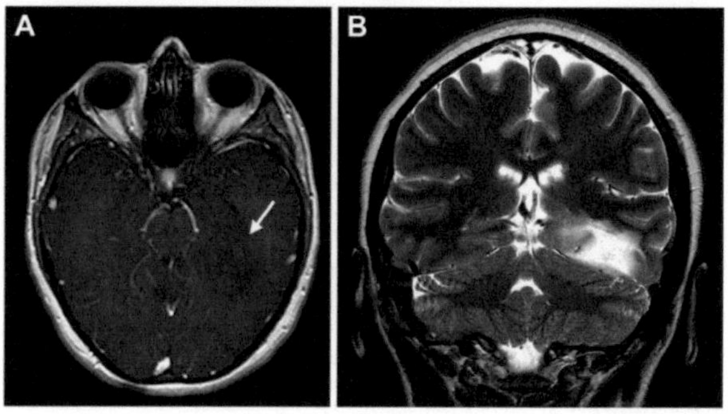

Figure 1. Magnetic resonance imaging (MRI) of 20-years old woman. A – OA, T1-weighted sequence after gadolinium contrast enhancement (arrow); B – Id, hyperintensity in T2-weighted sequence.

3. Histopathology

According to the current WHO classification system [1], OA was classified in two subtypes: grade II OA (OAII) and grade III OA (OAIII).

3.1. Macroscopic appearance

On gross pathology, OA was characterized by a soft, well-defined, grey-tan, mucoid or hemorrhagic, calcified mass with or without necrosis that may expand the gyrus, and cause blurring of the grey white matter junction.

3.2. Microscopic appearance

On histopathologic analysis, OA was characterized by highly cellular lesions composed of both tumor astrocytes and oligodendrocytes that could be separated or intermingled [5], *i.e.* the tumor could be defined as "biphasic" (**Figure 2A–C**) or "diffuse" (**Figure 2D**). Astrocytic tumor cells scattered within oligodendroglial cells had to be recognized as neoplastic and not reactive/ hypertrophic astrocytes.

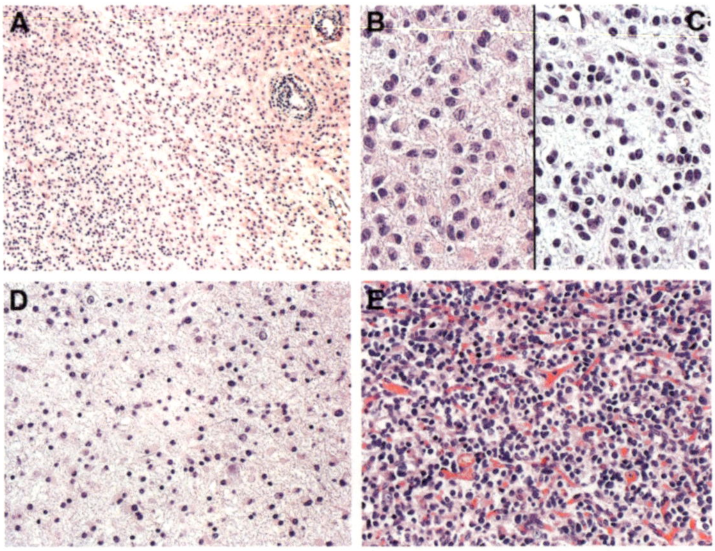

Figure 2. Histopathologic features of OA. A – OAII with separated astrocytic and oligodendroglial components, x100; B – Id, astrocytic component, x400; C – Id, oligodendroglial component, x400; D – OAII with intermingled astrocytic and oligodendroglial cells, x200; E – OAIII, x200. All hematoxylin and eosin (H&E).

OAII. The tumor showed a moderate cellularity with no or low mitotic activity. Microcalcifications and microcystic degeneration could occur.

Reactive astrocytes are present in all gliomas, OA included; in the latter, their distinction from tumor astrocytes was the most important problem since the protean appearance of reactive astrocytes, with large cytoplasms, and thick and long processes or with small cytoplasms with short processes and in variable number, did not allow a clear-cut distinction from tumor astrocytes.

An important bias was the occurrence of minigemistocytes, GFOC, and true gemistocytes. Both minigemistocytes and GFOC were regarded as either transitional forms between oligodendrocytes and astrocytes, corresponding to a bipotential glial progenitor cell [16], or as glial fibrillary acidic protein (GFAP) expressing oligodendrocytes [12], remnants of myelin forming glia of the developmental period [13].

A high frequency of minigemistocytes could confer an astrocytic aspect to the tumor.

OAIII. The tumor was mainly characterized by a significant or brisk mitotic activity (≥6 mitoses *per* 10 high power field [HPF]) and a high Ki-67/MIB-1 proliferation index, nuclear atypia, necrosis, and apoptotic cells (**Figure 2E**). The malignant transformation was considered as proceeding either from the one or the other cell component. In the differential diagnosis towards glioblastoma (GBM), the occurrence of circumscribed necroses was decisive; the presence of microvascular proliferations (MVPs) would indicate the grade III when occurring in the oligodendroglial part and the grade IV when in the astrocytic one.

3.3. Immunohistochemistry (IHC)

IHC was practically based only on GFAP expression. No specific immunohistochemical marker was available for oligodendrocytes [17, 18], although MAP2, OLIG2, Cyclin D1, and alpha-internexin (INA) immunopositivity could be found in the oligodendroglial component. Approximately one third of OAs showed nuclear p53 accumulation, more commonly in the astrocytic cells [19].

4. Molecular genetics

As in all gliomas, the origin of the tumor proceeds from the step-wise accumulation of genetic/epigenetic alterations. Thirty-fifty percent of OAs exhibited loss of heterozygosity (LOH) on chromosomes 1p and 19q [20, 21], while approximately 30% of them harboured TP53 mutations. In particular, OAs of the temporal lobe more frequently exhibited TP53 mutations, and less commonly, 1p and 19q losses [22, 23].

OAII typically exhibited the type and distribution of genetic alterations observed in grade II gliomas [22]. OAIII showed genetic alterations commonly involved in the progression of astrocytic and oligodendroglial tumors, including loss of 9p with homozygous deletion of the cyclin-dependent kinase inhibitor 2A (CDKN2A) ($p14^{ARF}$) gene, allelic loss on chromosome 10q and epidermal growth factor receptor (EGFR) gene amplification [24].

5. Treatment and prognosis

OAs responded less favourably to chemotherapy (CHT) due to the chemoresistance of their astrocytic components [25]. Studies have shown that the standard of care for 1p/19q co-deleted oligodendroglial tumors should be the combination of CHT and radiotherapy (RT). In OA, a favourable prognosis was associated to young age, grade II and extent of resection [26].

Compared to astrocytomas, OAs shared with oligodendrogliomas a more favourable prognosis and an improved response to adjuvant therapy. The NOA-04 prospective trial on anaplastic gliomas reported virtually identical outcomes for patients with oligodendrogliomas or OAs [27].

6. New criteria for glioma diagnosis after the "ISN-Haarlem Consensus"

Our knowledge on the nature of OA underwent a profound change after the "International Society of Neuropathology (ISN)-Haarlem *Consensus*" guidelines led to the official recognition of the indispensability of the genetic analysis in order to obtain an "integrated" diagnosis of gliomas [28]. Referred to grade II and III adult gliomas, this new approach would involve a combination of histologic and molecular data based on the 1p/19q, isocitrate dehydrogenase (IDH) 1/2 and α-thalassemia/mental retardation syndrome X-linked (ATRX) status.

6.1. 1p/19q chromosomal status

The genetic hallmark of oligodendroglial tumors is a combined chromosomal deletion of the short arm of the chromosome 1 (1p) and the long arm of the chromosome 19 (19q). Combined 1p and 19q losses were described in 80–90% of grade II and in 50–70% of grade III tumors [22, 24].

The 1p/19q chromosomal status was recognized as an important diagnostic biomarker in the clinical practice. The 1p/19q co-deletion was reported in 60–70% of oligodendrogliomas with a classical histologic phenotype (perinuclear "halo" and "chicken wire" vascular pattern). Partial 1p or 19q deletion occurred in approximately 75% of the cases [29, 30]. Oligodendroglial tumors with 1p/19q co-deletion were observed to typically arise at an extra-temporal location, whereas tumors with intact 1p/19q at the temporal lobe [22]. In contrast, childhood oligodendrogliomas only rarely exhibited chromosomal abnormalities.

Importantly, the occurrence of 1p/19q co-deletion supports the diagnosis of oligodendroglioma, especially when histology is atypical. However, its absence does not exclude this diagnosis, leaving unsolved the question of oligodendrogliomas with intact 1p/19q.

In OA, the frequency of the 1p/19q co-deletion was approximately 50% [22]. Virtually, it was mutually exclusive with LOH of chromosome 17p13 and TP53 mutations, both typical of astrocytic tumors. In OA, the 1p/19q co-deletion was referred to the oligodendroglial component, whereas TP53 mutations to the astrocytic one.

6.1.1. Mechanism of the combined loss of the chromosomes 1p and 19q

The mechanism of the combined loss of the two chromosomal arms is an unbalanced t(1;19)(q10;p10) translocation of 19p to 1q. A centromeric or pericentromeric translocation of chromosomes 1 and 19 results in two derivative chromosomes, der(1;19)(p10;q10) and der(1;19)(q10;p10), followed by the loss of the derivative chromosome containing the short arm of chromosome 1 and the long arm of chromosome 19 [31, 32].

The extent of the 1p/19q co-deletion has important diagnostic and prognostic implications. The chromosomal arm 1p is entirely deleted only in pure oligodendroglial tumors and the whole-arm 1p deletion has a strong favorable prognostic significance. Small telomeric (1p36) or interstitial 1p deletions are frequent as well, but with an opposite prognostic significance; they associate neither with deletion on the chromosomal arm 19q [33] nor with response to CHT [34].

While the total 1p/19q co-deletion is almost completely exclusive of oligodendrogliomas, partial 1p deletions are frequent in GBMs and isolated 19q loss in mixed and astrocytic gliomas in relation to the malignant transformation [35, 36].

Currently, there is a general agreement to diagnose the classical oligodendroglioma only in presence of a whole-arm 1p/19q co-deletion [37, 38].

Most oligodendrogliomas with 1p/19q co-deletion harbor IDH1/2, telomerase reverse transcriptase (TERT), homolog of the *Drosophila capicua* (CIC) and far upstream element-binding protein 1 (FUBP1) somatic mutations, and O^6-methylguanine-DNA methyltransferase (MGMT) or CDKN2A ($p14^{ARF}$) promoter hypermethylation [37, 39–41].

6.1.2. Methods for the detection of 1p/19q chromosomal status

Different methods for the detection of the 1p/19q chromosomal status are employed in the routine diagnostics. Fluorescent *in situ* hybridization (FISH) is a single-locus technique, limited to the 1p36 locus and thus not regarded as a suitable tool due to the high risk of false-positive results [34, 37, 42, 43]. On the other hand, LOH analysis is generally carried out with a low number of microsatellite markers covering only a small chromosomal region.

In contrast, multi-locus techniques, as comparative genomic hybridization (CGH) or multiplex ligation-dependent probe amplification (MLPA) detect gene copy number changes on the whole chromosome and distinguish whole-arm from partial 1p deletion [44]. Additionally, they can reveal putative gain of functions on both 1p and 19q chromosomes [45, 46].

In particular, MLPA has been validated as a high-resolution gene dosage assay for the screening of large deletions and duplication/amplification events in human cancers. In gliomas, three independent studies validated MLPA to assess the 1p/19q status by comparing MLPA data with CGH data obtained on the same tumor series, mainly composed of oligodendroglial tumors [47–49]. In the authors' experience, MLPA is a reliable and powerful tool to assess the 1p/19q status on formalin fixed and paraffin embedded tumor samples.

6.2. IDH1/2 mutations

IDHs catalyze the oxidative decarboxylation of isocitrate to α-ketoglutarate with production of NADH/NADPH and they are involved in the Krebs cycle.

Recurrent somatic point mutations affect the arginine (Arg) residue at codon 132 in the IDH1 gene on chromosome 2q33.3. Less frequently, they occur at the homolog Arg (R) residue at codon 172 in the IDH2 gene on chromosome 15q26.1. The IDH1/2 mutation rate is in the range of 70– 80% in OII and OIII [50–53] and less in OAII and OAIII, with a higher frequency in 1p/19q co-deleted tumors [37]. IDH1 mutations prevail in astrocytic tumors whereas IDH2 mutations are more common in oligodendroglial tumors [51, 54].

In low grade gliomas, they are prognostic favorable factors [53, 55, 56].

The c.395G>A (p.R132H) mutation can be easily detected by a anti-$IDH1^{R132H}$ mutation-specific antibody by immunohistochemical techniques [53, 57]. Tumor cells show $IDH1^{R132H}$ immunopositivity in their cytoplasms, whereas reactive astrocytes and normal glia cells are negative. This is particularly evident in the picture of cortical perineuronal satellitosis where positive (tumor) and negative (normal) satellites can be found, at the beginning of invasion.

6.2.1. ATRX mutations

The ATRX gene is located on chromosome Xq21.1, contains 35 exons, and encodes a 2,492 amino acid protein. ATRX belongs to the H3.3-ATRX-DAXX chromatin remodeling pathway, involved in chromatin stabilization [58]. ATRX and its binding factor death-associated protein 6 (DAXX) incorporates the histone protein H3.3 into the nucleosome at telomeres and pericentric heterochromatin [59, 60]. Alterations of this function lead to loss of structural integrity at telomeres leading to tumorigenesis. In fact, ATRX or DAXX protein loss is associated to the alternative lengthening of telomeres (ALT), a telomerase-independent mechanism of telomere lengthening [61–66].

Germline ATRX mutations give rise to a syndrome characterized by severe mental retardation [67] and to α-thalassemia.

Somatic ATRX mutations occur in gliomas of different types and histologic grades [38, 61–65, 68–70]. They are more frequent in grade II (67%) and in grade III (73%) astrocytic tumors and in secondary GBMs (57%), as well as in mixed gliomas (25% in grade II and 27–53.8% in grade III tumors) [64, 65, 69, 70]. In contrast, they are rare in primary GBMs (4%), pediatric GBMs (20%) and in pure oligodendroglial tumors (<10%) [63, 64, 68]. Very importantly, ATRX mutations do not affect pilocytic astrocytomas [64].

ATRX mutations occur in 70% of IDH mutant and intact 1p/19q low grade gliomas [62, 64, 65]. Restricted to IDH mutant tumors, they are significantly associated to TP53 mutations and nuclear p53 overexpression and to astrocytic differentiation; they are mutually exclusive with 1p/19q co-deletion [71, 72]. ATRX and IDH1/2 mutations occur in association and they may represent early genetic alterations in the development of gliomas affecting progenitors before their differentiation along the two lineages.

In pediatric gliomas, all ATRX mutations cluster near the C-terminal helicase domains; in adult tumors, they are evenly distributed across the gene, mainly as frameshift mutations leading to truncated proteins [63, 64, 69].

The relatively large size of the ATRX gene makes the mutation analysis difficult to be applied in the routine diagnostic procedures. The immunohistochemical evaluation of the ATRX protein expression could represent an alternative method to assess the ATRX status. Although studies reported concordant results between the mutation analysis and IHC [38, 72], tumor heterogeneity in the ATRX expression and concurrent normal non-tumor cells with constitutive ATRX expression may explain possible discrepancy. As a matter of fact, ATRX mutations/ATRX protein loss characterizes astrocytic gliomas, whereas retained ATRX immunoreactivity characterizes oligodendroglial gliomas. Referred to OA, the former is typical of the astrocytic component while the latter of the oligodendroglial one [71].

6.2.2. *ATRX and prognosis*

Patients harboring ATRX mutations would show a better outcome [65]. ATRX has important prognostic implications in anaplastic gliomas [65]. ATRX loss is a prognostic factor in IDH mutant and non 1p/19q co-deleted low grade gliomas [62, 65]. In GBMs, ATRX loss affects younger patients [72].

7. Nosograhic position of OA after the "ISN-Haarlem Consensus"

The "integrated" diagnosis provided for grade II and III adult gliomas covers the diagnostic uncertainties between astrocytoma and oligodendroglioma and, mainly, of OA.

It has been found that OAs more frequently exhibited the molecular signature of either pure oligodendroglioma (IDH1/2, 1p/19q co-deletion, CIC, FUB1, and TERT promoter mutations) or pure astrocytoma (IDH1/2, TP53, and ATRX mutations) with almost total exclusivity [71]. A recent study proved that most low grade gliomas (including 74 OAs) with IDH1/2 mutations and intact 1p/19q harbored a high frequency of TP53 mutations (94%) and ATRX mutations (86%) [73].

In 31 of 43 OAs (72.1%), the absence of ATRX mutations, associated with IDH1/2 mutations and total 1p/19q co-deletion, reclassified them as oligodendrogliomas; 11 of 43 (25.6%), with concurrent ATRX protein loss and TP53 mutations were reclassified as astrocytomas. The astrocytes within the tumor were, therefore, interpreted as reactive [71]. These results were similar to a previous one [64] and were confirmed in a large collection of cases [38]. The conclusion is that OA should be removed from the WHO classification as a distinct tumor entity, although rare instances of clearly biphasic OAs exhibiting morphologic and molecular heterogeneity have been described. Mixed areas of the tumor could show heterogeneous ATRX immunoreactivity with positive reactive astrocytes and negative tumor astrocytes [74, 75]. As ATRX is ubiquitously expressed in normal cells (endothelial cells, reactive astrocytes, microglia cells, and lymphocytes) [38, 71], the real problem in the diagnosis of OA according to the 2007 WHO classification seems to ascertain the occurrence of ATRX-negative and $IDH1^{R132H}$ -positive astrocytes in the tumor.

The astrocytic and oligodendroglial components have been found to share the same molecular signature, but with a sheer cell differentiation [71]. They should be regarded as "morphologically ambiguous" rather than "mixed" tumors, as conventionally referred. 1p/19q co-deletion and TP53 mutations represent distinct mechanisms of oncogenesis but they do not provide evidence for a genetic signature specifically related to OA [76].

The "ISN-Haarlem *Consensus*" suggested considering OA or tumors with ambiguous histology as diffuse astrocytoma when harboring IDH1/2 mutations, intact 1p/19q, and ATRX loss; as oligodendroglioma when harboring IDH1/2 mutations, 1p/19q co-deletion, and intact ATRX and as diffuse astrocytoma when harboring wild type IDH. In the absence of molecular data, the tumor should be diagnosed as oligodendroglioma or diffuse astrocytoma not otherwise specified (NOS). Finally, the denomination of OA would be only maintained when molecular testing does not solve tumor diagnosis [27].

Anyway, there is no doubt on the usefulness of the ATRX IHC [72] and of the double ATRX/$IDH1^{R132H}$ immunostaining [77] in the diagnosis of adult diffuse gliomas. Based on molecular data from the above mentioned markers on 54 OAs, it has been concluded that OA represents a morphological grey zone rather than a group of truly "mixed" or "intermediate" gliomas [78]. Importantly, it remains unsolved how to explain IDH mutant diffuse gliomas with ATRX expression and intact 1p/19q (neither merely astrocytic nor oligodendroglial lesions) or, more rarely, cases with loss of ATRX protein expression and total 1p/19q co-deletion (both astrocytic and oligodendroglial lesions).

8. Observations on personal OA series

Our analysis started from the established principles that 1p/19q co-deletion is typical of oligodendrogliomas, but that it occurs in a low percentage only of tumors with a classical oligodendroglial phenotype ("honeycomb" appearance and "chicken wire" vessels). Our 40 OA cases had been initially diagnosed according to stringent histologic criteria, so that their number is slightly lower compared to others' series. The current revision has been carried out on the basis of 1p/19q chromosomal status, as detected by MLPA, IDH1/2 mutation status by IHC and sequencing analysis, and ATRX expression by IHC. The key points were: 1) the retained expression of ATRX by tumor oligodendroglial nuclei and by reactive astrocyte, microglia/macrophage, endothelial cell, lymphocyte nuclei, and the ATRX protein loss in tumor astrocytic nuclei; 2) IDH1/2 mutations, present in low grade gliomas with a higher frequency in oligodendrogliomas than astrocytomas [52, 79] (**Figure 3A–D**); 3) therefore, although they reveal the tumor nature of cells, IDH1/2 mutations can lack both in oligodendroglial and astrocytic tumor cells. As, beside reactive astrocytes, ATRX is expressed in microglia/macrophage nuclei, Iba-1, CD68, CD16, and CD163 IHC has been performed on parallel serial tumor sections, as well as the double ATRX/GFAP, ATRX/Iba-1, and ATRX/$IDHR^{132H}$ immunostaining. Microglia/macrophages can reach in the tumor sections a frequency of 50–130 *x* 40 HPF (personal data); ATRX expressing nuclei could be, therefore, referred to tumor oligodendrocytes only if their number encompasses the number of microglia/macrophage nuclei. The occurrence of microglia/macrophages is, in our experience, the main bias to recognize the oligodendroglial component in OA (**Figure 4A–H**). Normal oligodendrocytes do not express ATRX and they can be distinguished in this way from tumor oligodendrocytes; moreover, they express Cyclin D1 that, in contrast, is not expressed by tumor oligodendrocytes unless they are cycling cells (**Figure 5A–D**) [80].

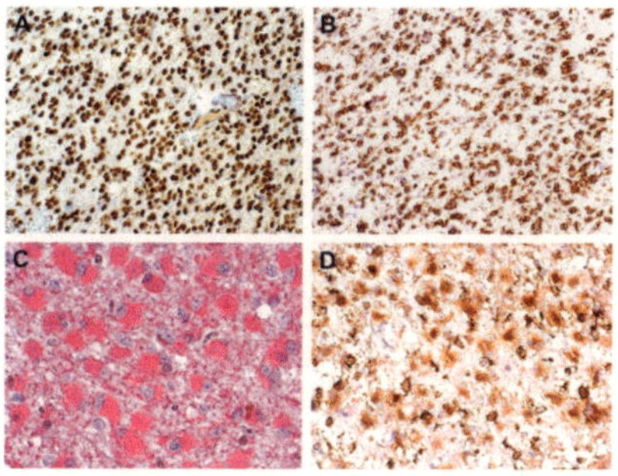

Figure 3. Immunohistochemistry (IHC). A – Oligodendroglioma, ATRX-positive cells, DAB, x200; B – Id, IDH1^{R132H} -positive perinuclear rim in tumor cells, DAB, x200. C – Gemistocytic astrocytoma, ATRX-negative and GFAP-positive tumor astrocytes, double IHC with DAB and *Fast Red*, respectively, x400; D – Id, IDH1^{R132H} -positive cells, DAB, x400. Anti-IDH1^{R132H} mouse monoclonal antibody (clone H09, Dianova GmbH, Hamburg, Germany) and anti-ATRX rabbit polyclonal antibody (HPA001906, Sigma Aldrich Co., St. Louis, MO, USA). DAB, 3,3'-Diaminobenzidine.

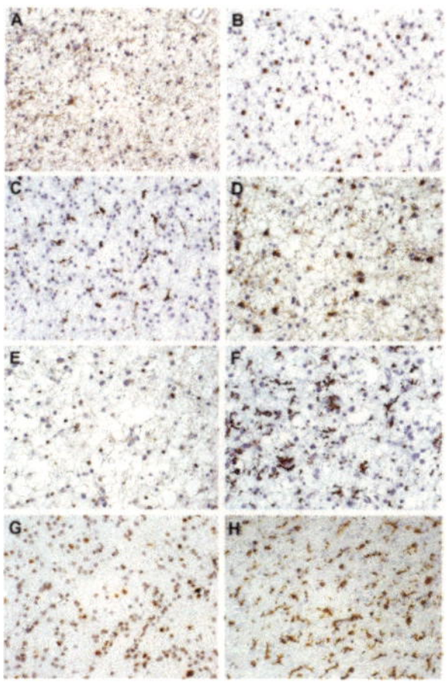

Figure 4. Immunohistochemistry (IHC). A – Diffuse astrocytoma, GFAP-positive cells, x200; B– Id, scattered ATRX-positive nuclei, the frequency of which corresponds to the frequency of CD68 positive-cells (C), both x200; D – Diffuse astrocytoma, apparent OA with GFAP-positive astrocytes and possible oligodendroglial nuclei, x200; E – Id, scattered ATRX-positive nuclei, x200; F – Id, Iba-1-positive cells covering the number of ATRX-positive nuclei, x200; G – Oligodendroglial infiltration, ATRX-positive and ATRX-negative nuclei, x200; H – Id, Iba-1-positive cells, x200 in 40 x high power field. All 3,3'-Diaminobenzidine (DAB).

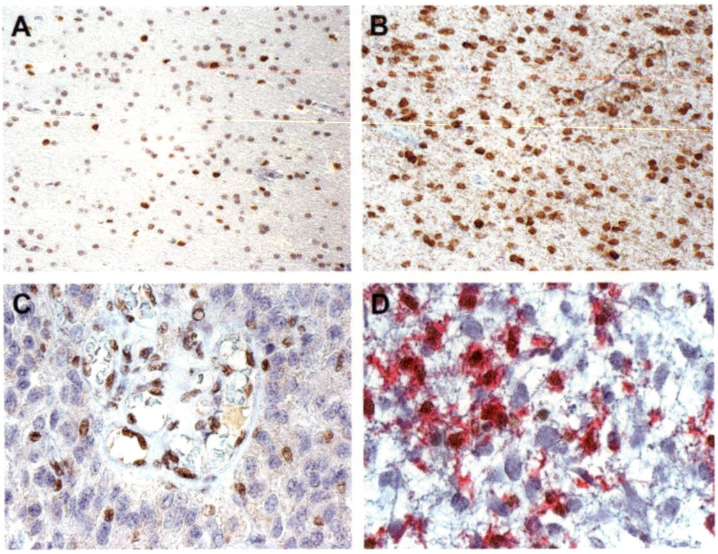

Figure 5. Immunohistochemistry (IHC). A – Oligodendroglioma, mild infiltration with several ATRX-negative normal oligodendrocytes and few ATRX-positive nuclei (tumor muclei or microglia/macrophage cells?), DAB, x200; B – Id, Cyclin D1-positive normal oligodendrocytes, DAB, x200; C – Oligodendroglioma, ATRX-positive endothelial cells, DAB, x400; D – Gemistocytic astrocytoma, microglia/macrophage cells, Iba-1- and ATRX-positive cells, double IHC with *Fast Red* and DAB, respectively, x400. DAB, 3,3'-Diaminobenzidine.

The diagnosis of the 40 OA cases changed in 87.5% of them (35/40): 22/40 (55%) were reclassified as astrocytomas due to the absence of total 1p/19q co-deletion, the occurrence of IDH1/2 mutations, and the loss of ATRX expression in GFAP-positive, phenotypically looking tumor astrocytes (**Figure 6A–D**); 11/40 (27.5%) were reclassified as oligodendrogliomas due to IDH1/2 mutations, retained ATRX expression, total 1p/19q in 2/11 (18.2%) cases and partial 1p or 19q deletions in 9/11 (81.8%) cases. In 2/40 (5%) cases the diagnosis changed into reactive gliosis due to retained ATRX expression in GFAP-positive reactive astrocytes and to the lack of ATRX-positive oligodendrocytes (**Figure 6E–F**). Among the remaining five cases, in one case with partial 1p/19q co-deletion, ATRX-negative and GFAP-positive astrocytes co-existed with a number of ATRX-positive and GFAP-negative oligodendrocytes; both cell components showed IDH^{R132H} immunopositivity by double ATRX/$IDH1^{R132H}$ immunostaining. Importantly, by the double ATRX/Iba-1 immunostaining, it was possible to verify that the number of ATRX-positive oligodendroglial nuclei was higher than the number of Iba-1-positive cells. The diagnosis of OA in this case was thus confirmed (**Figure 7A**). Two wild type IDH cases without total 1p/19q co-deletion and with heterogeneous ATRX expression were regarded as ambiguous since the tumor nature of the two cell components could not be ascertained. In the other two cases, one with partial 1p/19q deletion and one with intact 1p/19q, the diagnosis of OA could not be maintained since it was technically impossible to perform $IDH1^{R132H}$ IHC.

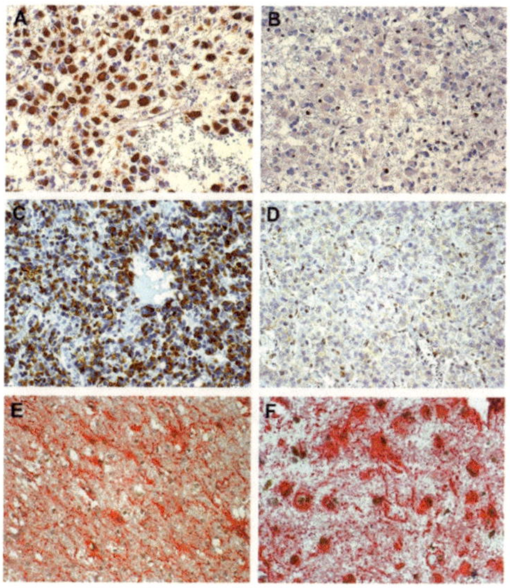

Figure 6. Immunohistochemistry (IHC). A – Gemistocytic astrocytoma, GFAP-positive cells, DAB, x200; B – Id, ATRX-negative cells, DAB, x200; C – Anaplastic astrocytoma, GFAP-positive cells, DAB, x200; D – Id, ATRX-negative cells, DAB, x200; E – Oligodendroglioma, reactive astrocytes with GFAP-positive thick cytoplasms and long processes and ATRX-positive nuclei, double IHC with *Fast Red* and DAB, respectively, x400. F – Reactive gliosis, reactive astrocytes with GFAP-positive large cytoplasms and short processes and ATRX-positive nuclei, double IHC with *Fast Red* and DAB, respectively, x400. DAB, 3,3'-Diaminobenzidine.

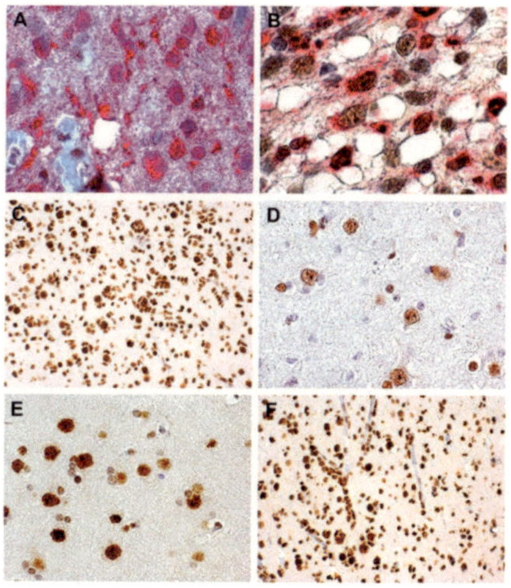

Figure 7. Immunohistochemistry (IHC). A – OA, ATRX- and $IDH1^{R132H}$ -positive astrocytes, double IHC with DAB and *Fast Red*, respectively, x630; B – Oligodendroglial minigemistocytes with ATRX-positive nuclei and GFAP-positive cytoplasms, double IHC with DAB and *Fast Red*, respectively, x1000; C – Oligodendroglioma, satellitosis with ATRX-positive nuclei, DAB, x200; D – Normal cortex, ATRX-positive neurons with ATRX-negative satellites, DAB, x400; E – Oligodendroglial cortical infiltration, ATRX-positive neurons with ATRX-positive and ATRX-negative satellites, DAB, x400; F – Id, ATRX-positive pericapillary tumor cells, DAB, x200. DAB, 3,3'-Diaminobenzidine.

The distinction of reactive from tumor astrocytes has always been a crucial point in the diagnosis of OA. Their recognition as reactive is a point of reference in denying the existence of such tumor category. Reactive astrocytes retain nuclear ATRX protein expression, as tumor oligodendrocytes, while tumor astrocytes lack ATRX expression.

By comparing our results with those of the literature, it is noteworthy that the change of diagnosis from the initial to the current analyses of cases, largely depends on the criteria used in the initial recognition of OAs. Upon the reclassification of the 35 cases as astrocytoma, oligodendroglioma, or reactive gliosis, only one could deserve the dignity of OA among the remaining five cases.

It must be incidentally remark that total 1p/19q co-deletion occurred in 43/113 (38.1%) of our oligodendroglioma series (selected by the typical morphology of honeycomb appearance and chicken wire vessel distribution); partial 1p and/or 19q deletions occurred in 36/82 (43.9%) of oligodendrogliomas and in 12/24 (50%) astrocytomas. Referring to the 40 cases with initial diagnosis of OA, two had total 1p/19q co-deletion, 14 partial 1p/19q deletion, 12 intact 1p/19q, and one a gain of function on the chromosome 19q. For the remaining 11 cases, the 1p/19q status was not available. It is widely accepted that partial 1p/19q deletions may occur in other gliomas, but one wonders how tumors with an oligodendroglial phenotype with partial deletions or intact 1p/19q can be classified.

9. Conclusions

By applying the "integrated" approach to the revision of our OA series, we conclude that, OA could no longer be regarded as a separate tumor entity. However, rare cases might retain the OA denomination [74, 75, our case], indicating that tumors can differentiate in oligodendroglial and astrocytic sense, even maintaining the same molecular genetics [71], or that they can arise from progenitors before differentiation in the two lineages.

Two points must be emphasized: one is the importance of the double immunostaining to recognize the astrocytic nature of tumor cells, especially the association between IDH and ATRX expression, considering that IDH1/2 mutations prevail in oligodendrogliomas in comparison to astrocytomas [52, 79]. In supposed mixed tumors with the two separate components, it has been observed that these share the same molecular asset and that astrocytes in the tumor are reactive cells [71]. However, in tumors with the two cell types intermingled, tumor cells can be distinguished from reactive astrocytes by the double ATRX/GFAP immunostaining. It must be remarked that in rare instances 1p/19q co-deletion can be associated with ATRX mutations/ATRX protein loss [64] and that, since a quota of astrocytomas do not harbor IDH1/2 mutations, tumor astrocytes with wild type IDH may be found.

Minigemistocytes show definitely the oligodendroglial nature due to their ATRX-positive nuclei (**Figure 7B**).

The other point is the great influence that microglia/macrophage occurrence may exert in the recognition of tumor oligodendrocytes due to their nuclear ATRX positivity. In cases where

http://dx.doi.org/10.5772/63240

the number of microglia/macrophages is very high to reach the number of ATRX-positive nuclei, if tumor astrocytes are demonstrable, the tumor should be reclassified as astrocytoma. In order to recognize an oligodendroglial tumor infiltration, often result of a biopsy, it is still mandatory that the number of ATRX-positive nuclei in a given area encompasses the number of microglia/macrophages (personal data). ATRX-negative nuclei in infiltration areas correspond to normal oligodendrocytes. Only the double ATRX/Iba-1 immunostaining can reveal the occurrence of normal oligodendrocytes, beside their Cyclin D1 expression. In $IDH1^{R132H}$ mutant cases, the double ATRX/$IDH1^{R132H}$ immunostaining unequivocally identifies oligodendroglial tumor cells. The coexistence of normal and tumor oligodendrocytes by ATRX IHC can be demonstrated in perineuronal satellitosis: in its initial phases, ATRX-positive and ATRX-negative nuclei are found around neurons; in later phases, all nuclei are ATRX-positive (**Figure 7C–E**). The same can be said for pericapillary satellitosis (**Figure 7F**).

The last point to be discussed is the possibility to find a false "honeycomb" appearance mimicking the typical perinuclear "halo" with ATRX-positive nuclei. This aspect cannot be interpreted as suggestive of an oligodendroglial origin of the tumor, being expressions of a water disturb/edema of unspecified nature, as it may happen for instance, in pilocytic astrocytoma [81].

Acknowledgements

We thank Dr. M.C. Valentini (Neuroradiology Department / Città della Salute e della Scienza Hospital, Turin, Italy) for providing the MRI figures.

We thank Fondazione Cassa di Risparmio di Vercelli (Vercelli, Italy) for the support to the elaboration of this chapter.

Disclosure of Potential Conflicts of Interest:

Authors declare no potential conflicts of interest.

Author details

Marta Mellai, Laura Annovazzi, Marta Mazzucco and Davide Schiffer*

*Address all correspondence to: davide.schiffer@unito.it

Research Center/Policlinico di Monza Foundation, Vercelli, (Italy)

References

[1] Louis DN, Ohgaki H, Wiestler OD, Cavenee WK. WHO Classification of Tumours of the Central Nervous System. 4th ed. Lyon, France: International Agency for Research on Cancer (IARC); 2007. p. 309.

[2] Von Deimling A, Reifenberger G, Kros JM, Louis DN, Collins VP. Oligoastrocytoma. In: Louis DN, Ohgaki H, Wiestler OD, Cavenee WK, editors. WHO Classification of Tumours of the Central Nervous System. 4th ed. Lyon, France: International Agency for Research on Cancer (IARC); 2007. pp. 63-65.

[3] Von Deimling A, Reifenberger G, Kros JM, Louis DN, Collins VP. Anaplastic oligoastrocytoma. In: Louis DN, Ohgaki H, Wiestler OD, Cavenee WK, editors. WHO Classification of Tumours of the Central Nervous System. 4th ed. Lyon, France: International Agency for Research on Cancer (IARC); 2007. pp. 63-67.

[4] Cooper ERA. The relation of oligocytes and astrocytes in cerebral tumours. J Pathol. 1935;41:259-266.

[5] Hart MN, Petito CK, Earle KM. Mixed gliomas. Cancer. 1974;33:134-140.

[6] Daumas-Duport C, Varlet P, Tucker ML, Beuvon F, Cervera P, et al. Oligodendrogliomas. Part I: Patterns of growth, histological diagnosis, clinical and imaging correlations: a study of 153 cases. J Neurooncol. 1997;34:37-59.

[7] Coons SW, Johnson PC, Scheithauer BW, Yates AJ, Pearl DK. Improving diagnostic accuracy and interobserver concordance in the classification and grading of primary gliomas. Cancer. 1997;79:1381-1393.

[8] Krouwer HG, van Duinen SG, Kamphorst W, van der Valk P, Algra A. Oligoastrocytomas: a clinicopathological study of 52 cases. J Neurooncol. 1997;33:223-238.

[9] Schiffer D. Brain Tumor Pathology: Current Diagnostic Hotspots and Pitfalls. Dordrecht, Netherlands: Springer Verlag; 2006. p. 272.

[10] de Armond SJ, Eng LF, Rubinstein LJ. The application of glial fibrillary acidic (GFA) protein immunohistochemistry in neurooncology. A progress report. Pathol Res Pract. 1980;168:374-394.

[11] van der Meulen JD, Houthoff HJ, Ebels EJ. Glial fibrillary acidic protein in human gliomas. Neuropathol Appl Neurobiol. 1978;4:177-190.

[12] Herpers MJ, Budka H. Glial fibrillary acidic protein (GFAP) in oligodendroglial tumors: gliofibrillary oligodendroglioma and transitional oligoastrocytoma as subtypes of oligodendroglioma. Acta Neuropathol. 1984;64:265-272.

[13] Choi BH, Kim RC. Expression of glial fibrillary acidic protein in immature oligodendroglia. Science. 1984;223:407-409.

[14] Fuller CE, Schmidt RE, Roth KA, Burger PC, Scheithauer BW, et al. Clinical utility of fluorescence in situ hybridization (FISH) in morphologically ambiguous gliomas with hybrid oligodendroglial/astrocytic features. J Neuropathol Exp Neurol. 2003;62:1118-1128.

[15] Maintz D, Fiedler K, Koopmann J, Rollbrocker B, Nechev S, et al. Molecular genetic evidence for subtypes of oligoastrocytomas. J Neuropathol Exp Neurol. 1997;56:1098-1104.

[16] Raff MC, Williams BP, Miller RH. The in vitro differentiation of a bipotential glial progenitor cell. EMBO J. 1984;3:1857-1864.

[17] Blümcke I, Becker AJ, Normann S, Hans V, Riederer BM, et al. Distinct expression pattern of microtubule-associated protein-2 in human oligodendrogliomas and glial precursor cells. J Neuropathol Exp Neurol. 2001;60:984-993.

[18] Matsumura N, Nobusawa S, Ikota H, Hirato J, Hirose T, et al. Coexpression of cyclin D1 and alpha-internexin in oligodendroglial tumors. Brain Tumor Pathol. 2015;32:261-267. DOI: 10.1007/s10014-015-0228-2.

[19] Yaziji H, Massarani-Wafai R, Gujrati M, Kuhns JG, Martin AW, et al. Role of p53 immunohistochemistry in differentiating reactive gliosis from malignant astrocytic lesions. Am J Surg Pathol. 1996;20:1086-1090.

[20] Kraus JA, Koopmann J, Kaskel P, Maintz D, Brandner S, et al. Shared allelic losses on chromosomes 1p and 19q suggest a common origin of oligodendroglioma and oligoastrocytoma. J Neuropathol Exp Neurol. 1995;54:91-95.

[21] Okamoto Y, Di Patre PL, Burkhard C, Horstmann S, Jourde B, et al. Population-based study on incidence, survival rates, and genetic alterations of low-grade diffuse astrocytomas and oligodendrogliomas. Acta Neuropathol. 2004;108:49-56.

[22] Mueller W, Hartmann C, Hoffmann A, Lanksch W, Kiwit J, et al. Genetic signature of oligoastrocytomas correlates with tumor location and denotes distinct molecular subsets. Am J Pathol. 2002;161:313-319.

[23] Eoli M, Bissola L, Bruzzone MG, Pollo B, Maccagnano C, et al. Reclassification of oligoastrocytomas by loss of heterozygosity studies. Int J Cancer. 2006;119:84-90.

[24] Reifenberger J, Reifenberger G, Liu L, James CD, Wechsler W, et al. Molecular genetic analysis of oligodendroglial tumors shows preferential allelic deletions on 19q and 1p. Am J Pathol. 1994;145:1175-1190.

[25] Smith JS, Perry A, Borell TJ, Lee HK, O'Fallon J, et al. Alterations of chromosome arms 1p and 19q as predictors of survival in oligodendrogliomas, astrocytomas, and mixed oligoastrocytomas. J Clin Oncol. 2000;18:636-645.

[26] Chen R, Ravindra VM, Cohen AL, Jensen RL, Salzman KL, et al. Molecular features assisting in diagnosis, surgery, and treatment decision making in low-grade gliomas. Neurosurg Focus. 2015;38:E2. DOI: 10.3171/2015.1.

[27] Wick W, Hartmann C, Engel C, Stoffels M, Felsberg J, et al. NOA-04 randomized phase III trial of sequential radio chemotherapy of anaplastic glioma with procarbazine, lomustine, and vincristine or temozolomide. J Clin Oncol. 2009;27:5874-5880. DOI: 10.1200/JCO.2009.23.6497.

[28] Louis DN, Perry A, Burger P, Ellison DW, Reifenberger G, et al. International Society Of Neuropathology-Haarlem consensus guidelines for nervous system tumor classification and grading. Brain Pathol. 2014;24:429-435. DOI: 10.1111/bpa.12171.

[29] Burger PC, Minn AY, Smith JS, Borell TJ, Jedlicka AE, Huntley, et al. Losses of chromosomal arms 1pand 19q on the diagnosis of oligodendroglioma. Study of paraffin-embedded sections. Mod Pathol. 2001;14:842-853.

[30] McDonald JM, See SJ, Tremont IW, Colman H, Gilbert MR, et al. The prognostic impact of histology and 1p/19q status in anaplastic oligodendroglial tumors. Cancer. 2005;104:1468-1477.

[31] Griffin CA, Burger P, Morsberger L, Yonescu R, Swierczynski S, et al. Identification of der(1;19)(q10;p10) in five oligodendrogliomas suggests mechanism of concurrent 1p and 19q loss. J Neuropathol Exp Neurol. 2006;65:988-994.

[32] Jenkins RB, Blair H, Ballman KV, Giannini C, Arusell RM, et al. A t(1;19)(q10;p10) mediates the combined deletions of 1p and 19q and predicts a better prognosis of patients with oligodendroglioma. Cancer Res. 2006;66:9852-9861.

[33] Idbaih A, Marie Y, Pierron G, Brennetot C, Hoang-Xuan K, et al. Two types of chromosome 1p losses with opposite significance in gliomas. Ann Neurol. 2005;58:483-487.

[34] Barbashina V, Salazar P, Holland EC, Rosenblum MK, Ladanyi M. Allelic losses at 1p36 and 19q13 in gliomas: correlation with histologic classification, definition of a 150-kb minimal deleted region on 1p36, and evaluation of CAMTA1 as a candidate tumor suppressor gene. Clin Cancer Res. 2005;11:1119-1128.

[35] Hartmann C, Johnk L, Kitange G, Wu Y, Ashworth LK, et al. Transcript map of the 3.7-Mb D19S112-D19S246 candidate tumor suppressor region on the long arm of chromosome 19. Cancer Res. 2002;62:4100-4108.

[36] von Deimling A, Bender B, Jahnke R, Waha A, Kraus J, et al. Loci associated with malignant progression in astrocytomas: a candidate on chromosome 19q. Cancer Res. 1994;54:1397-1401.

[37] Labussière M, Idbaih A, Wang XW, Marie Y, Boisselier B, et al. All the 1p19q codeleted gliomas are mutated on IDH1 or IDH2. Neurology. 2010;74:1886-1890. DOI: 10.1212/WNL.0b013e3181e1cf3a.

[38] Reuss DE, Sahm F, Schrimpf D, Wiestler B, Capper D, et al. ATRX and IDH1-R132H immunohistochemistry with subsequent copy number analysis and IDH sequencing as a basis for an "integrated" diagnostic approach for adult astrocytoma, oligodendroglioma and glioblastoma. Acta Neuropathol. 2015;129:133-146. DOI: 10.1007/s00401-014-1370-3.

[39] Bettegowda C, Agrawal N, Jiao Y, Sausen M, Wood LD, et al. Mutations in CIC and FUBP1 contribute to human oligodendroglioma. Science. 2011;333:1453-1455. DOI: 10.1126/science.1210557.

[40] Yip S, Butterfield YS, Morozova O, Chittaranjan S, Blough MD, et al. Concurrent CIC mutations, IDH1/2 mutations, and 1p/19q loss distinguish oligodendrogliomas from other cancers. J Pathol. 2012;226:7-16. DOI: 10.1002/path.2995.

[41] Sahm F, Koelsche C, Meyer J, Pusch S, Lindenberg K, et al. CIC and FUBP1 mutations in oligodendrogliomas, oligoastrocytomas and astrocytomas. Acta Neuropathol. 2012;123:853-860. DOI: 10.1007/s00401-012-0993-5.

[42] Ichimura K, Vogazianou AP, Liu L, Pearson DM, Bäcklund LM, et al. 1p36 is a preferential target of chromosome 1 deletions in astrocytic tumours and homozygously deleted in a subset of glioblastomas. Oncogene. 2008;27:2097-2108.

[43] Leeper HE, Caron AA, Decker PA, Jenkins RB, Lachance DH, et al. IDH mutation, 1p19q codeletion and ATRX loss in WHO grade II gliomas. Oncotarget. 2015;6:30295-30305. DOI: 10.18632/oncotarget.4497.

[44] Idbaih A, Kouwenhoven M, Jeuken J, Carpentier C, Gorlia T, et al. Chromosome 1p loss evaluation in anaplastic oligodendrogliomas. Neuropathology. 2008;28:440-443. DOI: 10.1111/j.1440-1789.2008.00863.

[45] Jeuken JW, Sprenger SH, Wesseling P, Macville MV, von Deimling A, et al. Identification of subgroups of high-grade oligodendroglial tumors by comparative genomic hybridization. J Neuropathol Exp Neurol. 1999;58:606-612.

[46] Jeuken JW, Sprenger SH, Boerman RH, von Deimling A, Teepen HL, et al. Subtyping of oligo-astrocytic tumours by comparative genomic hybridization. J Pathol. 2001;194:81-87.

[47] Jeuken J, Cornelissen S, Boots-Sprenger S, Gijsen S, Wesseling P. Multiplex ligation-dependent probe amplification: a diagnostic tool for simultaneous identification of different genetic markers in glial tumors. J Mol Diagn. 2006;8:433-443.

[48] Natté R, van Eijk R, Eilers P, Cleton-Jansen AM, Oosting J, et al. Multiplex ligation-dependent probe amplification for the detection of 1p and 19q chromosomal loss in oligodendroglial tumors. Brain Pathol. 2005;15:192-197.

[49] Franco-Hernández C, Martínez-Glez V, de Campos JM, Isla A, Vaquero J, et al. Allelic status of 1p and 19q in oligodendrogliomas and glioblastomas: multiplex ligation-

dependent probe amplification versus loss of heterozygosity. Cancer Genet Cytogenet. 2009;190:93-96. DOI: 10.1016/j.cancergencyto.2008.09.017.

[50] Yan H, Parsons DW, Jin G, McLendon R, Rasheed BA, et al. IDH1 and IDH2 mutations in gliomas. N Engl J Med. 2009;360:765-773. DOI: 10.1056/NEJMoa0808710.

[51] Hartmann C, Meyer J, Balss J, Capper D, Mueller W, et al. Type and frequency of IDH1 and IDH2 mutations are related to astrocytic and oligodendroglial differentiation and age: a study of 1,010 diffuse gliomas. Acta Neuropathol. 2009; 118: 469–474. DOI: 10.1007/s00401-009-0561-9.

[52] Balss J, Meyer J, Mueller W, Korshunov A, Hartmann C, et al. Analysis of the IDH1 codon 132 mutation in brain tumors. Acta Neuropathol. 2008;116:597-602. DOI: 10.1007/s00401-008-0455-2.

[53] Mellai M, Piazzi A, Caldera V, Monzeglio O, Cassoni P, et al. IDH1 and IDH2 mutations, immunohistochemistry and associations in a series of brain tumors. J Neurooncol. 2011;105:345-357. DOI: 10.1007/s11060-011-0596-3.

[54] Gravendeel LA, Kloosterhof NK, Bralten LB, van Marion R, Dubbink HJ, et al. Segregation of non-p.R132H mutations in IDH1 in distinct molecular subtypes of glioma. Hum Mutat. 2010;31:E1186-1199. DOI: 10.1002/humu.21201.

[55] Sun H, Yin L, Li S, Han S, Song G, et al. Prognostic significance of IDH mutation in adult low-grade gliomas: a meta-analysis. J Neurooncol. 2013;113:277-284. DOI: 10.1007/s11060-013-1107-5.

[56] Wang XW, Ciccarino P, Rossetto M, Boisselier B, Marie Y, et al. IDH mutations: genotype-phenotype correlation and prognostic impact. Biomed Res Int. 2014;2014:540236. DOI: 10.1155/2014/540236.

[57] Capper D, Reuss D, Schittenhelm J, Hartmann C, Bremer J, et al. Mutation-specific IDH1 antibody differentiates oligodendrogliomas and oligoastrocytomas from other brain tumors with oligodendroglioma-like morphology. Acta Neuropathol. 2011;121:241-252. DOI: 10.1007/s00401-010-0770-2.

[58] Clynes D, Higgs DR, Gibbons RJ. The chromatin remodeller ATRX: a repeat offender in human disease. Trends Biochem Sci. 2013;38:461-466. DOI: 10.1016/j.tibs.2013.06.011.

[59] Goldberg AD, Banaszynski LA, Noh KM, Lewis PW, Elsaesser SJ, et al. Distinct factors control histone variant H3.3 localization at specific genomic regions. Cell. 2010;140:678-691. DOI: 10.1016/j.cell.2010.01.003.

[60] Lewis PW, Elsaesser SJ, Noh KM, Stadler SC, Allis CD. Daxx is an H3.3-specific histone chaperone and cooperates with ATRX in replication-independent chromatin assembly at telomeres. Proc Natl Acad Sci U S A. 2010;107:14075-14080. DOI: 10.1073/pnas.1008850107.

[61] Heaphy CM, de Wilde RF, Jiao Y, Klein AP, Edil BH, et al. Altered telomeres in tumors with ATRX and DAXX mutations. Science. 2011;333:425. DOI: 10.1126/science.1207313.

[62] Kannan K, Inagaki A, Silber J, Gorovets D, Zhang J, et al. Whole-exome sequencing identifies ATRX mutation as a key molecular determinant in lower-grade glioma. Oncotarget. 2012;3:1194-1203.

[63] Schwartzentruber J, Korshunov A, Liu XY, Jones DT, Pfaff E, et al. Driver mutations in histone H3.3 and chromatin remodelling genes in paediatric glioblastoma. Nature. 2012;482:226-231. DOI: 10.1038/nature10833.

[64] Jiao Y, Killela PJ, Reitman ZJ, Rasheed AB, Heaphy CM, et al. Frequent ATRX, CIC, FUBP1 and IDH1 mutations refine the classification of malignant gliomas. Oncotarget. 2012;3:709-722.

[65] Wiestler B, Capper D, Holland-Letz T, Korshunov A, von Deimling A, et al. ATRX loss refines the classification of anaplastic gliomas and identifies a subgroup of IDH mutant astrocytic tumors with better prognosis. Acta Neuropathol. 2013;126:443-451. DOI: 10.1007/s00401-013-1156-z.

[66] Nguyen DN, Heaphy CM, de Wilde RF, Orr BA, Odia Y, et al. Molecular and morphologic correlates of the alternative lengthening of telomeres phenotype in high-grade astrocytomas. Brain Pathol. 2013;23:237-243. DOI: 10.1111/j.1750-3639.2012.00630.

[67] Villard L, Toutain A, Lossi AM, Gecz J, Houdayer C, et al. Splicing mutation in the ATR-X gene can lead to a dysmorphic mental retardation phenotype without alpha-thalassemia. Am J Hum Genet. 1996;58:499-505.

[68] Khuong-Quang DA, Buczkowicz P, Rakopoulos P, Liu XY, Fontebasso AM, et al. K27M mutation in histone H3.3 defines clinically and biologically distinct subgroups of pediatric diffuse intrinsic pontine gliomas. Acta Neuropathol. 2012;124:439-447. DOI: 10.1007/s00401-012-0998-0.

[69] Liu XY, Gerges N, Korshunov A, Sabha N, Khuong-Quang DA, et al. Frequent ATRX mutations and loss of expression in adult diffuse astrocytic tumors carrying IDH1/IDH2 and TP53 mutations. Acta Neuropathol. 2012;124:615-625. DOI: 10.1007/s00401-012-1031-3.

[70] Sahm F, Reuss D, Koelsche C, Capper D, Schittenhelm J, et al. Farewell to oligoastrocytoma: in situ molecular genetics favor classification as either oligodendroglioma or astrocytoma. Acta Neuropathol. 2014;128:551-559. DOI: 10.1007/s00401-014-1326-7.

[71] Ikemura M, Shibahara J, Mukasa A, Takayanagi S, Aihara K, et al. Utility of ATRX immunohistochemistry in diagnosis of adult diffuse gliomas. Histopathology. 2016. DOI: 10.1111/his.12927.

[72] Cryan JB, Haidar S, Ramkissoon LA, Bi WL, Knoff DS, et al. Clinical multiplexed exome sequencing distinguishes adult oligodendroglial neoplasms from astrocytic and mixed lineage gliomas. Oncotarget. 2014;5:8083-8092.

[73] Cancer Genome Atlas Research Network. Comprehensive, integrative genomic analysis of diffuse lower-grade gliomas. N Engl J Med. 2015;372:2481-2498.

[74] Huse JT, Diamond EL, Wang L, Rosenblum MK. Mixed glioma with molecular features of composite oligodendroglioma and astrocytoma: a true "oligoastrocytoma"? Acta Neuropathol. 2015;129:151-153. DOI: 10.1007/s00401-014-1359-y.

[75] Wilcox P, Li CC, Lee M, Shivalingam B, Brennan J, et al. Oligoastrocytomas: throwing the baby out with the bathwater? Acta Neuropathol. 2015;129:147-149. DOI: 10.1007/s00401-014-1353-4.

[76] Bai H, Zou Y, Lee AM, Tang X, Zhang P, et al. Does morphological assessment have a role in classifying oligoastrocytoma as "oligodendroglial" vs. "astrocytic"? Histopathology. 2015. DOI: 10.1111/his.12891.

[77] Cai J, Zhu P, Zhang C, Li Q, Wang Z, Li, et al. Detection of ATRX and IDH1-R132H immunohistochemistry in the progression of 211 paired gliomas. Oncotarget. 2016. DOI: 10.18632/oncotarget.7650.

[78] Hewer E, Vajtai I, Dettmer MS, Berezowska S, Vassella E. Combined ATRX/IDH1 immunohistochemistry predicts genotype of oligoastrocytomas. Histopathology. 2016;68:272-278. DOI: 10.1111/his.12743.

[79] Mellai M, Caldera V, Annovazzi L, Schiffer D. The distribution and significance of IDH mutation in gliomas. In: Lichtor T, editor. Evolution of the Molecular Biology of Brain Tumors and Therapeutic Implications. Rjieka, Croatia: InTech; 2013. pp. 299-342.

[80] Bosone I, Cavalla P, Chiadò-Piat L, Vito ND, Schiffer D. Cyclin D1 expression in normal oligodendroglia and microglia cells: its use in the differential diagnosis of oligodendrogliomas. Neuropathology. 2001;21:155-161.

[81] Prayson RA. Oligodendroglioma look-alikes: the histopathologic differential diagnosis. In: Reeves C, editor. Oligodendrogliomas (ODs): Diagnosis, Outcomes and Prognosis. New York: Nova Biomedical; 2016. pp. 83-118.

Chapter 15

Meningiomas' Management: An Update of the Literature

Giulia Cossu, Mahmoud Messerer, Fabrice Parker,
Marc Levivier and Roy Thomas Daniel

Additional information is available at the end of the chapter

http://dx.doi.org/10.5772/62929

Abstract

Meningiomas are the most common primary intracranial tumors in the adult population [1]. They are generally considered benign lesions but after the 2007 WHO classification, the proportion of atypical meningiomas has steeply increased. Surgery is considered the mainstay of the treatment and a complete resection is considered curative in WHO grade I meningiomas. The role of adjuvant treatments like radiotherapy (stereotactic radiosurgery or conventional external beam irradiation) and chemotherapy in more aggressive cases is still discussed, above all in WHO grade II meningiomas. We would like to expose the most important advances in meningiomas' management in accordance with the recent literature evidences.

Keywords: meningioma, management, benign meningiomas, atypical meningioma, anaplastic meningioma, malignant meningioma, surgery, radiotherapy, chemotherapy

1. Introduction

Meningiomas are the most common primary intracranial tumors[1]. Their origin from the arachnoid layer was first hypothesized by John Cleland in 1864 [2] and then reasserted by Cushing and Weed in 1915 [3]. Meningiomas are classified according to their dural attachment and histological grading. The 2000 WHO histological classification has been modified in 2007, and the epidemiology of more aggressive subtypes has thus recently changed [4]. Meningiomas may be incidental and asymptomatic, or they may present clinically with focal neurological deficit in accordance with a mass effect on an eloquent area or with epileptic seizures.

Surgery represents the mainstay of the treatment, but the management of more aggressive meningioma is challenging. The role of adjuvant therapies should thus be discussed in cases of more aggressive histological types, subtotal resection and recurrent diseases.

2. Epidemiology

Meningiomas account for 20 and 38% of all primary intracranial tumors, respectively, in males and in females, with an incidence of about five cases per 100,000 persons [5]. In an autoptic series about 2–3% of the general population had an incidental asymptomatic meningioma [6]. The female sex and estrogenic conditions seem to be a risk factor for developing meningiomas, with a female to male ratio of about 3:1 [7].

Hormonal therapy and hormone-dependent conditions such as breast cancer [8], pregnancy [9], or obesity [10] were in fact associated with a higher incidence of meningiomas. Cranial irradiation is also a recognized risk factor for developing meningiomas, usually with tumors having a more complex cariotype and a more aggressive behavior [11]. Head traumas have been for long associated with a higher meningioma incidence, but the causal effect was never demonstrated.

Some genetic conditions may favor the arising of meningiomas, such as neurofibromatosis type 2 (NF2), an autosomal dominant disorder characterized by mutation of the tumor suppressor gene NF2 coding for merlin in chromosome 22q12.2. Also multiple endocrine neoplasia type 1 (MEN1) is associated to a higher incidence of meningioma.

Meningiomas may derive from the dura of the cranial vault, of the skull base and at sites of dura reflection like the falx, the tentorium, and the dura recovering venous sinuses. Meningiomas may also arise from the optic-nerve sheath and from the choroid plexus. About 10% of them arise in the spine. In rare cases, meningiomas outside the craniospinal axis have been reported [12]. The preferential localization of intracranial meningiomas is summarized in **Figure 1**.

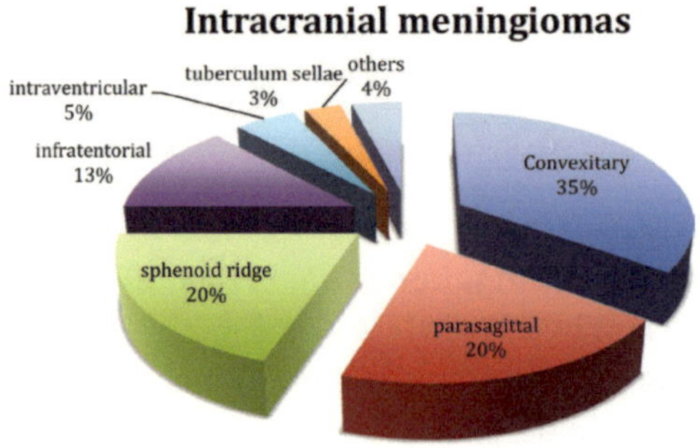

Figure 1. Graphic representation of the topographic distribution of intracranial meningiomas.

According to the 2007 World Health Organization (WHO) classification, meningiomas are divided in three categories: grade I or benign meningiomas, grade II or atypical meningiomas, and grade III or anaplastic meningiomas [11]. With this new grading system, which includes the brain invasion into the diagnostic criteria for aggressiveness, the percentage of atypical meningiomas grew to 20–35% of newly diagnosed meningiomas [13]. This classification is important because, together with the extension of resection, it may help in predicting the recurrence rate and thus the global prognosis [14, 15] (**Figure 2**).

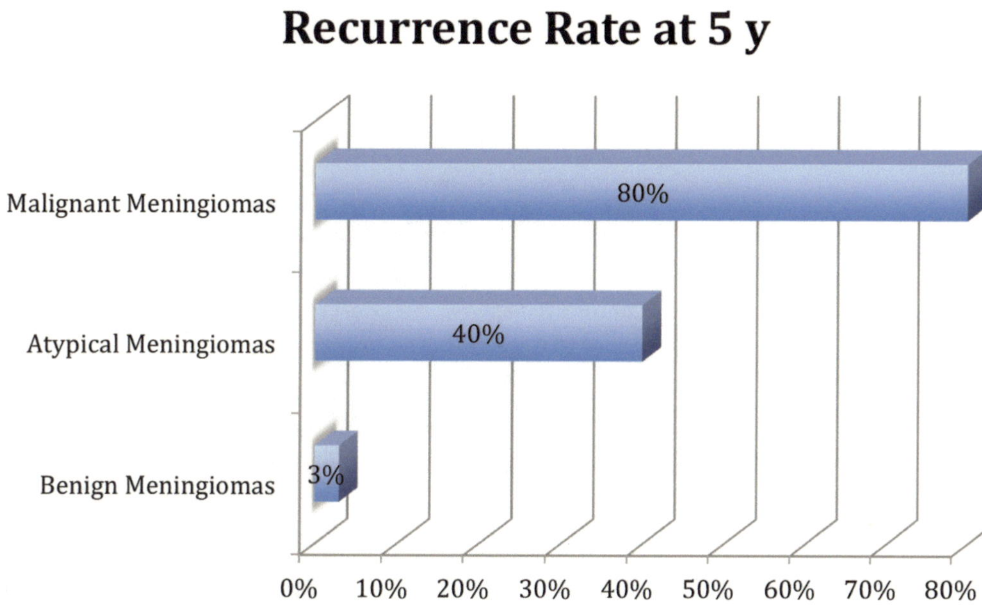

Figure 2. The recurrence rate at 5 years was stratified according to literature data: The recurrence after surgery is strictly related to the histologic grade of the lesion (WHO classification).

3. Clinical presentation

In many cases, meningiomas are asymptomatic and discovered in the context of investigations of unrelated symptoms [16]. When symptomatic they may determine epileptic seizures or focal neurological deficit according to the irritation or the compression of eloquent areas or vasculo-nervous structures. Hydrocephalus may be secondary to meningiomas obstructing the physiologic CSF flow. An increased intracranial pressure may be present in cases of voluminous lesions or with an associated peritumoral edema.

Focal neurological deficit is directly linked to the localization of the tumor, according to the compression of cranial nerves or specific hemispheric regions. Spinal tract compression is also typical for spinal meningiomas.

4. Radiology

Meningiomas present as well-defined extra-axial lesions with a typical peripheral CSF cleft. They present a homogeneous contrast enhancement on CT- and T1-weighted MRI with gadolinium administration. The tumor has a dural or bone implantation and a typical dural tail (contrast enhancement of the dura adjacent to meningioma implantation) (Figures 3 and 4). A reactive sclerosis of the underlying bone may be present in about half of skull-base meningiomas [17]. In rare cases, bone erosion is present (**Figure 5**). Calcifications or cystic portions may be present. Hyperintensity in T2-weighted MRI may denote a higher water content and thus an easily resectability during surgery.

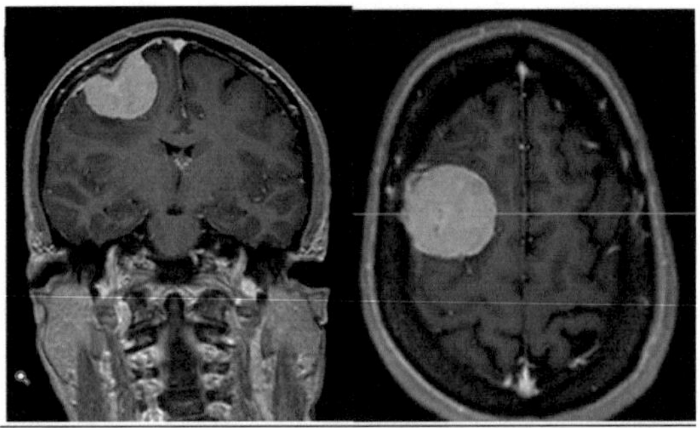

Figure 3. T1-weighted coronal (a) and axial (b) MRI with gadolinium administration showing a well-defined extra-axial lesion with an homogeneous enhancement and a contiguous dural enhancement (dural tail). A subtle CSF cleft is also visible between the lesion and the cerebral surface. These radiologic findings are typical for a convexitary meningioma.

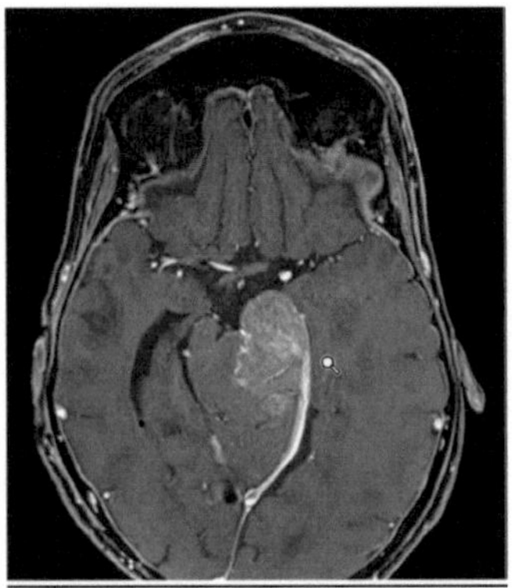

Figure 4. A tentorial meningiomas with less demarcated limits and probably infiltrating the adjacent brainstem. The dural tail is evident in this T1-weighted MRI post gadolinium administration. This 33-year-old patient was irradiated during infancy after the resection of an ependymoma of the IVth ventricle. This may help in explaining the atypical features of the lesion.

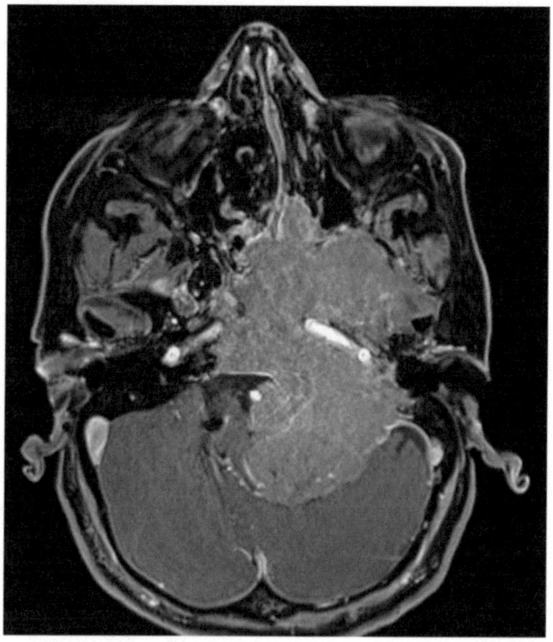

Figure 5. This skull base meningioma completely eroded the skull base and encased the internal carotid artery on the left side. Also the vertebral artery was surrounded by the tumor (not shown). The anatomy was completely modified by the lesion, and a preoperative study of the images was essential to plan the surgery.

Meningiomas may present an associated venous invasion and MRI venography may help in evaluating sinus thrombosis in the preoperative period.

An angiography may be performed in the preoperative period to assess the vascularization of the lesion and the relationship with important vascular structures. Meningiomas are in most of cases vascularized by the meningeal artery supplying the meninges at the tumor sites, and the angiographic blush is also called mother-in-law blush, because it comes early and leaves late. However, because of the risks linked to this invasive procedure, it is often performed in the context of the planning of a preoperative embolization.

5. Genetic and molecular profiles

More than a half of sporadic meningiomas of every histological grade have a mutation in NF2 gene on the chromosome 22q12, coding for merlin (moesin–ezrin–radixin-like protein), and it is considered an early event in tumorigenesis [18]. Merlin seems to interact with transmembranous proteins to activate pathways promoting cell proliferation. Its expression may vary, however, according to meningioma's subtype [19]. The product of the DAL-1 gene, a member of the protein 4.1 family, has also been supposed to be implicated in meningioma tumorigenesis and progression. The prevalence of mutations of protein 4.1B was not different among WHO grades, and it may be an early event in meningioma tumorigenesis [20].

Aside 22q deletions, multiple genetic mutations are observed in meningioma progression, such as loss of heterozygosis in 1p, 3p, 6q, 9p, 10q, and 14q [21] and are associated with histological progression [22].

Recently, the analysis of microRNAs (miRNAs) profiles was identified as a potential tool to define the natural history of different meningiomas. A low expression of miR-29c-3p and miR-219-5p was associated with more aggressive phenotypes and with a higher risk of recurrence [23]. On the contrary, high expression of miR-145 seems to be associated with a more indolent biological behavior.

Complex cariotypes were found in 34% of benign meningiomas, 45% of atypical, and 70% of anaplastic meningiomas [24].

Proliferative markers such as MIB-1 and Ki67 have been associated with a more aggressive biological behavior in some studies [25, 26]. The relationship between genetic and molecular alterations and recurrence is a matter of debate: According to Sandberg et al. [26], the recurrence rate seems to be associated to proliferative markers and Ki-67 and cyclin B1 genes were overexpressed in recurrent meningiomas [27, 28], with a significant association between Ki-67 and tumor recurrence [29]. Contrasting results exist, however, on this argument, as Aguiar et al. [30] did not find any association between MIB-1 and the histological grade. Other markers have also been investigated, such as p53, TGFalpha, and beta, PDGF [25, 31]. EGFRs are overexpressed in about 60% of meningiomas, while VEGF is also upregulated in meningioma cells but no association with the WHO histological grade was observed [32]. The invasiveness of meningioma cells has been linked to the expression of matrix-metalloproteinase-9 (MMP-9), and its expression may be a prognostic marker for recurrence [33].

In 1979, Donnell et al. [34] were the first to describe the role of estrogen receptors in meningiomas development. However, over the time, progesterone receptors showed to have a higher expression in meningioma cells and their level was correlated to a favorable clinical behavior [35]. Also the expression of E-cadherin was more elevated in benign meningiomas [36].

Furthermore, about 70–100% meningiomas express somatostatin receptors, predominantly the type 2a (hsst2a) [37].

6. Benign meningiomas or WHO grade I meningiomas

In most of cases, WHO grade I meningiomas are diagnosed. They present a benign clinical course, with rare mitoses and occasional pleomorphic nuclei. Various architectural patterns have been described, whose most frequent are meningothelial, fibroblastic, and transitional meningiomas. Meningothelial or syncytial meningiomas are characterized by a high cellular density with cells disposed in packed sheets. Fibroblastic meningiomas are similar to schwannomas, with elongated cells. Cellular whorls and psammoma bodies (mineralized whorls) are most common in the transitional type, which present intermediate features between the meningothelial and the fibroblastic subtype. Other rare variants are the psammomatous meningiomas, characterized by multiple psammoma bodies, the angiomatous meningiomas, which are extremely vascularized with scarce foci of meningothelial cells and the secretory meningiomas, with lumina formed by cytokeratin-immunoreactive cells and containing PAS positive material.

Benign meningiomas are considered cured, if a complete resection is performed. Thus, a simple surveillance is indicated in cases where a gross total resection is possible (Simpson grade 1 or 2) with serial cerebral MRI, without any complementary treatment. A very small portion of benign meningiomas progresses to more aggressive variants (<2%) [38], but when considering only recurrent tumors, the prevalence becomes significantly higher (14%) [39]. The clinical behavior and the malignant potential of meningioma are still matter of debate. Many authors applied the model of clonal progression to meningiomas with a progressive appearance of more aggressive cellular subpopulations according with the presence of genetic imbalances and molecular modifications [40, 41].

Meningiomas show immunohistochemical positivity for epithelial membrane antigen (EMA) in 80% of cases. They also express other epithelial markers such as vimentin and cytokeratin. Antileu 7 and glial fibrillary acidic protein (GFAP) stains, characteristics for schwannomas and gliomas, respectively, are uniformly negative. Immunohistochemistry may thus help in the differential diagnosis in difficult cases.

An elevated labeling for Ki-67 may denote a more aggressive lesion [42, 43].

7. Atypical meningiomas or WHO grade II

According to the WHO classification of 2007, a growing subset of lesions (about one third) has the histopathological characteristics to be defined atypical, thus showing a more aggressive behavior [13].

The criteria to define atypical meningiomas are independent from meningioma subtype.

Atypical meningiomas are in fact described as lesions with one or more of these characteristics:

- 4–19 mitoses per 10 high power fields (hpf) and/or brain invasion and/or at least three of the following features:

- necrosis
- macronucleoli
- loss of ordered architecture
- hypercellularity
- small cells

Four subtypes of WHO grade II meningiomas have been described [11]: The chordoid meningioma is histologically similar to chordoma, with a mucin-rich stroma and clear vacuoles in epithelioid cells. This pattern is mixed with meningothelial or transitional tumor areas, and it is usually supratentorial. Castleman's disease has been reported in association with this subtype [44]. The clear cell meningioma is composed by cells with glycogen-rich clear cytoplasm and extensive collagen deposition. This subtype typically occurs in the cauda equina region and in the posterior fossa. A high recurrence rate is characteristics. The atypical meningioma has atypical features and cannot be classified as chordoid or clear cell meningioma.

An association between the survival rate and the extent of resection for atypical meningiomas was confirmed by multiple studies [45, 46]. Even if a maximal resection is the first aim of the surgery, these lesions are often less well delimited and a safe resection is often incomplete because of bone infiltration and vascular invasion. Many studies are actually investigating the real role of adjuvant therapies. If fact both radiotherapy and eventually chemotherapy are not free of side effects and even if they are commonly adopted for malignant meningiomas, the balance benefits–risks is not yet assessed for atypical meningiomas.

8. Anaplastic or malignant meningiomas or WHO grade III

Anaplastic meningiomas may present directly as primary tumors or may derive from a malignant transformation of less aggressive lesions. Malignant meningiomas are characterized by the following [4]:

- 20 or more mitoses/10 hpf

- predominant rhabdoid or papillary morphology

Papillary meningiomas are rare and commonly found in children, characterized by a pseudopapillary architecture. Rhabdoid meningiomas are formed by cells with eccentric nuclei and paranuclear inclusions.

Anaplastic meningiomas are associated with a high risk of recurrence and distant metastases. The most common sites of extraneural metastases are the liver, lungs, pleura, and lymph nodes.

Surgery aiming to obtain gross total or near total surgical resection represents the first choice, and it is combined with different types of external beam radiotherapy (fractionated or stereotactic radiosurgery) [47, 48] Anaplastic meningiomas are malignant tumors with a survival limited to 1.5–3.5 years according to most of the series [49]. A better overall survival was observed in cases <60 years old and in patients receiving adjuvant radiotherapy [46]. The role of chemotherapic agents is still under investigation, and the debate is open in particular for somatostatine analogues [50, 51].

9. Management

9.1. Surgery

The mainstay of the treatment for symptomatic or enlarging meningiomas of every histological grade is the surgical excision. A complete surgical excision of the tumor and of the surrounding dural attachment is recommended and may be curative. Furthermore surgery allows a pathological diagnosis, may improve the symptoms, and relieve the mass effect. The extent of surgical resection was first classified by Simpson [52], and it is strongly associated to the recurrence rate (Table 1). The term "Simpson grade 0" was also coniated, to define a total resection of the tumor, of the infiltrated dura and of the hyperostotic bone, with a 2 cm of free margins [53]. A complete resection (Simpson I) may not always be performed because of the localization/size of the tumor and their relationship with neurovascular structures. Thus, the highest recurrence rate was described in patients with sphenoid wing meningiomas, followed by parasagittal meningiomas. En plaque meningiomas, with a flat extension in the subdural space, may also be difficult to resect completely. However, according to a recent study, patients with skull base meningiomas present at a younger age and lesions have often a more indolent behavior [54].

Simpson grade	Extent of resection	Recurrence rate at 5 years
0	Total removal of the tumor, dural attachment, and infiltrated bone with additional resection of a 2-cm dural margin	0%
1	Total removal of the tumor, dural attachment, and infiltrated bone	9%
2	Total removal of the tumor, dural attachment coagulated	19%
3	Total removal of the tumor, without resection nor coagulation of the dura/infiltrated bone	29%
4	Partial resection of the tumor	39%
5	Decompression (biopsy)	Ns

Modified according to Kinjo et al. [53].

Table 1. Simpson grade classifying the extent of resection for meningiomas.

More aggressive meningiomas may present with associated brain invasion, venous sinuses invasion or less defined limits, thus rendering the complete resection more challenging. The minimization of postoperative neurological deficit is one of the main goals of neurosurgeons, thus respecting neurovascular structures and the extent of resection should be balanced with the risk of postoperative disability. In the most complex cases, thus, a subtotal resection may be performed and a residue is left in place, which will be followed or treated with adjuvant radiotherapy, as fractionated external beam or stereotactic radiotherapy.

The extent of resection being a key predictor of recurrence, a long-term follow-up is essential, especially in cases of subtotal resection.

9.2. Radiotherapy

Radiotherapy has been advocated as primary therapeutic option in cases, where the surgical excision was judged too risky because of the considerable postoperative neurological morbidities or as complementary treatment after surgery [55]. Several options of radiation therapies are available to treat meningiomas, such as photon-based stereotactic radiosurgery and hypofractionated radiation therapy. Positive results with radiation therapy have been observed in cases of incomplete resection [56, 57] or recurrence [58].

Furthermore interesting results have been found with cavernous sinus meningiomas [59] or parasagittal meningiomas [60] involving the posterior third of the superior sagittal sinus. Patients treated with a combined approach (subtotal resection followed by stereotactic radiosurgery) experienced a progression-free survival similar to the subgroup where GTR was achieved.

To summarize the most recent literature evidences, the adjuvant use of radiotherapy after the resection of grade III meningiomas is well established, while it is still matter of debate after gross total resection of grade II meningiomas. Aghi et al. [61] showed how immediate adjuvant radiation therapy may improve overall survival and reduce local recurrence with atypical meningiomas. However, no randomized controlled or prospective studies exist and the level of evidence is thus low. Some authors suggest in fact that a close follow-up is sufficient after GTR of atypical meningiomas, thus avoiding the risk of side effects of radiotherapy. Sun et al. [47] suggested that the analysis of histopathological features of aggressiveness, such as brain invasion and the MIB-1 index, to decide of a complementary treatment should be administered.

A dose of 60 Gy is generally considered beneficial for fractionated radiotherapy after subtotal resections and many centers administer hypofractionated radiotherapy, with doses of 1, 8, or 2 Gy per fraction, to diminish the risk of long-term neurotoxicity. After gross total resections, some authors suggest the possibility to lower the doses to 54 Gy (RTOG trial N°0539). The EORTC trial N°22042-26042 is actually investigating the benefit of 60 Gy after GTR, with an additional boost of 10 Gy after STR. The same doses seem to be advantageous with proton-beam therapy [62].

Further indications for radiation therapy are as follows: As adjuvant treatment after the incomplete resection of a meningioma or with recurrent tumors whose surgical removal of the residue will bring important potential neurological morbidities or with inoperable lesions.

The limitation of fractionated radiotherapy and stereotactic radiosurgery are linked to the tumor size and to the radiation neurotoxicity, with a risk of necrosis, cerebral edema and damage of critical neurovascular structures with consequent cranial nerve palsy [48]. Recent progresses in the field of conformational radiotherapy and stereotactic radiotherapy allow a better definition of the target, thus limiting the dose to the normal tissue and delivering a more focused dose on the resection bed/residual meningioma.

Other radiation-induced complications described in literature are the risk of secondary malignancy or of tumor progression [63, 64].

9.3. Chemotherapy

The development of new medical options for recurrent or aggressive meningiomas is strongly dependent from progresses made in the understanding of molecular pathways. The role of classic chemotherapic agents is disappointing [65]. Temozolomide showed no efficacy on refractory meningiomas according to Chamberlain et al. [66], and its efficacy seems to be linked to the functionality of the enzyme O6-methylguanine-DNA-methyltransferase [67]. Hydroxyurea showed preliminary favorable results in recurrent and radiation refractory meningiomas [68], but the study was conducted in a limited number of patients. The study of Chamberlain et al. [69] on the contrary showed a limited efficacy. Contrasting results exist on the efficacy of irinotecan on preclinical studies [70].

Multiple targeted therapies have been tried in preclinical and clinical trials. In the animal model, the use of mTOR inhibitors such as temsirolimus and everolimus showed a reduced growth rate in meningioma cells [71]. On the contrary, the application of EGFR inhibitors (gefitinib and erlotinib) did not show a significant benefit in patients with refractory meningiomas [72]. The most famous monoclonal antibody binding VEGFB, bevacizumab, was also investigated by Lou et al. [73] in a population of recurrent/progressive meningiomas, and a positive response was obtained in recurrent meningiomas. The benefit of this therapy was, however, not clear in the study of Nunes et al. [74]. Two ongoing trials will evaluate the efficacy of bevacizumab in a phase II trial (NCT01125046) and its association with everolimus in a cohort of recurrent/progressive meningiomas (NCT00972335). In preclinical studies sunitinib, a PDGFRB inhibitor may inhibit cellular migration in vitro [75]. Encouraging results from the use of sunitinib were also obtained in a cohort of patients with malignant meningiomas [50].

Hormonal therapies have been widely investigated as cytostatic therapies after the discovery of the association between meningioma incidence and hyperestrogenic and hyperprogestinic conditions [18]. Mifepristone (RU-486) is an antagonist of progesterone receptors, and it is the most widely investigated agent in the oncologic field. Clinical studies on its efficacy show, however, contrasting results [7, 76, 77], and only minor evidences exist to recommend mifepristone with inoperable progressive meningiomas, after consideration of the histological grade of the tumor and progesterone receptor expression [78]. Positive preliminary results were obtained with diffuse meningiomatosis [79].

Immunohistochemical studies showed a high prevalence of somatostatin receptor (SSTR) expression in meningiomas, in particular of SSTR2A. The sandostatin LAR was tested in a prospective trial including recurrent menngiomas, with a partial radiological response in one third of patients [80]. However, pasireotide, an analogue with a wider affinity for multiple subtypes of SSTR, showed no benefit in recurrent meningiomas [51].

In conclusion, up to date chemotherapeutic agents and hormonal therapies shows a limited efficacy in the management of recurrent/progressive and more aggressive meningiomas and the field of investigation remains large. The nanotechnology, combined with the most recent targeted therapies, may actually represent a revolution in the targeting, transport and delivering of chemotherapeutic agents [81], thus opening new ways for the treatment of these tumors.

10. Conclusions

Meningiomas were classically considered benign tumors. However, according to the new WHO classification, the proportion of more aggressive variants has steeply increased and thus the management has become more challenging. Surgery represents the mainstay of the treatment and a complete resection may be considered curative in WHO grade I meningiomas. However, neurosurgeons have often to deal with the risk of postoperative neurological morbidities and the role of adjuvant treatments, such as radiotherapy and chemotherapy, after subtotal resection or after the pathological confirmation of WHO grade II or III meningiomas, is actually being defined. A huge literature dealing with adjuvant radiotherapy and new cytostatic agents is developing, with the aim of obtaining an optimal long-term control. Up to now, treatments are empirically based and many hopes reside in new prospective and randomized controlled trials to better define the role of each therapeutic strategy and the best way to combine them.

Author details

Giulia Cossu[1*], Mahmoud Messerer[1,2], Fabrice Parker[2], Marc Levivier[1] and Roy Thomas Daniel[1]

*Address all correspondence to: giulia.cossu@chuv.ch

1 Department of Clinical Neurosciences, Faculty of Medicine and Biology of Lausanne, Lausanne University Hospital, Lausanne, Switzerland

2 Department of Neurosurgery, Faculty of Medicine of Paris Sud, Kremlin-Bicêtre University Hospital, Le Kremlin-Bicêtre, France

References

[1] Claus EB, Bondy ML, Schildkraut JM, Wiemels JL, Wrensch M, Black PM. Epidemiology of intracranial meningioma. Neurosurgery. 2005;57(6):1088–95; discussion 95.

[2] Cushing H. The meningiomas (dural endotheliomas): their source, and favoured seats of origin. Brain: a Journal of Neurology. 1922;45:282.

[3] Cushing HW, Weed LH. Calcareous and osseous deposits in the arachnoidea. Studies in the cerebro-spinal fluid and its pathway. Bull Johns Hopkins Hosp 1915; No. IX. 26:367.

[4] Louis DN, Ohgaki H, Wiestler OD, Cavenee WK, Burger PC, Jouvet A, et al. The 2007 WHO classification of tumours of the central nervous system. Acta Neuropathologica. 2007;114(2):97–109.

[5] Longstreth WT, Jr., Dennis LK, McGuire VM, Drangsholt MT, Koepsell TD. Epidemiology of intracranial meningioma. Cancer. 1993;72(3):639–48.

[6] Nakasu S, Hirano A, Shimura T, Llena JF. Incidental meningiomas in autopsy study. Surgical Neurology. 1987;27(4):319–22.

[7] Grunberg SM, Weiss MH, Spitz IM, Ahmadi J, Sadun A, Russell CA, et al. Treatment of unresectable meningiomas with the antiprogesterone agent mifepristone. Journal of Neurosurgery. 1991;74(6):861–6.

[8] Schoenberg BS, Christine BW, Whisnant JP. Nervous system neoplasms and primary malignancies of other sites. The unique association between meningiomas and breast cancer. Neurology. 1975;25(8):705–12.

[9] Roelvink NC, Kamphorst W, van Alphen HA, Rao BR. Pregnancy-related primary brain and spinal tumors. Archives of Neurology. 1987;44(2):209–15.

[10] Bellur SN, Chandra V, Anderson RJ. Association of meningiomas with obesity. Annals of Neurology. 1983;13(3):346–7.

[11] Perry A, Louis DN, Scheiithauer BW, Budka H, Von Deiming A. The 2007 WHO classification of tumours of the central nervous system. Acta Neuropathologica. 2007;114(2):97–109.

[12] Falleni M, Roz E, Dessy E, Del Curto B, Braidotti P, Gianelli U, et al. Primary intrathoracic meningioma: histopathological, immunohistochemical and ultrastructural study of two cases. Virchows Archiv: an International Journal of Pathology. 2001;439(2): 196–200.

[13] Pearson BE, Markert JM, Fisher WS, Guthrie BL, Fiveash JB, Palmer CA, et al. Hitting a moving target: evolution of a treatment paradigm for atypical meningiomas amid changing diagnostic criteria. Neurosurgical Focus. 2008;24(5):E3.

[14] Nakasu S, Fukami T, Jito J, Nozaki K. Recurrence and regrowth of benign meningiomas. Brain Tumor Pathology. 2009;26(2):69–72.

[15] Yang SY, Park CK, Park SH, Kim DG, Chung YS, Jung HW. Atypical and anaplastic meningiomas: prognostic implications of clinicopathological features. Journal of Neurology, Neurosurgery, and Psychiatry. 2008;79(5):574–80.

[16] Nakamura M, Roser F, Michel J, Jacobs C, Samii M. The natural history of incidental meningiomas. Neurosurgery. 2003;53(1):62–70; discussion 1.

[17] Pieper DR, Al-Mefty O, Hanada Y, Buechner D. Hyperostosis associated with meningioma of the cranial base: secondary changes or tumor invasion. Neurosurgery. 1999;44(4):742–6; discussion 6–7.

[18] Chen JA, Coutin-Churchman PE, Nuwer MR, Lazareff JA. Suboccipital craniotomy for Chiari I results in evoked potential conduction changes. Surgical Neurology International. 2012;3:165.

[19] Stamenkovic I, Yu Q. Merlin, a "magic" linker between extracellular cues and intracellular signaling pathways that regulate cell motility, proliferation, and survival. Current Protein & Peptide Science. 2010;11(6):471–84.

[20] Gutmann DH, Donahoe J, Perry A, Lemke N, Gorse K, Kittiniyom K, et al. Loss of DAL-1, a protein 4.1-related tumor suppressor, is an important early event in the pathogenesis of meningiomas. Human Molecular Genetics. 2000;9(10):1495–500.

[21] Watson MA, Gutmann DH, Peterson K, Chicoine MR, Kleinschmidt-DeMasters BK, Brown HG, et al. Molecular characterization of human meningiomas by gene expression profiling using high-density oligonucleotide microarrays. The American Journal of Pathology. 2002;161(2):665–72.

[22] Cai DX, Banerjee R, Scheithauer BW, Lohse CM, Kleinschmidt-Demasters BK, Perry A. Chromosome 1p and 14q FISH analysis in clinicopathologic subsets of meningioma: diagnostic and prognostic implications. Journal of Neuropathology and Experimental Neurology. 2001;60(6):628–36.

[23] Zhi F, Zhou G, Wang S, Shi Y, Peng Y, Shao N, et al. A microRNA expression signature predicts meningioma recurrence. International Journal of Cancer. 2013;132(1):128–36.

[24] Cerda-Nicolas M, Lopez-Gines C, Perez-Bacete M, Barcia-Salorio JL, Llombart-Bosch A. Histopathological and cytogenetic findings in benign, atypical and anaplastic human meningiomas: a study of 60 tumors. Journal of Neuro-oncology. 2000;47(2):99–108.

[25] Amatya VJ, Takeshima Y, Sugiyama K, Kurisu K, Nishisaka T, Fukuhara T, et al. Immunohistochemical study of Ki-67 (MIB-1), p53 protein, p21WAF1, and p27KIP1 expression in benign, atypical, and anaplastic meningiomas. Human Pathology. 2001;32(9):970–5.

[26] Sandberg DI, Edgar MA, Resch L, Rutka JT, Becker LE, Souweidane MM. MIB-1 staining index of pediatric meningiomas. Neurosurgery. 2001;48(3):590–5; discussion 5–7.

[27] Bie L, Zhao G, Ju Y, Zhang B. Integrative genomic analysis identifies CCNB1 and CDC2 as candidate genes associated with meningioma recurrence. Cancer Genetics. 2011;204(10):536–40.

[28] Perez-Magan E, Rodriguez de Lope A, Ribalta T, Ruano Y, Campos-Martin Y, Perez-Bautista G, et al. Differential expression profiling analyses identifies downregulation

of 1p, 6q, and 14q genes and overexpression of 6p histone cluster 1 genes as markers of recurrence in meningiomas. Neuro-oncology. 2010;12(12):1278–90.

[29] Ho DM, Hsu CY, Ting LT, Chiang H. Histopathology and MIB-1 labeling index predicted recurrence of meningiomas: a proposal of diagnostic criteria for patients with atypical meningioma. Cancer. 2002;94(5):1538–47.

[30] Aguiar PH, Tsanaclis AM, Tella OI, Jr., Plese JP. Proliferation rate of intracranial meningiomas as defined by the monoclonal antibody MIB-1: correlation with peritumoural oedema and other clinicoradiological and histological characteristics. Neurosurgical Review. 2003;26(3):221–8.

[31] Nagashima G, Asai J, Suzuki R, Fujimoto T. Different distribution of c-myc and MIB-1 positive cells in malignant meningiomas with reference to TGFs, PDGF, and PgR expression. Brain Tumor Pathology. 2001;18(1):1–5.

[32] Barresi V, Tuccari G. Increased ratio of vascular endothelial growth factor to semaphorin3A is a negative prognostic factor in human meningiomas. Neuropathology. 2010;30(5):537–46.

[33] Barresi V, Vitarelli E, Tuccari G, Barresi G. MMP-9 expression in meningiomas: a prognostic marker for recurrence risk? Journal of Neuro-oncology. 2011;102(2):189–96.

[34] Donnell MS, Meyer GA, Donegan WL. Estrogen-receptor protein in intracranial meningiomas. Journal of Neurosurgery. 1979;50(4):499–502.

[35] Hsu DW, Efird JT, Hedley-Whyte ET. Progesterone and estrogen receptors in meningiomas: prognostic considerations. Journal of Neurosurgery. 1997;86(1):113–20.

[36] Schwechheimer K, Zhou L, Birchmeier W. E-Cadherin in human brain tumours: loss of immunoreactivity in malignant meningiomas. Virchows Archiv: an International Journal of Pathology. 1998;432(2):163–7.

[37] Schulz S, Pauli SU, Schulz S, Handel M, Dietzmann K, Firsching R, et al. Immunohistochemical determination of five somatostatin receptors in meningioma reveals frequent overexpression of somatostatin receptor subtype sst2A. Clinical Cancer Research. 2000;6(5):1865–74.

[38] Lamszus K, Kluwe L, Matschke J, Meissner H, Laas R, Westphal M. Allelic losses at 1p, 9q, 10q, 14q, and 22q in the progression of aggressive meningiomas and undifferentiated meningeal sarcomas. Cancer Genetics and Cytogenetics. 1999;110(2):103–10.

[39] Jaaskelainen J, Haltia M, Servo A. Atypical and anaplastic meningiomas: radiology, surgery, radiotherapy, and outcome. Surgical Neurology. 1986;25(3):233–42.

[40] Al-Mefty O, Kadri PA, Pravdenkova S, Sawyer JR, Stangeby C, Husain M. Malignant progression in meningioma: documentation of a series and analysis of cytogenetic findings. Journal of Neurosurgery. 2004;101(2):210–8.

[41] Nowell PC. Mechanisms of tumor progression. Cancer Research. 1986;46(5):2203–7.

[42] Hsu DW, Efird JT, Hedley-Whyte ET. MIB-1 (Ki-67) index and transforming growth factor-alpha (TGF alpha) immunoreactivity are significant prognostic predictors for meningiomas. Neuropathology and Applied Neurobiology. 1998;24(6):441–52.

[43] Cobb MA, Husain M, Andersen BJ, al-Mefty O. Significance of proliferating cell nuclear antigen in predicting recurrence of intracranial meningioma. Journal of Neurosurgery. 1996;84(1):85–90.

[44] Kepes JJ, Chen WY, Connors MH, Vogel FS. "Chordoid" meningeal tumors in young individuals with peritumoral lymphoplasmacellular infiltrates causing systemic manifestations of the Castleman syndrome. A report of seven cases. Cancer. 1988;62(2): 391–406.

[45] Palma L, Celli P, Franco C, Cervoni L, Cantore G. Long-term prognosis for atypical and malignant meningiomas: a study of 71 surgical cases. Journal of Neurosurgery. 1997;86(5):793–800.

[46] Durand A, Labrousse F, Jouvet A, Bauchet L, Kalamarides M, Menei P, et al. WHO grade II and III meningiomas: a study of prognostic factors. Journal of Neuro-oncology. 2009;95(3):367–75.

[47] Sun SQ, Hawasli AH, Huang J, Chicoine MR, Kim AH. An evidence-based treatment algorithm for the management of WHO Grade II and III meningiomas. Neurosurgical Focus. 2015;38(3):E3.

[48] Walcott BP, Nahed BV, Brastianos PK, Loeffler JS. Radiation Treatment for WHO Grade II and III Meningiomas. Frontiers in Oncology. 2013;3:227.

[49] Champeaux C, Wilson E, Brandner S, Shieff C, Thorne L. World Health Organization grade III meningiomas. A retrospective study for outcome and prognostic factors assessment. British Journal of Neurosurgery. 2015:1–6.

[50] Kaley TJ, Wen P, Schiff D, Ligon K, Haidar S, Karimi S, et al. Phase II trial of sunitinib for recurrent and progressive atypical and anaplastic meningioma. Neuro-oncology. 2015;17(1):116–21.

[51] Norden AD, Ligon KL, Hammond SN, Muzikansky A, Reardon DA, Kaley TJ, et al. Phase II study of monthly pasireotide LAR (SOM230C) for recurrent or progressive meningioma. Neurology. 2015;84(3):280–6.

[52] Simpson D. The recurrence of intracranial meningiomas after surgical treatment. Journal of Neurology, Neurosurgery, and Psychiatry. 1957;20(1):22–39.

[53] Kinjo T, al-Mefty O, Kanaan I. Grade zero removal of supratentorial convexity meningiomas. Neurosurgery. 1993;33(3):394–9; discussion 9.

[54] Mansouri A, Klironomos G, Taslimi S, Kilian A, Gentili F, Khan OH, et al. Surgically resected skull base meningiomas demonstrate a divergent postoperative recurrence

http://dx.doi.org/10.5772/62929

pattern compared with non-skull base meningiomas. Journal of Neurosurgery. 2016:1–10.

[55] Starke RM, Williams BJ, Jane JA, Jr., Sheehan JP. Gamma Knife surgery for patients with nonfunctioning pituitary macroadenomas: predictors of tumor control, neurological deficits, and hypopituitarism. Journal of Neurosurgery. 2012;117(1):129–35.

[56] Goldsmith BJ, Wara WM, Wilson CB, Larson DA. Postoperative irradiation for subtotally resected meningiomas. A retrospective analysis of 140 patients treated from 1967 to 1990. Journal of Neurosurgery. 1994;80(2):195–201.

[57] Barbaro NM, Gutin PH, Wilson CB, Sheline GE, Boldrey EB, Wara WM. Radiation therapy in the treatment of partially resected meningiomas. Neurosurgery. 1987;20(4): 525–8.

[58] Kokubo M, Shibamoto Y, Takahashi JA, Sasai K, Oya N, Hashimoto N, et al. Efficacy of conventional radiotherapy for recurrent meningioma. Journal of Neuro-oncology. 2000;48(1):51–5.

[59] Wang YC, Chuang CC, Wei KC, Hsu YH, Hsu PW, Lee ST, et al. Skull base atypical meningioma: Long term surgical outcome and prognostic factors. Clinical Neurology and Neurosurgery. 2015;128:112–6.

[60] Kondziolka D, Flickinger JC, Perez B. Judicious resection and/or radiosurgery for parasagittal meningiomas: outcomes from a multicenter review. Gamma Knife Meningioma Study Group. Neurosurgery. 1998;43(3):405–13; discussion 13–4.

[61] Aghi MK, Carter BS, Cosgrove GR, Ojemann RG, Amin-Hanjani S, Martuza RL, et al. Long-term recurrence rates of atypical meningiomas after gross total resection with or without postoperative adjuvant radiation. Neurosurgery. 2009;64(1):56–60; discussion.

[62] Boskos C, Feuvret L, Noel G, Habrand JL, Pommier P, Alapetite C, et al. Combined proton and photon conformal radiotherapy for intracranial atypical and malignant meningioma. International Journal of Radiation Oncology, Biology, Physics. 2009;75(2): 399–406.

[63] Kaido T, Hoshida T, Uranishi R, Akita N, Kotani A, Nishi N, et al. Radiosurgery-induced brain tumor. Case report. Journal of Neurosurgery. 2001;95(4):710–3.

[64] Sheehan J, Yen CP, Steiner L. Gamma knife surgery-induced meningioma. Report of two cases and review of the literature. Journal of Neurosurgery. 2006;105(2):325–9.

[65] Sherman WJ, Raizer JJ. Chemotherapy: What is its role in meningioma? Expert Review of Neurotherapeutics. 2012;12(10):1189–95; quiz 96.

[66] Chamberlain MC, Tsao-Wei DD, Groshen S. Temozolomide for treatment-resistant recurrent meningioma. Neurology. 2004;62(7):1210–2.

[67] de Robles P, McIntyre J, Kalra S, Roldan G, Cairncross G, Forsyth P, et al. Methylation status of MGMT gene promoter in meningiomas. Cancer Genetics and Cytogenetics. 2008;187(1):25–7.

[68] Schrell UM, Rittig MG, Anders M, Kiesewetter F, Marschalek R, Koch UH, et al. Hydroxyurea for treatment of unresectable and recurrent meningiomas. I. Inhibition of primary human meningioma cells in culture and in meningioma transplants by induction of the apoptotic pathway. Journal of Neurosurgery. 1997;86(5):845–52.

[69] Chamberlain MC, Johnston SK. Hydroxyurea for recurrent surgery and radiation refractory meningioma: a retrospective case series. Journal of Neuro-oncology. 2011;104(3):765–71.

[70] Gupta V, Su YS, Samuelson CG, Liebes LF, Chamberlain MC, Hofman FM, et al. Irinotecan: a potential new chemotherapeutic agent for atypical or malignant meningiomas. Journal of Neurosurgery. 2007;106(3):455–62.

[71] Pachow D, Andrae N, Kliese N, Angenstein F, Stork O, Wilisch-Neumann A, et al. mTORC1 inhibitors suppress meningioma growth in mouse models. Clinical Cancer Research. 2013;19(5):1180–9.

[72] Norden AD, Raizer JJ, Abrey LE, Lamborn KR, Lassman AB, Chang SM, et al. Phase II trials of erlotinib or gefitinib in patients with recurrent meningioma. Journal of Neuro-oncology. 2010;96(2):211–7.

[73] Lou E, Sumrall AL, Turner S, Peters KB, Desjardins A, Vredenburgh JJ, et al. Bevacizumab therapy for adults with recurrent/progressive meningioma: a retrospective series. Journal of Neuro-oncology. 2012;109(1):63–70.

[74] Nunes FP, Merker VL, Jennings D, Caruso PA, di Tomaso E, Muzikansky A, et al. Bevacizumab treatment for meningiomas in NF2: a retrospective analysis of 15 patients. Plos One. 2013;8(3):e59941.

[75] Pfister C, Pfrommer H, Tatagiba MS, Roser F. Vascular endothelial growth factor signals through platelet-derived growth factor receptor beta in meningiomas in vitro. British Journal of Cancer. 2012;107(10):1702–13.

[76] Grunberg SM, Weiss MH, Russell CA, Spitz IM, Ahmadi J, Sadun A, et al. Long-term administration of mifepristone (RU486): clinical tolerance during extended treatment of meningioma. Cancer Investigation. 2006;24(8):727–33.

[77] Lamberts SW, Tanghe HL, Avezaat CJ, Braakman R, Wijngaarde R, Koper JW, et al. Mifepristone (RU 486) treatment of meningiomas. Journal of Neurology, Neurosurgery, and Psychiatry. 1992;55(6):486–90.

[78] Cossu G, Levivier M, Daniel RT, Messerer M. The Role of mifepristone in meningiomas management: a systematic review of the literature. BioMed Research International. 2015;2015:267831.

[79] Touat M, Lombardi G, Farina P, Kalamarides M, Sanson M. Successful treatment of multiple intracranial meningiomas with the antiprogesterone receptor agent mifepristone (RU486). Acta Neurochirurgica. 2014;156(10):1831–5.

[80] Chamberlain MC, Glantz MJ, Fadul CE. Recurrent meningioma: salvage therapy with long-acting somatostatin analogue. Neurology. 2007;69(10):969–73.

[81] Caruso G, Elbabaa SK, Gonzalez-Lopez P, Barresi V, Passalacqua M, Caffo M. Innovative therapeutic strategies in the treatment of meningioma. Anticancer Research. 2015;35(12):6391–400.

Chapter 16

Medulloblastoma: Clinical Challenges and Emerging Molecular Discoveries

Eric Q. Trieu, Sherri Y. Huang and Jer-Yen Yang

Additional information is available at the end of the chapter

http://dx.doi.org/10.5772/63004

Abstract

Medulloblastoma is the most common type of malignant brain tumor in children, responsible for 25% of pediatric brain cancers. Conventional treatment methods, which include surgery, radiotherapy, and chemotherapy, have improved overall survival rates for patients with medulloblastoma to over 50%. A majority of survivors, however, suffer serious long-term side effects, including developmental, neurological, and psychosocial deficits. Now entering clinical trials for sonic hedgehog-driven medulloblastomas, Smoothened inhibitors have been FDA approved for the treatment of basal cell carcinomas. However, treatment efficacy endures only for a few months before lesion relapses and drug resistance occurs. Therefore, there is an urgent need for new therapies to reduce the significant problems associated with current drug-resistant treatments. In this chapter, we will illustrate the clinical presentation and current treatment methods for medulloblastoma and detail the molecular pathways within each of the four molecular subgroups of medulloblastoma, with an eye for possible candidates for novel combination therapies.

Keywords: medulloblastoma, Sonic hedgehog (SHH) pathway, pediatric tumors, CNS tumors, smoothened

1. Introduction: medulloblastoma as a clinical problem

Medulloblastoma is the most common malignant pediatric brain tumor, accounting for about 25% of pediatric brain tumor cases [1]. However, it is found in infants and adults as well. Arising from embryonal cells in the cerebellum, medulloblastoma is a highly invasive cancer which unfortunately manifests initially with subtle clinical symptoms [2]. While conventional treatments are able to control the tumor in the majority of patients, debilitating side effects along with drug resistance remain significant concerns. For the clinician, one of the challenges to treating medulloblastoma is its complexity as it may be grouped either histologically or molecularly. Currently, there are four molecular subgroups of medulloblastoma, each of which contains specific genetic or cytological backgrounds which may impact prognosis [3].

1.1. Origin and epidemiology of medulloblastoma

Medulloblastoma is classified as a primitive neuroectodermal tumor, typically occurring in the cerebellar vermis which is located in the posterior fossa of the skull (**Figure 1**) [1]. This tumor accounts for 40% of those arising from the posterior fossa [4]. Medulloblastoma is the most common malignant central nervous system (CNS) tumor of childhood, comprising 15–30% of pediatric CNS tumors and 1–3% of adult CNS tumors [5]. Medulloblastomas can affect any age group, although the majority (85%) occurs in childhood, and of those half occur between the ages of 4–9 [6]. Tumors most often arise sporadically, although they may arise as part of inherited disorders such as Li-Fraumeni, Turcot, or Gorlin syndrome [7]. The cellular origins of medulloblastoma differ by the tumor subgroup (described below). For example, medulloblastomas of the sonic hedgehog (SHH) subgroup arise from granule neuron progenitors (GNPs) that reside in the outermost layer of the cerebellum [8]. Wnt-subgroup medulloblastomas, on the other hand, arise from lower rhombic lip precursors in the brain-stem [9].

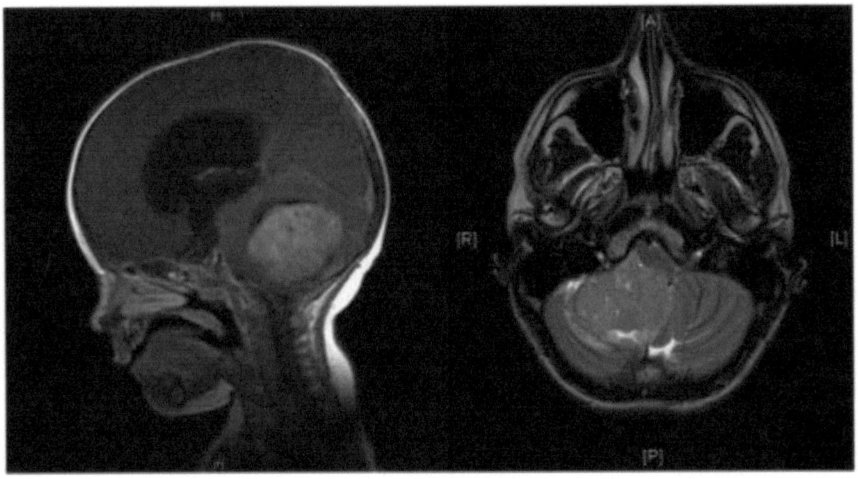

Figure 1. Medulloblastoma is a primitive neuroectodermal tumor commonly arising in the cerebellar vermis. The left image is a sagittal view of an MRI for a pediatric patient. The right image is a horizontal view of an MRI showing tumor growth towards the right cerebellar hemisphere, with displacement of the vermis. Copyright © 2014 from *Pediatric medulloblastoma—update on molecular classification driving targeted therapies* (DeSouza, Jones, Lowis and Kurian, Front. Oncol. 2014).

1.2. Clinical presentation and diagnosis

Given that the cerebellum is located against the fourth ventricle, tumors arising from it result in mass effect and hydrocephalus. Consequently, patients initially diagnosed with medulloblastoma present most commonly with symptoms of elevated intracranial pressure—chronic progressive nausea, vomiting, and headache [10]. These symptoms can progress to altered mental status, sensorimotor symptoms, and cerebellar symptoms if left untreated [10]. Children and infants may present instead with nonspecific lethargy and weakness. Neurological signs, often subtle, may be present for 3 or more months before diagnosis [11].

Medulloblastoma metastasizes most commonly to the spinal cord. In an international meta-analysis of medulloblastoma, metastatic disease was identified in 103 of 432 patients (24%) on initial diagnosis [6], although the incidence was much lower in adults (2%). Metastatic disease was most common in Group 3 and Group 4 medulloblastomas (30 and 31%, respectively), while much lower in the Wnt group (9% of children) [6].

Although a biopsy specimen is required for definitive diagnosis of medulloblastoma, brain magnetic resonance imaging (MRI) with gadolinium is the preferred imaging modality to best characterize lesions suspected to be medulloblastoma. Brain MRIs allow for greater resolution of soft tissue with less interference from bone compared to computed tomography [12]. MRI findings associated with medulloblastoma can have varying enhancement patterns and intensities. Imaging can also identify areas of hemorrhage, calcification, or findings that suggest leptomeningeal metastasis [12]. It has been suggested that certain MRI findings may be more associated with certain histopathological subtypes [12].

1.3. Current conventional treatments and treatment considerations

Once identification of suspected medulloblastoma has been made on imaging, a decision needs to be as to how tissue sample should be accessed. The current standard of care is to resect as much of the lesion as possible if able to do so in a safe manner [13]. If it is deemed unsafe to do so, a stereotactic biopsy of the suspected lesion would allow for a confirmatory pathologic diagnosis. Once tissue has been obtained, the patient must be reassessed and assigned to the standard-risk group or high-risk group which informs subsequent patient treatment regimen. The goal of this treatment regimen, which includes chemotherapy with or without chemoradiation, is to treat disease that may not have been fully resected by surgery.

In order to place patients into one of these groups, additional imaging is required postoperatively, as well as cerebrospinal fluid (CSF) analysis and adequate pathologic specimen. Specifically, these two risk classifications are defined by size of residual tumor following resection and status of metastasis [14]. Standard-risk groups are less likely to have tumor recurrence following resection, while high-risk groups are more likely to have tumor recurrence.

Standard-risk medulloblastoma occurs in 70% of patients [15]. Although prospective randomized trials comparing radiotherapy alone to combined chemoradiation for treatment of standard-risk medulloblastoma have not been performed, combined therapy is currently the standard of care of standard risk medulloblastoma [16]. Patients in this risk group are typically treated with a combination of chemotherapy followed by radiation, although radiation therapy alone has been used [15, 17, 18]. Multiple protocols exist for the chemotherapeutic treatment of medulloblastoma. One chemotherapeutic regimen includes treatment with a combination of vincristine, cisplastin, lomustine, and cyclophosphamide alongside radiation therapy over about a 1-year period [15]. High-risk or unresectable tumors are also treated with chemoradiation. Infants (<3 years old) are typically not treated with radiation owing to intolerability of side effects.

Risk stratification of medulloblastoma patients has improved cure rates for high-risk cases and limited radiation therapy exposure in treatment regimen for standard-risk patients, thereby reducing side effects. Nevertheless, even with improved cure rates for patients, long-term sequelae of treatment remain a concern. Radiation therapy has been associated with long-term neurocognitive deficits, cytopenias, opportunistic infections, and secondary malignancies [15, 19]. Children are especially sensitive to the adverse effects of radiation therapy, and as such radiation doses for treatment are lower for pediatric than for adult patients [15].

Long-term chemotherapy too has known side effects that have been described extensively elsewhere and include neurocognitive impairment, hearing loss, endocrine perturbations, cardiac and respiratory conditions, and secondary malignancies [15, 20]. Moving forward, further studies need to be performed to optimize current treatment or to identify new therapeutics to minimize side effect profile. Classification of medulloblastoma subgroups, for instance, focuses research toward drug targets within molecular pathways driving these subgroups. These subgroups are described in detail below.

1.4. Prognosis

In one trial of pediatric medulloblastoma, 10-year event free survival (EFS) and overall survival (OS) rates were 75 and 80%, respectively, for kids with standard-risk medulloblastoma treated with radiation followed by chemotherapy [21]. In another trial, 5-year EFS ranged from 65 to 70% in patients who received both chemotherapy and radiation following tumor resection [13]. Treatment with radiation therapy alone had survival rates 50–65% even with higher dose radiation [21, 22].

In comparison to pediatric medulloblastoma literature, studies assessing the treatment of adult medulloblastoma are rare. One retrospective study of adult medulloblastoma treated with chemotherapy and craniospinal radiation identified a 4-year EFS of 68% [18]. Other studies have identified survival rates of 40–80% [23].

Relapses most likely occur within the first 2 years of diagnosis, with one-third occurring within the first 3–5 years [21]. Earlier relapses are more likely to be associated with metastatic disease [21], while later relapses (>5 years after diagnosis) were more likely to be related to local disease. The posterior fossa is the most common site of relapse. Relapses must be distinguished from secondary tumors. Secondary tumors can occur following radiation, either at sites of prior irradiation or at extracranial sites near sites of primary radiation (thyroid, bone, etc.). One study identified a 4.2% 10-year cumulative incidence of secondary tumors following treatment with chemoradiation [21]. Increased use of mutagenic chemotherapy has also been suggested to play a role in the increasing incidence of secondary tumors following treatment of medulloblastoma.

Molecular subgrouping of medulloblastoma plays an important role in prognosis. In brief, the Wnt subgroup demonstrates the most favorable prognosis, whereas Group 3 medulloblastomas present the worst. Other factors that may affect prognosis include stage and complete or incomplete resection of tumors [18].

2. Molecular subgroups of medulloblastoma

The World Health Organization has subdivided medulloblastoma into five distinct histopathologic categories [24]: classic, desmoplastic/nodular, medulloblastoma with excessive nodularity, anaplastic medulloblastoma, and large cell medulloblastoma (**Figures 2** and **3**). Certain histological subtypes predominate patient age groups: 71% of pediatric cases classify as classic medulloblastoma, whereas 57% of infant cases exhibit desmoplastic/nodular histology [25]. Large cell and anaplastic medulloblastomas are associated with a poor prognosis, whereas desmoplastic/nodular medulloblastomas usually demonstrate an excellent outcome [25].

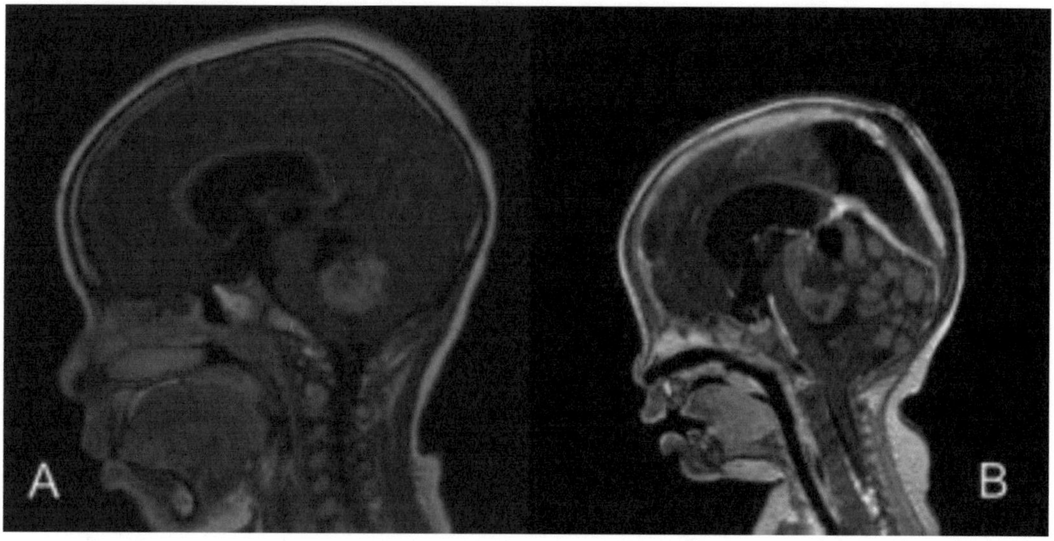

Figure 2. Medulloblastomas are grouped histologically or molecularly. Left image shows MRI of a pediatric patient with a classical medulloblastoma. Right image shows MRI of an infant with medulloblastoma with extensive nodularity. Copyright © 2014 Faculty of 1000 Ltd, from *Advances in managing medulloblastoma and intracranial primitive neuroectodermal tumors* (Adamski, Ramaswamy, Huang and Bouffet, F1000Prime Rep. 2014).

In addition to histological categories, retrospective molecular diagnostics have additionally allowed for medulloblastoma to be subdivided into four molecular subgroups (**Table 1**). The most well understood of these four subgroups are those medulloblastoma variants that involve the sonic hedgehog pathway (30% of patients with medulloblastoma and 60% of adults) and those involving the Wnt pathway (10% of all patients with medulloblastomas and 15% of adults) [26]. Molecular subgrouping may inform chemotherapy regimen, especially in light of emerging research about potential drug targets within involved molecular pathways.

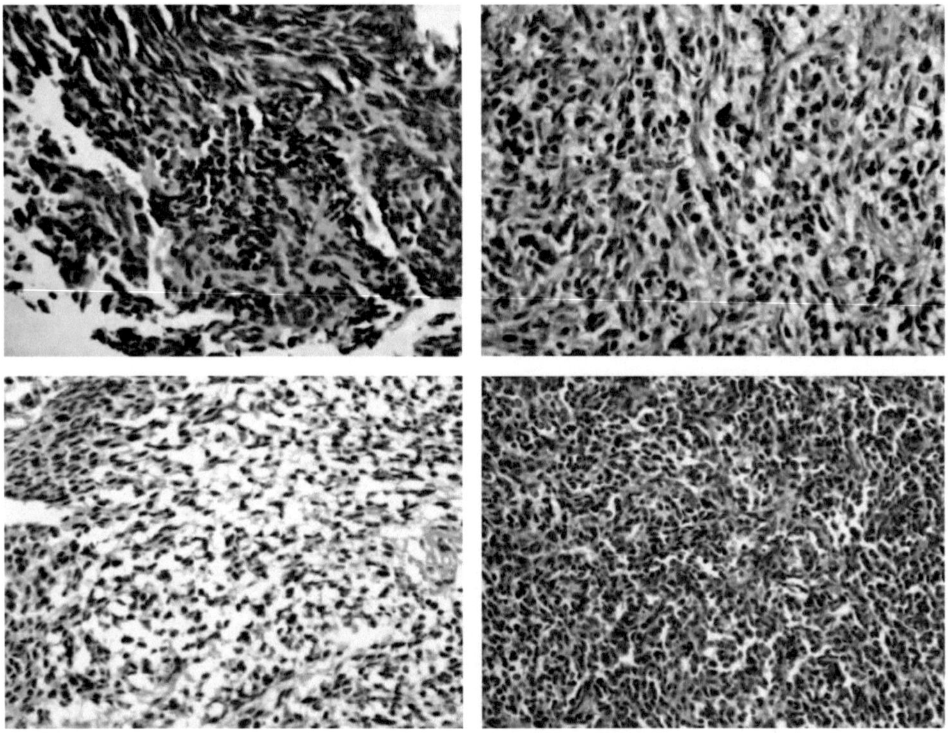

Figure 3. Histological slides stained with hematoxylin and eosin of medulloblastomas showing heterogeneity across patient tissue samples. Images obtained with permission from Dr. Kay Ka Wai Li (Prince of Wales Hospital, Department of Anatomical and Cellular Pathology, The Chinese University of Hong Kong).

2.1. Wnt pathway medulloblastoma

Wnt-type medulloblastoma is characterized by enhanced Wnt-β-catenin pathway activation [5] and tends to show classic histology rather than the poorer prognoses anaplastic or large cell type histology [6]. Among the medulloblastoma molecular subgroups, Wnt medulloblastoma is the least common, occurring in 10–15% of medulloblastomas [27]. It affects males 1.5 times more than females [6] and occurs rarely in infants (<3 years old).

For reasons that have yet to be elucidated, medulloblastoma tumors carrying Wnt mutations carry a better prognosis than other subtypes. In fact, meta-analysis of medulloblastoma subgroups found an overall 10-year survival rate of 95% in children with Wnt medulloblastoma and 100% 5-year survival rate among adult Wnt medulloblastoma [6].

2.1.1. Molecular basis of Wnt medulloblastomas

All medulloblastomas with heightened nuclear staining of β-catenin are grouped into Wnt-type. β-Catenin is a key promoter of the Wnt pathway, an evolutionarily conserved pathway involved in cellular homeostasis and embryogenesis. The pathway is involved in central nervous system development; indeed, derangements of Wnt signaling have been described in diseases of the CNS, including neural tube defects, Williams syndrome, Alzheimer's disease, and schizophrenia [28].

The Wnt pathway classifies into the canonical pathway and two separate noncanonical pathways. The noncanonical Wnt pathways appear to be independent of β-catenin. The canonical pathway is β-catenin dependent and is characterized by interaction of a Wnt ligand with the extracellular domain of Frizzled, a G-protein-coupled receptor. This interaction results in accumulation of intracellular β-catenin, promoting downstream gene activation [29, 30]. Multiple genes and proteins have been identified as regulatory factors for this pathway. β-Catenin is an unstable protein, and in the absence of Wnt ligand, it is broken down by a degradation complex composed of multiple proteins, the tumor suppressor protein APC and the scaffolding protein AXIN [31] are among them.

Ninety percent of the time, Wnt medulloblastoma is driven by mutation of β-catenin (*CTNNB1*), resulting in increased activation of MYC and MYCN oncogenes [5, 27]. A number of other frequently mutated genes have been identified in Wnt medulloblastoma [5, 27].

Alongside other evolutionarily conserved pathways [31] including the SHH and Notch pathways, the Wnt pathway has also been implicated in the development of cancer stem cells (CSCs), a subgroup of cancer cells defined by their pluripotency and capacity for self-renewal [29, 31]. The identification of cancer stem cells as a subgroup of pluripotent self-renewing cancer cells has led to the theory that they may be necessary for tumorigenesis. Aberrations in evolutionary conserved pathways, including the Wnt pathway, are frequently identified in cancer stem cells. The Wnt pathway therefore is an attractive means for targeting cancer stem cells, particularly in malignancies that are known to overexpress Wnt.

2.1.2. Drug targets in Wnt medulloblastoma

A number of molecules that interact with the Wnt pathway are currently being investigated as potential antitumor therapies in both preclinical studies and clinical trials. Tankyrase inhibitors have been identified that lead to downstream degradation of β-catenin [29]. JW55, a novel tankyrase inhibitor, has been shown in mice studies to reduce tumor development and colorectal cancer cell growth [32]. Inhibitors of Dishevelled, a protein that promotes downstream Wnt signal transduction, have also been shown to inhibit downstream Wnt signaling [33].

Interestingly, known nonsteroidal anti-inflammatory drugs (NSAIDs) have been found to have anti-Wnt pathway activity, possibly explaining in part their antineoplastic properties [27, 34, 35]. *In vitro* studies of colon cancer cells have shown that the NSAID sulindac inhibits canonical Wnt pathway activity via inhibition of cGMP hydrolysis [27]. Sulindac may also affect the Wnt pathway by affecting Dishevelled [34]. Celecoxib and diclofenac have been shown to decrease Wnt pathway signaling in *in vitro* glioblastoma cells [36]. Aspirin too affects the Wnt pathway [37]; in one study, aspirin diminished tumorigenesis in intestinal cells. The possible mechanism for aspirin in this study was downregulation of the expression of *PPAR-δ*, a growth and antiapoptotic promoting transcription factor that is a direct product of the Wnt pathway [38].

There are a number of ongoing trials using novel agents targeting the Wnt pathway. These agents include PRI-724, designed by Prism BioLab and which blocks the interaction of β-catenin with cotranscriptional coactivator CBP [29, 31]. A Phase I clinical on the molecule LGK-794, a porcupine inhibitor that inhibits Wnt protein secretion, is currently recruiting patients and will assess the safety profile in patients who carry malignancies that are dependent on Wnt ligands [29, 31]. It is important to note that these Wnt pathway-targeting compounds have not been tested in medulloblastomas, which would be the next direction for assessing their efficacy in Wnt medulloblastoma. However, although the Wnt pathway is a potential target for future medulloblastoma therapies, some authors have described potential theoretical barriers to the utilization of Wnt-targeted therapy in malignancy [28]. First, the Wnt pathway is crucial to organogenesis and homeostasis, begging the question as to whether altering the Wnt pathway may be detrimental to these processes. Second, some have contested the assumption that Wnt pathway antagonism would be desirable as anticancer therapy, given that the Wnt pathway is involved in neural regeneration after brain injury (such as surgery). The ongoing clinical trials using therapies targeting the Wnt pathway will help to better elucidate the safety and viability of targeting this pathway.

Clinical and molecular overview of medulloblastoma subgroups

Group	Patient epidemiology	Prognosis	Associated genetic aberration
SHH	Frequent in infants and in adults but not in pediatric and teenage patients	75% 5-year survival	*Ptch1, Smo, Gli1, Gli2*, and/or *SUFU*—hyperactivation of sonic hedgehog signaling
WNT	Rare in infants More common in males than in females	Best prognosis of all subgroups: 95% 10-year survival in children; 100% 5-year survival in adults	β-Catenin—increased MYC expression
Group 3	Infants and pediatric patients but rare in adults	Worst prognosis of all subgroups: 40–60% 5-year survival	MYC Photoreceptor-associated pathways
Group 4	Most prevalent subgroup, 34% of cases Found in all age groups	75% 5-year survival	17q chromosome Loss of X chromosome in female patients

Table 1. Summary of key aspects of the four molecular subgroups of medulloblastoma.

2.2. Sonic hedgehog (SHH) pathway medulloblastomas

Activation of the sonic hedgehog (SHH) pathway drives tumorigenesis in the SHH group of medulloblastomas. SHH medulloblastomas are frequently found in infant (ages 0–3) and adult (>16 years) but occur less commonly in pediatric cases [25]. The prognosis is similar to Group 4 medulloblastomas.

2.2.1. Molecular basis of SHH medulloblastomas

In sonic hedgehog signaling, the receptor Patch (specifically Ptch1) inhibits a G-protein-coupled receptor called Smoothened (Smo) in the absence of Hedgehog ligand. Hedgehog ligand binding to Patch results in disinhibition of Patch from Smo, allowing downstream signaling transduction and the activation of the Gli transcription factors, Gli1, Gli2, and Gli3 (**Figure 4**) [39, 40]. Mutations in Patch, Smo, Gli1, and Gli2 have been shown to initiate medulloblastoma in a variety of models [41–44]. Mutation in SUFU, a negative regulator of SHH signaling, is another initiating mutation [45].

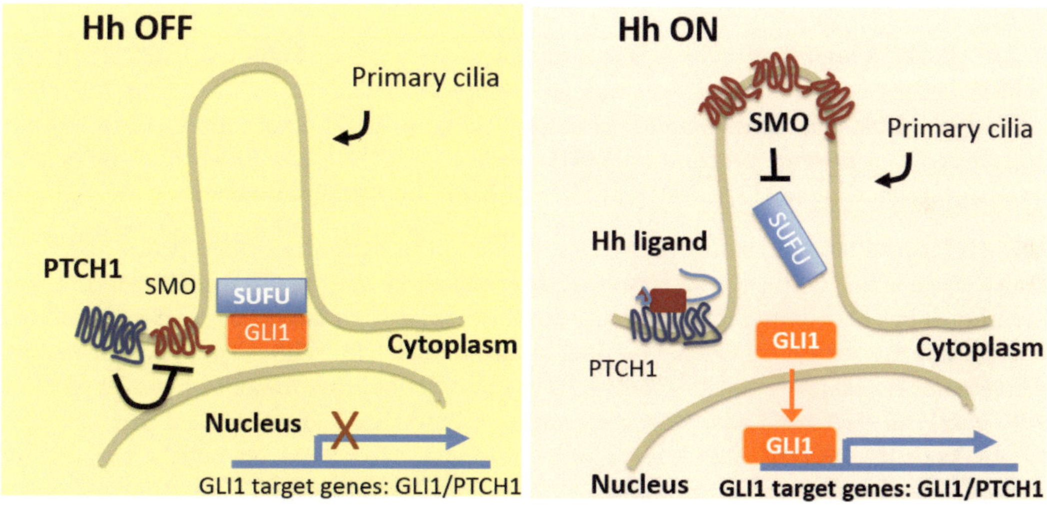

Figure 4. Schematic showing sonic hedgehog (SHH) signaling: in the absence of Hedgehog ligand, the Patch receptor (Ptch1) inhibits Smoothened (Smo). Hedgehog ligand binding to Patch results in the disinhibition of Smoothened, leading to downstream activation of the Gli transcription factors. Schematic illustrated by author JYY of this book chapter.

2.2.2. Drug targets in SHH medulloblastomas

Alkylating agents have long since served in chemotherapy for medulloblastoma, but for the SHH subgroup, inhibitors of Smo are also popular. The compound cyclopamine launched initial interest in targeting SHH signaling which was responsible for the developmental defects found in sheep that ingested corn lilies in which cyclopamine was originally discovered [46]. 2004 marked the year that Genentech identified the drug vismodegib in a screen for compounds that inhibit the SHH pathway [46]. Studies assessed vismodegib initially in advanced basal cell carcinoma and were also launched to assess the drug for other cancers [46]. Vismodegib was approved in 2012 by the Food and Drug Administration (FDA) for the treatment of metastatic or recurring BCC [46]. A Phase I study has been undertaken to assess the safety, safe dosing range, and side effects of vismodegib in a population of children with recurrent or refractory medulloblastoma [47]. Out of the 20 patients enrolled for flat-dosage testing (150 mg for smaller body area and 300 mg for larger), only two dose-limiting toxicities were observed. The study concluded that vismodegib is well tolerated in pediatric patients with recurrent or refractory medulloblastoma and recommended 150 or 300 mg dosage for Phase II trials.

Consequently, a Phase II trial was conducted at this recommended dosage with adult and pediatric patient groups. The study found that vismodegib increased progression-free survival in SHH medulloblastoma group but not in the non-SHH medulloblastoma group. Vismodegib exhibited activity against adult SHH medulloblastoma. However, inadequate sampling size for the pediatric group precluded conclusions about vismodegib efficacy in this group [48]. Therefore, vismodegib appears promising for adult medulloblastoma patients but remains to be further examined for pediatric patients.

In 2015, the FDA approved another Smo inhibitor, sonidegib (also known as LDE225), for use in treating basal cell carcinoma [49]. Sonidegib has been tested in a variety of cancers, including medulloblastoma [50]. Other Smo inhibitors are being tested in other cancers. GANT61 has been tested in a prostate cancer model [51], while BMS-833923 was tested in a gastric and esophageal cancer model [52]. Both remain to be tested in medulloblastoma.

For SHH medulloblastoma, targeting SHH signaling is a more direct therapeutic approach than the use of alkylating agents; however, drug resistance may pose a realistic concern. For example, it has been found that drug resistance can arise from amino acids changes in Smo which leads to a deficiency in drug binding to vismodegib [53]. With the approval of sonidegib, researchers then investigated whether its usage might improve tumor response in patients with basal cell carcinoma who were resistant to vismodegib. They concluded that, unfortunately, patients with advanced basal cell carcinoma, who were previously resistant to vismodegib, also experienced resistance with sonidegib treatment [54]. So, drug resistance with novel Smo inhibitors remains an ongoing concern.

Toward the goal of developing combination therapies and limiting drug resistance, recent research has progressed to investigating the molecular regulation of proteins within the SHH pathway as potential drug targets. For example, several kinases have been shown to control the activity of Gli1: ribosomal protein S6 activates Gli1 through phosphorylation on its serine 84 [55], while protein kinase A phosphorylation inhibits Gli1's activity [56].

AMP kinase (AMPK), a regulator of cell energy allocation during stress conditions, has been shown to modulate Gli1 activity. Specifically, overexpression of AMPK leads to a decrease in Gli1 expression, while downregulation of AMPK activity increases Gli1 expression [57].

http://dx.doi.org/10.5772/63004

Therefore, suppression of SHH signaling through downregulation of Gli1 may serve as a venue of targeting SHH medulloblastomas. Our group has demonstrated how direct regulation of SHH signaling through AMPK function impacts tumorigenesis. We found that AMPK regulates Gli1 activity by phosphorylating the transcription factor at serines 102 and 408 and threonine 1074. Mutation of these phosphorylation sites to nonphosphorylatable alanine increases Gli1 protein stability, transcriptional activity, and oncogenic potency, suggesting that AMPK phosphorylation reduces Gli1 activity (**Figure 5**). Another group has supported our finding that AMPK phosphorylates and may regulate Gli1 through serine 408. This group found that AMPK promotes Gli1 degradation upon its phosphorylation of serine 408 on Gli1 [58]. Further studies illustrating the effect of modulating the activity of Gli1 regulators on medulloblastoma tumorigenesis in *in vivo* systems will inform whether they are potential drug targets.

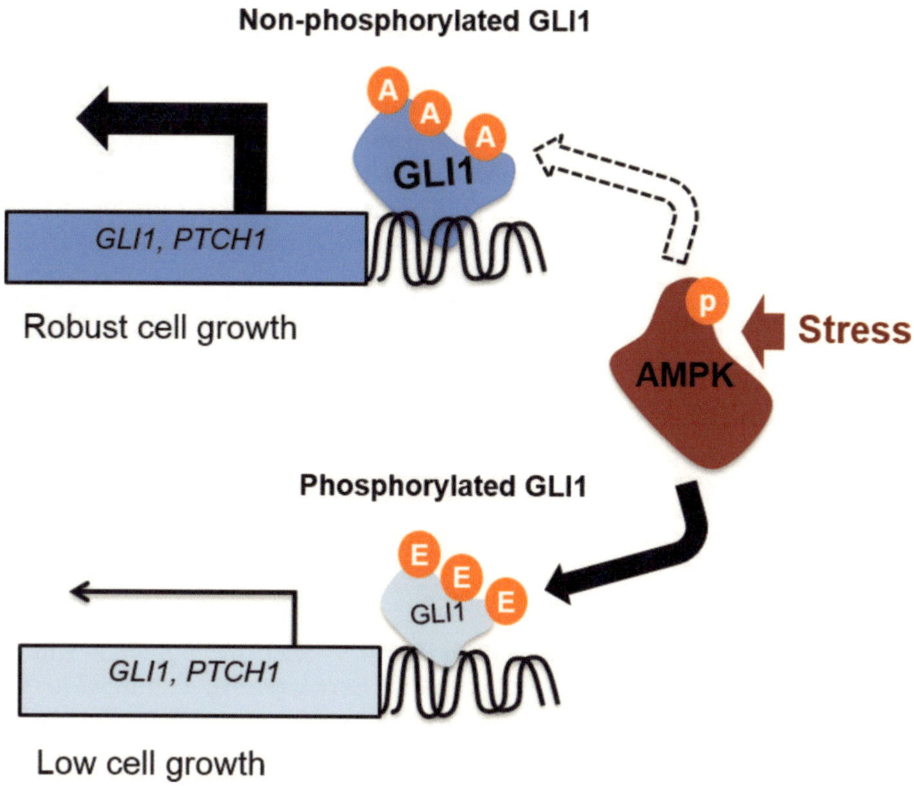

Figure 5. AMPK phosphorylation on Gli1 reduces Gli1 activity. During stress conditions, AMPK phosphorylation on Gli1 results in decreased cell growth. Uncontrolled Gli1 activity, which can arise from downregulating AMPK, leads to uncontrolled cell growth such as in medulloblastoma. Schematic adapted from author JYY's work, *AMP-activated protein kinase directly phosphorylates and destabilizes hedgehog pathway transcription factor GLI1 in medulloblastoma* (Li et al., Cell Rep. 2015).

Another approach to developing combination drug therapies has been to identify additional signaling pathways that impact SHH-driven medulloblastoma. Research has demonstrated that these pathways play a role in medulloblastoma development:

- p53: Tumor suppressor p53 is highly mutated in pediatric medulloblastomas and is a significant factor in determining prognosis [6]. A cohort study found that 5-year survival rates differed between 41 and 82%, respectively, for SHH medulloblastoma cases with and without p53 mutations [59]. In mice, the incidence of medulloblastoma increases to nearly 100% with p53 loss [60]. Therefore, regulators of p53 activity might serve as highly attractive drug candidates for combination therapy with Smo inhibitors. For example, driving down levels of MDM2, a negative regulator of p53, has been shown to decrease expression of Gli1 and Gli2 [61].

- cAMP: In general, researchers have discovered that the levels of second messenger cAMP are inversely correlated with tumor grade and growth. Ablation of the G protein Gαs is sufficient to initiate SHH medulloblastoma, and mice harboring the *GNAS* mutation demonstrate decreased tumor proliferation when cAMP levels are elevated [62].

- TGF-β: Expression analysis of Ptch1 heterozygous and Smo/Smo mouse medulloblastoma tumors of varying clinical severities found a correlation between TGF-β expression levels and medulloblastoma progression. In general, it was found that activation of the TGF-β pathway correlated with better prognosis with patients [63]. For instance, positive nuclear staining of SMAD3, a downstream component of TGF-β signaling, was associated with longer patient survival [63]. Therefore, regulation of the TGF-β signaling pathway in conjunction with SHH signaling may be another venue of combination therapy.

- Basic FGF: Overall, basic FGF (bFGF) signaling appears to have an inhibitory role on SHH-induced proliferation. The addition of bGFG to tumor cultures has been shown to limit tumor formation and proliferation and to inhibit expression of the transcriptional products of SHH signaling, namely *Gli1, Nmyc*, and *cyclin D1* [64].

While these intersecting pathways contain possible targets, determining the exact mechanism by which they impact SHH medulloblastoma is the limiting step to uncovering the best candidates to target.

2.3. Group 3 medulloblastomas

While Wnt and SHH medulloblastomas have been identified by mutations within these pathways, more comprehensive biological pathways have not been delineated for Group 3 and Group 4 medulloblastomas. Hence, these have been so named until the underlying biology is further elucidated.

Conventional diagnosis of Group 3 medulloblastomas is accomplished through transcriptional profiling [3]. Group 3 medulloblastoma is associated with increased MYC expression and enrichment for photoreceptor pathway-associated genes; these genes are overexpressed in Group 3 [3]. In addition, Group 3 can be divided into subtype based on MYC expression. In Group 3α subtype, all patients contain MYC amplification and this is associated with poor prognosis with increased recurrence and mortality, while the Group 3β subtype contains no MYC amplification and has a prognosis similar to Group 4 medulloblastomas [3]. Medulloblastomas of this group are found in both infants and children, but rarely in adults, and are found more in males than in females [3]. Histologically, Group 3 medulloblastomas frequently have large anaplastic cell pathology [3].

2.3.1. *Molecular basis of Group 3 medulloblastomas*

While many details about the molecular makeup of Group 3 medulloblastomas remain unresolved, recent literature therapeutically targeting Group 3 medulloblastoma may reveal clues to the molecular pathways driving this subgroup. The folate synthesis inhibitor pemetrexed and nucleoside analog gemcitabine demonstrated a synergistic effect in increasing the survival of mice bearing MYC-overexpressing tumors [65]. The same drug combination had little effect on mice medulloblastomas of the SHH subgroup [65]. These observations are supported by gene set enrichment analysis showing that Group 3 medulloblastomas are enriched in the folate and purine metabolism pathways compared to Group 4 and SHH medulloblastoma [65].

The antihelmintic drug, mebendazole, has been shown to inhibit angiogenesis in medulloblastoma [66]. While it acts as a microtubule synthesis inhibitor in worms, studies with medulloblastoma models suggest that it can inhibit vascular endothelial growth factor receptor 2 (VEGFR2) [66]. Targeting class I histone deacetylase 2 has also been shown to impact Group 3 medulloblastoma tumor cell viability [67].

The International Cancer Genome Consortium (ICGC) PedBrain Tumor Project published in 2014 the analyses of deep sequencing of Group 3 and Group 4 tumors. This study uncovered novel information about the biology between this subgroup. Tetraploidy was a common event for both Group 3 and Group 4 tumors, respectively, and tetraploid tumors displayed signs of genomic instability [68]. With Group 3, the most frequently mutated gene was SMARCA4 [68]. Together, both *in vitro* drug assays and genome-wide mining of Wnt medulloblastomas introduce molecular pathways for further exploration in uncovering Group 3 medulloblastoma biology and which may reveal possible drug targets.

2.4. Group 4 medulloblastomas

Group 4 is the most prevalent medulloblastoma subgroup, accounting for about 34% of all medulloblastomas [6]. A high frequency (66%) of isochromosome 17q is associated with Group 4 medulloblastomas [6]. Strikingly, 80% of women with Group 4 medulloblastoma also have X chromosome loss [6]. Group 4 medulloblastomas have a prognosis comparable to SHH group medulloblastomas [6].

2.4.1. *Molecular basis of Group 4 medulloblastomas*

The ICGC PedBrain Project found that KDM64, a histone 3 lysine 27 demethylase, was mutated in 10% of Group 4 tumors [68]. These mutations reveal the genetic and molecular pathways that go awry in Group 3 and Group 4 tumors. For example, the ICGC PedBrain uncovered an association between TBR1 and Group 4 medulloblastomas [68]. TBR1 is a T-box transcription factor shown to play a role in brain development. Of particular interest is the gene CTDNEP1, found mutated in 10% of Group 4 tumors and which is located on 17q [68]. CTDNEP1 encodes a nuclear membrane phosphatase and in mammals is shown to play a role in nuclear membrane biogenesis and in lipid activation. As 66% of Group 4 medulloblastomas contain 17q, mutations found on this isochromosome are particularly important for study.

2.5. Future clinical and basic science directions for medulloblastoma

Clearly, with respect to Group 3 and Group 4 medulloblastomas, further studies about the molecular basis for these subgroups are needed. These two subgroups pose great clinical challenges: Group 4 is the most prevalent group, while Group 3 has the poorest diagnosis. Yet a dearth of knowledge about the molecular basis behind each group limits drug targeting. The growing body of studies which include genome-wide mining for enrichments within each subgroup along with *in vitro* studies for Group 3 and Group 4 may soon intersect to reveal a broader picture of the molecular pathways behind these subgroups.

Currently, there are a number of clinical trials evaluating the safety and efficacy of Wnt-targeted therapies in patients with other malignancies that overexpress the Wnt pathway; however, none of these are being tested in medulloblastomas. The efficacy of these agents in treating Wnt medulloblastoma remains to be assessed. Additionally, in light of the high survival rates of standard risk patients with Wnt medulloblastoma, additional studies would be helpful to identify optimal treatment regimens that will maintain these high survival rates while minimizing treatment side effects. With respect to SHH-driven medulloblastoma, identification of novel targets especially for combination drug therapy will address the concern for drug resistance and limited efficacy of current treatments. For example, the identification and assessment of novel Gli inhibitors for SHH-mediated cancers should be evaluated in the context of medulloblastoma. In addition, the effects of the crosstalk of intersecting pathways on medulloblastoma tumorigenesis should be further studied.

Author details

Eric Q. Trieu[1], Sherri Y. Huang[2] and Jer-Yen Yang[3*]

*Address all correspondence to: jyyang@purdue.edu

1 Cedars-Sinai Medical Center, Los Angeles, LA, USA

2 Department of Pharmacology and Toxicology, Indiana University School of Medicine, Indianapolis, IN, USA

3 Department of Basic Medical Sciences, Center for Cancer Research, Purdue University College of Veterinary Medicine, West Lafayette, IN, USA

References

[1] Koeller K, Rushing E. From the archives of the AFIP. RadioGraphics. 2003;23(6):1613–1637.

[2] Ali-Osman F. Brain tumors. Totowa, N.J.: Humana Press; 2005.

[3] Taylor M, Northcott P, Korshunov A, Remke M, Cho Y, Clifford S, et al. Molecular subgroups of medulloblastoma: the current consensus. Acta Neuropathologica. 2011;123(4):465–472.

[4] Kleihues P, Cavenee W. Pathology and genetics of tumours of the nervous system. Lyon: IARC Press; 2000.

[5] Brandes A, Bartolotti M, Marucci G, Ghimenton C, Agati R, Fioravanti A, et al. New perspectives in the treatment of adult medulloblastoma in the era of molecular oncology. Critical Reviews in Oncology/Hematology. 2015;94(3):348–359.

[6] Kool M, Korshunov A, Remke M, Jones D, Schlanstein M, Northcott P, et al. Molecular subgroups of medulloblastoma: an international meta-analysis of transcriptome, genetic aberrations, and clinical data of Wnt, SHH, Group 3, and Group 4 medulloblastomas. Acta Neuropathologica. 2012;123(4):473–484.

[7] Sandberg A, Stone J. The genetics and molecular biology of neural tumors. Totowa, N.J.: Humana Press; 2008.

[8] Spassky N, Han Y, Aguilar A, Strehl L, Besse L, Laclef C, et al. Primary cilia are required for cerebellar development and Shh-dependent expansion of progenitor pool. Developmental Biology. 2008;317(1):246–259.

[9] Gibson P, Tong Y, Robinson G, Thompson M, Currle D, Eden C, et al. Subtypes of medulloblastoma have distinct developmental origins. Nature. 2010;468(7327):1095–1099.

[10] Tonn J. Neuro-oncology of CNS tumors. Berlin: Springer; 2006.

[11] Smee R, Williams J. Medulloblastomas—primitive neuroectodermal tumours in the adult population. Journal of Medical Imaging and Radiation Oncology. 2008;52(1):72–76.

[12] Yeom K, Mobley B, Lober R, Andre J, Partap S, Vogel H, et al. Distinctive MRI features of pediatric medulloblastoma subtypes. American Journal of Roentgenology. 2013;200(4):895–903.

[13] Tarbell N, Friedman H, Polkinghorn W, Yock T, Zhou T, Chen Z, et al. High-risk medulloblastoma: a Pediatric Oncology Group randomized trial of chemotherapy before or after radiation therapy (POG 9031). Journal of Clinical Oncology. 2013;31(23): 2936–2941.

[14] Fisher P. Biologic risk stratification of medulloblastoma: the real time is now. Journal of Clinical Oncology. 2004;22(6):971–974.

[15] Martin A, Raabe E, Eberhart C, Cohen K. Management of pediatric and adult patients with medulloblastoma. Current Treatment Options in Oncology. 2014;15(4):581–594.

[16] Sirachainan N, Nuchprayoon I, Thanarattanakorn P, Pakakasama S, Lusawat A, Visudibhan A, et al. Outcome of medulloblastoma in children treated with reduced-dose radiation therapy plus adjuvant chemotherapy. Journal of Clinical Neuroscience. 2011;18(4):515–519.

[17] [Internet]. 2016 [cited 2 February 2016]. Available from: https://www.nccn.org/store/login/login.aspx?ReturnURL=http://www.nccn.org/professionals/physician_gls/pdf/cns.pdf

[18] Friedrich C, von Bueren A, von Hoff K, Kwiecien R, Pietsch T, Warmuth-Metz M, et al. Treatment of adult nonmetastatic medulloblastoma patients according to the paediatric HIT 2000 protocol: a prospective observational multicentre study. European Journal of Cancer. 2013;49(4):893–903.

[19] Mulhern R, Merchant T, Gajjar A, Reddick W, Kun L. Late neurocognitive sequelae in survivors of brain tumours in childhood. The Lancet Oncology. 2004;5(7):399–408.

[20] Fossati P, Ricardi U, Orecchia R. Pediatric medulloblastoma: toxicity of current treatment and potential role of protontherapy. Cancer Treatment Reviews. 2009;35(1):79–96.

[21] Packer RJ, Macdonald T, Vezina GI, Keating RO, Santi MA. Medulloblastoma and primitive neuroectodermal tumors. Handb Clin Neurol. 2012; 105:529–48.

[22] Thomas P, Deutsch M, Kepner J, Boyett J, Krischer J, Aronin P, et al. Low-stage medulloblastoma: final analysis of trial comparing standard-dose with reduced-dose neuraxis irradiation. Journal of Clinical Oncology. 2001;5(2):210–211.

[23] Brandes A, Franceschi E, Tosoni A, Blatt V, Ermani M. Long-term results of a prospective study on the treatment of medulloblastoma in adults. Cancer. 2007;110(9):2035–2041.

[24] Louis D, Ohgaki H, Wiestler O, Cavenee W, Burger P, Jouvet A, et al. The 2007 WHO classification of tumours of the central nervous system. Acta Neuropathologica. 2007;114(2):97–109.

[25] Gururangan S, Schroeder K. Molecular variants and mutations in medulloblastoma. Pharmacogenomics and Personalized Medicine. 2014;7:43–51.

[26] Northcott P, Dubuc A, Pfister S, Taylor M. Molecular subgroups of medulloblastoma. Expert Review of Neurotherapeutics. 2012;12(7):871–884.

[27] Li K, Lau K, Ng H. Signaling pathway and molecular subgroups of medulloblastoma. International Journal of Clinical and Experimental Pathology. 2013;6(7):1211–1222.

[28] Kahn M. Can we safely target the Wnt pathway? Nature Reviews Drug Discovery. 2014;13(7):513–532.

[29] Takebe N, Miele L, Harris P, Jeong W, Bando H, Kahn M, et al. Targeting Notch, hedgehog, and Wnt pathways in cancer stem cells: clinical update. Nature Reviews Clinical Oncology. 2015;12(8):445–464.

[30] Komiya Y, Habas R. Wnt signal transduction pathways. Organogenesis. 2008;4(2):68–75.

[31] Duchartre Y, Kim Y, Kahn M. The Wnt signaling pathway in cancer. Critical Reviews in Oncology/Hematology. 2016;99:141–149.

[32] Waaler J, Machon O, Tumova L, Dinh H, Korinek V, Wilson S, et al. A novel tankyrase inhibitor decreases canonical wnt signaling in colon carcinoma cells and reduces tumor growth in conditional APC mutant mice. Cancer Research. 2012;72(11):2822–2832.

[33] Grandy D, Shan J, Zhang X, Rao S, Akunuru S, Li H, et al. Discovery and characterization of a small molecule inhibitor of the PDZ domain of dishevelled. Journal of Biological Chemistry. 2009;284(24):16256–16263.

[34] Lee H, Wang N, Shi D, Zheng J. Sulindac inhibits canonical Wnt signaling by blocking the PDZ domain of the protein dishevelled. Angewandte Chemie International Edition. 2009;48(35):6448–6452.

[35] Barker N, Clevers H. Mining the Wnt pathway for cancer therapeutics. Nature Reviews Drug Discovery. 2006;5(12):997–1014.

[36] Sareddy G, Kesanakurti D, Kirti P, Babu P. Nonsteroidal anti-inflammatory drugs diclofenac and celecoxib attenuates Wnt/β-catenin/Tcf signaling pathway in human glioblastoma cells. Neurochemical Research. 2013;38(11):2313–2322.

[37] Gala M, Chan A. Molecular pathways: aspirin and Wnt signaling—a molecularly targeted approach to cancer prevention and treatment. Clinical Cancer Research. 2014;21(7):1543–1548.

[38] Ouyang N. NO-donating aspirin isomers downregulate peroxisome proliferator-activated receptor (PPAR)delta expression in APCmin/+ mice proportionally to their tumor inhibitory effect: implications for the role of PPARdelta in carcinogenesis. Carcinogenesis. 2006;27(2):232–239.

[39] Merchant M, Vajdos F, Ultsch M, Maun H, Wendt U, Cannon J, et al. Suppressor of fused regulates Gli activity through a dual binding mechanism. Molecular and Cellular Biology. 2004;24(19):8627–8641.

[40] Chen W. Activity-dependent internalization of smoothened mediated by beta-arrestin 2 and GRK2. Science. 2004;306(5705):2257–2260.

[41] Dey J, Ditzler S, Knoblaugh S, Hatton B, Schelter J, Cleary M, et al. A distinct smoothened mutation causes severe cerebellar developmental defects and medulloblastoma in a novel transgenic mouse model. Molecular and Cellular Biology. 2012;32(20):4104–4115.

[42] Hatton B, Villavicencio E, Tsuchiya K, Pritchard J, Ditzler S, Pullar B, et al. The Smo/Smo model: hedgehog-induced medulloblastoma with 90% incidence and leptomeningeal spread. Cancer Research. 2008;68(6):1768–1776.

[43] Zurawel R, Allen C, Chiappa S, Cato W, Biegel J, Cogen P, et al. Analysis of PTCH/SMO/SHH pathway genes in medulloblastoma. Genes Chromosome Cancer. 2000;27(1):44–51.

[44] Zurawel R, Allen C, Wechsler-Reya R, Scott M, Raffel C. Evidence that haploinsufficiency of Ptch leads to medulloblastoma in mice. Genes Chromosome Cancer. 2000;28(1):77.

[45] Taylor M, Liu L, Raffel C, Hui C, Mainprize T, Zhang X, et al. Mutations in SUFU predispose to medulloblastoma. Nature Genetics. 2002;31(3):306–310.

[46] Gene.com. Genentech: Erivedge® (vismodegib) Development timeline [Internet]. 2016 [cited 3 February 2016]. Available from: http://www.gene.com/media/product-information/erivedge-development-timeline

[47] Gajjar A, Stewart C, Ellison D, Kaste S, Kun L, Packer R, et al. Phase I study of vismodegib in children with recurrent or refractory medulloblastoma: a pediatric brain tumor consortium study. Clinical Cancer Research. 2013;19(22):6305–6312.

[48] Robinson G, Orr B, Wu G, Gururangan S, Lin T, Qaddoumi I, et al. Vismodegib exerts targeted efficacy against recurrent sonic hedgehog-subgroup medulloblastoma: results from phase II pediatric brain tumor consortium studies PBTC-025B and PBTC-032. Journal of Clinical Oncology. 2015;33(24):2646–2654.

[49] National Cancer Institute. Sonidegib approved for advanced basal cell carcinoma [Internet]. 2016 [cited 27 February 2016]. Available from: http://www.cancer.gov/news-events/cancer-currents-blog/2015/sonidegib-BCC

[50] Rodon J, Tawbi H, Thomas A, Stoller R, Turtschi C, Baselga J, et al. A phase I, multicenter, open-label, first-in-human, dose-escalation study of the oral smoothened inhibitor sonidegib (LDE225) in patients with advanced solid tumors. Clinical Cancer Research. 2014;20(7):1900–1909.

[51] Lauth M, Bergstrom A, Shimokawa T, Toftgard R. Inhibition of GLI-mediated transcription and tumor cell growth by small-molecule antagonists. Proceedings of the National Academy of Sciences. 2007;104(20):8455–8460.

[52] Zaidi A, Komatsu Y, Kelly L, Malhotra U, Rotoloni C, Kosovec J, et al. Smoothened inhibition leads to decreased proliferation and induces apoptosis in esophageal adenocarcinoma cells. Cancer Investigation. 2013;31(7):480–489.

[53] Yauch R, Dijkgraaf G, Alicke B, Januario T, Ahn C, Holcomb T, et al. Smoothened mutation confers resistance to a hedgehog pathway inhibitor in medulloblastoma. Science. 2009;326(5952):572–574.

[54] Danial C, Sarin K, Oro A, Chang A. An investigator-initiated open-label trial of sonidegib in advanced basal cell carcinoma patients resistant to vismodegib. Clinical Cancer Research. 2016;22(6):1325–1329.

[55] Wang Y, Xia W, Lang J, Hsu J, Wang H, Ajani J et al. Abstract 989: the crosstalk of mTOR/S6K1 and hedgehog pathways. Cancer Research. 2012;72(8 Suppl):989–989.

[56] Sheng T, Chi S, Zhang X, Xie J. Regulation of Gli1 Localization by the cAMP/protein kinase A signaling axis through a site near the nuclear localization signal. Journal of Biological Chemistry. 2005;281(1):9–12.

[57] Li Y, Luo J, Mosley Y, Hedrick V, Paul L, Chang J, et al. AMP-activated protein kinase directly phosphorylates and destabilizes hedgehog pathway transcription factor GLI1 in medulloblastoma. Cell Reports. 2015;12(4):599–609.

[58] Di Magno L, Basile A, Coni S, Manni S, Sdruscia G, et al. The energy sensor AMPK regulates hedgehog signaling in human cells through a unique Gli1 metabolic checkpoint. Oncotarget. 2016;7(8):9538–49

[59] Zhukova N, Ramaswamy V, Remke M, Pfaff E, Shih D, Martin D, et al. Subgroup-specific prognostic implications of TP53 mutation in medulloblastoma. Journal of Clinical Oncology. 2013;31(23):2927–2935.

[60] Wetmore C, Eberhart D, Curran T. Loss of p53 but not ARF accelerates medulloblastoma in mice heterozygous for patched. Cancer Research. 2001;61(2):513–516.

[61] Malek R, Matta J, Taylor N, Perry M, Mendrysa S. The p53 inhibitor MDM2 facilitates sonic hedgehog-mediated tumorigenesis and influences cerebellar foliation. PLoS One. 2011;6(3):e17884.

[62] He X, Zhang L, Chen Y, Remke M, Shih D, Lu F, et al. The G protein α subunit Gαs is a tumor suppressor in Sonic hedgehog-driven medulloblastoma. Nature Medicine. 2014;20(9):1035–1042.

[63] Aref D, Moffatt C, Agnihotri S, Ramaswamy V, Dubuc A, Northcott P, et al. Canonical TGF-β pathway activity is a predictor of SHH-driven medulloblastoma survival and delineates putative precursors in cerebellar development. Brain Pathology. 2012;23(2): 178–191.

[64] Fogarty M, Emmenegger B, Grasfeder L, Oliver T, Wechsler-Reya R. Fibroblast growth factor blocks sonic hedgehog signaling in neuronal precursors and tumor cells. Proceedings of the National Academy of Sciences. 2007;104(8):2973–2978.

[65] Morfouace M, Shelat A, Jacus M, Freeman B, Turner D, Robinson S, et al. Pemetrexed and gemcitabine as combination therapy for the treatment of Group 3 medulloblastoma. Cancer Cell. 2014;25(4):516–529.

[66] Bodhinayake I, Symons M, Boockvar J. Repurposing mebendazole for the treatment of medulloblastoma. Neurosurgery. 2015;76(2):N15–N16.

[67] Ecker J, Oehme I, Mazitschek R, Korshunov A, Kool M, Hielscher T, Kiss J, Selt F, Konrad C, Lodrini M, Deubzer HE. Targeting class I histone deacetylase 2 in MYC amplified group 3 medulloblastoma. Acta neuropathologica communications. 2015;3(1):1

[68] Jones D, Jäger N, Kool M, Zichner T, Hutter B, Sultan M, et al. Dissecting the genomic complexity underlying medulloblastoma. Nature. 2012;488(7409):100–105.

Chapter 17

Diffuse Intrinsic Pontine Glioma: A Therapeutic Challenge

Heloisa H. Moser, Eshini Panditharatna,
Roger J. Packer and Javad Nazarian

Additional information is available at the end of the chapter

http://dx.doi.org/10.5772/63066

Abstract

Diffuse intrinsic pontine glioma (DIPG) is a tumor of the brainstem, specifically in the pons, accounting for 10–20% of all of central nervous system (CNS) tumors in children. Unfortunately, DIPG is the leading cause of death in children with CNS cancers. Clinical interventions trying to effectively treat children with DIPG have failed despite 40 years of clinical trials. The critical location of these tumors eliminates extensive surgical resection as an option. Radiation therapy (RT) is the standard of care, and although it improves the clinical symptoms of most patients, the results are temporary, with tumor progression typically occurring months post radiation. Given the dismal prognosis associated with this disease and the challenge to find chemotherapeutic agents, especially molecularly targeted drugs that improve the survival of the patients, there is a strong incentive to move new treatments forward into clinical trials. The more effective treatment would potentially involve combinatory therapeutic regimens with new epigenetic drugs that can offer synergistic benefits and potentially increase therapeutic efficacy. The increasing knowledge of genomic, epigenomic, and proteomic characteristics of DIPG is opening doors to new therapeutic avenues and provides hope and promise for this devastating childhood cancer.

Keywords: diffuse intrinsic pontine glioma (DIPG), brainstem glioma, high-grade glioma (HGG), targeted therapy, combinatory mutations, precision medicine

1. Introduction

Diffuse intrinsic pontine glioma (DIPG) is a tumor that arises in the pons and diffusely infiltrates the brainstem. It is believed that DIPG originates from a dysregulation of a postnatal neurodevelopmental process. It usually affects middle childhood, with a peak onset of 6–9 years of age. High-grade gliomas (HGGs) typically have a predilection for the ventral pons, a finding that would reflect the presence of a cell of origin as well as a signaling microenvironment favorable for tumor formation [1–3]. A study using early postmortem DIPG tumor tissue has shown that the Sonic Hedgehog (Shh) signaling pathway in DIPG tumor cells is involved in many developmental and oncogenic processes, such as neural embryogenesis and oligodendrogenesis. The dysregulation of this molecular system in DIPG leads to hypertrophy of the ventral pons and suggests a potential molecular origin for this poorly understood cancer [4]. According to the lessons learned from other pediatric brain tumors, such as medulloblastoma, neural stem or precursor cells would be the most likely cell type that could transform and give rise to DIPG [4–6].

In the United States, 200–300 children are diagnosed each year with DIPG [7]. Unfortunately, being the pediatric brain tumor with the highest mortality rate, DIPGs have poor prognosis with a less than 1-year survival, where less than 10% and 2% of patients survive after 2 and 5 years post-diagnosis, respectively [8]. The grim outcome first and foremost is due to the tumor's delicate anatomical location and significant infiltration. Extensive surgical resection is not a treatment option, leaving radiation therapy (RT) and chemotherapy as the only remaining therapies.

RT is the standard treatment for children with DIPG and results in improvement of symptoms in more than 80% of the patients; however, it rarely results in a cure. The conventional treatment consists of 1.8 Gy fractions delivered once daily, 5 days a week, for about 6 weeks to a total cumulative target dose of 54 Gy. Hyperfractionated doses up to 72 Gy have not shown improved efficacy in children and resulted in increased morbidity. On the other hand, hypofractionated RT may lead to similar outcomes as standard treatment. The median survival of patients treated with RT is only 10 months [9,10]. When RT is associated with standard chemotherapeutic agents, no survival benefit was shown, in neither the event-free survival (EFS) nor the overall survival (OS) of patients [11].

Another reason of poor prognosis is associated with the ineffective results using chemotherapeutic agents. Despite decades of research and use of different chemotherapeutic strategies, no survival advantage has been achieved. In the last 30 years, several clinical trials were done using various adjuvant chemotherapeutic drugs utilized prior to, during, or after radiotherapy in DIPG patients. The results were bleak: none of these clinical trials showed any improvement in survival of this pediatric cancer, leaving DIPG as the number one cause of brain tumor-related death in children [12]. In addition to the difficulty associated with finding effective therapeutics, it is also speculated that the tumor biology changes between the primary and recurrent tumors, leading to another problem—resistance to therapy. Furthermore, an additional challenge includes ways of overcoming the restrictive ability of the intact blood–brain barrier (BBB) in patients with DIPG.

The lack of reliable models along with poor knowledge of the biological basis of DIPG has been critical elements in failure to make progress in this disease. In the pre-CT and magnetic resonance imaging (MRI) eras, histological assessment of biopsies was routinely conducted to diagnose DIPGs. However, this standard of care was discontinued in the early 1990s, due to

http://dx.doi.org/10.5772/63066

the high rate of morbidity and improvement of imaging techniques [13]. Recently, the increase in availability for biopsy and acquisition of autopsy specimen for experimental purposes, as well as the insight gleaned from recent studies, is beginning to unravel the genetic and epigenetic drivers of DIPG. Stereotactic biopsies in well-trained neurosurgical teams are a safe procedure [14] and are being incorporated for patients with DIPG. Improved methods of modeling DIPGs by mimicking genetic and epigenetic changes, preclinical testing, and translational studies will bring a strong incentive to move new treatments forward into clinical trials.

Given the different molecular subgroups within the disease and the combinatory mutations found through gene expression, mutational, and epigenetic analysis, the key for an effective treatment relies on combinatory therapy. Studies using deep sequencing analysis, comprehensive methylation, copy number, and mRNA expression profiling show that these subgroups are characterized by upregulation of MYCN (N-Myc), Shh signaling, and H3-K27M mutations [15–18]. The combinatory genomic aberrations have introduced one more challenge for designing therapeutic regiments—most of the combinatory mutations are novel and thus there is a deficit of preclinical data on combinatory drug regimens. However, the increase in knowledge of DIPG and development of novel *in vitro* and *in vivo* approaches is a promise for effectively targeting driver mutations with the use of combinatory drugs.

New promising approaches provide a glimpse of hope for patients who are battling this devastating tumor. Among the many devastating childhood cancers, DIPG patients desperately need access to new treatments. Increased availability of tumor tissue for preclinical investigation and the development of experimental model systems now provide important tools to guide future clinical trials. Advances in the knowledge of the molecular biology of DIPG are key to developing new therapeutic testing.

2. Diagnosis: clinical presentation, radiographic findings, and stereotactic biopsy

2.1. Clinical presentation

Cerebellar signs (e.g., ataxia, dysmetria, and dysarthria), pyramidal tract signs (e.g., hyperreflexia, clonus, increased tone, and presence of a Babinski reflex), and cranial nerve palsies (unilateral or bilateral) are the classic triad clinical presentation in DIPG. As the tumor grows, the pons become diffusely infiltrated and enlarged, the basilar artery is encased, and crucial nuclei of cranial nerve tracts V, VI, VII, and VIII within the pons are compressed. The symptom onset is acute, with a fast progression, where children typically experience 1 month or less of neurologic manifestations before they are diagnosed. Symptom duration greater than 6 months prior to presentation should prompt a search for an alternate diagnosis. The most common reported symptoms are abnormal or limited eye movements, diplopia, asymmetric smile, clumsiness, difficulty walking, loss of balance, and weakness [19,20]. Obstructive hydrocephalus presenting with headaches, nausea, and vomiting may be present due to increased intracranial pressure, resulting from expansion of the pons. Other less common symptoms may occur, including behavioral changes, night terrors, and scholarly difficulties [8]. Among the rare symptoms are urinary retention and other voiding abnormalities without spinal cord lesions, which can be due to disruption of the pontine micturition center [21].

2.2. Radiographic findings

Advances in imaging technology over the last few decades and the development of MRI have significantly improved the accurate diagnosing of DIPG. MRI scan is the best noninvasive method to determine the size and the characteristics of the tumor. Thus, the comprehensive diagnosis of DIPG is based on MRI findings combined with the clinical presentation.

On MRI, the boundaries of a DIPG are hard to determine, as the tumor cells invade the surrounding tissue of the pons—the tumor appears as a large expansible brainstem mass. The epicenter of DIPG lies within the pons and the lesion involves the majority of its structure. Tumors typically show diffuse hyperintense bright signal on T2-weighted and are hypo- or isointense on T1 (**Figure 1**).

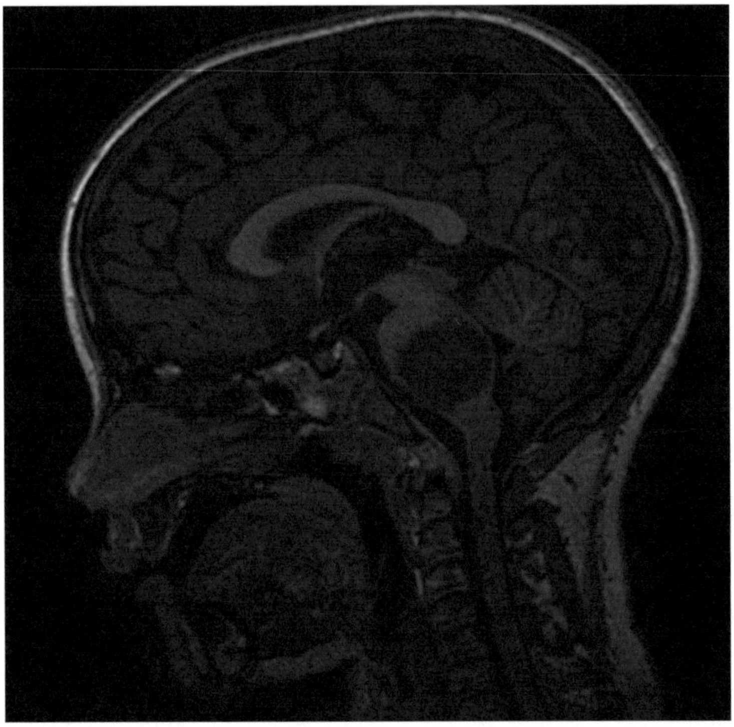

Figure 1. Precontrast sagittal volume T1 MRI of the brain of a DIPG patient showing diffusely infiltrating pontine mass.

On fluid-attenuated inversion recovery (FLAIR) imaging sequences, the tumor frequently appears homogeneous. MRI can also show pinpoint intratumoral hemorrhages, ventral involvement of the pons, encasement of the basilar artery, and possible sites of tumor extension [8,22,23].

One classification system developed by Choux et al. [24] classifies brainstem gliomas into diffuse, intrinsic focal, extrinsic focal, and cervicomedullary based on MRI. DIPGs are classified as type I tumors—those that diffuse throughout the brainstem. Type II, III, and IV tumors are characterized by more focal lesions and may have a more favorable outcome.

Compared to computed tomography (CT), MRI provides superior imaging of the posterior fossa of the brain and has a superior contrast resolution of soft tissue. Other advanced imaging techniques include magnetic resonance spectroscopy (MRS), perfusion imaging, and positron emission tomography (PET). These imaging methods show improved advantages such as tumor differentiation. However, MRI appearance is uncertain and stratification of patients based on the aggressiveness of their tumors could be helpful in deducing a more accurate diagnosis, leading to an improved understanding of these tumors.

2.3. Differential diagnosis in MRI

A universally diagnostic criterion has not yet been defined for DIPGs. Currently, the criteria that are typically accepted include symptom duration less than 6 months, at least two or three symptoms related to brainstem dysfunction, and pontine enlargement with evidence of diffusely infiltrative tumor centered in and involving greater than 50–66% of the pons [25].

In MRI, DIPGs present with distinct characteristics from pilocytic astrocytoma; for example, MRI shows the following aspects: (A) focal, well defined on T1 and T2 weighting, (B) minimum brainstem swelling, and (C) brainstem location without extension. The two most common types of pediatric brainstem tumors, DIPGs and pilocytic astrocytoma, can be accurately identified by MRI alone in most cases. Although MRI is not 100% specific, the vast majority of children diagnosed with DIPG by MRI do have a diffuse infiltrative glioma.

Patients with diffuse brainstem gliomas associated with neurofibromatosis type 1 (NF1) may mimic DIPG on imaging. However, they are usually low-grade gliomas (LGG—World Health Organization (WHO) grades I–II) which can be asymptomatic and present with a simple differential diagnosis based on family history and clinical examination [26].

In the context of an atypical presentation of DIPG (presentation with clinical features and circumscribed MRI characteristics), it is important to rule out potential differential diagnosis. These include embryonic tumors such as ATRT, PNET, and nonmalignant lesions such as infections, neurodegenerative conditions, and hemangioblastomas [27].

2.4. Stereotactic biopsy

Before the advent of effective imaging techniques, surgical biopsies played an important role in DIPG diagnosis. However, with improved radiologic capabilities—primarily MRI—until recently, stereotactic biopsies are only performed in the rare cases, where the diagnosis is uncertain based on MRI findings. Nonetheless, as neurosurgical experience with stereotactic biopsies of DIPGs grew and was proven to be safer, as well as neuropathologic expertise to identify molecular subtypes increased, biopsy has been increasingly performed to not only identify the type of tumor present but to delineate potential molecular targets that could be therapeutically explored. In experienced hands, the permanent morbidity after stereotactic biopsy has been found to be less than 5%.

In histologic diagnosis, DIPGs are defined as a fibrillary astrocytoma, WHO grades II–IV, and in most of the cases resemble malignant gliomas in other locations [28]. However, the prognosis for DIPGs is not associated with the histological classification. DIPGs harboring the histone 3 mutation classified as WHO II and III have a poor OS, similar to WHO IV patients [29]. In addition, significant histopathological variability has been reported in DIPGs, where a single biopsy may not be representative of the histological classification of the entire tumor [23,29,30].

Important biological information obtained from biopsies may be used in future clinical trials, guiding new treatment regimens and allowing for advances in surgical and molecular analytical techniques [31]. The use of tissue obtained from pretreatment biopsies combined with antibodies to detect driver mutations gives the opportunity to identify the genomic mutational landscape of DIPG and provides opportunities to improve diagnosis, prognosis, and better understanding of the potential drug targets.

3. New advances: the future of genomics, epigenomics, and proteomics

Taking into consideration that DIPG may represent a biologically distinct subclass of glioma, there is a great need for the comprehensive investigation of tumor biology. Therefore, studies in this rare type of cancer cannot be performed without the knowledge of genomics and proteomics. The development of new technologies that can rapidly analyze DNA, RNA, and proteins and the progress in bioinformatics area are substantial advances that have largely been achieved in the past years. Analysis of mRNA, methylation, and proteomic profiling of DIPGs compared to healthy brain tissue identified two distinct subgroups characterized by upregulation of N-Myc and Hedgehog signaling pathways [15]. Combinatory analysis of whole-genome and whole-exome sequencing, copy number alterations, methylation, and gene expression profiling revealed three molecular subgroups in DIPG, highlighting novel therapeutic targets [18]. The three molecular subgroups consisted of upregulation of N-Myc (histone 3 wild-type DIPGs), silent genomes with fewer copy number alterations, and histone 3 K27M mutant DIPGs with *ACVR1* and *TP53* mutations. DIPGs of silent and H3-K27M molecular subtypes would benefit from therapies targeting altered histone modifications, while patients of the N-Myc subtype would benefit from therapy targeting N-Myc or ID2. Furthermore, DIPGs of the N-Myc and silent subgroups lacked amplification of receptor tyrosine kinases, indicating the inefficacy of inhibitors targeting these kinase pathways [18]. Therefore, numerous combinatory analyses of DIPG have identified the importance of the synergistic genetic and epigenetic basis of this fatal childhood cancer.

3.1. DIPG and tissue donation

A primary requirement for genomic analysis of cancer is tumor material. Much of the histological and prognostic information that we have about DIPG is from biopsies that were frequently performed until the early 1970s, before any of the current genomic techniques were available, and when CT/MRI were not widely accessible. After this period, the frequency of biopsies significantly decreased and histological information from pretreatment samples has not been available. Over the past 40 years, most DIPG patients participated in clinical trials without prior genomic profiling of their tumors. Therefore, the reason why these treatments failed is not clear.

Over the years, the lack of tissue samples and biological information on DIPG caused many research groups to explore other ways to collect tissue samples. Among these, autopsy procurement of brain samples began to have a great meaning in the understanding of DIPG. Programs for postmortem specimen donations from research groups throughout the world in a variety of tumors had positive results. The contribution of autopsy tissue donation in DIPG is relatively new and yields promise to facilitate genome-wide studies in this disease.

A variety of research teams have been working in the recent years with postmortem tissue collection and several important publications show a number of potential targets for new treatments [18,32–35]. These studies also revealed that DIPG cannot be considered a single entity, and according to the underlying biology of the tumor, different types of treatment may be needed. Findings from preclinical drug testing conducted on accurate *in vitro* and *in vivo* models of DIPG will provide direction to future clinical trials.

3.2. Preclinical models

In vitro and *in vivo* models of pontine gliomas are helping to guide the understanding of DIPG and key genomic changes that help maintain the tumor's growth and resistance to therapy. Different approaches have been used to generate primary neurosphere cultures and allograft and xenograft mouse models to elucidate the biology of DIPG; however, they are unlikely to provide all the answers. Allograft models mimicking brainstem gliomas have been used to unravel expression signatures and to serve as a platform to test the efficacy of novel therapeutic agents, such as small molecule multi-kinase inhibitors [36,37]. Primary neurosphere cultures and xenograft models from DIPG tissue obtained at autopsy have provided remarkable advances in understanding tumor biology. Some of these include the identification of a cell of origin, methods of effective drug delivery, and identification of potential therapeutic targets [4,38–41]. A pitfall in these models is the exposure of autopsied tissue to chemotherapeutic agents. Therefore, research groups are increasingly focusing on deriving preclinical models from biopsied tissue [42]. Biopsy-derived preclinical models have been utilized for identification of genomic expression profiles and for testing potential therapeutic agents [40,43,44].

Effectively treating cancer in mouse models may not always yield similar results in humans. On the other hand, animal models can represent an alternative for screening of novel agents and combination of drugs, leading to the discovery of the most promising drugs for human

DIPG trials. A recent study identified a FDA-approved epigenetic drug, Panobinostat, to be a leading therapeutic candidate by testing a plethora of promising anticancer drugs in biopsy- and autopsy-derived preclinical models of DIPG [44].

A better knowledge of the genomic aberrations that are considered drivers in DIPG is essential to treat accurate animal models. Research is improving and several studies are focusing on the discovery of these important mutations and agreeing that novel combinations should be tested in genetically and histologically accurate preclinical models prior to their translation to the clinic [5,42]. This collaborative effort will elucidate many of the unanswered questions in DIPGs.

4. Molecular basis of DIPG: major driver mutations

4.1. Histone mutations

Recent studies and advances in DIPG and biopsy specimens available at the time of the diagnosis have permitted researchers to identify the mutations encoding for histones H3.1 (*HIST1H3B* and *HIST1H3C*), H3.2 (*HIST2H3C*), and H3.3 (*H3F3A*)—proteins known for packaging DNA into chromatin. Histone mutations are found in nearly 80% of children with DIPG, and its high frequency strongly suggests its potential as a driver mutation [45,46]. Clear evidence also indicates that the molecular pathogenesis of DIPG is distinct from non-brain-stem HGGs [46].

The *K27M* (lysine replaced by methionine at amino acid 27) or *K27I* (lysine replaced by isoleucine at amino acid 27) mutations result from a gain of function and have the potential to lower overall amounts of wild-type H3 with trimethylated lysine 27 (*H3K27me3*). This results in a loss of methylation at this site. Also, sequestration of the polycomb repressive complex 2 (*PRC2*) further results in overall histone hypomethylation. Normally, the *PRC2* complex represses gene expression through histone methylation. In the absence of *PRC2* complex member *EZH2*, genes that should be silent by methylation are expressed and transcriptionally active, leading to the mechanism of *K27M*/*K27I* tumorigenicity [47].

Studies analyzing the differences between H3.3 and H3.1 subgroups are showing that they can have distinct cells of origin [48]. A distinct genomic expression pattern between these two subgroups, in addition to the higher frequency of H3.1 mutation in a younger age, could imply that H3.3 and H3.1 mutations target distinct progenitors. Another interesting finding is that *PDGFRA* amplification is seen mainly in combination with H3.3 mutation, while *ACVR1* is only seen mainly in combination with mutant H3.1 [18,48].

It is known that the type of histone H3 mutation can predict the prognosis and OS of DIPG patients in a more accurate way than clinical, histological, or radiological characteristics of the tumor [29]. The discovery of the histone mutations and its importance are an incentive to the reintroduction of biopsy at the time of diagnosis, permitting to identify the genomic landscape of the patient and determination of a better treatment plan.

4.2. Partner mutations

Studies have shown that although about 80% DIPGs harbor histone mutation as expected, nearly all H3 mutant DIPGs also harbor partner mutations that vary across patients [23,34,46, 49]. Histone 3 mutations can be seen in combination with a variety of genomic alterations, such as *ACVR1, TP53,* and *PDGFRA* (**Table 1**).

Gene	Alteration	Possible targeted therapy
H3F3A/HIST1H3B and *HIST1H3C*	Mutations	Panobinostat
TP53	Mutations	Sertraline Thioridazine Wee1 inhibitors
ACVR1	Mutations	ALK2 inhibitors
ATRX	Mutations	Cisplatin Fluorouracil Carboplatin Oxaliplatin
PIK3CA/PIK3R1	Mutations	Temsirolimus Metformin everolimus Chlorpromazine Sirolimus
PDGFRA	Amplification	Axitinib Dasatinib Pazopanib Ponatinib Sorafenib Mebendazole Sunitinib
PPM1D	Mutations	Arsenic trioxide

Table 1. Specific mutations and copy number abnormalities and possible target treatments in DIPG.

Recent whole-genome sequencing studies reveal that 20–30% of DIPGs—usually patients less than 5 years old—contain mutations in the *ACVR1* gene, which encodes the type 1 bone morphogenetic protein (BMP) receptor, *ALK2* [18,50,51]. The high percentage of *ACVR1* mutation in DIPG provides strong evidence that it is an oncogenic driver in this cancer. Almost always *ACVR1* mutation occurs in combination with *HIST1H3B K27M,* encoding mutant histone H3.1, which is also associated with a younger age. When a HGG arises early in development and affect infants, usually the prognosis is better and the mutation burden is lower, suggesting that the tumor would be generated with fewer mutations [46,52].

Mutations in *ACVR1* gene activate the *ALK2* receptor, increase phosphorylation of SMAD proteins, and up-regulate genes in BMP developmental signaling pathway. These mutations are also described in patients with fibrodysplasia ossificans progressiva (FOP), although amino acid substitutions that occur in DIPGs have not been found in FOP patients [51]. Because FOP is not associated with cancer predisposition, it is likely that *ACVR1* mutations provide a selective advantage in the presence of other critical partner mutations, rather than driving tumor initiation [52].

Pathways common in a variety of tumor types occur also in DIPG. One example is *TP53* checkpoint, harmed by *TP53* mutations, which occurs in approximately 55% of patients with HGGs and is associated with *H3F3A*, *ATRX*, and *DAXX* mutations [45]. Mutant p53 proteins have an extended half-life and can be detected by immunohistochemistry (IHC) due to their protein accumulation [53]. In 9–23% of DIPGs, there are also mutually exclusive mutations in the *TP53* target gene *PPM1D*, which plays a role downstream of p53 in the DNA damage response [51,54].

Also, the association of p53 abnormalities in the context of *PDGFRA* amplification or *PI3K* mutations raises the possibility that the *PI3K* signaling pathway constitutes a major component of the pathogenesis of DIPG [49]. *PDGFRA* is known to be expressed in malignant gliomas and plays a role during embryonic development, suggesting an embryonic origin for DIPG, given the incidence of this disease in middle childhood [55].

Other important genomic alterations include ATRX, TERT, MYCN, and PTEN. The identification of driver mutations in DIPG helps more than to confirm the diagnosis at a molecular level: it provides relevant clinical and prognostic information, leading to the improvement in the genomic and epigenetic knowledge of DIPG. The combination of different mutations in a singular patient elucidates the fact that DIPG is a complex and varied pathology comprised of different molecular subgroups that share the same clinical features as well as a grim prognosis.

5. Challenges in the treatment: BBB and combinatory mutations

5.1. The blood–brain barrier

The infiltrative nature of DIPG makes effective therapy extremely difficult and characterizes this tumor as one of the most, if not the most challenging childhood cancer. The successful and efficient delivery of effective therapy to the DIPG tumor is the major challenge that contributes to the poor treatment options in children with this disease. For the effectiveness of a therapy, the agent needs to have certain important characteristics: (A) it has to be active and reach its molecular target in the tumor cell in adequate concentrations, (B) it has to reach the target for an adequate amount of time, and (C) the tumor cells need to be sensitive to the compound. Many factors can affect the level of a drug in the brain tumor site, including the concentration of this drug in the bloodstream, amount of protein to tissue binding, and the degree of central nervous system (CNS) penetration [8]. In DIPG, the BBB is often intact and has the ability to restrict the delivery of chemotherapeutic agents. Even for drugs that are capable of crossing the cerebral capillary bed, it is difficult to achieve optimal concentrations due to systemic toxicity.

Strategies have been used to overcome the BBB and to direct those agents to the specific anatomic region or tumor mass, reducing the disturbance of normal neurological functions. Among these strategies are the temporary disruption of the BBB, modification of drugs to enhance their ability to permeate the BBB, and local delivery methods such as the convection-enhanced delivery (CED) to deliver drugs directly into the extracellular space [38,56].

Also known as interstitial infusion, CED is a technique designed to deliver high concentrations of drugs directly into the tumor, allowing intratumoral injection of novel therapeutic agents. The use of hydrostatic pressure allows the distribution of a homogeneous concentration of molecules over large distances by displacing extracellular fluid with the infusate. Several clinical trials in patients with neurodegenerative disorders and malignant gliomas have been done with the use of CED, including ongoing phase I/II clinical trials in DIPG, and published studies have shown CED in DIPG to be feasible and safe [57–60]. The use of CED into murine brainstem had been well tolerated by mice with and without brainstem tumors, increasing median survival in preclinical models [38]. However, it is necessary to develop novel therapeutic agents for delivery via CED and also to improve the technique of CED in order to provide a better outcome and a new hope of treatment for children with DIPG.

5.2. Combinatory mutations

Novel genome-wide studies and increasing availability of tumor tissue, from autopsy and surgical biopsy samples, show that each individual tumor harbors multiple mutations, as well as copy number abnormalities, gene expression, and methylation patterns. While there are several ongoing clinical trials using target therapies, targeting only specific mutations in a patient has rarely been effective. Studies are showing that using chemotherapy alone or in combination with RT does not lead to any additional survival benefit [8,10,11].

In this context, multi-targeting combinatory regimens are the new promise for DIPG. Considering that DIPG is not a single disease and that HGGs harbor distinct genomic aberrations compared to adult glioblastomas, the heterogeneity of DIPG can be correlated with age of onset and the range of genomic mutations particular to each subtype. It is also believed that DIPG heterogeneity partially accounts for its resistance to current targeted therapies.

The main challenge is to combine different molecularly targeted chemotherapeutics that in a mutual mechanism of action would target the distinct driver mutations of each patient. For this purpose, it is essential to deeply investigate the mechanism of action of these drugs, as well as the pathway of each mutation found in DIPG. Preclinical studies conducted *in vitro* and *in vivo* are crucial to gain a perspective of what can be done in the clinic. Also, it is necessary to discover proper drug concentrations, study the ability of the agent to overcome the BBB, and minimize the possible adverse effects.

Hopefully, a better understanding of the molecular landscape of DIPG patients will lead to the use of combinatory therapy not only in preclinical models but also in clinical trials, aiming for an optimal personalized drug combination that can be used in children with DIPG.

5.3. Clinical trials

Clinical trials are the best way to evaluate treatment for DIPG and to test if the therapeutic agents are effective or not. While determining the origin of DIPG is important, it is also essential to evaluate new drug targets, biological agents, and immunotherapeutic strategies in clinical trials to determine if they can be used in the clinic. Numerous molecularly targeted chemotherapeutic agents have been tested in the past year with and without RT (**Table 2**).

Title	**Clinical trial ID**	**Chemotherapy**	**Radiotherapy**
Study of suberoylanilide hydroxamic acid (SAHA) with temsirolimus in children with DIPG	NCT0242061	Vorinostat; temsirolimus	Single daily fractions of 1.8 Gy for 30 treatments over 6–7 weeks. Total dose of radiation 54 Gy
Intra-arterial chemotherapy for the treatment of progressive DIPGs	NCT01688401	Melphalan hydrochloride intra-arterially	No
Study of the combination of crizotinib and dasatinib in pediatric research participants with DIPG and HGG	NCT01644773	Crizotinib; dasatinib	No
Biological medicine for DIPG eradication (BIOMEDE)	NCT02233049	Erlotinib; dasatinib; everolimus	No
Lenalidomide and radiation therapy in HGGs or DIPGs	NCT01222754	Lenalidomide	Five days per week to a prescription dose of 54–59.4 Gy
Molecular profiling for individualized treatment plan for DIPG	NCT02274987	Individualized treatment plan for each patient and different approaches depending on the molecular profile of the patient's tumor (specialized tumor board recommendations)	Standard radiation therapy followed by molecular based therapy with FDA-approved drugs
Anti PD1 antibody in DIPG	NCT01952769	MDV9300 (pidilizumab); cyclophosphamide	Yes
A phase I study of mebendazole for the treatment of pediatric gliomas	NCT01837862	Mebendazole; bevacizumab; irinotecan	No

Title	Clinical trial ID	Chemotherapy	Radiotherapy
DIPG reirradiation (ReRT)	NCT01469247	No	Starting dose 24 Gy in 2 Gy fractions
Safety and efficacy of cabazitaxel in pediatric patients with refractory solid tumors including central nervous system tumors	NCT01751308	Cabazitaxel (XRP6258)	No
WEE1 inhibitor MK-1775 and local radiation therapy in treating younger patients with newly diagnosed DIPGs	NCT01922076	WEE1 inhibitor AZD1775	Yes. Five days a week for 6 weeks (up to 30 fractions)
Convection-enhanced delivery of 124I-8H9 for patients with non-progressive diffuse pontine gliomas previously treated with external beam radiation therapy	NCT01502917	No	Radioactive iodine-labeled monoclonal antibody 8H9
Valproic acid and radiation followed by maintenance valproic acid and bevacizumab in children with HGGs or DIPG	NCT00879437	Valproic acid; bevacizumab	Total dose of between 54.0 and 59.4 Gy in 30–33 fractions over 6–7 weeks
Erivedge (vismodegib) in the treatment of pediatric patients with refractory pontine glioma	NCT01774253	Erivedge (vismodegib)	No

Table 2. Clinical trials conducted for patients with DIPG in 2015.

Although clinical trials are a big hope in finding a treatment that could lead to a better prognosis, it also has its own challenges—not all the patients qualify for participation; the families have a crucial responsibility in the decision to participate or not; the length of time to complete a trial can be long, given the rarity of this cancer; and finally, there are strict guidelines that need to be followed in order to guarantee the patient safety and minimize the risk.

Every time that a clinical trial is formulated, it has great potential, but not a guarantee of benefit. However, it is important to recall the example of so many other pediatric cancers, such as leukemia, lymphoma, and Wilms' tumor, which obtained their success in treatment because of the persistence of the researchers and physicians in clinical trials.

The biggest hope is that in the future, patients can be divided into subgroups according to their genetic, epigenetic, and proteomic molecular particularities through a biopsy of their tumor. This way, targeted therapy could be individualized—however, the only way to achieve this goal is through improvement of research and investment in more clinical trials.

5.4. What to expect?

Although DIPG still remains a lethal cancer with an abysmal prognosis, scientists and physicians have for the first time the appropriate tools and knowledge to change the outcome of this disease in children affected with DIPG. The new generation of DIPG clinical trials will focus on new studies of the molecular landscape diversity of children affected with this cancer and will aim to assess the tumor, identify tumor targets, select appropriate agents, and determine the adequate dosing for a treatment selection.

Finally, it is also crucial that the collaborative efforts in this disease continue, given the small number of patients and the difficulty to obtain tumor tissue. The historical tragedy of DIPG should not discourage researchers and physicians from continuing forward. The recent data show improved knowledge that we never previously had about this devastating childhood cancer—and this improvement is a substantial step in opening novel avenues for promising approaches.

Acknowledgements

The authors would like to thank the following funding institutions: the Smashing Walnuts Foundation, the Musella Foundation, Goldwin Foundation, CTSI UL1TR000075 and KL2TR000076 from the NIH National Center for Advancing Translational Sciences, Lilabean Foundation, Kisses for Kayla Foundation, Matthew Larson Foundation, and Kaminsky Foundation.

Author details

Heloisa H. Moser[1*], Eshini Panditharatna[1,2*], Roger J. Packer[3*] and Javad Nazarian[1,4*]

*Address all correspondence to: HMoser@childrensnational.org, EPanditharatna@childrensnational.org, RPacker@childrensnational.org, and JNazarian@childrensnational.org

1 Center for Genetic Medicine Research, Children's National Health System, Washington, DC, USA

2 Institute for Biomedical Sciences, George Washington University School of Medicine and Health Sciences, Washington, DC, USA

3 Brain Tumor Institute, Center for Neuroscience and Behavioral Medicine, Children's National Health System, Washington, DC, USA

4 Department of Integrative Systems Biology, George Washington University School of Medicine and Health Sciences, Washington, DC, USA

References

[1] Gilbertson RJ, Gutmann DH. Tumorigenesis in the brain: location, location, location. Cancer Res. 2007;67(12):5579–82. Epub 2007/06/19.

[2] Calabrese C, Poppleton H, Kocak M, Hogg TL, Fuller C, Hamner B, et al. A perivascular niche for brain tumor stem cells. Cancer Cell. 2007;11(1):69–82. Epub 2007/01/16.

[3] Gilbertson RJ, Rich JN. Making a tumour's bed: glioblastoma stem cells and the vascular niche. Nat Rev Cancer. 2007;7(10):733–6. Epub 2007/09/21.

[4] Monje M, Mitra SS, Freret ME, Raveh TB, Kim J, Masek M, et al. Hedgehog-responsive candidate cell of origin for diffuse intrinsic pontine glioma. Proceedings of the National Academy of Sciences of the United States of America. 2011;108(11):4453–8. Epub 2011/03/04.

[5] Becher OJ, Hambardzumyan D, Walker TR, Helmy K, Nazarian J, Albrecht S, et al. Preclinical evaluation of radiation and perifosine in a genetically and histologically accurate model of brainstem glioma. Cancer Res. 2010;70(6):2548–57. Epub 2010/03/04.

[6] Goodrich LV, Milenković L, Higgins KM, Scott MP. Altered neural cell fates and medulloblastoma in mouse patched mutants. Science. 1997;277(5329):1109–13.

[7] CBTRUS (2010). CBTRUS Statistical Report: Primary Brain and Central Nervous System Tumors Diagnosed in the United States in 2004-2006. Source: Central Brain Tumor Registry of the United States (CBTRUS), Hinsdale, IL. website: www.cbtrus.org.

[8] Warren KE. Diffuse intrinsic pontine glioma: poised for progress. Front Oncol. 2012;2:205. Epub 2013/01/08.

[9] Janssens GORJ, Gidding CEM, Van Lindert EJ, Oldenburger FR, Erasmus CE, Schouten-Meeteren AYN, et al. The role of hypofractionation radiotherapy for diffuse intrinsic brainstem glioma in children: a pilot study. Int J Radiat Oncol Biol Phys.73(3): 722–6.

[10] Kebudi R, Cakir F. Management of diffuse pontine gliomas in children: recent developments. Pediatr Drugs. 2013;15(5):351–62.

[11] Bailey S, Howman A, Wheatley K, Wherton D, Boota N, Pizer B, et al. Diffuse intrinsic pontine glioma treated with prolonged temozolomide and radiotherapy—results of a United Kingdom phase II trial (CNS 2007 04). Eur J Cancer. 2013;49(18):3856–62. Epub 2013/09/10.

[12] Buczkowicz P, Hawkins C. Pathology, molecular genetics and epigenetics of diffuse intrinsic pontine glioma. Front Oncol. 2015;5(147):1–9.

[13] Albright AL, Packer RJ, Zimmerman R, Rorke LB, Boyett J, Hammond GD. Magnetic resonance scans should replace biopsies for the diagnosis of diffuse brain stem gliomas:

a report from the Children's Cancer Group. Neurosurgery. 1993;33(6):1026–9; discussion 9-30. Epub 1993/12/01.

[14] Puget S, Blauwblomme T, Grill J. Is biopsy safe in children with newly diagnosed diffuse intrinsic pontine glioma? American Society of Clinical Oncology educational book/ASCO American Society of Clinical Oncology Meeting. 2012:629–33. Epub 2012/01/01.

[15] Saratsis AM, Kambhampati M, Snyder K, Yadavilli S, Devaney JM, Harmon B, et al. Comparative multidimensional molecular analyses of pediatric diffuse intrinsic pontine glioma reveals distinct molecular subtypes. Acta Neuropathol. 2014;127(6): 881–95. Epub 2013/12/04.

[16] Panditharatna E, Yaeger K, Kilburn LB, Packer RJ, Nazarian J. Clinicopathology of diffuse intrinsic pontine glioma and its redefined genomic and epigenomic landscape. Cancer Genet. 2015;208(7):367–73.

[17] Khuong-Quang DA, Buczkowicz P, Rakopoulos P, Liu XY, Fontebasso AM, Bouffet E, et al. K27M mutation in histone H3.3 defines clinically and biologically distinct subgroups of pediatric diffuse intrinsic pontine gliomas. Acta Neuropathol. 2012;124(3):439–47. Epub 2012/06/05.

[18] Buczkowicz P, Hoeman C, Rakopoulos P, Pajovic S, Letourneau L, Dzamba M, et al. Genomic analysis of diffuse intrinsic pontine gliomas identifies three molecular subgroups and recurrent activating ACVR1 mutations. Nat Genet. 2014;46(5):451–6. Epub 2014/04/08.

[19] Fisher PG, Breiter SN, Carson BS, Wharam MD, Williams JA, Weingart JD, et al. A clinicopathologic reappraisal of brain stem tumor classification. Identification of pilocystic astrocytoma and fibrillary astrocytoma as distinct entities. Cancer. 2000;89(7): 1569–76.

[20] Schroeder KM, Hoeman CM, Becher OJ. Children are not just little adults: recent advances in understanding of diffuse intrinsic pontine glioma biology. Pediatr Res. 2014;75(1–2):205–9.

[21] Soler D, Borzyskowski M. Lower urinary tract dysfunction in children with central nervous system tumours. Arch Dis Child. 1998;79(4):344–7.

[22] Robison NJ, Kieran MW. Diffuse intrinsic pontine glioma: a reassessment. J Neurooncol. 2014;119(1):7–15.

[23] Hoffman LM, DeWire M, Ryall S, Buczkowicz P, Leach J, Miles L, et al. Spatial genomic heterogeneity in diffuse intrinsic pontine and midline high-grade glioma: implications for diagnostic biopsy and targeted therapeutics. Acta Neuropathol Commun. 2016;4:1.

[24] Choux M, Lena G, Do L. Brainstem tumors. In: Choux M, Di Rocco C, Hockley A, editor. Pediatric Neurosurgery. New York, NY: Churchill Livingstone; 2000. p. 471–91.

[25] Hargrave D, Bartels U, Bouffet E. Diffuse brainstem glioma in children: critical review of clinical trials. Lancet Oncol. 2006;7(3):241–8. Epub 2006/03/03.

[26] Vanan MI, Eisenstat DD. DIPG in children—what can we learn from the past? Front Oncol. 2015;5:237.

[27] Sufit A, Donson AM, Birks DK, Knipstein JA, Fenton LZ, Jedlicka P, et al. Diffuse intrinsic pontine tumors: a study of primitive neuroectodermal tumors versus the more common diffuse intrinsic pontine gliomas. J Neurosurg Pediatr. 2012;10(2):81–8. Epub 2012/07/04.

[28] Martin Schumacher, Jürgen Schulte-Mönting, Peter Stoeter, Monika Warmuth-Metz, Laszlo Solymosi. Magnetic resonance imaging compared with biopsy in the diagnosis of brainstem diseases of childhood: a multicenter review. J Neurosurg Pediatr. 2007;106(2):111–9.

[29] Buczkowicz P, Bartels U, Bouffet E, Becher O, Hawkins C. Histopathological spectrum of paediatric diffuse intrinsic pontine glioma: diagnostic and therapeutic implications. Acta Neuropathol. 2014;128(4):573–81. Epub 2014/07/23.

[30] Caretti V, Bugiani M, Freret M, Schellen P, Jansen M, van Vuurden D, et al. Subventricular spread of diffuse intrinsic pontine glioma. Acta Neuropathol. 2014;128(4):605–7.

[31] Roujeau T, Machado G, Garnett MR, Miquel C, Puget S, Geoerger B, et al. Stereotactic biopsy of diffuse pontine lesions in children. J Neurosurg Pediatr. 2007;107(1):1–4.

[32] Broniscer A, Baker JN, Baker SJ, Chi SN, Geyer JR, Morris EB, et al. Prospective collection of tissue samples at autopsy in children with diffuse intrinsic pontine glioma. Cancer. 2010;116(19):4632–7. Epub 2010/07/01.

[33] Paugh BS, Broniscer A, Qu C, Miller CP, Zhang J, Tatevossian RG, et al. Genome-wide analyses identify recurrent amplifications of receptor tyrosine kinases and cell-cycle regulatory genes in diffuse intrinsic pontine glioma. J Clin Oncol. 2011;29(30):3999–4006. Epub 2011/09/21.

[34] Zarghooni M, Bartels U, Lee E, Buczkowicz P, Morrison A, Huang A, et al. Whole-genome profiling of pediatric diffuse intrinsic pontine gliomas highlights platelet-derived growth factor receptor alpha and poly (ADP-ribose) polymerase as potential therapeutic targets. J Clin Oncol. 2010;28(8):1337–44. Epub 2010/02/10.

[35] Kambhampati M, Perez JP, Yadavilli S, Saratsis AM, Hill AD, Ho CY, et al. A standardized autopsy procurement allows for the comprehensive study of DIPG biology. Oncotarget. 2015;6(14):12740–7. Epub 2015/03/10.

[36] Misuraca KL, Barton KL, Chung A, Diaz AK, Conway SJ, Corcoran DL, et al. Pax3 expression enhances PDGF-B-induced brainstem gliomagenesis and characterizes a subset of brainstem glioma. Acta Neuropathol Commun. 2014;2(1):134. Epub 2014/10/22.

[37] Halvorson KG, Barton KL, Schroeder K, Misuraca KL, Hoeman C, Chung A, et al. A high-throughput in vitro drug screen in a genetically engineered mouse model of diffuse intrinsic pontine glioma identifies BMS-754807 as a promising therapeutic agent. PLoS One. 2015;10(3):e0118926.

[38] Sewing ACP, Caretti V, Lagerweij T, Schellen P, Jansen MHA, van Vuurden DG, et al. Convection enhanced delivery of carmustine to the murine brainstem: a feasibility study. J Neurosci Methods 2014;238:88–94.

[39] Yadavilli S, Scafidi J, Becher OJ, Saratsis AM, Hiner RL, Kambhampati M, et al. The emerging role of NG2 in pediatric diffuse intrinsic pontine glioma. Oncotarget. 2015;6(14):12141–55. Epub 2015/05/20.

[40] Mueller S, Hashizume R, Yang X, Kolkowitz I, Olow AK, Phillips J, et al. Targeting Wee1 for the treatment of pediatric high-grade gliomas. Neuro Oncol. 2014;16(3):352–60.

[41] Caretti V, Hiddingh L, Lagerweij T, Schellen P, Koken PW, Hulleman E, et al. WEE1 kinase inhibition enhances the radiation response of diffuse intrinsic pontine gliomas. Mol Cancer Ther. 2013;12(2):141–50.

[42] Hashizume R, Smirnov I, Liu S, Phillips JJ, Hyer J, McKnight TR, et al. Characterization of a diffuse intrinsic pontine glioma cell line: implications for future investigations and treatment. J Neurooncol. 2012;110(3):305–13. Epub 2012/09/18.

[43] Chan KM, Fang D, Gan H, Hashizume R, Yu C, Schroeder M, et al. The histone H3.3K27M mutation in pediatric glioma reprograms H3K27 methylation and gene expression. Genes Dev. 2013;27(9):985–90. Epub 2013/04/23.

[44] Grasso CS, Tang Y, Truffaux N, Berlow NE, Liu L, Debily M-A, et al. Functionally defined therapeutic targets in diffuse intrinsic pontine glioma. Nat Med. 2015;21(6): 555–9.

[45] Schwartzentruber J, Korshunov A, Liu XY, Jones DT, Pfaff E, Jacob K, et al. Driver mutations in histone H3.3 and chromatin remodelling genes in paediatric glioblastoma. Nature. 2012;482(7384):226–31. Epub 2012/01/31.

[46] Wu G, Broniscer A, McEachron TA, Lu C, Paugh BS, Becksfort J, et al. Somatic histone H3 alterations in pediatric diffuse intrinsic pontine gliomas and non-brainstem glioblastomas. Nat Genet. 2012;44(3):251–3. Epub 2012/01/31.

[47] Lewis PW, Müller MM, Koletsky MS, Cordero F, Lin S, Banaszynski LA, et al. Inhibition of PRC2 activity by a gain-of-function H3 mutation found in pediatric glioblastoma. Science (New York, NY). 2013;340(6134):857–61.

[48] Castel D, Philippe C, Calmon R, Le Dret L, Truffaux N, Boddaert N, et al. Histone H3F3A and HIST1H3B K27M mutations define two subgroups of diffuse intrinsic pontine gliomas with different prognosis and phenotypes. Acta Neuropathol. 2015;130(6):815–27.

[49] Grill J, Puget S, Andreiuolo F, Philippe C, MacConaill L, Kieran MW. Critical oncogenic mutations in newly diagnosed pediatric diffuse intrinsic pontine glioma. Pediatric Blood Cancer. 2012;58(4):489–91. Epub 2011/12/23.

[50] Fontebasso AM, Papillon-Cavanagh S, Schwartzentruber J, Nikbakht H, Gerges N, Fiset PO, et al. Recurrent somatic mutations in ACVR1 in pediatric midline high-grade astrocytoma. Nat Genet. 2014;46(5):462–6. Epub 2014/04/08.

[51] Taylor KR, Mackay A, Truffaux N, Butterfield YS, Morozova O, Philippe C, et al. Recurrent activating ACVR1 mutations in diffuse intrinsic pontine glioma. Nat Genet. 2014;46(5):457–61. Epub 2014/04/08.

[52] Wu G, Diaz AK, Paugh BS, Rankin SL, Ju B, Li Y, et al. The genomic landscape of diffuse intrinsic pontine glioma and pediatric non-brainstem high-grade glioma. Nat Genet. 2014;46(5):444–50. Epub 2014/04/08.

[53] Badhe PB, Chauhan PP, Mehta NK. Brainstem gliomas—a clinicopathological study of 45 cases with p53 immunohistochemistry. Indian J Cancer. 2004;41(4):170–4. Epub 2005/01/22.

[54] Zhang L, Chen LH, Wan H, Yang R, Wang Z, Feng J, et al. Exome sequencing identifies somatic gain-of-function PPM1D mutations in brainstem gliomas. Nat Genet. 2014;46(7):726–30. Epub 2014/06/02.

[55] Chojnacki A, Weiss S. Production of neurons, astrocytes and oligodendrocytes from mammalian CNS stem cells. Nat Protocols. 2008;3(6):935–40.

[56] Bredlau AL, Dixit S, Chen C, Broome AM. Nanotechnology applications for diffuse intrinsic pontine glioma. Curr Neuropharmacol. 2016;[Epub ahead of print]. Epub Feb 23. Volume 14:1–1.

[57] Murad GJA, Walbridge S, Morrison P.F., Szerlip N, Butman JA, Oldfield E.H., et al. Image-guided convection-enhanced delivery of gemcitabine to the brainstem. J Neurosurg. 2007;106(2):351–6.

[58] Anderson RCE, Kennedy B, Yanes CL, Garvin J, Needle M, Canoll P, et al. Convection-enhanced delivery of topotecan into diffuse intrinsic brainstem tumors in children. J Neurosurg Pediatr. 2013;11(3):289–95.

[59] Barua NU, Lowis SP, Woolley M, O'Sullivan S, Harrison R, Gill SS. Robot-guided convection-enhanced delivery of carboplatin for advanced brainstem glioma. Acta Neurochir (Wien). 2013;155(8):1459–65.

[60] Saito R, Sonoda Y, Kumabe T, Nagamatsu K, Watanabe M, Tominaga T. Regression of recurrent glioblastoma infiltrating the brainstem after convection-enhanced delivery of nimustine hydrochloride. J Neurosurg Pediatr. 2011;7(5):522–6.

Chapter 18

Minimally Invasive Surgery for Treatment of Patients with Advanced Cancer and Thoraco-lumbar Spine Metastases

Massimo Miscusi, Stefano Forcato and
Antonino Raco

Additional information is available at the end of the chapter

http://dx.doi.org/10.5772/63125

Abstract

Spinal metastases are common in patients with cancer. Spinal cord compression is the initial symptom of 5–10% of patients with diffuse cancer, and about 70% of lesions are found in the thoracic vertebrae. Patients with advanced cancer are generally excluded from major spine surgery, to reduce postoperative morbidity and mortality. Minimally invasive spine surgery (MISS) has recently been advocated as a useful approach for spinal metastases, especially in advanced cancer patients, seeking to decrease the morbidity of more traditional open spine surgery; furthermore, reducing the recovery time, MISS permits the post-operative chemotherapy and radiotherapy to begin sooner.

A series of 29 cancer patients, with a short life expectancy, presenting acute myelopathy due to vertebral thoracic metastases, underwent MISS, with simple laminotomy and percutaneous stabilization; results from such series were compared to those retrospectively obtained from an homogenous series of patients operated with traditional open surgery.

No significant differences between two groups were demonstrated in terms of surgical complications and neurological recovery. Nevertheless, patients operated with MISS appear to have an earlier recovery and better quality of life in the immediate post-operative period, which is a fundamental aim for patients who have a short life expectancy.

Keywords: minimally invasive spine surgery, cancer, thoracic metastases, myelopathy, quality of life

1. Introduction

Spinal cord involvement due to vertebral metastases is a frequent complication in cancer patients and metastatic lesions of spine can significantly condition their quality of life, potentially producing untreatable pain, vertebral fractures, or even neurological deficit due to spinal cord or radicular involvement [1, 2]. Spinal metastases are likely to increase their incidence because patients with cancer today can live longer, due to early detection, as well as to improvements in cancer treatment and care [3]. These lesions should be considered and treated both medically or surgically to prevent undesired sequelae, and to preserve or, whenever possible, improve the quality of their residual life [4, 5].

The spine is the third most common site for cancer cells to metastasize, following the lungs and the liver. Almost 70% of cancer patients are expected to have spinal metastasis. In case of symptomatic lesions, the majority (60–70%) are found in the thoracic region, while of the remainder, 20% are found in the lumbar region, and 10% are found in the cervical spine. More than 50% of patients with spinal metastasis have more than one level involved [6, 7].

Surgery of spinal metastases cannot be curative, but only palliative, aimed to preserve or, whenever possible, improve quality of life for patients with short- or mid-term life expectancy. In such cases, surgery is indicated for the stabilization of involved segments, for spinal cord or root decompression, and for tissue diagnosis.

In the optic of reducing post-operative morbidity and accelerate the post-operative recovery, minimally invasive spine surgery (MISS) may represent the best option to achieve equivalent or superior outcomes to those of traditional open spine surgery, and to reduce the impact of surgery on critical patients with poor general and neurological conditions with short- or mid-term life expectancy.

2. Patients with advanced cancer and thoraco-lumbar spine metastases

2.1. Management and surgical indication

The evaluation of clinical general and neurological conditions of patients with advanced cancer and spinal metastases is performed with the Karnowsky performance scale (KPS) and the American Spinal Injury Association (ASIA) scores. Total spine MRI and total body CT scan is mandatory in order to update the stadium of the disease and to planning the most correct treatment.

Approximately 90% of cancer patients with spinal metastases have bone and/or back pain, followed by radicular pain. Half of these patients have sensory and motor dysfunction, and more than half have bowel and bladder dysfunction. Five to 10% of cancer patients present with cord compression as their initial symptom; among these, 50% are non-ambulatory at diagnosis, and 15% are paraplegic [8].

The initial functional neurological score, evaluated with ASIA score, is the most important prognostic factor for the neurological recovery of patients undergoing surgery. Surgery, in the majority of spinal metastasis cases, does not have a curative aim, but only palliative, to assure stability, pain control, and maintenance of neurologic integrity [3]. Surgery is also important to confirm the primary diagnosis, to debulk or remove the tumor mass for a more effective adjuvant therapy, and permit a patient's mobilization.

The main indications for surgery in case of spinal metastases are the progressive neurologic deficit before, during, or after chemo- and radiotherapy, the intractable pain unresponsive to conservative treatment, the need for histological diagnosis, the treatment of radio-resistant tumor histology (e.g., RCC, melanoma), and to restore the spinal stability.

Numerous grading systems has been proposed, like the modified Bauer Scoring System (mBS), in order to give an indication to a conservative, palliative or more aggressive surgical treatment to a metastatic spine disease. The modified Bauer classification results equal or inferior then 3 points in case of patients with short- or mid-term life expectancy (**Figure 1**).

Modified Bauer Scoring System	
Points	**Positive prognostic factors**
1	no visceral metastases
1	no lung cancer
1	primary tumour = breast, kidney, lymphoma, multiple myeloma
1	one solitary skeletal metastasis

Prognostic Score	Treatment Goal	Surgical Strategy
0-1	Supportive care	no surgery
2	short term palliation	dorsal
3-4	middle term local control	ventral-dorsal

Figure 1. Modified Bauer Scoring System and the prognostic score.

To improve outcomes for patients with metastatic spine disease, many aggressive surgical strategies have been proposed. Nevertheless, an aggressive strategy is frequently associated with high morbidity and complication rates, and is not generally indicated in patients with poor general conditions and a limited life expectancy [9, 10].

These patients, in fact, often suffer from co-morbidities, malnourishment, diminished immunity, considerable pain, and they cannot face major surgery. Thus extensive surgical procedures or prolonged hospital stays are neither acceptable nor feasible in many of such patients.

Therefore, surgical risks must be weighed against life expectancy and quality of life, in order to justify standard surgical interventions.

2.2. The role of MISS

Recent advances in surgical techniques and percutaneous instrument placement have led to the development of minimally invasive approaches for the treatment of spinal metastases; these result in less post-operative pain, shorter overall hospital stays, less intra-operative blood loss, and an earlier start of adjuvant therapy [2, 11–14].

The reported advantages of these techniques include smaller incisions, which limit wound complications, and the avoidance of back muscles detachment and retraction that causes post-operative pain and profuse bleeding, thus, reducing the need of intra or post-operative blood transfusion. These advantages are crucial for maintaining and improving the quality of life of cancer patients with short- or mid-term life expectancy [15–17].

MISS technique has the aim to perform (1) percutaneous insertion of pedicle screws and rods; (2) small exposure and detachment of the para-spinal muscles, to avoid their denervation and devascularization; (3) a mini-open midline approach to decompress the spinal cord, reducing bleeding and post-operative pain.

Standard open techniques require the full exposure of the posterior elements of the involved segments, with complete exposure of facet joints, thus resulting in much more aggressive damage to the back muscles and soft tissues.

Our procedure is first based on the placement of purely percutaneous pedicle screws; using a double x-ray arch, a four-handed surgery was performed, in order to reduce the operation time and minimize the radiation exposure.

A mini-open median posterior approach to expose only spinous process and laminae of the involved segments is then performed. A laminotomy, without the removal of the spinous process, just in case it was not infiltrated, is performed; the posterior joints are not exposed and removed to reduce the muscle detachment and retraction (which produces an excessive bleeding).

The advantage of MISS techniques, in achieving an early better quality of life, seems to be related to their ability to reduce post-operative pain for both surgical-related and spinal metastasis-related components.

Criticism remains, regarding the reported difficulty of MISS to decompress enough spinal cord in case of spinal canal invasion; this persuasion is due to the erroneous conviction that the larger the surgical exposure, the better results achieved. On the contrary, in fact, MISS techniques permit an easy access to the spinal canal and complete spinal cord decompression and roots if needed.

2.3. Comparative study to traditional open surgery—materials and methods

Two series of cancer patients, with a mBS 1 or 2, presenting acute myelopathy due to vertebral thoracic metastases have been compared. The first group were composed of patients prospectively enrolled from May 2010 to December 2013 and treated with MISS procedures (MISS) (n=29); the second group was composed of retrospectively collected patients treated

http://dx.doi.org/10.5772/63125

with a traditional open surgery (OS) (n=25). Patients with complete neurological deficit (ASIA A) for more than 24 hours and a mBS >2 were excluded from present study.

For both groups (n = 48, 32 women and 16 men, with a mean age of 54.6 yrs), the primitive tumors were: lung cancer (n = 17, 35.4%), breast cancer (n = 15, 31.2%), myeloma (n = 4, 8.3%), clear cell renal carcinoma (n = 3, 6.2%), melanoma (n = 3, 6.2%), prostate cancer (n = 2, 4%), ovarian cancer (n = 1, 2%), and thyroid cancer (n = 1, 2%) (**Table 1**).

Group	OPEN	MISS	Total	p value
Demographic data				
Patients	19	29	48	
Sex ratio (M/F)	7:12	9:20	16:32	
Mean Age	51.74	57.60	54.65	
Clinical data				
Karnowsky	57.89%	55.36%	56.09%	0.94
Modified Bauer	2.6	2.3	2.4	0.135
Spinal metastases				
Single level	14 (73.6%)	18 (62.0%)	32 (66.6%)	
Two or more level	5 (26.3%)	11 (37.9%)	16 (33.3%)	
One column	10 (52.6%)	9 (31.0%)	19 (39.5%)	
Two or more column	9 (47.4%)	20 (68.9%)	29 (60.4%)	
Primary cancer				
Lung	8 (42%)	9 (31.0%)	17 (35.4%)	
Breast	6 (31.6%)	9 (31.0%)	15 (31.2%)	
Mieloma		4 (17.4%)	4 (8.3%)	
Kidney	2 (10.5%)	3 (10.3%)	3 (6.2%)	
Melanoma		3 (10.3%)	3 (6.2%)	
Prostate	2 (10.5%)		2 (4%)	
Ovary	1 (5.3%)		1 (2.0%)	
Thyroid		1 (3.4%)	1 (2.0%)	

Table 1. The clinical and oncological data of all the patients and divided by group.

Thirty two patients had one single level involved (66.6%), while 16 patients had a diseases extended to two or more segments (33.3%). In 19 patients (39.5%), the fracture involved a single column (OS: 52.6%, MISS: 31.0%), while two or three columns were substituted by cancer in 60.4% (**Table 1**).

The two groups were homogeneous, in terms of general and neurological conditions. All patients preoperatively presented an overall mean KPS of 56%, with 57.89 and 55.36% in the OS and MISS groups, respectively (p = 0.9); the mean overall mBS was 2.4 (2.6 and 2.3 in the OS and MISS group, respectively, p = 0.18) (**Table 1**). Pre- and post-operative ASIA scores for both groups are reported in **Table 2**.

	Group	OPEN	MISS	Total	P value
ASIA					
Pre-op					
	A	3	3	6	
	B	2	4	6	
	C	6	9	15	
	D	8	13	21	
	E	0	0	0	
Post-op					
	Improved	12 (63%)	18 (62.0%)	30 (62.5%)	
	Stable	6 (31%)	9 (31.0%)	15 (31.2%)	
	Worse	1 (5%)	2 (6.7%)	3 (6.2%)	
P value				0.001	0.54
EORTC					
QLQ-C30					
QoL					
	Pre-op	16.00%	16.90%	16.60%	
	Post-op	25.80%	32.10%	28.90%	
P value				0.01	
Functional scales					
	Pre-op	59.10%	55.10%	57.10%	
	Post-op	72.60%	70.90%	71.70%	
P value				0.04	
Symptom scales					
	Pre-op	33.00%	34.10%	33.50%	
	Post-op	15.80%	15.10%	15.40%	
P value				0.009	
QLQ-BM22					
	Functional scales b				
	Pre-op	75.15%	72.90%	74.00%	
	Post-op	79.80%	85.10%	82.45%	
P value				0.025	
	Symptom scales b				

http://dx.doi.org/10.5772/63125

	Group	OPEN	MISS	Total	P value
	Pre-op	16.65%	18.10%	17.37%	
	Post-op	8.20%	5.90%	7.05%	
P value				0.001	

Table 2. The pre-operative and post-operative neurological data (ASIA) and the quality of life data (EORTC QLQ-C30 and QLQ-BM22) of all the patients and divided by group.

The pre-operative neurological assessment showed a prevalence of ASIA D in both groups.

2.4. Comparative study to traditional open surgery—results

Thirty patients (62.5%) showed an improvement of neurological status, while 15 patients were stable (31.2%), and only 3 patients (6.2%) worsened. No statistically significant differences in terms of neurological improvement were demonstrated between the two groups ($p = 0.54$). The neurological conditions for only three patients (7.1%) (1 from the OS group, and 2 from the MISS group) worsened; these results were not due to surgical-related complications, but to bad general conditions.

Surgical and hospitalization data are given in **Table 3**.

Group	OPEN	MISS	
Surgery data			
Operative time	3.2 h (2.5–4.5 h)	2.1 h (1.5–3 h)	
Blood loss	900 ml (350–1500 ml)	140 ml (50–250 ml)	
Hospitalization			
Blood supply	12 pts	0 pt	
Complication	0 pt	1 pt	
Post-op bed-rest	4 d (2–10 d)	2 d (1–3 d)	
Discharge	9.25 d (5–14 d)	7.3 d (4–9 d)	
Death	1 pt	0 pts	
			P value < 0.01

Table 3. Surgical and hospitalization data divided by group.

There were no serious peri-operative complications, in the MISS group; only one patient developed a post-operative urinary infection. In the OS group, 1 patient died on the 14th post-operative day, due to metastatic hepatic failure. The mean operation length was 3.2 h and 2.1 h respectively in the OS group and in the MISS group ($p < 0.01$).

The mean intra-operative blood loss was 900 mL in the OS group and 140 mL in the MISS group ($p < 0.01$). Twelve patients in the OS group required post-operative RBC transfusions, while no one in the MISS group required additional blood supply. The mean post-operative bed-rest time was 4 days with a mean length of hospitalization of 9.25 days in the OS group, while the mean post-operative bed-rest time was 2 days with a mean length of hospitalization of 7.3 days in the MISS group ($p < 0.01$).

Pre-operative scoring for quality of life (QoL) was homogeneous in both groups, according to the EORTC QLQ-C30 and EORTC QLQ-BM22 scales (**Table 2**). At follow-up, the analysis of EORTC QLQ-C30 questionnaire showed a mean overall improvement of 12.3% in QoL score (OS: 9.8%, MISS: 15.2%, $p = 0.01$), 14.6% in the functional scale score (OS: 13.5%, MISS: 15.8%, $p = 0.04$), and 18.1% for the symptoms scale score (OS: 17.2%, MISS 19%, $p = 0.009$). The evaluation of QLQ-BM22 scale showed a mean overall improvement at follow-up of 8.45% in the functional scale score (OS: 4.65%, MISS: 12.2%, $p = 0.025$), and 10.32% in symptoms scale score (OS: 8.45%, MISS: 12.2%, $p = 0.001$). The pre-operative VAS scores did not significantly differ between the groups ($p > 0.015$) (**Table 4**).

	Group	OPEN	MISS	Total
VAS				
Pre-op				
	0–20	2	3	5
	40	4	4	8
	60	6	11	17
	80	3	6	9
	100	4	5	9
Post-op				
	Improved	10 (53%)	21 (72%)	31 (65%)
	Stable	7 (37%)	7 (24%)	14 (29%)
	Worse	2 (10%)	1 (4%)	3 (6%)
P value				0.015
ANTALGIC				
Pre-op				
	Ad lib.	2	3	5
	NSAID	10	14	24
	Morphine	7	12	19
Post-op				
	Ad lib.	10	18	28
	NSAID	4	8	12
	Morphine	5	3	8
P value				0.01

Table 4. The pre-operative and post-operative clinical data (VAS) and drug data (ANTALGIC) of all the patients and divided by group.

At follow-up, 31 patients (65%) showed an improvement of VAS score (OS: 53%, MISS: 72%), while 14 patients (29%) were stable (OS: 37%, MISS: 24%), and 3 patients (6%) worsened (OS: 10%, MISS: 4%) (p = 0.007).

In the pre-operative period, five patients received ad libitum administration of antalgic drugs, and 28 patients received it at follow-up (OS: 10, MISS: 18). 24 patients were pre-operatively administered NSAIDs, while 12 patients received NSAIDs at follow-up (OS: 4, MISS: 8). Nineteen patients were pre-operatively administered morphine, while eight patients were administered morphine at follow-up (OS: 5, MISS: 3) (p = 0.01).

2.5. Illustrative case 1

A 75-year-old with a two-year history of white cell renal carcinoma, already treated with chemo- and radio-therapy, presented with sudden leg weakness, hyper-reflexia, and urge-

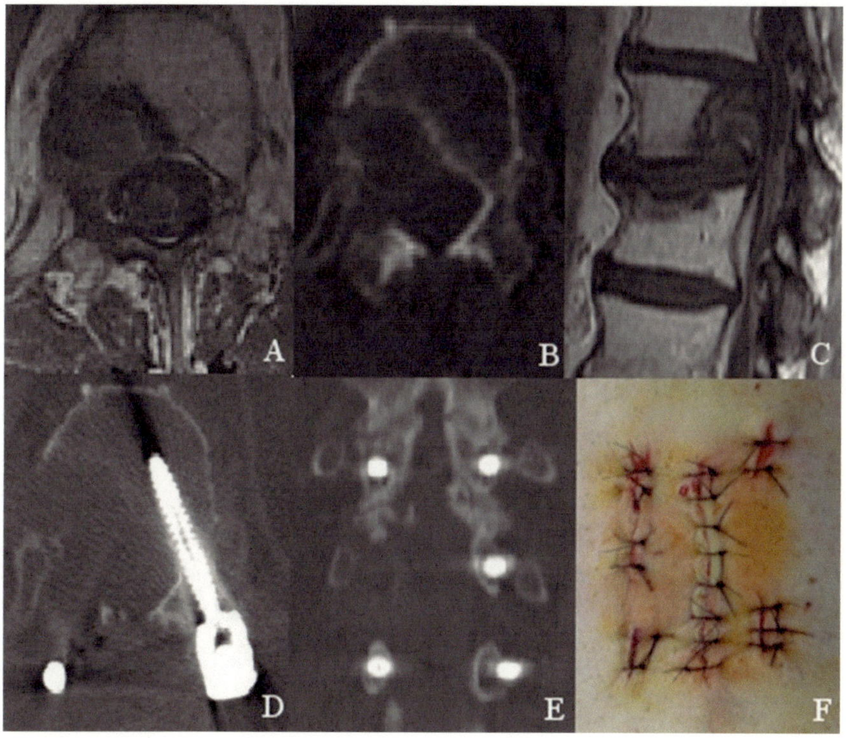

Figure 2. Clinical case #1. Pre-operative MRI axial, CT axial and MRI sagittal scan (A, B and C) showed an osteolytic lesion which substituted the T12 body and its right pedicle, with initial invasion of the spinal canal. In the D and E images it is shown the postoperative CT scan in the axial and coronal plane which documented the percutaneous short fixation with transpedicular screws at T11, L1, and at the left pedicle of T12, followed by a mini-open access, centered at the level of T12, with a decompressive right laminotomy. Skin incisions in the F image.

incontinence (ASIA C, KPS 60, mBS 2), after a one-month history of severe thoracic spinal pain (VAS 90/100), unresponsive to common analgesics. Imaging showed a lesion which substituted the T12 body and its right pedicle, with initial invasion of the spinal canal. He then underwent a pure percutaneous short fixation with transpedicular screws at T11, L1, and at the left pedicle of T12, followed by a mini-open access, centered at the level of T12, with a decompressive laminotomy.

The patient was mobilized in the first post-operative day, with an almost complete resolution of thoracic pain (VAS 20/100). Intraoperative blood loss was 200 cc, and RBC transfusion was not necessary. No opioids were administered in the post-operative period, and the patient was discharged on the fourth post-operative day. A post-operative CT scan showed the complete decompression of the spinal cord, with segmental fixation. At the follow-up, the patient presented a complete restoration of neurological deficit (ASIA E), and antalgic therapy with non-steroidal anti-inflammatory drugs (NSAID) was only administered ad libitum (**Figure 2**).

2.6. Illustrative case 2

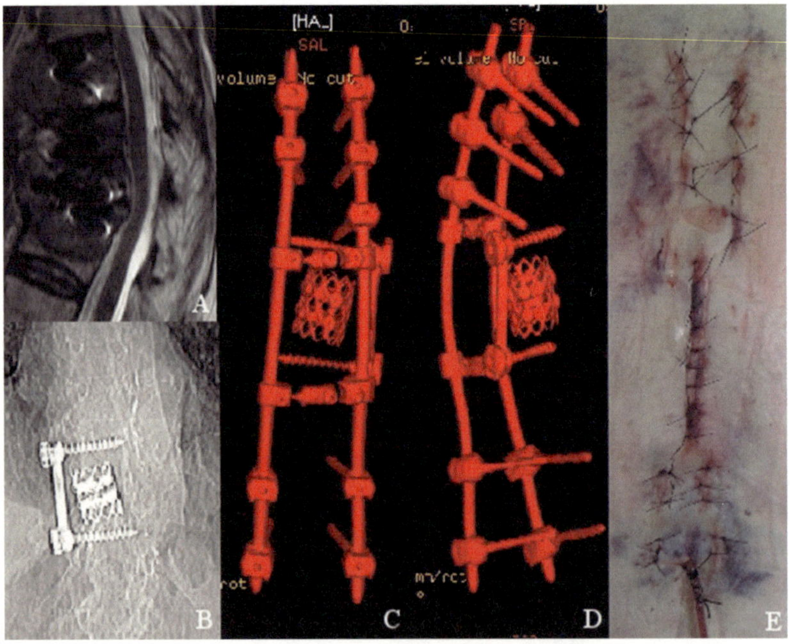

Figure 3. Clinical case 2. Pre-operative MRI sagittal scan and coronal thoraco-lumbar X-ray (A and B images) showed diffuse spinal metastatic localizations with pathologic fractures of T9, T10 and T11, severe kyphosis and medullary compression in patient with a previous right partial T10 corpectomy with T9-T11 antero-lateral fixation. In the C and D images it is shown the postoperative CT scan 3D reconstruction which documented the percutaneous fixation with transpedicular screws at T7, T8, left pedicle of T9, L1 and L2, followed by a mini-open access, centered at the level of T10-T11, with a decompressive laminotomy and double cross-link. Skin incisions in the F image.

http://dx.doi.org/10.5772/63125

A 77-year-old woman, with a seven-year history of follicular thyroid cancer and previous lung and spine metastases that were treated with left inferior pulmonary lobectomy and right partial T10 corpectomy with T9-T11 antero-lateral fixation, respectively, came to our attention, having a new onset of severe thoraco-lumbar pain (VAS 90/100) with leg weakness (ASIA C). The free interval of disease was three years, after the conclusion of adjuvant chemo- and radio-therapy. Imaging showed diffuse spinal metastatic localizations with pathologic fractures of T9, T10 and T11; a severe kyphosis of the dorsal spine was evident. MRI results also showed spinal cord compression at T10-T11 levels, due to extradural metastatic tissue and progressive kyphosis (ASIA C, KPS 60, mBS 2).

The patient underwent a pure percutaneous fixation by transpedicular screws at T7, T8, L1 and L2, while at T9 only on the left pedicle was screwed; a mini-open access, centered at the level of T10-T11, was performed with decompressive laminotomy and positioning of two cross-links. The patient was mobilized in the first post-operative day. Intraoperative blood loss was only 350 cc. No opioids were administered in the post-operative period, and the patient was discharged on the eighth post-operative day. A CT scan, performed at the discharge, showed the complete decompression of the spinal cord and the final fixation. At follow up, the neurological conditions improved (ASIA D), and opioids were stopped, in order to start antalgic therapy with NSAID (**Figure 3**).

2.7. Discussion

Results of our comparative study demonstrate that standard open techniques and the MISS techniques are equivalent, in terms of the ability to achieve an early neurological improvement in patients with acute myelopathy due to spinal cord compression. Nevertheless, MISS approach has a clear and significant advantage over standard open techniques, in terms of blood loss, operation length, and hospital stay; they also confirm its safety, with no patients presenting peri-operative surgical-related complications.

The study consisted of 48 patients with advanced cancer from different primary tumors, presenting a low Karnowsky score and acute myelopathy due to spinal-cord compression; All of them had low modified Bauer scores, which indicate only a short or middle term surgical palliation through posterior decompression and spinal segmental fixation [18]. Surgery was instrumented in all patients, to treat a preoperative instability or to prevent post-surgical instability. A gross total or complete resection of metastases was never attempted because clearly not indicated for any of the patients in the series.

According to the biological behavior of the lesion (i.e., osteolytic or osteoblastic), the number of segments involved, and the columns involved for each segment, the implant for fixation was as shortest as possible, and, in cases where the lesion was partially invading the vertebra, pedicle screws are also inserted in the fractured vertebrae.

We have been interested in comparing the quality of life at an early follow-up, since, in patients with advanced metastatic cancer, the late follow-up is generally conditioned by the progression of the primary disease, and this can produce a bias when evaluating the surgical results for neurological restoration alone or the quality of life. Considering an equivalent neurological recovery, at 30 days follow-up, patients in the MISS group presented a better outcome in terms of quality of life: in our opinion this is the final aim of surgical treatment in case of patients with short- to mid-term life expectancy.

Interestingly some patients of our series aged over 60 years presented an early worsening of neurological symptoms, confirming that age is a key prognostic factor which must to be considered before choosing the surgical strategy in treating advanced cancer patients.

Finally, MISS seem to significantly reduce the post-operative pain. In fact, in our series, VAS reduced and the need for opioids was significantly lower in patients of the MISS group. The reduction in opioids administration improves the quality of life of such patients, avoiding severe constipation or alterations in consciousness.

In our experience, metastatic patients operated with MISS techniques, compared to those operated with traditional open surgery techniques, presented a significant improvement in term of blood loss, operation time, and bed rest length, which is associated to a more rapid functional recovery and discharge from hospital. The post-operative pain and the need of opioids administration were also significantly less pronounced, and these effects appear to translate to a better quality of life of such patients, which is a primary aim in case of patient with a short life expectancy.

Author details

Massimo Miscusi[1*], Stefano Forcato[2] and Antonino Raco[3]

*Address all correspondence to: massimo.miscusi@uniroma1.it

1 Department of Medico-Surgical Sciences and Biotechnologies, Sapienza University of Rome, Italy

2 Department NESMOS, Sapienza University of Rome, Italy

3 Department NESMOS, Sapienza University of Rome, Full Professor of Neurosurgery, Italy

References

[1] Ibrahim A, Crockard A, Antonietti P, Boriani S, Bünger C, Gasbarrini A, et al. Does spinal surgery improve the quality of life for those with extradural (spinal) osseous metastases? An international multicenter prospective observational study of 223 patients. Invited submission from the joint section meeting on disorders of the spine and peripheral nerves, March 2007. J Neurosurg Spine. 2008;8:271–278.

[2] Ofluoglu O. Minimally invasive management of spinal metastases. Orthop Clin North Am. 2009;40:155–168.

[3] Bhatt AD, Schuler JC, Boakye M, Woo SY. Current and emerging concepatients in non-invasive and minimally invasive management of spine metastasis. Cancer Treat Rev. 2013;39:142–152. DOI: 10.1016/j.ctrv.2012.08.002.

[4] Weber MH, Burch S, Buckley J, Schmidt MH, Fehlings MG, Vrionis FD, et al. Instability and impending instability of the thoracolumbar spine in patients with spinal metastases: a systematic review. Int J Oncol. 2011;38:5–12.

[5] Winstead ER. After treatment: the needs of cancer survivors. NCI Cancer Bull. 2005;2:1–2.

[6] Rose PS, Buchowski JM. Metastatic disease in the thoracic and lumbar spine: evaluation and management. J Am Acad Orthop Surg. 2011;19:37–48.

[7] Zairi F, Marinho P, Allaoui M, Assaker R. New advances in the management of thoracolumbar spine metastasis. Bull Cancer. 2013;100:435–441. DOI: 10.1684/bdc.2013.1748.

[8] Chow E, Nguyen J, Zhang L, Tseng LM, Hou MF, Fairchild A, et al. International field testing of the reliability and validity of the EORTC QLQ-BM22 module to assess health-related quality of life in patients with bone metastases. Cancer. 2012;118:1457–65.

[9] Harel R, Angelov L. Spine metastases: current treatments and future directions. Eur J Cancer. 2010;46:2696–2707. DOI: 10.1016/j.ejca.2010.04.025.

[10] Miscusi M, Domenicucci M, Polli FM, Forcato S, De Giorgio F, Raco A. Spondylectomy of T-2 according to the Tomita technique via an extended Fessler approach: a cadaveric study. J Neurosurg Spine. 2011;16:22–26. DOI: 10.3171/2011.9.SPINE10834.

[11] Huang TJ, Hsu RW, Li YY, Cheng CC. Minimal access spinal surgery (MASS) in treating thoracic spine metastasis. Spine. 2006;31:1860–1863.

[12] Logroscino CA, Proietti L, Tamburrelli FC. Minimally invasive spine stabilisation with long implants. Eur Spine J. 2009;18:75–81.

[13] McLain RF, Lieberman IH. Endoscopic approaches to metastatic thoracic disease. Spine. 2000;25:1855–1858.

[14] Rosenthal D, Marquardt G, Lorenz R, Nichtweiss M. Anterior decompression and stabilization using a microsurgical endoscopic technique for metastatic tumors of the thoracic spine. J Neurosurg. 1996;84:565–572.

[15] Hsieh PC, Koski TR, Sciubba DM, Moller DJ, O'Shaughnessy BA, Li KW, et al. Maximizing the potential of minimally invasive spine surgery in complex spinal disorders. Neurosurg Focus. 2008;25:E19.

[16] Kan P, Schmidt MH. Minimally invasive thoracoscopic approach for anterior decompression and stabilization of metastatic spine disease. Neurosurg Focus. 2008;25:E8.

[17] Mobbs RJ, Sivabalan P, Li J. Technique, challenges and indications for percutaneous pedicle screw fixation. J Clin Neurosci. 2011;18:741–749. DOI: 10.1016/j.jocn.2010.09.019.

[18] Leithner A, Radl R, Gruber G, Hochegger M, Leithner K, Welkerling H, et al. Predictive value of seven preoperative prognostic scoring systems for spinal metastases. Eur Spine J. 2008;17:1488–1495.

Chapter 19

The Role of Exercise in Chemotherapy-Induced Peripheral Neuropathy

Karen Y. Wonders and Brittany Stout

Additional information is available at the end of the chapter

http://dx.doi.org/10.5772/62839

Abstract

Chemotherapy-induced peripheral neuropathy (CIPN) is the most common neurological side effect of chemotherapy and is characterized by damage to the nervous system that is a direct result of the medications associated with chemotherapy. Often, this damage to the central nervous system pain pathways results in neuropathic pain described as burning, paroxysmal, stabbing, or elective shock-like and accompanied by pins-and-needles sensations and itching. The presence and severity of neuropathic pain is often shown to be associated with impairments in walking, general activities, sleep, work, mood, enjoyment of life, and relationships with others. Treatment of neuropathic pain due to CIPN often requires a multidisciplinary approach due to the broad variety of symptoms and their negative impact on quality of life. To provide treatment strategies that are effective for patients, they should include a combination of pharmacological agents and exercise rehabilitation. Exercise rehabilitation programs should be designed in order to help patients familiarize themselves to changes in physical functioning. The goals of the program should target three main areas: maximize functional capacities, prolong or maintain independent function, and improve quality of life.

Keywords: Cancer, Exercise, Neuropathy, Chemotherapy, Rehabilitation

1. Introduction

Treating cancer requires an understanding of cellular kinetics [1]. DNA mutations that occur during DNA replication can aide in the development of cancer cells. Activation for DNA repair in a normal cell cycle uses checkpoints to facilitate the repair; however, checkpoint integrity is lost in tumor cells and DNA repair is bypassed [2]. The resulting mutations impact the regulatory mechanisms the restrict cell proliferation in a normal cell [3].

The use of chemotherapeutic agents works by disrupting the cell cycle to prevent cell proliferation before it begins [4]. The negative of systemic chemotherapeutic agents is that normal cells, as well as malignant cells, are disrupted. This leads to untoward effects and long-term morbidities [4] that negatively impact functional ability and quality of life. Chemotherapy-induced peripheral neuropathy (CIPN) is the most common neurological side effect of chemotherapy [5]. This condition is characterized by damage to the nervous system that is a direct result of the medications associated with chemotherapy. Often, this damage to the central nervous system pain pathways results in neuropathic pain [6], frequently described as burning, paroxysmal, stabbing, or elective shock-like [7], accompanied by pins-and-needles sensations and itching. The presence and severity of neuropathic pain is often shown to be associated with impairments in walking, general activities, sleep, work, mood, enjoyment of life, and relationships with others [2, 8].

Little is known about the mechanisms responsible for the development of CIPN [4]. The peripheral toxicity involved with CIPN is specific to each chemotherapy drug class and appears to be dose and duration dependent. However, it can evolve even after a single-drug application [9]. The type and cause of neuropathy are dependent on the chemotherapy agent administered, with vincristine, paclitaxel, and cisplatin being the most neurotoxic [10].

Currently, prophylactic and symptomatic treatments have been ineffective because the neurobiology underpinning CIPN is not fully understood [11]. Thus, the purpose of this chapter was to outline the differences in treatment options available to patients with CIPN and analyze the benefits of exercise in the management of symptoms related to this disorder.

2. Etiology of CIPN

In healthy individuals, peripheral and central nervous system pain pathways function in a protective and adaptive manner [12]. The transduction, conduction, and transmission of nociceptor activity involve these pathways when carrying out activity within the cell. Whether induced by cancer or its treatments, damage to these pathways can result in neuropathic pain [13]. Discontinuation of treatment can result in the development of acute and chronic neurotoxic effects, and these effects can be seen immediately or within weeks or months after discontinuation. Symptoms seen immediately following the first course of treatment can often be contributed to vincristine and oxaliplatin-based regimens. Though both regimens typically produce symptoms immediately following treatment, these symptoms vary between treatments. Vincristine use typically involves the cranial nerve and can lead to symptoms such as seizures, quadriparesis, and numbness. In contrast, oxaliplatin use often produces acute sensory symptoms seen in the mouth or throat that can be intensified by exposure to cold [14]. Regimens that do not present symptoms for up to several weeks after the final treatment may induce a length-dependent neuropathy on small fibers [15].

Incidence of CIPN is estimated to range anywhere from 10 to 100%, depending on the antineoplastic agent, dose, and other factors as presented by the patient [16]. Patients previously affected by diabetes, alcoholism, or inherited neuropathies may be at an increased risk for CIPN [1, 16]. Clinical diagnosis of CIPN is complex, as there is often more than one contributing mechanism [17]. Therefore, testing is multi-faceted and includes neurological examination, quantitative sensory testing, nerve conduction studies, and toxicity grading. Positive symptoms include hypersensitivity to innoculous and noxious stimuli, such as gentle and/or blunt pressure and pinprick [18, 19].

3. Impact on quality of life

Neuropathic pain negatively affects health-related quality of life. Specifically, decrements to physical [20–22], emotional [20, 21, 23], and social functioning [21, 22, 24] are noted in patients with CIPN. In addition, sleep [20, 21, 24, 25] and global quality of life [3, 26] are disturbed. The presence and severity of pain was reported to cause depression and anxiety in patients [20, 21, 23].

4. Treatment strategies

Treatment of neuropathic pain due to CIPN often requires a multidisciplinary approach due to the broad variety of symptoms and their negative impact on quality of life. To provide treatment strategies that are effective for patients, they should include a combination of pharmacological agents and exercise rehabilitation.

4.1. *Pharmacological agents*

There has been much effort put into exploring pharmacological therapies to effectively reduce CIPN. To date, research has shown that some of these therapies provide modest improvements in neurological function. Unfortunately, in some cases, these agents have been shown to have additional negative side effects for cancer patients. The following text provides a discussion of some of these agents, their mechanism of action, and possible side effects.

Alpha-lipoic acid is a cyclic disulfide broad-spectrum antioxidant [27] that has been recently used in research for treatment of CIPN. It has been shown to be effective in animal subjects of CIPN treated with oxaliplatin, cisplatin, and vincristine. Alpha-lipoic acid has the ability to enter all parts of a nerve because it displays the unique capability of functioning in both water and fat. They utilize this ability and other mechanisms by involving the regulation of acetyl-CoA, acetylation of tubulin, and increasing NGF-induced histone acetylation [28]. Alpha-lipoic acid also increases the formation of glutathione and is involved in the recycling of antioxidants such as glutathione, vitamin C, and vitamin E [29]. A few possible side effects of the treatment includes headache, tingling, pins-and-needles sensation, rash, and muscle cramps.

Another possible treatment for CIPN is carbamazepine; a sodium-channel inhibitor prescribed in the treatment of epilepsy. Sodium channel dysfunction is linked to oxaliplatin-induced peripheral neuropathy [30] and carbamazepine has been reported to be an effective treatment against certain forms of pain associated with oxaliplatin. The reported areas of effectiveness with carbamazepine have been against the lancing and shooting pain components with less effectiveness seen in burning pain sensations [31]. Side effects of using carbamazepine include dizziness, drowsiness, and headache, as well as cardiac conduction defects, abnormalities in antidiuretic hormone secretion, loss of balance, and diplopia [9].

Another solution used in the treatment of epilepsy that has been recently acknowledged for its role in treating neuropathic pain is gabapentin. Gabapentin has been found to be effective in painful diabetic neuropathy [32] by binding with subunits of the calcium channel [33]. It was originally developed as a γ-aminobutyric acid (GABA) analogue and has been associated with symptoms such as fatigue, blurred or double vision, muscle pain, swelling in extremities, tremor, and drowsiness [34].

Previously, it has been reported that individuals with cancer more often than not have shown reduced levels of glutamine. Glutamine is an amino acid that functions as the primary energy source for rapidly proliferating cells. It also plays a significant role in the upregulation of nerve growth factor, mRNA [35]. Additionally, studies involving human subjects report reduced levels of nerve growth factor during therapy [36]. Together, these findings provide support the use of glutamine as a neuroprotective agent in individuals with cancer.

Glutathione is an antioxidant and antiviral tripeptide. It has been reported that concurrent administration of glutathione and cisplatin results in a reduction of CIPN. This is thought to be due to a reduction in platinum deposits, as glutathione has a high affinity for heavy metals [37, 38]. However, increased levels of glutathione have been linked to chemotherapy resistance in bone marrow, breast, colon, larynx, and lung cancers [39].

Lamotrigine is a neuroprotective agent that stabilizes sodium channels. In vitro studies suggest that lamotrigine modulates the release of glutamate. Studies examining its efficacy have reported positive effects on diabetic neuropathy [40] and neuropathic pain in the elderly [41]. Adverse effects include loss of balance, dizziness, fatigue, memory and cognitive problems, and drowsiness [40].

Phenytoin is an anticonvulsant drug that works as a sodium channel stabilizer, which works to reduce neuronal excitability. Phenytoin has recently been seen to be effective at decreasing visual analogue scale pain scores [42]; however, excessive use of the drug has been associated with neurological problems such as horizontal gaze. Other associated problems include loss of balance, drowsiness, dizziness, and inhibited insulin release.

Valproic acid has been used quite extensively in the management of neuropathic pain [43]; however, there is little evidence to support its clinical use currently. It is believed to increase levels of GABA in the brain, yet its mechanism of action is unknown. Side effects reported with use of the drug include a decrease in blood clotting mechanisms, which may lead to excessive bleeding. Valproic acid has also been associated with side effects such as drowsiness, dizziness, nausea, vomiting, and tremors [43].

Venlafaxine is a drug that has traditionally been used as an antidepressant, but is currently being looked at for its beneficial effects in cancer patients. Venlafaxine works in the selective reuptake of serotonin and norepinephrine and has been recently found to lessen the hyperexcitability of peripheral nerves [44]. However, reported side effects with venlafaxine can include headaches, anxiety, drowsiness, and increased blood pressure.

Vitamins have also been studies as a possible means of controlling symptoms of neuropathy. Vitamin E is a fat-soluble antioxidant that prevents the peroxidation of polyunsaturated fatty acids. Typically in patients with peripheral neuropathy, there is usually an accompanied deficiency of vitamin E [45] and a greater chance of developing fat-malabsorption disorders. Vitamin E supplementation during treatment with paclitaxel or cisplatin [46, 47] has demonstrated evidence of neuroprotection in clinical trials. These same trials have indicated that Vitamin E supplementation may reduce mortality rates associated with certain forms of cancer [48].

Other prophylactic agents that have been identified as potential neuroprotective agents in CIPN include amifostine, corticosteroids, diethyldihiocarbamate, electrolyte infusions, recombinant human leukemia inhibitory factor, nimodipine, and ORG-2766. These agents have only been tested in animal populations; however, human studies have shown little or no evidence of neuroprotection [49–55].

4.2. *Exercise rehabilitation*

Most preventative and treatments option thus far have come accompanied with a variety of side effects. Due to this, options other than the use of pharmacological interventions that target CIPN should be considered. Exercise rehabilitation is a potential avenue for preventative measures as well as alleviating CIPN symptoms in cancer patients. Many previous research trials have shown beneficial effects of exercise in offsetting countless cancer treatment-related toxicities as well as enhancing the quality of life of the patients. However, clinical trials examining the role of exercise in preserving neurological function following chemotherapy are limited. One recent investigation on the current exercise behaviors of breast cancer patients diagnosed with CIPN patients reported that those individuals who met the amount of recommended physical activity levels reported a significantly higher quality of life and experienced significantly less pain than their sedentary counterparts [56]. A follow-up investigation examined the effect of 12 weeks of supervised exercise training on symptoms of CIPN and found that exercise training positively impacted neurological function. Specifically, unpleasant skin sensations and sensitivity related to neuropathic pain were attenuated following chronic exercise training [57].

While the mechanisms underlying the role of exercise in neuroprotection are unclear, several theories have been circulated. With neuropathy, muscle mass atrophies cause significant decreases in muscular strength [24]. This decline in strength appears to be slow and progressive. It also appears to affect distal muscle groups more so than proximal muscles. Researchers have indicated that this muscle weakness translates into impaired motor performance skills and a reduced exercise capacity [29]. However, several studies have reported improvements in muscular strength following moderate resistance exercise programs in patients with hereditary motor and sensory neuropathies [20, 21], as well as diabetic neuropathies, and those associated with fibromyalgia and chronic fatigue [3, 26–28, 39, 40]. In light of these findings, many researchers recommend that exercise training serve as an important component in the comprehensive treatment plan for patients with peripheral neuropathy [3, 23, 27]. Moderate to intense strength training and aerobic exercise appears to be well tolerated by these patients [23] and is associated with improvements in motor function and nerve conduction velocity [26, 28], as well as improved muscle reinnervation and increased axon regeneration [22]. In addition, one investigation reported that low intensity treadmill exercise promoted Schwann cell proliferation in the injured peripheral nerve [25]. In light of these findings, it is feasible to assume that an individual who has experienced a reduction in muscular strength and functional ability due to CIPN may experience similar improvements following an exercise program.

Those affected by CIPN typically experience large amounts of pain associated with peripheral neuropathy and can be severe enough that it interferes with an individual's quality of life [13]. This type of pain has long been recognized as one of the more difficult types of pain to treat; however, exercise rehabilitation may be able to reduce the amount of pain accompanying peripheral neuropathy. In healthy individuals, studies have shown that acute exercise can temporarily decrease pain perception; a condition known as exercise-induced hypoalgesia (EIH). Specifically, there have been reported increases in pain thresholds and pain tolerance levels both during and after exercise. Even further, there appears to be a decrease in intensity ratings of pain following exercise. To date, research in these areas has yet to determine the optimal intensity of aerobic exercise needed to produce a hypoalgesic effect [58–63]. Typically, exercising at intensities between 60 and 75% of maximum heart rate has been found to produce EIH [58, 59]. Thus far, it has been reported that women tended to experience hypoalgesia following aerobic exercise at 85% HR_{max} [60]. In most research that has been performed, subject has self-selected their aerobic exercise intensities in which they reported EIH following the exercise bout [61, 62]. EIH has also been observed following resistance exercise training, though reports are limited in this area. In a study conducted by Koltyn and Arbogast [63], it was shown that following 45 min of resistance exercise at 75% of the subject's 1-RM, increases in pain thresholds were observed.

Exercise rehabilitation programs should be designed in order to help patients familiarize themselves to changes in physical functioning. Further, goals of the program should target three main areas: maximize functional capacities, prolong or maintain independent function, and improve quality of life. For example, studies performed using populations with hereditary motor and sensory neuropathy have shown that a minimum of 12 weeks of low to moderate resistance training (approximately 30% overload) resulted in strength gains [64–66] that improved function ability [67]. An important area of concern for resistance training is watching for signs that indicate the muscles are being over-worked or exhausted. Symptoms of muscle exhaustion include, but are not limited to, muscle weakness within a half hour of completion of the exercise and excessive muscle soreness between 24 and 48 h after exercise [76, 77]. Training programs should also target aerobic exercise due to its associated benefits with cardiovascular performance and pain tolerance as well as decreased fatigue and depression scores. Currently, research suggests that endurance-based programs should be low impact or utilize approximately 50% of the patient's heart rate reserve [68, 69]. Studies in this area also suggest including a proper warm up and cool down component.

5. Summary

In closing, CIPN is a dose-limiting effect of cancer therapy that has negative implications on a patient's quality of life. While much effort has been made to explore pharmacological therapies aimed at cancer patients. However, exercise rehabilitation is one lifestyle modification that positively impacts the lives of patients with CIPN.

Author details

Karen Y. Wonders[1,2*] and Brittany Stout[2]

*Address all correspondence to: karen.wonders@wright.edu

1 Department of Kinesiology and Health, Wright State University, 316 Nutter Center, Colonel Glenn Hwy, Dayton, USA

2 Maple Tree Cancer Alliance, 425 N Findlay St, Dayton, USA

References

[1] Quasthoff S, Hartung HP (2002) Chemotherapy-induced peripheral neuropathy. J Neurol 249: 9–17.

[2] Rieger PT (2006) Cancer biology and implications for treatment. Clin J Oncol Nurs, 10(4): 457–460.

[3] Jensen MP, Smith DG, Edhe DM, Robinson LR (2001) Pain site and the effects of amputation pain: further clarification of the meaning of mild, moderate, and severe pain. Pain 91: 317–22.

[4] Honea N, Brant J, Beck SL (2007) Treatment-related symptom clusters. Sem Oncol Nurs, 23(2): 142–151.

[5] Quasthoff S, Hartung HP (2002) Chemotherapy-induced peripheral neuropathy. J Neurol, 249: 9–17.

[6] American Cancer Society (2009) Cancer Facts & Figures 2009. Atlanta, GA: Author.

[7] National Heart, Lung, and Blood Institute (2008) NHLBI Fact Book, Fiscal Year 2007. Bethesda, MD: Author.

[8] Lind J (1992) Tumor cell growth and cell kinetics. Sem Oncol Nurs, 8(1): 3–9.

[9] Goodman LS, Limbird LE, Milinoff PB, et al., ed. (1996) Goodman and Gilman's: The Pharmacological Basis of Therapeutics. 9th edn. New York, NY: McGraw-Hill Professional.

[10] Antonine JC, Camdessanche JP (2007) Peripheral nervous system involvement in patients with cancer. Lancet Neurol 6: 75–86.

[11] Kaley TJ, DeAngelis LM (2009) Therapy of chemotherapy-induced peripheral neuropathy. Br J Haematol, 145; 3–14.

[12] Woolf CJ (2004) Pain: moving from symptom control toward mechanism-specific pharmacologic management. Ann Intern Med 140: 441–5.

[13] Horowitz SH (2007) The diagnostic workup of patients with neuropathic pain. Med Clin N Am 91: 21–30.

[14] Grothey A (2007) Oxaliplatin-safety profile: neurotoxicity. Sem Oncol 30(suppl 15): 5–13.

[15] Quastoff S, Hartung HP (2002) Chemotherapy-induced peripheral neuropathy. J Neurol 249: 9–17.

[16] Bakitas MA, Smith E, Cohen J, Fadul C (2004) Measurement issues in chemotherapy-induced peripheral neuropathy. Paper presented at the International Conference on the Mechanisms and Treatment of Neuropathic Pain, Bermuda, November 4–6, 2004.

[17] Wolf CJ, Mannion RJ (1999) Neuropathic pain: aetiology, symptoms, mechanisms, and management. Lancet 353: 1959–64.

[18] Scadding JW, Kiltzenburg M (2006) Painful peripheral neuropathies. In: McMahon SB, Koltzenburg M, ed. Wall and Melzacks, Textbook of Pain 5th edn. Philadelphia, PA, Elsevier Churchill Livingstone, pp. 973–99.

[19] Jensen TS, Baron R (2003) Translation of symptoms and signs into mechanisms of neuropathic pain. Pain 102: 13–8.

[20] Tolle T, Zu Z, Sadosky AB (2006) Painful diabetic neuropathy: a cross-sectional survey of health state impairment and treatment patterns. J Diabetes Complicat 20: 26–33.

[21] Zelman D, Core M, Dukes E, Tai K, Brandenburg N (2005) Validation of a modified version of the brief pain inventory for painful diabetic peripheral neuropathy. J Pain Symptom Manag 29: 401–10.

[22] Turner J, Cardenas D (1999) Chronic pain problems in individuals with spinal cord injuries. Sem Clin Neuropsychiatry 4: 186–94.

[23] Bergbom-Engberg I, Grondahl G, Thibom K (2005) Patients' experiences of herpes zoster and postherpetic neuralgia. J Adv Nurs, 21: 427–33.

[24] Galer B, Gianas A, Jensen M (2000) Painful diabetic polyneuropathy: epidemiology, pain, description, and quality of life. Diabetes Res Clin Pract 47: 123–8.

[25] Jensen MP, Hoffman AJ, Cardenas DD (2005) Chronic pain in individuals with spinal cord injury: a survey and longitudinal study. Spinal Cord 43: 1–9.

[26] Tasmuth T, von Smitten K, Hietanen P, et al. (1995) Pain and other symptoms after different treatment modalities of breast cancer. Ann Oncol 6: 453–59.

[27] Flier J, Van Muiswinkel FL, Jongenen CA, et al. (2002) The neuroprotective antioxidant alpha-lipoic acid induces detoxication enzymes in cultured astroglail cells. Free Radic Res 36: 695–99.

[28] Bianchi G, Vitali G, Caraceni A, et al. (2005) Symptomatic and neurophysiological responses of paclitaxel- or cisplatin-induced peripheral neuropathy to oral acetyl-L-carnitine. Eur J Cancer 41: 1746–50.

[29] Tankova T, Cherninkova S, Koev D (2005) Treatment for diabetic mononeuropathy with alpha-lipoic acid. Int J Clin Pract 59: 645–50.

[30] Eckel F, Schmelz R, Adelsberger H, et al. (2002) Prevention of oxaliplatin-induced neuropathy by carbamazepine. A pilot study. Dtsch Med Wochenchr 127: 78–82.

[31] Sindrup S, Jensen T (1999) Efficacy of pharmacological treatments of neuropathic pain: an update and effect related to mechanism of drug action. Pain 83: 389–400.

[32] Backonja M, Beydoun A, Edwards KR, et al. (1978) Gabapentin for the symptomatic treatment of painful neuropathy. J Assoc Physicians India 26(5): 403–6.

[33] Jensen TS (2002) Anticonvulsants in neuropathic pain. Eur J Pain 6(Suppl A): 61–8.

[34] Gatti G, Bonomi I, Jannuzzi G, et al. (2000) The new antiepileptic drugs: pharmacological and clinical aspects. Curr Pharm Des 6: 839–60.

[35] Gwag BJ, Sessler FM, Robine V, et al. (1997) Endogenous glutamate levels regulate nerve growth factor mRNA expression in the rat denate gyrus. Mol Cells 7: 425–30.

[36] DeSantis S, Pace A, Bove L, et al. (2000) Patients treated with antitumor drugs displaying neurological deficits are characterized by a low circulating level of nerve growth factor. Clin Cancer Res 6: 90–5.

[37] Smyth JF, Bowman A, Parren T, et al. (1997) Glutathione reduces the toxicity and improves quality of life of women diagnosed with ovarian cancer treated with cisplatin: results of a double-blind, randomized trial. Ann Oncol 8: 569–73.

[38] Cascinu S, Cordella L, Del Ferro E, et al. (1995) Neuroprotective effect of reduced glutathione on cisplatin-based chemotherapy in advanced gastric cancer: a randomized double-blind placebo-controlled trial. J Clin Oncol 13: 26–32.

[39] Balendiran GK, Dabur R, Fraser D (2004) The role of glutathione in cancer. Cell Biochem Funct 22(6): 343–52.

[40] Eisenberg E, Lurie Y, Braker C, et al. (2001) Lamotrigine reduces painful diabetic neuropathy: a randomized, controlled study. Neurology 57: 505–9.

[41] Canavero S, Bonicalz V (1996) Lamotrigine control of central pain. Pain 68: 179–81.

[42] Saudek CD, Werns S, Reidenberg MM (1977) Phenytoin in the treatment of diabetic symmetrical polyneuropathy. Clin Pharmacol Ther 22(2): 169–9.

[43] XXX.

[44] Wilson RH, Lehky T, Thomas RR, et al. (2002) Acute oxaliplatin-induced peripheral nerve hyperexcitability. J Clin Oncol 20: 1767–74.

[45] Traber MG. (2006) Vitamin E. In: Shils ME, Shike M, Ross AC, Caballero B, Cousins R, eds. Modern Nutrition in Health and Disease. 10th edn. Baltimore, MD: Lippincott Williams & Wilkins, pp. 396–411.

[46] Argyriou AA, Chroni E, Koutras A, et al. (2005) Vitamin E for prophylaxis against chemotherapy-induced neuropathy: a randomized controlled trial. Neurology 64: 26–31.

[47] Pace A, Savarese A, Picardo M, et al. (2003) Neuroprotective effect of vitamin E supplementation in patients treated with cisplatin chemotherapy. J Clin Oncol 21: 927–31.

[48] Jacobs EJ, Henion AK, Briggs PJ, et al. (2002) Vitamin C and vitamin E supplement use and bladder cancer mortality in a large cohort of US men and women. Am J Epidemiol 156: 1002–10.

[49] Moore DH, Donnelly J, McGuire WP, et al. (2003) Limited access trial using amifostine for protection against cisplatin- and three-hour paclitaxel-induced neuropathy: a phase II study of the Gynecologic Oncology Group. J Clin Oncol 21: 4207–13.

[50] Nelson DF, Gillespie BW, Diener MD, et al. (1984) Is misonidazole neurotoxicity altered by the use of phenytoin and/or dexamethasone in ROTG 79–18 and RTOG 79-16? Int J Radiat Oncol Biol Phys 10: 1731–4.

[51] Bergouignan FX, Vital C, Henry P, et al. (1988) Disulfiram neuropathy. J Neurol 235: 382–3.

[52] Lehky TJ, Leonard GD, Wilson RH, et al. (2004) Oxaliplatin-induced neurotoxicity: acute hyperexcitability and chronic neuropathy. Muscle Nerve 29: 387–92.

[53] Davis ID, Kiers L, MacGregor L, et al. (2005) A randomized, double-blinded, placebo-controlled phase II trial of recombinant human leukemia inhibitory factor (rhuLIF, emfilermin, AM424) to prevent chemotherapy-induced peripheral neuropathy. Clin Cancer Res 11: 1890–98.

[54] Hamers FP, van der Hoop RG, Steerenburg PA, et al. (1991) Putative neurotrophic factors in the protection of cisplatin-induced peripheral neuropathy in rats. Toxicol Appl Pharmacol 111: 514–22.

[55] Roberts JA, Jenison EL, Kim K, et al. (1997) A randomized, multicenter, double-blind, placebo-controlled, dose-finding study of ORG 2766 in the prevention or delay of

cicplatin-induced neuropathies in women with ovarian cancer. Gynecol Oncol 67: 172–7.

[56] Wonders KY & Drury DG (2012). Current exercise behaviors of breast cancer patients diagnosed with chemotherapy-induced peripheral neuropathy. J Integr Oncol 1(1): 103–107.

[57] Wonders KY (2014). The effect of supervised exercise training on chemotherapy-induced peripheral neuropathy. Int J Phys Med Rehabil. 2(4): 210–215.

[58] Koltyn KF, Wertz AL, Gardiner RL, et al. (1996) Perception of pain following aerobic exercise. Med Sci Sports Exerc 28: 1418–21.

[59] Gurevich M, Kohn PM, Davis C (1994) Exercise-induced analgesia and the role of reactivity in pain sensitivity. J Sports Sci 12: 549–59.

[60] Sternberg WF, Bokat C, Kass L, et al. (2001) Sex-dependent components of the analgesia produced by athletic competition. Pain 94: 65–74.

[61] Sternberg WF, Bailin D, Grant M, et al. (1998) Competition alters the perception of noxious stimuli in male and female athletes. Pain 76: 231–8.

[62] Haier RJ, Quaid K, Mills JSC (1981) Naloxone alters pain perception after jogging. Psychiatry Res 5: 231–2.

[63] Koltyn KF, Arbogast RW (1998) Perception of pain after resistance exercise. Br J Sports Med 32: 20–4.

[64] Lindeman E, Leffers P, Spaans F, Drukker J, Reulen J, Kerckhoffs M, Koke A (1995) Strength training in patients with myotonic dystrophy and hereditary motor and sensory neuropathy: a randomized clinical trial. Arch Phys Med Rehabil 76(7): 612–20.

[65] Kilmer DD, McCroy MA, Wright NC, Aitkens SG, Bernauer EM (1994) The effect of a high resistance exercise program in slowly progressive neuromuscular disease. Arch Phys Med Rehabil 75(5): 560–3.

[66] Aitkens SG, McCrory MA, Kilmer DD, Bernauer EM (1993) Moderate resistance exercise program: its effect in slowly progressive neuromuscular disease. Arch Phys Med Rehabil 74(7): 711–5.

[67] Lindeman E, Leffers P, Reulen J, Spaans F, Drukker J (1998) Quadriceps strength and timed motor performances in myotonic dystrophy, Charcot-Marie-Tooth disease, and healthy subjects. Clin Rehabil 12(2): 127–35.

[68] Breslin E, Booth J, Lord B, et al. (1993) Respiratory responses to unsupported arm exercise (UAE) in Charcot Marie Tooth (CMT) [abstract]. *Am Thorac Soc Am Rev Respir Dis* 147: A532.

[69] Balducci S, Iacobellis G, Parisi L, Di Biase N, Calandriello E, Leonetti F, Fallucca F (2006) Exercise training can modify the natural history of diabetic peripheral neuropathy J Diabetes Complicat 20: 216–23.

[70] Carter GT, Kikuchi N, Abresch RT, Walsh SA, Horasek S, Fowler WM (1994) Effects of exhaustive concentric and eccentric exercise on murine skeletal muscle. Arch Phys Med Rehabil 75: 555–59.

[71] Carter GT, Abresch RT, Fowler WM (2002) Adaptations to exercise training and contraction-induced muscle injury in animal models of neuromuscular disease. Am J Phys Med Rehabil 81(suppl): S151–S161.

Chapter 20

Pediatric Neuro-Oncology in Low-/Middle-Income Countries

Mohamed S. Zaghloul

Additional information is available at the end of the chapter

http://dx.doi.org/10.5772/63111

Abstract

Pediatric cancer is becoming increasingly important in low-/middle-income countries (LMICs), due to the improvement in controlling communicable diseases, decrease infant, and early childhood mortalities associated with infection and malnutrition.

Worldwide, although much improvement was encountered in many pediatric tumors particularly acute leukemia that represents the commonest type of cancer in children, this was not so obvious in CNS tumors, the second most common tumor type. Slow advances have been achieved to improve treatment end results in pediatric neuro-oncology. This was largely related to disease under diagnosis, incorrect clinical assessment, improper staging, and lack of the availability of appropriate radiologic, neurosurgical, and radiotherapeutic services in LMICs. Moreover, the need for multidisciplinary team working together to embalmment unified approved management guidelines, highly specific care level within a widely accepted quality control measures are of utmost importance to raise the treatment outcome levels to that of high-income countries (HICs).

Much effort is needed in LMICs to improve the management of pediatric CNS tumors, decrease the gap, and reach good results already attained by the dedicated centers in HICs. There are many international organizations and societies that can and are willing to help in this matter.

In this chapter, an illustration of the obstacles faced by LMIC neuro-oncologists will be discussed. The different ways and procedures are recommended to improve the general situation to attain good results similar to that in HICs.

Keywords: neuro-oncology, children, low-/middle-income countries, LMIC, CNS tumors, brain, late sequelae

1. Introduction

Pediatric central nervous system (CNS) tumors represent the second most common cancer in childhood after leukemias. Pediatric cancer is the leading cause of disease-related childhood mortality in high-income countries (HICs). Furthermore, it is becoming increasingly important in low-/middle-income countries (LMICs) because of the continuing success to decrease the infant and childhood mortality associated with malnutrition and communicable disease. Unfortunately, the 80% cure rate for HIC children suffering from cancer does not apply to many of pediatric patients in LMIC [1]. The barriers to optimize the management of children with cancer in LMICs to reach the same level as that in HICs were investigated in many situations; however, minimal advances have been made to improve the treatment and clinical end results of children especially those with brain tumors. Many factors were identified as responsible for this failure to achieve such an acceptable level of cure. These were underdiagnosis, abandonment of therapy, incorrect assessment, lack of appropriate radiological, histopathologic, neurosurgical, radiotherapeutic, and pediatric oncologic services. More important is the deficiency of the real concept of multidisciplinary care and the team management that definitely contributes negatively to the results of treatment [2]. In many LMICs, a significant portion of pediatric brain tumors remains undiagnosed and the patients subsequently die of their malignancy. Many others abandoned effective treatment due to different reasons: financial, social, long distance from the treating center, or being treated with herbal and unconventional therapy. The identification of these findings will help the development of targeted strategies, such as increased training and tools for neuropathology, improved access to neuroimaging and radiotherapy, improve early diagnosis, and optimal collaborate therapy. Interventions to implement and increase family support may positively contribute on improvement of outcome.

1.1. Magnitude of the PROBLEM

Underdiagnosis, treatment abandonment, improper assessment, lack of appropriate medical imaging, histopathologic, neurosurgical, radiotherapeutic pediatric oncologic services deficiencies, and the deficiency of the multidisciplinary care concept and the team management are well-known barriers that hinder successful neuro-oncologic management that leads to the obtainment of equivalent clinical end results already achieved in HICs. In addition, in many patients, treatment may be negatively affected because of poor general health, with the comorbidity of malnutrition and infections such as human immunodeficiency virus (HIV) and tuberculosis. Furthermore, the lack of adequate supportive drugs and supplements that ameliorate the oncologic treatment side effects and preserve a tolerable general condition may contribute not only in intolerance of therapy but also in lowering the survival rates and quality of life (QoL) of such patients. The applied treatment protocols have to take these factors and conditions into account. Protocols applied in HICs may not be optimum and may be even dangerous in LMICs especially whenever the supportive care is deficient [3]. The aggregation of the necessary facilities and properly trained staff in one referral center serving an LMIC or a large sector of it may be the proper way to serve these children and to raise the standard of care to reach the acceptable level of cure attained in HICs [4]. It is obvious that it is easier, more convenient, and cheaper to arrange for establishing a referral pediatric neuro-oncologic center to be responsible for the welfare of such children. The tremendous improvements in imaging, surgical approaches, pathological diagnosis, radiotherapy techniques, and chemotherapy drugs in the last three decades have improved survival rates in children with brain tumors and are attained in such referral centers. Innovations in radiation techniques, including the three-dimensional (3D) radiation therapy (RT) and different forms of intensity-modulated radiation therapy (IMRT) such as static IMRT, volumetric modulated arc therapy (VMAT), tomotherapy, cyberknife, and all forms of image-guided radiotherapy, have contributed to the precise and extremely accurate delivery of the radiation dose to the target while reducing the dose to the normal brain tissue. These techniques minimize RT-related toxicities through decreasing the dose to the surrounding functioning structures while increasing tumor control probability [5].

1.2. Diagnosis delay in CNS tumors

Despite advances in neuroimaging, timely diagnosis of CNS tumors remains a problem even in HICs. It is obvious that the issue of late diagnosis of CNS tumors is more obvious and more intense in LMICs. Beyond the usual challenges of nonspecific symptoms, the access to neuroimaging facilities is the main obstacle that patients and families face. The limited number of computerized tomography (CT) or magnetic resonance imaging (MRI) scans in LMICs; prolonged waiting lists, especially in children needing sedation; and high cost of these tests are among the reasons that delay the diagnosis of brain tumor. Furthermore, in many places, the imaging study is limited to the brain, regardless of the state-of-art recommendation. It is exceptional to have preoperative imaging of the spine when a malignant brain tumor such as medulloblastoma is suspected. Most developing countries lack specialized centers presenting the complete multidisciplinary service equipped with the necessary diagnostic and treatment tools in hands of experienced staff [6].

The adoption of unified management protocols represents a major drawback. A single referral neuro-oncologic center in each LMIC that is fully equipped and adequately staffed could serve the patients in a more professional and efficient way that decrease the cost and improve the clinical outcome. Aggregation of the needed staff, equipment, and experience together with standardizing policies, treatment protocols, and managements may be the best way to overcome the difficulties facing LMIC challenges in pediatric neuro-oncology practice [4]. The obstacles of long distance and financial needs to access these specialized centers will remain as a problem that needs effort to be solved. The diagnosis of brain tumor in some LMIC cultures has a negative perception and stigmatization. Families may abundant treatment and even referred to cancer center, for the fear of marginalization associated with brain tumor. Stigma of the false belief that cancer means death or mental and physical disability may influence parental or family decisions including treatment abandonment. Some cultural preferences such as treating boys over girls have to be strongly faced.

Radiotherapy evolved tremendously in the last three to four decades, depending upon the advances in physics, atomic sciences, materials, engineering, computer science, and telecommunication. Linear accelerator-based RT became the backbone technology. This phase represented a megavoltage (MV) power race, which would have skin-sparing properties, while delivering a high dose of radiation at depth. Linear accelerators initiated the new technologies of 3D conformal RT, IMRT, and image-guided radiotherapy including the helical tomotherapy and others [7]. The technique of radiosurgery was developed through combined efforts of multiple specialties, where multiple cobalt-60 sources were fitted into a helmet-like configuration with precision beam collimation to produce remarkably tiny and accurate beams, resulting in the concept of using single-fraction radiation doses for the purposes of target ablation, which expanded the clinical utility beyond neoplasms into the field of benign and functional indications.

1.3. Neuroimaging

Neuroimaging is a key tool in the diagnosis and follow-up of neuro-oncologic patients. MRI and CT are the main imaging modalities involved in neuroimaging diagnosis of these patients. Nevertheless, in pediatric neuro-oncology MRI ranked superior not only due to lack of radiation exposure provided by CT but also due to the more significant details of the brain parenchyma offered by MRI. The standard MRI sequences (T1- and T2-weighted spin-echo in three planes; axial, coronal, and sagittal). Fluid attenuation inversion recovery (FLAIRE) sequences followed by post-contrast are usually adopted. These sequences are usually enough for an accurate differential diagnosis. However, newer sequences and techniques provide additional information for both the diagnosis and treatment management of difficult and/or atypical cases [8]. Although gadolinium-based contrast media is not nephrotoxic yet, it is not advisable for children younger than 2 years [8].

Ideally, post-surgery studies should be performed within the first 48 h after neurosurgical procedure in order to avoid misinterpretations of residual tumor enhancement with blood leakage across the blood-brain barrier. Diffusion study, describing the random thermal motion of the water molecule in tissues, detects the tissue cellularity. It gives a clue about the grade of the tumor and its cellularity. Diffusion tensor imaging (DTI) allows determination of fiber bundle directionality (tractography) study [9].

In neuro-oncology, 3D imaging is used for stereotaxy, a technique creating a coordinate system to guide lesion localization in a surgical procedure or radiotherapy treatment. In order to reduce morbidity in CNS tumor resection, this technique is usually supplemented by other maneuvers and techniques such as functional MRI and direct cortical stimulation [8].

MR spectroscopy (MRS) is a technique widely used to assess metabolites in the brain parenchyma and lesions. The results of an MRS acquisition are typically displayed in a graphic of metabolite peaks. The assessed metabolites are choline, creatine, N-acetylaspartate (NAA), and lactate. Perfusion technique can be applied with both MRI and CT. Nevertheless, there is a new MRI sequence called arterial spin labeling (ASL) that can be used to study brain perfusion without the use of contrast media [10]. The perfusion images are frequently interpreted

http://dx.doi.org/10.5772/63111

in a color map. The red zones usually demonstrate increased perfusion and the blue zones decreased perfusion. The perfusion technique differentiates between low- and high-grade tumors. It is helpful in the differentiation of radiation necrosis (decreased perfusion) from tumor recurrence (normal to elevated perfusion) and in defining the ideal area for surgical biopsy, avoiding areas of necrosis.

1.3.1. PET scan and future molecular imaging

Positron emission tomography (PET) and molecular imaging are rapidly developing as new techniques to evaluate brain tumor. The results provided by PET and molecular imaging appear to corroborate the findings of MRI studies for decision making in the treatment and follow-up. The use of a PET scan is often carried out together with low-dose CT images or MRI to improve the anatomical localization. Common radiopharmaceuticals applied in brain imaging are fludeoxyglucose (FDG), L-[methyl-11 C] methionine ([11 C]MET), and 3′-deoxy-3′- [18 F]fluorothymidine ([18 F]FLT). However, FDG applicability in clinical practice is low as the normal gray matter also demonstrates increased glucose metabolism, effacing lesions [11].

1.4. Neuropathological services

Experienced pathologists able to differentiate subtypes of pediatric neurological tumors are deficient in many LMICs. Some diagnoses can be promptly made on standard hematoxylin and eosin stains based on classic architectural features alone, while more challenging cases often require ancillary studies including immunohistochemistry, electron microscopy, cytogenetics, and/or molecular studies. The lack of trained personal and inadequate technical equipment is therefore limiting the possibility to achieve an accurate diagnosis in many places. It is likely that a significant number of children are treated without an adequate diagnosis that may lead to inadequate or even improper treatment. Microscopic examination combined with molecular signatures of these tumors continues to identify and define features specific to CNS tumor subtypes mostly of great importance, to reach to the proper diagnosis or the appropriate subtype [12]. Neuro-oncologic telepathology and twinning between centers in both LMICs and HICs can improve the capacity of accurate histopathological diagnosis with little burden on centers shared in these programs [13].

1.5. Radiotherapy services

RT is one of the main critical components of treatment of many pediatric CNS tumors; however, limited radiotherapy machines and personnel in LMICs make them available only at large centers with long waiting lists. Delay in starting radiotherapy has a negative impact on survival. Radiation indications, treatment volumes, and doses are determined according to the extent of disease, magnitude of excision, tumor histology, pattern of spread, and pattern of failure in each tumor type and grade. In malignant CNS tumors such as medulloblastoma and ependymoma, excellent clinical end results have been reported, particularly in patients with features denoting standard risk (complete resection, absence of metastatic disease, and no anaplastic features). The overall survival rates are above 90% in patients with pure germinoma, regardless of metastatic stage, with a combination of chemotherapy and radiation. However, access to radiation oncology services and the number of functioning radiotherapy machines available in most LMICs is the main barrier to optimal patient care. It is obvious that pediatric neuro-oncology programs cannot be implemented in countries, which have no radiation oncology services. Based on World Bank classification, 139 countries are defined in the category of LMICs. Out of these, only four (2.9%) have the requisite number of teletherapy units and 55 (39.5%) have no RT facilities. It is also worth mentioning that LMICs have 0.71 teletherapy units per million population in contrast to 7.62 teletherapy units per million population for HICs [14]. A survey of radiotherapy equipment in Africa reported that 52% (29/56) of their countries had no radiotherapy at all and two-thirds of the MV equipment available in the continent were located in two countries (Egypt and South Africa) [15]. Moreover, many countries rely on machines that are more than 20 years old, which questions their functionality and reliability. The available radiation oncology equipment in the continent represented 18% of the estimated needs, at time of reporting. The needs increased more due to rapid increase in the population in many African countries without simultaneous increase in the facilities. Furthermore, appropriate maintenance of the radiation equipment is a major, problematic issue in countries wherever only one radiotherapy machine is the case. The treatment could get interrupted for an undetermined period of time and the waiting times can be prolonged considerably with the machine going out of service. It was estimated that the LMIC deficit in the teletherapy units was 61.4%, in radiation oncologists 38.9%, radiation physicists 68.4%, and RT technologists was 66.5% to reach the requirement applied in HICs [14]. As a consequence, access to radiation and delay in initiation and/or continuation of radiation treatment are a major problematic issue in most LMICs.

In several situations, pediatric oncologists on trying to overcome the problem of availability of radiotherapy design protocols that offer postoperative chemotherapy prior to radiation, in particular for medulloblastoma patients. Although this is not the sound or ideal option, it may delay or decrease recurrence or dissemination following initial surgery. Another limiting factor in the management is the number of experienced, well-qualified personnel with an experience in CNS radiation techniques. Several medulloblastoma trials showed that the quality of craniospinal radiotherapy (CSI) affects outcome. Therefore, the deficiency of adequate human resources is another major contributing factor for poor RT capacity in LMICs. Most reports on radiation oncology personnel availability and training confirm the unavailability of enough physicians and staff to deal with the number of patients needing radiation treatment. This lack of trained personnel with the high patient volume often leads to long waiting list, disease progression, and poor outcome [16]. In Latin America, a survey reported the major obstacles for provision of adequate RT as insufficient number of specialists, rather than a lack of equipment [17]. The insufficient number of radiation oncologists, medical physicists, and radiation technologists training programs contributed negatively to efficient number of personnel needed for a decent service. To add to the gloomy picture, it is well estimated that within the next 10 years, 70% of newly diagnosed cancer patients will be living in countries that collectively have only 5% of the global resources for cancer control. It is estimated that approximately 60% of the world's patients with cancer, including the pediatric neuro-oncology patients, do not have access to a complete cancer systemic therapy regimen, and the percentage is higher for radiotherapy [18].

National cancer control programs, large national or international meetings, or even national treatment guidelines though of extreme importance, were not adequate to improve the current situation of neuro-oncology in LMICs. A survey in 167 countries performed by the WHO found that almost half of these countries had a sort of plan for improving treatment, but national guidelines are generally lacking while the accessibility and affordability of treatment remained low in LMICs. In many countries, the national cancer control plans had been designed according to WHO plan without tailoring it to the local conditions, needs, and challenges [19, 20].

Engaging in innovative strategic thinking and finding new ways to mobilize and enforcing local resources to improve the availability and accessibility of cancer care are essential to overall and balanced cancer control in underserved countries. Most LMICs have some local resources; however, they may not be adequately mobilized or used in the appropriate manner. LMICs should not rely entirely on external financial donations. Instead, what is needed is win-win support and adequate assistance from the affluent organizations or countries, as well as the pharmaceutical and radiology industrial companies. Assistance better take the form of technical support for building local capacity, staff training, management guidance, and research cooperation. Other types of support may include provision of information and communication technologies, help with obtaining local funds or international grants, and instructions on how to collaborate on international work in their own countries. (The Win-Win Initiative of ICEDOC's Experts in Cancer Without Borders [21].)

Conducting more clinical trials in LMICs, which have the major bulk of pediatric cancer and neuro-oncologic patients, could shorten the total time needed for conducting clinical trials, may reduce costs, and could enrich the scientific aspects of those trials with more variability. It could also help initiate more cost-effective ways in medical services in LMICs that can be applied even in HICs and could establish a better value cancer care. This may serve double purposes: improve the quality of both health care and research and prevent the brain drain experienced by LMICs when their most highly qualified people immigrate to HICs. Hypofractionation for glioblastoma multiforme (GBM) and diffuse intrinsic pontine glioma (DIPG) are treatment approaches to improve regional tumor control. This has several advantages over conventional RT via increased cell death due to the used higher doses per fraction and reduced tumor repopulation effect consequent to shortening of the overall treatment time. Haas-Kogan et al. [22] assumed that the α/β ratio equals 2 Gy in p53-mutated GBM, and not 7–10 as suggested in other malignant tumor types. Shortened treatment time has additional significant benefit for patients and their families, because patients with GBM or DIPG have a limited survival time after the completion of treatment. Shortening treatment time allows for a better QoL for the patients saving them and their families the burden of prolonged treatment with all its consequent suffering. However, there may be a risk of enhanced radioresistance. Hypofractionated radiation has become a frequent choice in the treatment of GBM and DIPG patients [23–27].

2. Neuro-oncologic treatment modalities

2.1. Neurosurgery

Neuro-oncology multidisciplinary team discussion allows for a non-bias, more appropriate decision, evident-based, and tailored according to local situation. The option between observation, surgical intervention, radiotherapy, chemotherapy, or a combination of these depends on many factors: tumor type, location, invasiveness as well as the patient's age and overall medical condition. Generally, if a tumor is accessible and the morbidity risk is acceptable, resection should be considered. Neurosurgeons should also actively follow up patients even if a nonsurgical approach is preferred since their interference might be required for treating unsuccessful cases or complications of the chosen modality.

Thorough evaluation of the patient should be performed before a precise neurosurgical opinion including the clinical condition, neuroimaging studies, and case-specific pertinent investigations (e.g., serum hormone levels, tumor markers, genetic syndrome features, etc.). Imaging of the entire neuraxis should be performed, especially for tumors with a tendency for CNS dissemination such as medulloblastomas, germ cell tumors, ependymomas, and primitive neuroectodermal tumors (PNETs).

The main objectives of the neurosurgeons are as follows:

– Maximal safe tumor resection when possible

– Histopathological diagnosis

– Treatment of associated conditions (e.g., hydrocephalus)

2.2. Tumor resection

Maximum safe resection can be performed for a lesion that significant neurological impairments can be avoided after its surgical removal. The patient's prognosis often correlates with the extent of resection.

2.3. Histopathological diagnosis

When pediatric CNS tumors are not amenable to surgical resection, a biopsy is required except in certain situation. Various biopsy techniques have been described and the choice of the appropriate method mainly depends on tumor location.

A) Stereotactic biopsy

Stereotactic coordinates are used for precise guidance of a needle inside the tumor. This is the method of choice for deeply located tumors. Stereotactic biopsy may be performed through a frameless via frameless neuro-navigation device or a metallic head frame-based system. The

http://dx.doi.org/10.5772/63111

coordinates for adequate placement of the burr hole, the angulation, and depth of the needle are determined by preoperative images.

B) Open biopsy

Open biopsy can be performed through a small craniotomy that allows for direct access to the tumor. This method is traditionally used for superficial tumors near or within the cerebral cortex or when leptomeningeal lesions are identified. Neuro-navigation can help in precise localization of the tumor in relation to the skull surface.

C) Endoscopic endonasal biopsy

Anterior skull base, sellar region, and tumors invading sinuses can sometimes be accessed through an endoscopic endonasal approach under general anesthesia.

D) Endoscopic intraventricular biopsy

Tumors located adjacent to or within the ventricular system may be amenable to an endoscopic transventricular approach. This procedure has the advantage of allowing treatment of associated hydrocephalus via endoscopic venticulostomy and obtaining intraventricular cerebrospinal fluid (CSF) sample.

2.4. Treatment of hydrocephalus

Due to the mass effect of the tumor causing partial obstruction of the pathway of CSF, hydrocephalus may develop. The main mechanism of hydrocephalus in the context of CNS tumors is obstruction of the ventricular system by tumors in the posterior fossa and that located around the third ventricle [28].

Unstable patients with clinical evidence of elevated ICP should undergo urgent surgery, inserting external ventricular drain (EVD). The anterior horn of the lateral ventricle is accessed through an inserted catheter through a skull burr hole and CSF flow is ensured. The EVD is connected to an external collecting device and allows the excess CSF to be drained [29]. Endoscopic third ventriculostomy (ETV) is another option in hydrocephalus resulting from posterior fossa or pineal region tumors. An ETV creates a communication between the third ventricle and the interpeduncular cistern under endoscopic guidance within the ventricular system [29, 30]. Many patients need permanent diversion of CSF ventriculoperitoneal shunt (VPS). A proximal catheter is inserted inside the lateral ventricle and is then connected to a distal catheter tunneled subcutaneously till it reaches the peritoneum. A valve is commonly inserted between the proximal and the distal catheter and allows for one-way drainage control. One of the disadvantages of VPSs includes the theoretical risk of intraperitoneal seedling of neoplastic cells.

2.5. Spinal cord neoplasms

Intramedullary spinal cord tumors are rare in the pediatric population, representing around 4% of all CNS tumors. Complete surgical excision if feasible or debulking is the general approach for spinal cord tumors. This procedure often leads to favorable outcome besides providing sufficient materials for histological diagnosis.

2.6. Management of cystic tumors

Many pediatric CNS tumors are composed of a cystic component or having both cystic and solid parts. The potential space of the cystic portion creates an isolated microenvironment that may hinder local treatment (radiotherapy or local chemotherapy). Simple aspiration of the fluid that composes the cyst may sometimes be a sufficient treatment. Moreover, surgical resection can be considered for most cystic tumors. Local treatment may be applied including the insertion of a device in which medical therapy will be administered. Specifically, the use of intracystic radioisotope (radioactive iodine-125 or phosphorus 32) and intracavitary chemotherapy may be used in selected cases [31]. The main advantage of this treatment is the low rate of long-term sequelae. Intracystic chemotherapy has been advocated to delay aggressive treatment such as radical resection or irradiation. This method allows for administration of effective therapy (commonly bleomycin or interferon) and abolishes the systemic toxicity of the systemic chemotherapy and the morbidity of surgical resection. Ommaya reservoir and instillations of single or multiple doses of active drugs remain the method of choice for intracystic chemotherapy.

2.7. Management of tumor recurrence

The decision to reoperate on a recurred tumor must be taken in the light of the patient's life expectancy and QoL, tumor histology, time length between initial resection and recurrence, the risks and benefits of a second surgery, and the potential for adjuvant therapy such as radiotherapy and chemotherapy. Each case should be individually evaluated through multidisciplinary discussion taking into consideration the patient's family opinion and preference. It is worth emphasizing that surgical treatment of recurrent tumors should be seriously considered as reoperation has improved survival for many tumors such as choroid plexus tumors, ependymomas, and cerebellar astrocytomas [32–34].

3. Radiotherapy

RT is an essential treatment for most of the neuro-oncology patients. It is frequently used together with either surgery or chemotherapy or both as a curative treatment. Furthermore, its use in the palliative setting is vital in many situations for symptom relieving [35]. There are two types of RT: 1. teletherapy (external beam therapy) treating patients with MV energy, such as cobalt units and linear accelerators (Linacs), and 2. brachytherapy (internal application of radioactive sources). It is worth noting that providing effective, reliable, and safe RT is a

http://dx.doi.org/10.5772/63111

complex, tedious, and expensive procedure. It requires specialized building structures (bankers) for radiation protection, investment in expensive machinery, dosimetric measurements, and verification devices used by trained staff capable of efficiently using and optimally maintaining such equipment. Furthermore, it requires continuously ongoing quality assurance and training programs for allocated staff. For these reasons, RT infrastructure in general may be poor in LMICs, to the extent that only four countries in Africa treat more than 100 children per year with RT, due to lack of radiation oncology staff, infrastructure, and services [36]. All RT programs require trained medical physicists and technical engineer staff to maintain their machines and to provide quality assurance of the treatment machines and planning programs. Highly trained radiation therapy technicians (RTT) responsible for planning RT treatment and for operating the machines are extremely needed for the appropriate therapy procedures. Unfortunately, skilled staff is frequently attracted away to better-resourced countries providing them with superior payment and better standard of living representing a major issue that needs serious challenge.

Accommodation for the patient and accompanying adult are frequently problematic. In some countries, accommodation and transport for these patients are frequently offered by charity organizations. The major challenge that staff face when dealing with pediatric patients in RT department is the length of time that is needed. Children (and their parents) are more likely to be cooperative when they are not being rushed, and when the team takes the time to explain all the details with patience and when accommodating their fears and anxieties.

In general, it is essential to

1. Allocate sufficient time and experienced staff for the daily workflow.
2. Have all the required clinical information at hand.
3. Get the patient's sedation history from other departments so that it is known beforehand whether the child is likely to cooperate, and how easily they can be sedated.
4. It is always helpful to get the child in for a "play" appointment prior to markup day, so that they familiarize themselves with staff and the machines. A round tour in the departments may be helpful in getting the patient confident that the procedure is not painful.
5. Children of 6 years and older will generally cooperate without sedation, especially if the parents help to prepare them. They should always be told the precise steps of what will happen to them during the process. The best person to convince the child is a colleague child patient who receives RT without anesthesia.
6. Children under 5 years of age usually need sedation. Between 5 and 6 years is variable.
7. Obtaining an anesthetist on a daily basis for radiotherapy treatments may be very difficult in many institutions [37].

Anesthesia may be oral or intravenous. The American Society of Anesthesiologists has proposed a grading system for sedation use as follows: [38].

1. Minimal sedation/anxiolysis.

2. Moderate sedation/analgesia.
3. Deep sedation/analgesia.
4. General anesthesia.

For the two-dimensional (2D) RT, the procedure is a clinical anatomical decision-making process, determining the tumor location as well as the proximity of critical normal tissues. Setting up two orthogonal radiation beam fields on an X-ray simulator with bony anatomy provides the bulk of the guidance. The target was identified on a planar X-ray, and areas not to be treated were blocked, originally with lead or cerrobend alloy, converting a square or a rectangular beam offered by the machine into an irregularly shaped beam, at least in two directions. Bony anatomy visualized on plain radiographs was the primary method of determining field placement using orthogonal, and occasionally oblique or vertex fields. The uncertainty in target determination with this rudimentary method mandated the incorporation of error as a significant element in the radiation field design, generally resulting in large volumes being irradiated [37]. The tremendous advancement in computers and telecommunication allowed more complex treatment planning systems (TPS). Technical advances such as multileaf collimation (MLC), digitally reconstructed radiographs (DRRs), and electronic portal imaging (EPI) greatly contributed to the integration of three-dimensional conformal radiation therapy (3DCRT) effective delivery. The planning process for 3DCRT is significantly more complex than for conventional RT. Therefore, multiple well-coordinated steps are taken by the different categories of radiation oncology team; radiation technologist, dosimetrist, physicist, and radiation oncologist. With the advancement in CT technology, it became possible to incorporate 3D data for both normal organ at risk and tumor into treatment planning systems. This results not only to delineate targets accurately but also to calculate radiation doses efficiently from multiple beams through multiple directions, and to block out (and save) normal tissue more effectively, thus yielding a more conformal 3D radiation plan.

3.1. Immobilization and imaging

The initial step of the planning process is to place the patient in a reproducible position that optimizes treatment of the entire tumor volume while sparing surrounding critical structures. Variable customizable immobilization devices may be used, including thermoplastic facemasks, alpha cradles, and vacuum mattresses. It is important to ensure that these devices are comfortable, reproducible, and sustainable along the whole radiotherapy treatment. Upon the optimal position of the patient, localization (determining points of origin through a laser device) is determined and marks are placed. With the patient in the treatment position, CT images of the area of interest are obtained and the data are transferred to the planning system. At this stage, the clinician will be able to define the target volumes as well as critical structures. Other modalities such as MRI can be co-registered with the CT data for better determination of the target volumes. Two main basic issues are essential for treatment planning: the identification of the topography and geometry of the diseased tissue and the correct segmentation of the anatomy of normal tissues. The International Commission on Radiation Units and

http://dx.doi.org/10.5772/63111

Measurements (ICRU) has defined evolving standard definitions for radiotherapy target volumes. Their recent recommendations [39] include:

- The gross tumor volume (GTV), being gross demonstrable extend and location of the malignant growth, irrespective of the method used for its detection.
- The clinical target volume (CTV), being a volume that contains a demonstrable GTV and/or subclinical malignant disease that must be eliminated.
- The planning target volume (PTV) including the CTV and the surrounding geometrical margin to ensure that the prescribed dose is actually delivered to the CTV with a clinically acceptable probability.
- The organs-at-risk (OAR) tissues that need to be avoided to decrease the morbidity and determine the exact dose to be delivered to each and to be adjusted according to the knowledge of tolerance and normal tissue complication probability (NTCP). This OAR dose determination may influence the treatment planning and/or the dose prescription. An acceptable plan is the one taking in consideration both tumor coverage and OAR dose distribution. Upon target volumes and critical structures definition, each beam geometry and weighting are determined to calculate the final dose distribution. Beam angles selection is performed using either the isodose distribution in axial images or the beam's eye view (BEV). BEV visualizes the relationship of tumor volumes to those of critical OAR, as if looking from the origin of the beam. Once an initial plan has developed, the resulting dose distributions are calculated and evaluated by the clinician. Accurate quantification of radiation doses to the normal structures will allow the choice of the prescribed maximum dose to the target simultaneously with minimum dose to the normal structures to produce a better therapeutic ratio. Consequently, more accurate shielding of normal structures is ensured using MLC. These data are represented graphically on a dose–volume histogram (DVH), presenting information pertinent to the adequacy of tumor dose and maintaining the normal tissue doses below safe thresholds. Conformal RT is the most common treatment used for primary brain tumors; however, the use of IMRT is rapidly increasing. Plans whether conformal or IMRT are evaluated by viewing isodose curves on serial images of a CT scan, as well as by the generation of DVH for tumor volume as well as other normal tissues or organ of interest. This allows the radiation oncologist to evaluate the dose delivered to the total volume (tumor volume and OAR). DVHs are graph percent volume of a given tissue on the *Y*-axis and dose on the *X*-axis allowing the visualization of the percentage of a defined structure receiving a given dose. These data allow plans to be modified as needed to either increase dose delivered to tumor or decrease dose to a nearby critical structure.

Once a satisfactory plan is generated, digital reconstructive radiograms (DRRs) corresponding to the planned radiation fields are obtained. These DRRs typically display field shapes and tumor volumes and the standard radiographic anatomical information. Using a complex 3D plan, MLC allows for rapid change of field shape under computer control, dramatically shortening the time needed to treat a patient. A verification simulation can be performed to check the validity and accuracy of the fields. This can be performed with the use of an electronic portal-imaging device (EPID) or a cone beam CT (CBCT). CBCT generates an image of the tumor and all surrounding normal structures using the same linear accelerator with which the patient is being treated. Linear accelerators produce the images of CBCT through either the same treating megavoltage beams (MV-CBCT) or built-in kilovoltage device (KV-CBCT). Appropriate adjustments of the exact treatment position can then be made daily to ensure that the tumor is receiving the prescribed dose of radiation, and normal tissues are receiving doses within their tolerance range. Recently, there are different devices for setup accuracy using either ultrasonography, infrared, radiofrequency for verification or setup positioning and to deal with intra-fractional movements.

The major hypothesized benefits of IMRT are a reduction in the dose to normal structures, as well as the potential for dose escalation. In IMRT, radiation beam is subdivided into a very large number of optimized small beamlets each with a unique intensity of radiation, influenced by the patient's anatomy in the path of the beamlet allowing tailored radiation dose distributions, to both the tumor and normal tissues. Three-dimensionally concave or convex shape configuration is one of the important characteristics of IMRT, resulting in a dramatic reduction of high doses of radiation to normal structures near the target. Moreover, it allows for differential doses to be delivered within the same target, giving the component at higher risk of recurrence higher dose while the rest of the target is being treated to a conventional dose. This technique is called simultaneous integrated boost (SIB). This is attractive in certain situations, in that it allows a higher dose per fraction to the target, while giving a lower dose per fraction to normal structures. Biologically effective dose (BED), which is calculated based on the linear-quadratic (LQ) model, is commonly used on trial to relate the unconventional dose to that for the well-known conventional fractionation.

The main disadvantage of IMRT, in some instances, is the increase in low doses to normal tissues leading to increase in the body integral dose (i.e., higher total dose of a large volume). Other challenges of IMRT are the rapid fall-off of dose; therefore, patient immobilization and daily setup verification become critical. Slight motion or setup error may result in a geographic miss; the high dose is deposited in the critical structure designated for avoidance. Therefore, it is always stated that daily setup verification better precedes IMRT especially if proximity of a nearby critical structure is a concern. Fortunately, the brain moves minimally, and standard immobilization devices yield relatively high daily setup accuracy. Because IMRT dose distributions are highly complex, it is not unusual to see unanticipated toxicities in low-dose areas, such as alopecia or mucositis, in the exit-beam regions [7]. Increased incidence of second malignancy was postulated as a serious late side effect. However, it remains unclear whether second malignancies are a real or a hypothetical risk [40]. Intensity-modulated radiotherapy has several potential benefits in specific CNS tumors. Medulloblastoma represents a good example that is treated after surgery with radiotherapy and cisplatin-based chemotherapy, and radiation. Both platinum and radiotherapy significantly contribute to the occurrence of ototoxicity. However, the use of IMRT can spare the auditory apparatus (cochlea) while still maintaining full dose to the target. Reduction in cochlear dose from 54.2 to 36.7 Gy leads to reduction of grade 3 or 4 hearing loss from 64 to 13% with the use of IMRT, compared with conventional RT [41]. Furthermore, decreasing the cumulative dose of *cis*-platinum or usage of efficient less ototoxic drug is preferable for better hearing integrity.

3.2. Image-guided radiation therapy

Image-guided radiation therapy (IGRT) is the technique of using imaging technology at the time of each treatment to verify accurate positioning.

There are several types of IGRT including CBCT, MV CT (helical tomotherapy), CT-on-rails, the use of electronic portal imaging devices (EPIDs), ultrasound guidance radiofrequency, and fiducial monitoring. Advances in IGRT have allowed selective boost of dose to some targets while at the same time selectively sparing normal structures more aggressively.

3.3. Stereotactic radiosurgery and stereotactic fractionated radiotherapy

The term *radiosurgery* was selected because of its similarity to stereotactic neurosurgery. Radiosurgery technology has become increasingly more available, and its application has widened. Its current indications include arteriovenous malformations, benign brain tumors, malignant brain tumors, and functional disorders. Delivery of radiosurgery is complex and coordination of care by the neurosurgeon, radiation oncologist, and medical physicist is essential. Appropriate coordination leads to improved quality of care, reduction in practice variation, and improved patient satisfaction [42].

Radiosurgery entails a single treatment, whereas conventional RT used multiple treatments. Further, in conventional fractionation regimens, normal brain tissue adjacent to the target receives a considerable dose of radiation. Taking into consideration late toxicity, radiosurgery is able to treat with considerably high-dose gradients adjacent to a nonmobile target that makes its use in the brain ideal. The use of a very large number of beams (significantly modulated beams) ensures that the geometry provides ideal physical dose distribution for targets less than 4 cm in greatest dimension with maximally low dose to surrounding tissues. Beyond this limit, it is difficult to achieve a rapid fall-off in these normal tissues. Radiosurgery can be performed using various devices, including the gamma knife, particle beam devices, or modified linear accelerators (X-knife, cyberknife). With the great technologic advances in software and hardware, there is no clear advantage of one technology over the other [43]. The linear accelerator-based units can serve to treat non-radiosurgery patients.

Radiosurgery and neurosurgical approaches are often complementary, with the advantage that radiosurgery does not require a craniotomy, nor general anesthesia and patients are usually discharged the same day.

3.4. Charged particles

Proton beam therapy gained great interest in the radiation oncology community especially the pediatric one. This is related mainly to the dosimetric advantages of protons. Proton beam deposits its energy rapidly in what is known as the Bragg peak, a narrow range energy deposition where at the end of its path length the particle slows and. delivers radiation with a rapid fall-off. This confines the radiation to a smaller volume (clinical tumor volume) and extremely reduces the exit dose. The beam stops at a given depth that depends on their initial energy. Therefore, the possibility of wide low doses of radiation to normal tissues is minimal; different from IMRT. The dose fall-off beyond the Bragg peak is very rapid, reaching zero within a few millimeters beyond the maximum [44–46]. Despite the lack of Level 1 evidence, retrospective studies do exist to support its use in pediatric intracranial lesions. Traditional proton therapy and intensity-modulated proton therapy (IMPT) resulted in more efficient sparing of normal tissue compared to photon-based IMRT [47]. A model was designed to predict neurocognitive dysfunction after RT. The reduction in lower-dose volumes and mean dose afforded by proton therapy might reduce the incidence of late-term sequelae in children with medulloblastomas, craniopharyngiomas, and optic-pathway gliomas [48].

4. Chemotherapy

Chemotherapy is an essential modality in the treatment of many childhood malignancies including brain tumors. A wide variety of chemotherapeutic agents proved to be effective for most types of brain tumors. The role of chemotherapy varies from delaying the RT timing to allow further development of brain functions in the young, stabilizing tumors, reducing radiation doses, or even avoiding RT altogether. Effective agents include many alkylating agents, vinca alkaloids, topoisomerase inhibitors, antimetabolites, and angiogenesis inhibitors.

Chemotherapy for brain tumors can be given by various routes, including orally, intravenously, intrathecally, and via an Ommaya reservoir. Furthermore, chemotherapy may be given as an adjuvant or as concomitant with radiotherapy, improved survival for many pediatric brain tumors including medulloblastoma, germ cell tumor, high-grade astrocytoma, and others. In other conditions, like ependymoma, chemotherapy may be used to increase resect ability of the tumor [49].

The blood-brain barrier is a dynamic interface separating the brain from the circulatory system. The blood-brain barrier regulates the transport of essential molecules from the circulation to the brain, protecting the brain from harmful chemicals. It limits the ability of many chemotherapy agents to penetrate into the CNS. There are mechanisms such as blood-brain barrier disruption, intra-arterial chemotherapy injection, intrathecal chemotherapy administration, or intratumoral chemotherapy administration which were utilized to overcome the blood–brain barrier.

4.1. Intrathecal chemotherapy

Intrathecal administration of chemotherapy is another method of bypassing the blood-brain barrier to deliver chemotherapy within the CNS. Many agents have been investigated for a variety of brain tumors. Intrathecal liposomal cytarabine, mafosfamide, and etoposide were used in children with ependymoma, primitive neuroectodermal tumor, medulloblastoma, and atypical teratoid rhabdoid tumor [50].

4.2. Intra-ommaya therapy

Ommaya reservoirs were placed directly into the lateral ventricle to prevent repeated lumbar punctures for intrathecal chemotherapy. These provide easy access to the intrathecal space. Ommaya reservoirs have also been placed into the cysts of craniopharyngiomas in order to deliver chemotherapy agents intratumorally. The two agents that have previously been successfully utilized using this method of drug delivery are bleomycin and alpha interferon [51, 52].

5. Supportive care

Supportive care describes the multidisciplinary care required to fulfill the needs of the patient and family in order to meet the physical, informational, psychosocial, emotional, practical, and spiritual needs during all phases of their cancer care [53]. The treatment of pediatric brain and spinal cord tumors is complex and every family is different, with variable needs throughout treatment. This requires a collaborative and multidisciplinary health-care team to effectively assess and address the required supportive care early during the stage of diagnosis or initial therapy [53, 54].

The supportive care needs of pediatric patients and their families include the physical (physiotherapy, occupational therapy, speech pathology, dietician, medical, pharmacy), education/informational (often met by nursing and medical team members), as well as psychosocial (social work, psychology, child life, psychiatry). It is important to reassure the family that the intense emotional reactions (including fear, powerlessness, denial, guilt, sadness, anger, confusion, anxiety, and depression) are normal responses to the child's illness and that the team is there to support and not judge them. Complete family assessment including psychosocial and practical resources, employment, socioeconomic status, as well as an assessment of marital-parental and sibling relationships should be studied and managed [54]. Misunderstanding may influence care [54].

5.1. Informational needs

Good communication by the health-care team, repetition of information, opportunities to ask questions, and written materials are important for assisting families. Gaining information about their child's condition allows parents to feel some control over the situation and regain some peace of mind. Psychosocial providers can assist families to manage feelings of information overload and problem solving according to the demands.

Parents may require guidance from the team regarding how and when to talk to their children, to do it so honestly and at an age-appropriate level, yet in a way that decreases anxiety and increases trust in the treatment process and team.

Normalizing activities as much as possible can be of great help in restoring a sense of safety and normalcy for children. Child life specialists can help to normalize daily activities. Once the child is discharged from the hospital, encourage parents to allow the child to live life as normal as possible. Social and medical staff have to help the parents to overcome their own fears, and to allow patients to return to pre-illness activities within the restrictions of the illness with no overindulging or overprotecting [54].

5.2. Nutritional support

It is well established that children and adolescents with cancer experience malnutrition due to their underlying malignancy and treatment-related factors. Diminished nutritional status contributes in poor wound healing, increased infection risk, and decreased tolerance to chemotherapy. It is established that poor nutrition affects the QoL, response to treatment, and overall cost of care. This may be attributed to their limited energy stores and increased nutritional requirements to attain their appropriate growth and neurodevelopment [57–58].

Nutritional strategies should be integrated as a fundamental feature of supportive care for all pediatric neuro-oncology patients. The goals of nutritional supportive care include the maintenance of body stores, minimization of weight loss, promotion of appropriate growth, and providing excellent QoL [58].

5.3. Endocrinopathy at diagnosis and during treatment of brain tumor

Tumors of suprasellar and pineal region show various endocrine abnormalities even before the start of any treatment. Endocrinal symptoms in midline tumors include diabetes insipidus; changes in weight, height, and growth velocity; precocious puberty; or delayed sexual development. These symptoms less often lead to diagnosis, despite being present long before diagnosis [59]. Hypothalamic and pituitary endocrinopathies occur commonly in children following ≥24 Gy whole brain or localized cranial RT that included these structures in the radiation field. Hypothalamic-pituitary axis dysfunction gives rise to endocrinal abnormalities. This could be permanent or transient and the pituitary gland may regain its ability to secrete hormones after treatment. Therapeutic modalities, including surgery and radiotherapy, can damage pituitary cells leading to worsening of preexisting hypopituitarism [60]. Careful history and clinical examination, as well as timely reevaluation of children with abnormal body mass index (BMI) or BMI progression, as the presence of other neurological, ophthalmologic, and endocrine signs and symptoms may be indicative of the presence of an underlying hypothalamic-pituitary lesion [59, 60].

6. Long-term sequelae

The high cure rate achieved in pediatric CNS tumors is greatly attributable to refined neurosurgical procedures, the advancement in RT as well as chemotherapy and the multidisciplinary team decisions for treatment. However, with prolonged survival and on reaching adulthood, the incidence of late effects becomes more apparent. A majority of long-term survivors have at least one chronic medical sequelae [61]. These complications include endocrinopathy, osteoporosis, cerebrovascular disease, neurological and neurosensory dysfunction, secondary neoplasms, as well as psychological consequence and neurocognitive impacts.

6.1. Growth

Radiation-induced growth deficiency is due to damage to either hypothalamus or pituitary gland or local radiation to the spine. Cranial irradiation has an immediate suppressive effect on the hypothalamic-pituitary axis. According to the total cranial dose received, it reduces growth hormone (GH) level and alters the normal pubertal rise in GH secretions. The size and the number of radiation fractions influence growth hormone levels. Early diagnosis of mild hypothyroidism and/or GH deficiency permits early intervention to improve growth velocity and QoL [62]. Craniospinal irradiation and/or disruption of the pituitary-hypothalamic axis can lead to more global changes in physical appearance such as short stature or obesity [62, 63].

Spinal radiation will affect vertebral body growth, especially in the younger ages. Chemotherapy may impair gonadal function, usually more in males than in females. Cyclophosphamide-induced testicular damage is dose dependent. In general, prepubertal patients tend to be more resistant to gonadal adverse effects of RT and chemotherapy than postpubertal patients [62].

6.2. Osteoporosis

Brain radiation, corticosteroids, poor nutrition, restricted weight-bearing exercise, and the developed endocrinopathies interact and all affect bone mineral density (BMD) during a crucial period for bone growth and skeletal growth. Depending on the magnitude of the BMD deficit and the potential for recovery, the pediatric neuro-oncology survivors are at increased risk for osteoporosis that may lead to osteoporotic fractures later in life.

These survivors should be assessed for low BMD and referred for potential bone health assessment and treatment as well as maximizing nutrition, exercise, and calcium and vitamin D intake [64].

6.3. Sleep disorder

Neuro-oncology patients may suffer from sleep disorders including disturbed sleep-wake rhythm, increased sleep duration, disturbed sleep timing, and daytime sleepiness that significantly affect their daily performance and their QoL. Disturbed pattern of sleep is more often experienced in children suffering from hypothalamic, pituitary, or brain stem lesions as well as in those treated with craniospinal radiotherapy. Excessive somnolence and psychosocial functioning with fatigue are common complaints of such patients. Routine evaluation of sleep habits during may help better understanding the mechanisms underlining these disorders and present possible interventions (e.g., melatonin, cognitive therapy, bright light therapy, medications, and/or physical activities) [65].

6.4. Vascular malformations

An increased risk of vascular malformations was noticed with radiotherapy. Radiation can weaken the vessel wall and result in cerebral cavernous malformation, telangiectasias of capillaries, and aneurysms. Radiation is believed to stimulate angiogenesis factors leading to these vascular malformations. Cerebral cavernous malformations were experienced six times higher in those treated with radiotherapy than in the control population. Most of these lesions are asymptomatic, but a subset may be presented with seizures, headaches, and hemorrhages that may require surgical intervention.

Telangiectasias are commonly found in brain tissue obtained from patients treated with radiotherapy, with thin-walled, dilated tortuous vascular channels, associated with perivascular leukocyte infiltration. These abnormalities may become symptomatic after bleeding but are usually considered as benign finding [66].

Small vessel vasculopathy with mineralizing microangiopathy of the basal ganglia and subcortical white matter has also been reported months to years after completion of radiation of the brain [67]. Most patients are asymptomatic, but some investigators have correlated their presence with behavioral disorders, neurological deterioration, and dementia.

Moyamoya vasculopathy was reported in pituitary and chiasmatic tumor patients treated with and without radiation. This vasculopathy is a progressive stenosis of the supraclinoid internal carotid arteries leading to the development of collateral blood vessel formation. Radiation to the circle of Willis and neurofibromatosis type I (NF1) have been identified as risk factors [28].

6.5. Seizures

Childhood Cancer Survivor Study (CCSS) reported the prevalence of epilepsy in long-term survivors of childhood brain tumors as 25%. Many of them had their first seizure more than 5 years after diagnosis of their cancer [68]. Seizures were more frequent in patients treated with RT >30 Gy to any cortical area and more frequent in children treated at young age or who underwent repeated brain tumor excisions. Methotrexate has also been related to late seizure onset, especially with the resulted necrotizing leukoencephalopathy.

6.6. Ototoxicity

High doses of platinum have been reported to cause irreversible early- or delayed-onset hearing loss. Platinum targets the outer hair cells in the organ of Corti and the cochleal wall epithelium. These late complications create hearing affection and hence affect speech development, learning, communication, school performance, social interaction, and overall QoL. Platinum ototoxicity is characterized by a dose-dependent high-frequency sensorineural hearing loss with tinnitus. The magnitude of ototoxicity was influenced by the young age at the start of treatment, the high cumulative doses of platinum compounds (>400 mg/m^2 for cisplatin and carboplatin), and the use of concomitant ototoxic treatments including CNS RT [69]. Genetic polymorphisms in enzymes responsible for platinum metabolism (e.g., gluta-

http://dx.doi.org/10.5772/63111

thione S-transferase, thiopurine methyltransferase, catechol O-methyltransferase) may contribute to the severity of hearing loss [70, 71].

RT to the cochlea or cranial nerve VIII can also cause sensorineural hearing loss. Cranial RT used alone results in ototoxicity when cochlear dosage exceeds 32 Gy. Young age, presence of a brain tumor, and/or hydrocephalus can increase susceptibility to hearing loss. When used concomitantly with platinum, RT can have a synergistic effect and it substantially exacerbates the hearing loss associated with chemotherapy, especially in the high-frequency speech range. RT to temporal lobe (>30 Gy) and to posterior fossa (≥50 Gy) was reported to be associated with an increased risk of tinnitus, and hearing loss.

Early detection of ototoxicity in children is of extreme importance in the prevention of severe hearing impairment that may affect speech recognition. Various strategies have been considered to minimize platinum ototoxicity. Radiation reduction dose to the cochlea has been investigated, including the use of 3D conformal RT, IMRT, and proton therapy [72]. Once treatment is completed, long-term audiometric monitoring should continue.

6.7. Visual affection

CCSS reported in adult survivors of childhood brain tumors, blindness in one or both eyes in 13%, cataracts in 3%, and double vision in 17% [68]. Although cataracts are known complication of RT, prolonged use of corticosteroid such as dexamethasone can also contribute to the development of posterior subcapsular cataracts. Ophthalmologic complications were reported in optic pathway glioma and craniopharyngioma in 20–70% of patients. Poor visual outcome has been frequently reported in the posterior chiasmatic area. Long-standing obstructive hydrocephalus can lead to severe optic atrophy and blindness.

6.8. Secondary neoplasms

The increase in survival in childhood tumors was accompanied with the emergence of secondary neoplasms as a long-term complication of treatment reaching up to 3–4% at 20 years post treatment [73]. Leukemia and primary CNS tumors have a tendency to develop into a subsequent CNS tumor. Armstrong et al. [74] reported 20 (1.1%) second CNS tumors out of 1877 survivors of CNS malignancies. They also observed 171 (9.1%) neoplasms classified as "benign" tumors including 59 meningiomas and 112 nonmelanoma skin cancers in these long survivors. The overall cumulative incidence of a subsequent neoplasm at 25 years was estimated to be 10.7%. Generally, the most common malignancies are malignant astrocytomas, followed by sarcomas and occasionally supratentorial primitive neuroectodermal tumors (sPNET). The cumulative incidence of secondary CNS such as glioblastomas plateaued at 15 years, whereas the cumulative incidence of meningiomas continues to increase beyond 35 years post treatment [75]. Although these secondary tumors have similar histological appearance to the primary tumors, they typically behave more aggressively and are resistant to treatment [76]. Moreover, the meningiomas have also been found to be more often atypical and prone to relapse. The development of secondary CNS tumors is most likely multifactorial, but RT certainly contributes to this process. The vast majority of secondary malignant neoplasm (SMN) appears within the radiation field. The cumulative incidence of SMNs at 25 years was 7.1% for children who received more than 50 Gy to the cranium compared to 1% for children who did not receive cranial irradiation. A linear dose response could be illustrated with an increased relative risk of 0.33% for gliomas and 1.06% for meningiomas per Gy. The chemotherapy contribution to the development of secondary CNS malignancy is more difficult to assess partly due to the use of combination chemotherapy regimens. Alkylating drugs, especially cyclophosphamide and epipodophyllotoxins, such as etoposide, have been reported to increase the cumulative incidence of second malignancies [77]. The presence of accompanying somatic mutations may predispose for the development of second malignancy. Patients with p53 (Li-Fraumeni syndrome) are more likely to develop SMN including sarcoma, primary brain tumor, and acute lymphoblastic leukemia (ALL).

Therapy may be tailored in order to avoid or reduce the combination of RT and certain chemotherapy agents. Alkylating drugs, especially cyclophosphamide and epipodophyllotoxins, such as etoposide, have been reported to increase the cumulative incidence of second malignancies up to 4% [77]. Other somatic mutations such as the ataxia telangiectasia mutated gene (ATM) known to be involved in DNA repair may possibly play a role. Finally, metabolism and detoxification might also be involved in the development of second malignancy especially in those with acute nonlymphocytic leukemia (ANLL) and acute myeloid leukemia (AML).

7. Palliative care

Palliative care for children has evolved, over the last two decades, as separate specialized entity. Its delivery encompasses the total care of children with life-limiting diseases, regardless of outcome. It is worth noting that palliative care is applicable from the time of diagnosis, through active and curative treatment, and afterwards. Timing is further complicated by the perceived sharp division between curative therapy and palliative care among pediatric oncologists and parents who view palliative care as giving up hope and representing failure.

Palliative care service includes improved communication and continuity of care across different disease and management stages. This care deals with assessment of physical, psychosocial, emotional, and spiritual needs, provision of comprehensive specialized pain and symptom management, and support with complex and ethical decision making. It is also concerned with enhanced awareness of diverse cultural beliefs about dying and death, specialized care of the dying patient, and provision of bereavement care. Education and staff support to improve delivery of care and respond to moral distress are additional important role [78, 79]. Palliative care services must better be organizationally situated within a pediatric oncology program. Without early integration of palliative care, the focus of care then centers on life-prolonging measures, which may result in painful and invasive procedures, additional unnecessary suffering, and futile resuscitation. Care may be missed if not addressed early in the trajectory of a cancer illness when death is expected. However, the pediatric brain tumor palliative care introduction time remains unclear and controversial, and has little evidence for practice guidelines [78].

8. Conclusion

Although the gap between the neuro-oncology services in HICs and LMICs is still huge, yet the continuous efforts performed by the LMICs assisted by different international organization, medical and scientific societies, and other international medical bodies can decrease and overcome this gap. Pediatric neuro-oncology service is a delicate art and science that is presented by a multidisciplinary team aimed at taking care of pediatric CNS tumors from the day of suspicion of the disease till long way across the adulthood life. The welfare of these patients is the concern of the multidisciplinary team along the journey of diagnosis, treatment, and prolonged extended follow-up. The team is concerned also with dealing with disease and treatment complications together with palliation of the symptoms faced by the patients. Much success was achieved; however, much effort is needed for more improvement of the quality of their life. Very long-term effects 30–40 years after treatment still need to be thoroughly investigated. Cerebrovascular diseases such as stroke, cognitive dysfunction leading to early dementia, secondary neoplasms, and peripheral neuropathy are likely to form real problem in the coming years.

The balance between survival and long-term side effects will certainly be a challenge for several decades. Tailored therapy to reduce and limit the need for radiation and chemotherapy will hopefully lead to improved outcomes with fewer adverse effects and morbidity.

Author details

Mohamed S. Zaghloul

Address all correspondence to: mszagh@yahoo.com

Children's Cancer Hospital, Cairo, Egypt & National Cancer Institute, Cairo University, Cairo University Rd, Oula, Giza, Giza Governorate, Egypt

References

[1] Wagner HP, Antic V. The problem of pediatric malignancies in the developing world. Ann N Y Acad Sci. 1997;824:193–204.

[2] Reutfors J, Kramárová E, Weiderpass E, Monge P, Wesseling C, Ahlbom A. Paediatric central nervous system tumours in children in Costa Rica, 1981-96. Perinat Epidemiol. 2002;16(3):219–25.

[3] Bouffet E, Amayiri N, Fonseca A, Scheinemann K. Pediatric neuro-oncology in countries with limited resources. In Pediatric Neuro-oncology, K. Scheinemann and E. Bouffet (eds.). New York, NY: Springer Science + Business Media; 2015, pp: 299–307.

[4] Zaghloul MS. Single pediatric neuro-oncology center may make difference in low/middle-income countries. Child's Nervous System. 2016;32(2):241–2.

[5] Miyakawa A, Shibamoto Y, Otsuka S, Iwata H. Applicability of the linear-quadratic model to single and fractionated radiotherapy schedules: an experimental study. J Radiat Res. 2013;55(3):451–4.

[6] El Fiki M. African neurosurgery, the 21st century challenge. World Neurosurgery. 2010;73(4):254–8.

[7] Mohan R, Wu Q, Manning M, Schmidt-Ullrich R. Radiobiological considerations in the design of fractionation strategies for intensity- modulated radiation therapy of head and neck cancers. Int J Radiat Oncol Biol Phys. 2000;46:619–30.

[8] ACR Manual on Contrast Media - Version 8. ACR Committee on Drugs and Contrast Media. Reston, VA: American College of Radiology; 2012.

[9] Assaf Y, Pasternak O. Diffusion tensor imaging (DTI)-based white matter mapping in brain research: a review. J Mol Neurosci. 2008;34(1):51–61.

[10] Rao P. Role of MRI in paediatric neurooncology. Eur J Radiol. 2008;68(2):259–70.

[11] Petrirena GJ, Goldman S, Delattre JY. Advances in PET imaging of brain tumors: a referring physician's perspective. Curr Opin Oncol. 2011;23(6):617–23.

[12] Burger P, Scheithauer BW. Diagnostic Pathology: Neuropathology. 1st ed. Salt Lake City, UT: Lippincott Williams & Wilkins and Amirsys; 2011.

[13] Szymas J, Wolf G, Papierz W, Jarosz B, Weinstein RS. Online Internet-based robotic telepathology in the diagnosis of neuro-oncology cases: a teleneuropathology feasibility study. Hum Pathol. 2001;32(12):1304–8.

[14] Datta NR, Samiei M, Bodis S. Radiation therapy infrastructure and human resources in low- and middle-income countries: present status and projections for 2020. Int J Radiat Oncol Biol Phys. 2014;89(3):448–57.

[15] Abdel-Wahab M, Bourque JM, Pynda Y, Iżewska J, Van der Merwe D, Zubizarreta E, Rosenblatt E. Status of radiotherapy resources in Africa: an international atomic energy agency analysis. Lancet Oncol. 2013;14(4):e168–75.

[16] Levin CV, et al. Radiationtherapy services in South Africa. S Afr Med J. 1994;84(6):349–51.

[17] Zubizarreta EH, Poitevin A, Levin CV. Overview of radiotherapy resources in Latin America: a survey by the International Atomic Energy Agency (IAEA). Radiother Oncol. 2004;73(1):97–100.

[18] Grover S, et al. A systematic review of radiotherapy capacity in low- and middle-income countries. Front Oncol. 2015;4: Article 380.

[19] Mellstedt H. Cancer initiatives in developing countries. Ann Oncol. 2006;17:viii24–31.

[20] World Health Organization (WHO). National Cancer Control Programmes: Policies and Managerial Guidelines. Geneva, Switzerland: WHO; 2002.

[21] Available from: http://www.icedoc.org/winwin.htm

[22] Haas-Kogan DA, et al. P53-dependent G1 arrest and P53- independent apoptosis influence on the radiobiologic response of glioblastoma. Int J Radiat Biol Phys. 1996;36:95–103.

[23] Reddy K, Damek D, Gaspar LE, Ney D, Waziri A, Lillehei K, Stuhr K, Kavanagh BD, Chen C. Phase II trial of hypofractionated IMRT with temozolomide for patients with newly diagnosed glioblastoma multiforme. Int J Radiat Oncol Biol Phys. 2012;84:655–60.

[24] Chen C, Damek D, Gaspar LE, Waziri A, Lillehei K, Kleinschmidt-DeMasters BK, Robischon M, Stuhr K, Rusthoven KE, Kavanagh BD. Phase I trial of hypofractionated intensity- modulated radiotherapy with temozolomide chemotherapy for patients with newly diagnosed glioblastoma multiforme. Int J Radiat Oncol Biol Phys. 2011;81:1066–74.

[25] Floyd NS, Woo SY, Teh BS, Prado C, Mai WY, Trask T, Gildenberg PL, Holoye P, Augspurger ME, Carpenter LS, Lu HH, Chiu JK, Grant WH 3rd, Butler EB. Hypofractionated intensity-modulated radiotherapy for primary glioblastoma multiforme. Int J Radiat Oncol Biol Phys. 2004;58:721–6.

[26] Zaghloul MS, Eldebawy E, Ahmed S, Mousa AG, Amin A, Refaat A, Zaky I, Elkhateeb N, Sabry M. Hypofractionated conformal radiotherapy for pediatric diffuse intrinsic pontine glioma (DIPG): a randomized controlled trial. Radiother Oncol. 2014;111(1):35–40.

[27] Zaghloul MS. Has hypofractionated radiotherapy become the standard of care in pediatric DIPG? Child's Nervous System. 2015;31(8):1221–2.

[28] Ullrich NJ, Robertson R, Kinnamon DD, Scott RM, Kieran MW, Turner CD, Chi SN, Goumnerova L, Proctor M, Tarbell NJ, Marcus KJ, Pomeroy SL. Moyamoya following cranial irradiation for primary brain tumors in children. Neurology. 2007;68(12): 932–8.

[29] Maher CO, Raffel C. Neurosurgical treatment of brain tumors in children. Pediatr Clin North Am. 2004;51:327–57.

[30] Crawford JR, MacDonald TJ, Packer RJ. Medulloblastoma in childhood: new biological advances. Lancet Neurol. 2007;6:1073–85.

[31] Kobayashi T, Kageyama N, Ohara K. Internal irradiation for cystic craniopharyngioma. J Neurosurg. 1981;55(6):896–903.

[32] Lapras C, Patet JD, Mottolese C, Vitale G. Cerebellar astrocytomas in children. Prog Exp Tumor Res. 1987;30:128.

[33] Winn HR, editor. Youman's Neurological Surgery. Philadelphia, PA: Elsevier; 2011.

[34] Obaid S, Champagne P, Mercier C, Crevier L. Neurosurgery. In Pediatric Neuro-Oncology, K. Scheinemann and E. Bouffet (eds.). New York, NY: Springer Science Business Media; 2015, pp: 31–39.

[35] Sullivan R, Kowalczyk JR, Agarwal B, Ladenstein R, Fitzgerald E, Barr R, Steliarova-Foucher E, Magrath I, Howard SC, Kruger M, Valsecchi MG, Biondi A, Grundy P, Smith MA, Adamson P, Vassal G, Pritchard-Jones K. Improving cancer care for children and young people 4. New policies to address the global burden of childhood cancers. Lancet Oncol. 2013;14(3):e125–35.

[36] Magrath I, Steliarova-Foucher E, Epelman S, Ribeiro RC, Harif M, Li CK, Kebudi R, Macfarlane SD, Howard SC. Paediatric cancer in low-income and middle-income countries. Lancet Oncol. 2013;14(3):e104–16.

[37] Parkes J, Wetter J. Pediatric radiotherapy. In Pediatric Hematology-Oncology in Countries with Limited Resources: A Practical Manual, D.C. Stefan and C. Rodriguez-Galindo (eds.). New York, NY: Springer Science Business Media; 2014, pp: 181–206.

[38] Practice Guidelines for Sedation and Analgesia by Non-Anesthesiologists. An Updated Report by the American Society of Anesthesiologists Task Force on Sedation and Analgesia by Non-Anesthesiologists. Anesthesiology 2002;96: 1004–1017.

[39] Gregoire V, Mackie TR. State of the art on dose prescription, reporting and recording in intensity-modulated radiation therapy (ICRU report No. 83). Cancer Radiother. 2011;15 (6–7):555–9.

[40] Hall EJ. Intensity-modulated radiation therapy, protons, and the risk of second cancers. Int J Radiat Oncol Biol Phys. 2006;65:1–7.

[41] Huang E, Teh BS, Strother DR, Davis QG, Chiu JK, Lu HH, Carpenter LS, Mai WY, Chintagumpala MM, South M, Grant WH 3rd, Butler EB, Woo SY. Intensity-modulated radiation therapy for pediatric medulloblastoma: early report on the reduction of ototoxicity. Int J Radiat Oncol Biol Phys. 2002;52:599–605.

[42] Larson DA, Bova F, Eisert D, Kline R, Loeffler J, Lutz W, Mehta M, Palta J, Schewe K, Schultz C. Task force on stereotactic radiosurgery, American Society for Therapeutic Radiology and Oncology. Current radiosurgery practice: results of an ASTRO survey. Int J Radiat Oncol Biol Phys. 1994;28:523–6.

[43] Stieber VW, Bourland JD, Tome WA, Mehta MP. Gentlemen (and ladies), choose your weapons: gamma knife vs. linear accelerator radiosurgery. Technol Cancer Res Treat. 2003;2:79–86.

[44] Hug EB, Slater JD. Proton radiation therapy for pediatric malignancies: status report. Strahlenther Onkol. 1999;175(Suppl. 2):89–91.

[45] Hug EB, Sweeney RA, Nurre PM, Holloway KC, Slater JD, Munzenrider JE. Proton radiotherapy in management of pediatric base of skull tumors. Int J Radiat Oncol Biol Phys. 2002;52:1017–24.

[46] Khuntia D, Tomé WA, Mehta MP. Radiation techniques in neuro-oncology. Neurotherapeutics 2009;6(3):478–499.

[47] MacDonald SM, Safai S, Trofimov A, Wolfgang J, Fullerton B, Yeap BY, Bortfeld T, Tarbell NJ, Yock T. Proton radiotherapy for childhood ependymoma: initial clinical outcomes and dose comparisons. Int J Rad Oncol Biol Phys. 2008;71:979–86.

[48] Merchant TE, Hua CH, Shukla H, Ying X, Nill S, Oelfke U. Proton versus photon radiotherapy for common pediatric brain tumors: comparison of models of dose characteristics and their relationship to cognitive function. Pediatr Blood Cancer 2008;51:110–7.

[49] Lee J, Johnston DL. Chemotherapy. In Pediatric Neuro-oncology, K. Scheinemann and E. Bouffet (eds). New York, NY: Springer Science + Business Media; 2015, pp: 207–215.

[50] Lassaletta A, Lopez-Ibor B, Mateos E, Gonzalez-Vicent M, Perez-Martinez A, Sevilla J, Diaz MA, Madero L. Intrathecal liposomal cytarabine in children under 4 years with malignant brain tumours. J Neurooncol. 2009;95:65–9.

[51] Dastoli PA, Nicácio JM, Silva NS, Capellano AM, Toledo SR, Ierardi D, Cavalheiro S. Cystic craniopharyngioma: intratumoural chemotherapy with alpha interferon. Arq Neuropsiquiatr. 2011;69:50–5.

[52] Mottolese C, Stan H, Hermier M, Berlier P, Convert J, Frappaz D, Lapras C. Intracystic chemotherapy with bleomycin in the treatment of craniopharyngiomas. Childs Nerv Syst. 2001;17:724–30.

[53] Kerr LM, Harrison MB, Medves J, Tranmer JE, Fitch MI. Supportive care needs of parents of children with cancer: transition from diagnosis to treatment. Oncol Nurs Forum. 2004;31(6):E116–26.

[54] PDQ Supportive and Palliative Care Editorial Board. Pediatric Supportive Care (PDQ®): Health Professional Version. PDQ Cancer Information Summaries [Internet]. Bethesda, MD: National Cancer Institute (US); 2002–2016.

[55] Lanskowksy P. Manual of Pediatric Hematology and Oncology: Psychosocial Aspects of Cancer for Children and their Families. 5th ed. Burlington, VT: Elsevier; 2011.

[56] Co-Reyes E, Li R, Huh W, Chandra J. Malnutrition and obesity in pediatric oncology patients: causes, consequences, and interventions. Pediatr Blood Cancer. 2012;59(7): 1160–7.

[57] Pizzo PA, Poplack DG. Principles and Practices of Pediatric Oncology: Nutritional Supportive Care. 6th ed. Philadelphia, PY: Lippincott Williams & Wilkins; 2011.

[58] Bauer J, Jürgens H, Frühwald MC. Important aspects of nutrition in children with cancer. Adv Nutr. 2011;2(2):67–77.

[59] Taylor M, Couto-Silva AC, Adan L, Trivin C, Sainte-Rose C, Zerah M, Valteau-Couanet D, Doz F, Chalumeau M, Brauner R. Hypothalamic-pituitary lesions in pediatric patients: endocrine symptoms often precede neuro-ophthalmic presenting symptoms. J Pediatr. 2012;161(5):855–63.

[60] Jorsal T, Rorth M. Intracranial germ cell tumours. A review with special reference to endocrine manifestations. Acta Oncol. 2012;51(1):3–9.

[61] de Boer AG, Verbeek JH, van Dijk FJ. Adult survivors of childhood cancer and unemployment: a meta-analysis. Cancer. 2006;107(1):1–11.

[62] Turner CD, Rey-Casserly C, Liptak CC, Chordas C. Late effects of therapy for pediatric brain tumor survivors. J Child Neurol. 2009;24(11):1455–63.

[63] Nathan PC, Jovcevska V, Ness KK, Mammone D'Agostino N, Staneland P, Urbach SL, Barron M. The prevalence of overweight and obesity in pediatric survivors of cancer. J Pediatr. 2006;149(4):518–25.

[64] Cohen LE, Gordon JH, Popovsky EY, Sainath NN, Feldman HA, Kieran MW, Gordon CM. Bone density in post-pubertal adolescent survivors of childhood brain tumors. Pediatr Blood Cancer. 2012;58(6):959–63.

[65] Verberne LM, Maurice-Stam H, Grootenhuis MA, Van Santen HM, Schouten-Van Meeteren AY. Sleep disorders in children after treatment for a CNS tumour. J Sleep Res. 2012;21(4):461–9.

[66] Burn S, Gunny R, Phipps K, Gaze M, Hayward R. Incidence of cavernoma development in children after radiotherapy for brain tumors. J Neurosurg. 2007;106(Suppl. 5): 379–83.

[67] Price RA, Birdwell DA. The central nervous system in childhood leukemia. III. Mineralizing microangiopathy and dystrophic calcification. Cancer. 1978;42(2):717–28.

[68] Packer RJ, Gurney JG, Punyko JA, Donaldson SS, Inskip PD, Stovall M, Yasui Y, Mertens AC, Sklar CA, Nicholson HS, Zeltzer LK, Neglia JP, Robison LL. Long-term neurologic and neurosensory sequelae in adult survivors of a childhood brain tumor: childhood cancer survivor study. J Clin Oncol. 2003;21(17):3255–61.

[69] Whelan K, Stratton K, Kawashima T, Leisenring W, Hayashi S, Waterbor J, Blatt J, Sklar CA, Packer R, Mitby P, Robison LL, Mertens AC. Auditory complications in child-

hood cancer survivors: a report from the childhood cancer survivor study. Pediatr Blood Cancer. 2011;57(1):126–34.

[70] Mukherjea D, Rybak LP. Pharmacogenomics of cisplatin- induced ototoxicity. Pharmacogenomics. 2011;12(7):1039–50.

[71] Ross CJ, Katzov-Eckert H, Dubé MP, Brooks B, Rassekh SR, Barhdadi A, Feroz-Zada Y, Visscher H, Brown AM, Rieder MJ, Rogers PC, Phillips MS, Carleton BC, Hayden MR; CPNDS Consortium. Genetic variants in TPMT and COMT are associated with hearing loss in children receiving cisplatin chemotherapy. Nat Genet. 2009;41(12):1345–9.

[72] Paulino AC, Lobo M, Teh BS, Okcu MF, South M, Butler EB, Su J, Chintagumpala M. Ototoxicity after intensity modulated radiation therapy and cisplatin-based chemotherapy in children with medulloblastoma. Int J Radiat Oncol Biol Phys. 2010;78(5): 1445–50.

[73] Inskip PD, Curtis RE. New malignancies following childhood cancer in the United States, 1973–2002. Int J Cancer. 2007;121(10):2233–40.

[74] Armstrong GT. Long-term survivors of childhood central nervous system malignancies: the experience of the Childhood Cancer Survivor Study. Eur J Paediatr Neurol. 2010;14(4):298–303.

[75] Hijiya N, Hudson MM, Lensing S, Zacher M, Onciu M, Behm FG, Razzouk BI, Ribeiro RC, Rubnitz JE, Sandlund JT, Rivera GK, Evans WE, Relling MV, Pui CH. Cumulative incidence of secondary neoplasms as a first event after childhood acute lymphoblastic leukemia. JAMA. 2007;297(11):1207–15.

[76] Sobowale OA, McCabe M, Pal P, Soh C, Karabatsou K. Radiotherapy-induced supratentorial primitive neuroectodermal tumour in a 17-yearold female: a case report and review of the literature. Acta Neurochir. 2011;153(2):413–7.

[77] Borgmann A, Zinn C, Hartmann R, Herold R, Kaatsch P, Escherich G, Möricke A, Henze G, von Stackelberg A; ALL-REZ BFM Study Group. Secondary malignant neoplasms after intensive treatment of relapsed acute lymphoblastic leukaemia in childhood. Eur J Cancer. 2008;44(2):257–68.

[78] Waldman E, Wolfe J. Palliative care for children with cancer. Nat Rev Clin Oncol. 2013;10(2):100–7.

[79] Epelman CL. End-of-life management in pediatric cancer. Curr Oncol Rep. 2012;14(2): 191–6.